Pathobiology of the
Human Atherosclerotic Plaque

Seymour Glagov   William P. Newman, III
Sheldon A. Schaffer
Editors

Pathobiology of the Human Atherosclerotic Plaque

With 273 Figures, 16 in Full Color

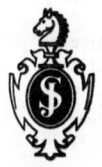

Springer-Verlag
New York Berlin Heidelberg
London Paris Tokyo Hong Kong

Seymour Glagov, MD
Professor of Pathology, The University of Chicago Hospital
Chicago, Illinois 60637, USA

William P. Newman III, MD
Department of Pathology, Louisiana State University
New Orleans, Louisiana 70112-1393, USA

Sheldon A. Schaffer, PhD
Colestech Corporation, Hayward, California 94545, USA

Library of Congress Cataloging-in-Publication Data
Pathobiology of the human atherosclerotic plaque / [edited by] Seymour
  Glagov, William P. Newman III, Sheldon A. Schaffer.
    p. cm.
  Contains nearly all the papers which were presented at a workshop
held in Rockville, Md., Sept. 20–23, 1986.
  Includes bibliographical references.

  ISBN-13: 978-1-4612-7968-6   e-ISBN-13: 978-1-4612-3326-8

  DOI: 10.1007/978-1-4612-3326-8

  1. Atherosclerosis—Pathophysiology—Congresses.
2. Atherosclerosis—Etiology—Congresses. I. Glagov, Seymour.
II. Newman, William P. III. Schaffer, Sheldon A.
  [DNLM: 1. Arteriosclerosis—pathology—congresses. 2. Ultrasonic
Diagnosis—congresses.   WG 550 P297 1986]
RC692.P353 1989
616.1'3607—dc20
DNLM/DLC
for Library of Congress   89-21674

© 1990 Springer-Verlag New York Inc.
Softcover reprint of the hardcover 1st edition 1990

Camera-ready copy provided by the editors.

9 8 7 6 5 4 3 2 1

Dedication

Colin B. Schwartz and Robert W. Wissler, for the Committee

Although the present volume is dedicated to those investigators who have made the study of the human atherosclerotic plaque their central focus of interest, two scientists whose efforts have been particularly noteworthy in this regard were honored during the deliberations which form the basis of this volume. They are <u>Drs. M. Daria Haust</u> and <u>Elspeth Smith</u>.

The following appreciations of their contributions were delivered during a special session of the workshop.

M. DARIA HAUST

About 60 years ago, I dare not be more specific, Dr. Haust made her debut in Central Europe. Her early years were disrupted by the turmoil of the second world war, but with rare determination, and an early sense of destiny, she made her way to Heidelberg where she graduated in 1951 with the Degree of Doctor of Medicine. Some of you may not know that she has an excellent voice, doubtless trained in the cellars of roten Ochsen in Heidelberg, the legendary inn of the student prince. There she met and married her prince, a charming friend of many of us, Dr. Heinz Haust, and together they settled in Kingston, Ontario, Canada, where her career both as an outstanding pathologist and biomedical scientist had its beginnings.

In the years 1955-1959 she was a resident in Pathology at Queens University, and in these years her work in

atherosclerosis commenced, in association with Robert H.
More and Henry Movat. Bob More was one of Daria's outstand-
ing mentors, and remains a lifelong friend and colleague. Dr.
Haust progressed rapidly up the rungs of the academic ladder,
and in 1968 was appointed Professor of Pathology at the
University of Western Ontario, where the late Jim Paterson,
one of the founding fathers of the American Society for the
Study of Atherosclerosis, later to become the AHA Council on
Arteriosclerosis, was a close friend and colleague.

Her early papers were landmarks in the field, and
emphasized the role of thrombosis in atherogenesis, and
later provided the first definitive report on the participation of smooth muscle cells in the human plaque. It is fair
to say that Dr. Haust was and is a first class Electronmicro-
scopist, and that she pioneered the application of this research
tool to the atherosclerosis arena. Other outstanding scientific contributions have included the early application of
fluorescent antibody techniques to the study of atherosclerosis, and in later years, the characterization of the roles
of connective tissue elements in the pathogenic sequence.
Her scientific productivity has never wained, and she has
over 200 publications to her credit.

She has played a key role in numerous professional and
scientific societies, including the Council on Arteriosclerosis,
the International Academy of Pathology, the International
Atherosclerosis Society, and the Canadian Atherosclerosis
Society, which was founded because of her efforts, and in
which she has held the honored position of President. In 1982
she was the recipient of the Alexander von Humboldt award for
Distinguished Service, in "Recognition of her dedicated
leadership, counsel, and service in the field of Atherosclerosis". It has been a personal pleasure and honor for me to
have this opportunity, on your behalf, to review only too
briefly a few of the many highlights of her outstanding
scientific career. Dr. Haust has truly dedicated her
scientific life to the study of arteriosclerosis, and also
to helping her colleagues and associates in their endeavors.
We wish you, Daria, good health, and continuing success and
fulfillment in the years ahead. This award is presented to

you on behalf of your colleagues, and in recognition of
your outstanding achievements. May you continue to inspire
us to probe the nature of the human manifestations of this
complex disease process.

CBS

ELSPETH B. SMITH

We now honor a pioneering, innovative and highly
productive contributor to our knowledge about the chemical
components of the atherosclerotic process in humans. Elspeth
Smith received most of her higher education, including her
biochemical training, in London and Cambridge. Her first
attention-demanding discoveries about human atherosclerosis
were made in London during the decade or more when she worked
at the Courtauld Institute of Biochemistry, under the sponsor-
ship and in close association with Sir Charles Dodds.

In 1967 she published what has become a very famous
paper in the Biochemical Journal on the immunological assay
of beta-lipoproteins from human aortic tissue. In 1973, after
she moved to Aberdeen, her highly useful contribution to the
Ciba Foundation Symposium, with the title "Lipids and Low
Density Lipoproteins in the Intima in Relation to its
Morphological Characteristics", appeared, and in 1977 her
most comprehensive overview in the American Journal of
Pathology entitled "Molecular Interactions in Human Atherosclerotic Plaques" was published. She has recently completed
two outstanding chapters on lipoproteins and atherosclerosis
and the relationship between lipids and atherosclerosis. In
between she has provided over 80 data filled publications,
almost all on macromolecules and their involvement in human
atherosclerotic lesions.

Although several of us were using immunological approaches
to study the human disease in the early 1960's, she recognized
the value of quantitating a number of the lipid, apo-protein
and other blood protein components and relating these results
in an enlightened way to each other, to the different types
of lesions and to various parts of the larger lesions. From
this work came some remarkable insights into the human

atherosclerotic process. These include the recognition that:

1. Substantial amounts of Apo B are localized in the human atherosclerosis lesion.

2. The lipid in the fatty streak is rich in oleic acid and poor in Apo B, which she interpreted as indicating that LDL had probably been altered by the lipid filled cells to convert it to cholesteryl esters with a predominance of oleic acid.

3. The lipid in the atheromatous core and that in fibrous caps and the shoulder regions of the advanced plaque is likely to be especially rich in polyunsaturated fatty acids, and rich in Apo B--probably indicating that the lipoproteins had not been metabolically altered by cells.

As she continued her investigations in Aberdeen she carried out and shared many other quantitative studies of arteries. These included some challenging concepts that the progressive atherosclerotic plaques are derived from gelatinous streaks, and that fibrinogen as well as albumin are noteworthy plasma protein components found in the developing atheromatous lesion. She also produced evidence that we need to search further for the true explanation for atherosclerotic plaque initiation and plaque progression.

I have had the honor and privilege of being involved in many meetings where Elspeth was a star participant and I have never failed to gain immensely from her stimulating findings and concepts. It gives me great pleasure to be the one chosen to present her with this richly deserved honor, a special award from the American Heart Association through its Council on Atherosclerosis and its Committee on Lesions.

RWW

Preface

Seymour Glagov

The last meeting, devoted exclusively to an examination of the atherosclerotic plaque, took place in Chicago 25 years ago under the joint auspices of the Council on Arteriosclerosis of the American Heart Association and the Chicago Heart Association. The proceedings were published subsequently in a volume entitled "Evolution of the Atherosclerotic Plaque", edited by Richard J. Jones (1). Both experimental and human lesions were considered and several provocative new approaches to the disorder were discussed.

The electron microscope was being applied systematically to the study of blood vessels at that time, so that details of the infrastructure and cellular composition of the artery wall and of atherosclerotic lesions were presented in some detail. There was, as one result of these explorations, considerable discussion of morphologic evidence suggesting that the principal cell involved in the atherogenic process was neither the fibroblast nor the macrophage, as had been supposed, but the smooth muscle cell. In particular, the findings indicated that this cell could incorporate lipid and become a foam cell.

A session devoted to plaque constituents included presentations dealing with fatty acids, phospholipids, lipoproteins, mucopolysaccharides and enzymes. Consideration of factors modifying plaque development included the roles of mechanical stress, platelet accretion and thrombosis, lipid

deposition, mesenchymal activation and mural collagen
metabolism. The fate of the plaque and the consequences of
plaque formation were addressed in papers on artery wall
vascularization, calcium deposition, thrombotic occlusion,
plaque ulceration and embolization. It is especially noteworthy that one of the presentations, from the laboratories
of Drs. Louis Katz and Ruth Pick, dealt with the potential
reversibility of lesions and emphasized, largely on the basis
of clinical findings associated with wartime undernutrition
and data from animal experiments, that one could no longer
consider atherosclerosis to be an inexorably progressive
disease but was instead a process which might be slowed,
arrested or reversed by modification of such factors as diet
and hormones. Arterial catheterization and angiography were
on the scene by then, but no papers were presented which
dealt with lesion visualization, *in vivo* lesion quantitation,
or the relationship between lesion localization and hemodynamic conditions.

In his preface to the published proceedings, Dr. Jones
wrote, "This symposium was dedicated to an evaluation of the
current concepts of the origin, growth and focal morbid
disposition of the atherosclerotic plaque. The reader needs
no reminder that it is this lesion of arteriosclerosis which,
at the same time that it provides the greatest threat to life,
allows the most hope for its reversal. Knowledge of the cause
of this pathological entity is essential to its rational
treatment or prevention".

Since the 1963 meeting, there has been a marked acceleration in the use of animal models designed to identify and
reproduce the clinical risk factors and to probe the pathobiologic processes by which these lead to plaque formation.
Tissue culture methods are now widely used to characterize
the metabolic responses and molecular biology of the cells
which comprise both the artery wall and the atherosclerotic
plaque. The smooth muscle cell, still presumed to be a
principal actor in the atherogenic sequence of events continues
to receive a great deal of attention, particularly with respect
to the modulation of its proliferative, biosynthetic and contractile responses. The macrophage has however reentered the

scene and has to some degree upstaged the smooth muscle cell,
at least in some of the scenes of the atherogenic drama.
The factors which regulate intimal ingress and egress of
these cells, modify their state of activity with regard to
lipid metabolism and matrix composition and determine their
interactions with smooth muscle cells have become major fields
of study. The latest cell to receive detailed and concentrated
critical scrutiny in relation to atherogenesis is the endothelial cell. Previously relegated to relatively passive
roles as a diffusional and convective barrier and as an antithrombotic lining, it has now moved to center stage as a major
participant with prominent interactive, metabolic, biosynthetic
and selective transport functions. It seemed at first that
endothelial injury to the point of detachment was required
to permit mitogens to gain access to the media and in so
doing to induce a primary, focal, smooth muscle proliferative
response. Depending on associated conditions, such a focal
initial reaction could conceivably resolve, stabilize or
evolve into a manifest plaque. Recent findings have however
indicated that the integrity and continuity of the endothelial
monolayer is conserved during the initiating phase of lesion
induction. Current approaches tend therefore to focus upon
humoral, cellular and hemodynamic mediators which result in
modified endothelial function rather than in necrosis or
sloughing. Such disturbances, affecting one or more of the
complex of metabolic, biosynthetic or transport functions,
are thought to contribute significantly to the conditions
necessary for induction and progression of atherosclerosis.

Although much of this work has been experimental, the
relevance to human atherosclerotic disease of some of the
findings can now be tested directly. Several of the participants in the present workshop have studied the human plaque
for some time and continue to provide valuable information
on plaque composition and morphology, while others are
applying recently developed experimental techniques of cell
and molecular biology to human lesions. In addition, methods
for detection and characterization of human plaques *in situ*
in the living subject have developed rapidly in conjunction
with quantitative methods for assessing the effects of plaques
on flow and of flow on plaques. These findings are being

related to clinical symptomatology and to attempts at risk factor control. Long-term effects on plaques of pharmacologic agents, modifications of diet and life style and the effects of exposure to factors such as cigarette smoking and hypertension are under close examination. Actual lesion size, configuration and composition, in addition to the presence of symptomatic disease or the occurrence of a catastrophic cardiovascular event are widely used to follow the disease process.

Furthermore, we are intervening directly on the plaque. No longer limited to open operative procedures to bypass stenoses or to remove plaques by endarterectomy, we may now disrupt, sear, aspirate, shear and displace plaques and lyse occluding thrombi forming on or about plaques by manipulating intravascular devices introduced percutaneously. The natural history of the human plaque and its clinical manifestations can therefore be studied and related directly to metabolic, hematologic and hemodynamic factors as never before. Plaque morphogenes and complication are no longer mainly the domain of the anatomic pathologist. The acquisition of new and clinically useful knowledge in these areas now depends on the close collaboration of cardiologists, surgeons, radiologists, hemodynamicists, pathologists and cell biologists.

Because of the rapid progress in the development of the various diagnostic modalities for the evaluation of human plaques *in vivo*, the Committee on Vascular Lesions of the American Heart Association sponsored a workshop at Silver Spring, Maryland, in 1982 (2). The objective was to assess the diagnostic methods then available and under consideration and to attempt to identify better methods for validation of the findings. In his preface to the volume which appeared after that conference, Dr. A. Bleakley Chandler wrote, "Against the background of current pathologic and clinical knowledge of atherosclerosis, invasive and non-invasive evaluation methods then in use and under development were surveyed in considerable depth". The deliberations revealed that adequate validation of these methods required a more complete knowledge of the natural history of the human atherosclerotic plaque in each of the vascular beds at high risk than was apparent at the meeting.

The new approaches to the study of the arterial lesions along with the concerns raised at the Silver Spring meeting stimulated the members of the Committee on Vascular Lesions of the American Heart Association to plan a second workshop meeting dealing exclusively with the human atherosclerotic plaque. The workshop took place at Rockville, Maryland on September 20 to 23, 1986 with the specific goal of surveying the current state of knowledge concerning the evolution of the human plaque. The participants were asked to review current information on the pathobiology of the human lesion as revealed by each of the various modes of study which have thus far been applied. They were asked further to identify those areas where information is absent or inadequate and to indicate where, in their best judgement, future efforts should be concentrated.

The present volume contains nearly all the papers which were presented at the Rockville workshop. Most of the manuscripts were submitted after the meeting, during 1987 and 1988 and some include additional newer material not presented at the conference. The papers in this volume bring up-to-date current perceptions of the human plaque and advances in the application of modern methods of imaging, fluid dynamic measurement and plaque analysis. It is the hope of the editors that the contents of the papers will, at the very least, indicate the directions in which research on the human plaque is headed and stimulate further interdisciplinary collaborative efforts.

Much of the credit for the planning and implementation of the conference and for the editing of many of the manuscripts is due to the members of the Committee on Vascular Lesions of the American Heart Association. The committee members at the time of the workshop meeting were: Mark L. Armstrong, David H. Blankenhorn, M. Gene Bond, A. Bleakley Chandler, J. Fredrick Cornhill, Assaad S. Daoud, Seymour Glagov, William Insull, Jr., William P. Newman, Sheldon A. Schaffer, Colin J. Schwartz, and Robert W. Wissler. The advice and unstinting efforts of Mr. Leonard Cook and of the other members of the administrative staff of the American Heart Association before and during the meeting were indispensable.

Thanks are due to the Directors of the Merck, Sharp and Dohme Company for their generosity in underwriting the publication of this volume and to the American Heart Association for the financial support and encouragement which enabled the Committee to plan and publicize the meeting.

Educational grants which helped defray the expenses of the meeting were furnished by the following groups,without whose support it could not have taken place:

Abbott Laboratories

American Cyanamid Company

Berlex Laboratories, Inc.

Burroughs Wellcome Company

CIBA-GEIGY Corporation

Diasonics, Inc.

E.I. duPont de Nemours & Company

Hoffman-La Roche, Inc.

Horizons Research Laboratories, Inc.

Marion Laboratories, Inc.

Merck Sharpe & Dohme Research Laboratories

Merrell Dow Pharmaceuticals

Pfizer, Inc.

Proctor & Gamble Company

Sandoz Research Institute

Schering Corporation

G.D. Searle & Co.

Smith Kline and French Laboratories

Squibb Institute for Medical Research

Thomae

Wyeth Laboratories

The editors wish also to express their gratitude to Philip Pizzolato of McAllen, Texas for his careful attention to accuracy of this typescript, to Mr. Eugene Wolfe for his contribution to the photographic reproductions and to Mss Kathy Fisher and Wanda Townsend for their care in the preparation of the camera-ready copy.

REFERENCES

1. Evolution of the Atherosclerotic Plaque (1963) R.J. Jones, (ed) University of Chicago Press, Chicago
2. Clinical Diagnosis of Atherosclerosis (1982) M. G. Bond, W. Insull, Jr., S. Glagov, A.B. Chandler and J.F. Cornhill (eds) Springer-Verlad, New York

Contents

Tissue Organization and Architecture

Pathobiologic Processes

Evaluation of Lesion Status in Major Arterial Beds

Current and Prospective Methods for Detecting Plaque Change

Summary

Contributors

Adams, Wendy A., University of Washington, Seattle, Washington, USA

Albers, John A., University of Washington, Seattle, Washington, USA

Anderson, H.C., University of Kansas, Kansas City, Missouri, USA

Ang, A.H., University of Melbourne, Melbourne, Australia

Angelo, J., Bowman-Gray School of Medicine, Winston-Salem, North Carolina, USA

Antonov, Alexander S., Cardiology Research Center, Moscow, USSR

Aretz, Thomas, Lahey Clinic, Boston, Massachusetts, USA

Armstrong, Mark L., University of Iowa, Iowa City, Iowa, USA

Arntzenius, A.C., Leiden University, Leiden, The Netherlands

Augustyn, Joan M., Albany Medical College, Albany, New York, USA

Azen, Stanley P., University of Southern California, Los Angeles, California, USA

Ball, Marshall, Bowman-Gray School of Medicine, Winston-Salem, North Carolina, USA

Ball, Richard Y., University of Cambridge, Cambridge, UK

Barger, A. Clifford, Harvard Medical School, Boston, Massachusetts, USA

Barnes, R.W., Bowman-Gray School of Medicine, Winston-Salem, North Carolina, USA

Barth, J.D., Leiden University Hospital, Leiden, The Netherlands

Beeuwkes, Reinier III, Harvard Medical School, Boston, Massachusetts, USA

Berenson, Gerald S., Louisiana State University, New Orleans, Louisiana, USA

Berson, Alan, National Institutes of Health, Bethesda, Maryland, USA

Blankenhorn, David H., University of Southern California, Los Angeles, California,USA

Bolson, Edward L., University of Washington, Seattle, Washington, USA

Bond, M. Gene, Bowman-Gray School of Medicine, Winston-Salem, North Carolina, USA

Born, Gustav V.R., Kings College, London, U.K.

Bradley, William A., Baylor College of Medicine, Houston, Texas, USA

Brown, B. Gregory, University of Washington, Seattle, Washington, USA

Bryan, Fred A., Jr., Research Triangle Institute, Research Triangle Park, North Carolina, USA

Calderon-Ortiz, Mauricio, Miami Heart Institute, Miami, Florida, USA

Campbell, G.R., University of Melbourne, Melbourne, Australia

Campbell, I.L., University of Melbourne, Melbourne, Australia

Campbell, J.H., University of Melbourne, Melbourne, Australia

Campeau, Lucien, Institut de Cardiologie de Montreal, Montreal, Canada

Caputo, Gary, University of California, San Francisco, California, USA

Carpenter, Keri L.H., University of Cambridge, Cambridge, UK

Chandler, A. Bleakley, Medical College of Georgia, Augusta, Georgia, USA

Choi, Hong Y., Johns Hopkins Medical Institutions, Baltimore, Maryland, USA

Clouse, Melvin E., New England Deaconess Hospital, Boston, Massachusetts, USA

Constantinides, Paris, Louisiana State University, Shreveport, Louisiana, USA

Cornhill, J. Fredrick, Ohio State University, Columbus, Ohio, USA

Crooks, Lawrence, University of California, San Francisco, California, USA

Dalferes, E.R., Jr., Louisiana State University, New Orleans, Louisiana, USA

Daoud, Assaad S., Veterans Administration Medical Center, Albany, New York, USA

DeBakey, Michael E., Baylor College of Medicine, Houston, Texas, USA

DeWeese, James A., University of Rochester, Rochester, New York, USA

DeWood, Marcus A., Deaconess and Sacred Heart Medical Centers, Spokane, Washington, USA

Dodge, Harold T., University of Washington, Seattle, Washington, USA

Dunn, Rosalie A., National Institutes of Health, Bethesda, Maryland, USA

Earle, Nan, Baylor College of Medicine, Houston, Texas, USA

Eckholm, Sven, University of Rochester, Rochester, New York, USA

Edwards, Ellen H., University of Texas, Austin, Texas, USA

Erikson, Uno, Linkoping University, Linkoping, Sweden

Faxon, David P., Boston University, Boston, Massachusetts, USA

Fischman, Alan J., New England Deaconess Hospital, Boston, Massachusetts, USA

Fishel, Jean, Bowman-Gray School of Medicine, Winston-Salem, North Carolina, USA

Franzblau, Carl, Boston University, Boston, Massachusetts, USA

Friedman, Morton H., Ohio State University, Columbus, Ohio, USA

Fry, Donald L., Ohio State University, Columbus, Ohio, USA

Gabbiani, G., University of Geneva, Geneva, Switzerland

Gerrity, Ross G., St. Vincent Hospital, Cleveland, Ohio, USA

Gianturco, Sandra H., University of Alabama, Birmingham, Alabama, USA

Giddens, Don P., Georgia Institute of Technology, Atlanta, Georgia, USA

Glagov, Seymour, University of Chicago, Chicago, Illinois, USA

Goldberg, Barry B., Jefferson Medical College, Philadelphia, Pennsylvania, USA

Goodison, Marta W., Miami Heart Institute, Miami, Florida, USA

Gould, Lance, University of Cincinnati, Cincinnati, Ohio, USA

Gown, Allen M., University of Washington, Seattle, Washington, USA

Gramiak, Raymond, University of Rochester, Rochester, New York, USA

Gustafson, Nancy F., Research Triangle Institute, Research Triangle Park, North Carolina, USA

Hale, James, University of California, San Francisco, California, USA

Harrison, David G., University of Iowa, Iowa City, Iowa, USA

Haudenschild, Christian C., Boston University, Boston, Massachusetts, USA

Haust, M. Daria, University of Western Ontario, London, Ontario, Canada

Heiss, Gerardo, University of North Carolina, Chapel Hill, North Carolina, USA

Heistad, Donald D., University of Iowa, Iowa City, Iowa, USA

Helmius, Gunnar, Linkoping University, Linkoping, Sweden

Hemmingsson, Anders, Linkoping University, Linkoping, Sweden

Henry, Philip D., Baylor College of Medicine, Houston, Texas, USA

Herson, Jay, Applied Logic Associates, Houston, Texas, USA

Higgins, Millicent, National Institutes of Health, Bethesda, Maryland, USA

Holen, Tarle, University of Rochester, Rochester, New York, USA

Hollander, William, Boston University, Boston, Massachusetts, USA

Holme, Ingar, Linkoping University, Linkoping, Sweden

Horrigan, S., University of Melbourne, Melbourne, Australia

Insull, William Jr., Baylor College of Medicine, Houston, Texas, USA

Kane, Robert A., New England Deaconess Hospital, Boston, Massachusetts, USA

Kaufman, Leon, University of California, San Francisco, California, USA

Kelley, Jim L., University of Texas, San Antonio, Texas, USA

Kelsey, Sheryl F., University of Pittsburgh, Pittsburgh, Pennsylvania, USA

Kim, D.N., Albany Medical College, Albany, New York, USA

Kirkeeide, Richard L., University of Texas, Houston, Texas, USA

Kromhout, D., Leiden University Hospital, Leiden, The Netherlands

Kurtz, Alfred, Jefferson Medical College, Philadelphia, Pennsylvania, USA

Lainey, Lewis L., Institute of Circadian Physiology, Boston, Massachusetts, USA

Lamkin, Glenn, Christ Hospital Cardiovascular Research Center, Cincinnati, Ohio, USA

Lawrie, Gerald M., Baylor College of Medicine, Houston, Texas, USA

Lazzari, Antonio, Boston University, Boston, Massachusetts, USA

Lees, Ann M., New England Deaconess Hospital, Boston, Massachusetts, USA

Lees, Robert S., New England Deaconess Hospital, Boston, Massachusetts, USA

Leimgruber, Pierre P., Spokane Cardiology, Spokane, Washington, USA

Lin, Jiin, University of Washington, Seattle, Washington, USA

Lopez, J. Antonio, University of Iowa, Iowa City, Iowa, USA

Lukashev, Matvey E., Cardiology Research Center, Moscow, USSR

Malinow, M. Rene, Oregon Health Sciences University, Portland, Oregon, USA

Mandel, Gretchen, Veterans Administration Medical Center, Milwaukee, Wisconsin, USA

Manderson, J.A., University of Melbourne, Melbourne, Australia

McCartney, Michael L., Research Triangle Institute, Research Triangle Park, North Carolina, USA

McGill, Henry C., Jr., University of Texas, San Antonio, Texas, USA

McGregor, D.H., Veterans Administration Hospital, Kansas City, Missouri, USA

McWhorter, J.M., Bowman-Gray School of Medicine, Winston-Salem, North Carolina, USA

Megan, Margorie B., University of Iowa, Iowa City, Iowa, USA

Mitchinson, Malcolm J., University of Cambridge, Cambridge, UK

Morris, George C., Jr., Baylor College of Medicine, Houston, Texas, USA

Morrisett, Joel D., Baylor College of Medicine, Houston, Texas, USA

Mosse, P.R.L., University of Melbourne, Melbourne, Australia

Nadeau, Parise, Institut de Cardiologie de Montreal, Montreal, Canada

Newman, W.P. III, Louisiana State University, New Orleans, Louisiana, USA

Nishikawa, Akira, University of Texas Medical School, Houston, Texas, USA

Nunn, Cathy, Bowman-Gray School of Medicine, Winston-Salem, North Carolina, USA

O'Leary, Daniel H., New England Deaconess Hospital, Boston, Massachusetts, USA

Olsson, Ansers G., Linkoping University, Linkoping, Sweden

Pignoli, Paolo, Ospedale di' Merate, Merate, Italy

Radhakrishnamurthy, B., Louisiana State University, New Orleans, Louisiana, USA

Raines, Jeff, University of Miami, Miami, Florida, USA

Rapp, Joseph, University of California, San Francisco, California, USA

Rennick, R.E., University of Melbourne, Melbourne, Australia

Richardson, Peter D., Brown University, Providence, Rhode Island, USA

Ricotta, John J., University of Rochester, Rochester, New York, USA

Rifkin, Matthew D., Jefferson Medical College, Philadelphia, Pennsylvania, USA

Riley, Ward A., Jr., Autrec Research Design and Development, Winston-Salem, North Carolina, USA

Romanov, Yuri A., Cardiology Research Center, Moscow, USSR

Romeo, Rosemarie, Albany Medical College, Albany, New York, USA

Rosenfeld, Michael E., University of California School of Medicine–San Diego, LaJolla, California, USA

Ross, Russell, University of Washington, Seattle, Washington, USA

Ruhn, Gunnar, Linkoping University, Linkoping, Sweden

Sanborn, Timothy A., Mount Sinai Hospital, New York, New York, USA

Schaffer, Sheldon A., Cholestech Corporation, Hayward, California, USA

Schenk, Eric, University of Rochester, Rochester, New York, USA

Schwartz, Colin J., University of Texas, San Antonio, Texas, USA

Selzer, Robert H., California Institute of Technology, Pasadena, California, USA

Sharrett, A. Richey, National Institutes of Health, Bethesda, Maryland, USA

Sheldon, Phil, University of California, San Francisco, California, USA

Silverman, Kenneth J., Beth Israel Hospital and Harvard Medical School, Boston, Massachusetts, USA

Small, Donald M., Boston University, Boston, Massachusetts, USA

Smirnof, Vladimir N., Cardiology Research Center, Moscow, USSR

Smith, Elspeth B., University of Aberdeen, Aberdeen, Scotland, UK

Smullens, Stanton N., Jefferson Medical College, Philadelphia, Pennsylvania, USA

Solymoss, B. Charles, Institut de Cardiologie de Montreal, Montreal, Canada

Sprague, Eugene A., University of Texas, San Antonio, Texas, USA

Srinivasan, S.R., Louisiana State University, New Orleans, Louisiana, USA

Stary, H.C., Louisiana State University, New Orleans, Louisiana, USA

Stein, Evan A., University of Cincinnati, Cincinnati, Ohio, USA

Steinberg, Daniel, University of California at San Diego, La Jolla, California, USA

Stifter, William F., Spokane Heart Clinic, Spokane, Washington, USA

Strandness, D. Eugene, Jr., University of Washington, Seattle, Washington, USA

Strauss, H. William, Massachusetts General Hospital and Harvard Medical School, Boston, Massachusetts, USA

Suenram, C. Allen, Cone Biotechnology, Seguin, Texas, USA

Tanimura, A., Kurume University School of Medicine, Kurume, Japan

Thomas, Wilbur A., Albany Medical College, Albany, New York, USA

Tinalski, Thomas, Miami Heart Institute, Miami, Florida, USA

Titus, Jack L., United Hospitals, St. Paul, Minnesota, USA

Toole, James F., Bowman-Gray School of Medicine, Winston-Salem, North Carolina, USA

Tsukada, Toyohiro, Tokyo Medical and Dental University, Tokyo, Japan

Valente, Anthony, Cleveland Heart Institute, Cleveland, Ohio, USA

Vijayagopal, P., Louisiana State University, New Orleans, Louisiana, USA

Wagner, William D., Bowman-Gray School of Medicine, Winston-Salem, North Carolina, USA

Weilbaecher, Donald G., Baylor College of Medicine, Houston, Texas, USA

Wheeler, Hugh G., New England Deaconess Hospital, Boston, Massachusetts, USA

Wilmoth, Sharon, Bowman-Gray School of Medicine, Winston-Salem, North Carolina, USA

Wissler, Robert W., University of Chicago, Chicago, Illinois, USA

York, B.J.G., Bowman-Gray School of Medicine, Winston-Salem, North Carolina, USA

Zarins, Christopher K., University of Chicago, Chicago, Illinois, USA

Introduction

1
Questions About the Natural History of Human Atherosclerosis

Henry C. McGill, Jr.

Criteria for a Good Question

It is much easier to ask questions than to answer them, but selecting the right questions is a difficult task. A good question, first, is answerable. There is not much use in trying to answer questions when methods to answer them are not adequate. Second, the answer to a good question makes a difference in future actions. I will review some of the current questions about the pathogenesis of atherosclerosis and atherosclerotic disease with these two criteria in mind.

Ischemic Injury

The clinically manifest events that make atherosclerosis so important in our population are predominantly the immediate results of ischemic injury to the heart, the brain, or the legs. Not too many years ago, we accepted ischemic injury as a rather simple process that was determined exclusively by the location and severity of arterial occlusion. More recently, investigators have identified a number of processes involved in ischemic injury, and they have shown that the size of an infarct can be modulated by manipulation of these processes. Most attention has been directed toward myocardial infarction. Factors identified include those that affect myocardial oxygen demand and supply, myocardial anaerobic metabolism, stability of membranes, homeostasis of ionic calcium, and acute inflammation (1).

An example of how the acute inflammatory reaction affects infarct size, and how it can be modified, is provided by the experiments reviewed by Pinckard et al. (2). Complement is bound to injured, but not necrotic, myocardial fibers at the periphery of standardized 24 hour experimental infarcts. Activation of the complement results in recruitment of leukocytes to the area, release of lysosomal enzymes, and necrosis of muscle. Blocking the activation of complement by cobra venom inhibits leukocyte recruitment and reduces the size of the infarct. Other types of interventions in the early period after arterial occlusion also show promise of significantly reducing the size of the infarct after arterial occlusion has occurred.

Questions about the control of infarct size can be studied in easily produced experimental models by ligating a coronary artery. Basic knowledge of cell biology and immunology make it possible to propose a variety of testable hypotheses. Consequently, questions about the control of infarct size can be answered readily. The answers may not be of great interest to the participants in this workshop, but they offer considerable potential benefit for the many persons who evade our programs of primary prevention. The questions about control of ischemic injury, although obviously concerned with end stage disease, seem to be good ones when evaluated by our two criteria.

Terminal Occlusive Event

Most investigators consider thrombosis the major occlusive event in atherosclerotic disease, but others cite plaque ulceration or hemorrhage (perhaps followed by thrombosis) as important mechanisms, and some suggest vasoconstriction as an occasional possibility. There are studies demonstrating a role for each of these in the occlusive events leading to infarction, and "all of the above" may turn out to be the correct answer.

The question of mechanisms involved in the terminal occlusive event is important because of the enormous potential for preventing occlusion in the many persons in our population with advanced atherosclerosis. On the other hand, it is very difficult to study this event. Animal models that simulate the process are not sufficiently reliable to be useful. The naturally occurring event in humans is episodic and unpredictable. Observations on occlusive lesions in human subjects necessarily are limited to those who die as a result of occlusion and who also are autopsied. The observations are confounded by the length of survival of the patient.

We need new techniques to study this occlusive event more effectively. Until a new approach to the problem is devised, the question of what happens in this process is important but not answerable. An encouraging development is the finding, for the first time, that an element of the hemostatic system, plasma fibrinogen, predicts the occurrence of myocardial infarction (3).

The Fibrous Plaque

The Fibrous plaque is widely accepted as the most common precursor of occlusive lesions and the major determinant of risk of clinical disease. The familiar appearance of the fibrous plaque is the logo for atherosclerosis. Its structure, composition, and topography are well defined. Fibrous plaques are now known to be associated with the major risk factors for clinical disease, particularly with hyperlipidemia and hypertension, and possibly also with smoking. The correlations with some risk factors are so strong that they seem likely to be causal.

The major question about the fibrous plaque is not its structure or composition, but its precursor. The conventional idea is that the fibrous plaque originates by a gradual increase in intimal lipid deposits to form a core of extracellular lipid and necrotic debris, covered by a fibromuscular cap. This concept is logical and attractive, but it has been extraordinarily difficult to prove. Fibrous plaques often, but not always, correspond topographically with fatty streaks, and the discrepancies have led to some skepticism about the relationship.

There is little question that the fibrous plaque is important in the pathogenesis of atherosclerosis because of its close relationship to clinical disease. The mature lesion is easy to study because there are many lesions, they

remain for a long time, and they now can be visualized in
some arteries by non-invasive methods. It is important to
know how and when it arises in humans, because this represents one critical stage in atherogenesis at which preventing progression would be most effective.

Determining the origin of the fibrous plaque in humans
requires reconstructing a process by examining multiple
still-picture frames. These frames must come from certain
sites in the arteries of young adults where the process is
likely to be taking place. Death rates in this age group
are low and cases are principally traumatic deaths autopsied
in medical examiners' laboratories. Consequently, securing
proper and sufficient material for study is difficult; and
obtaining data on risk factors is even more difficult. I
will return to this problem later.

The Transitional Lesion

I have proposed that there is a transitional lesion,
the missing link between the fatty streak and the fibrous
plaque. This lesion grossly resembles a fatty streak, but
microscopically shows a core of necrotic debris and extracellular lipid that causes it to resemble a fibrous plaque.
The transitional lesion occurs predominantly in 20 to 30
year old men, members of populations in which middle aged
men have severe atherosclerosis and high risk of atherosclerotic disease. It is found at sites where fibrous
plaques are known to occur in older persons, as in the
proximal portion of the left anterior descending coronary
artery, or in the abdominal aorta. Fatty streaks occur at
these same sites in younger persons. Compared to the
fibrous plaque, its life history is relatively brief,
perhaps a year or less. The extent and frequency of transitional lesions should be associated with the conditions
identified as risk factors for clinical disease, principally
hyperlipidemia and hypertension. More likely, they will be
associated with the upper percentiles of the frequency
distributions of these variables in young adults. These
higher percentiles may not be as high as those usually
considered elevated among middle-aged persons.

Because the transitional lesion is expected to share characteristics of both the fatty streak and the fibrous plaque, we may have difficulty in defining it by strict morphologic and biochemical criteria. The definition may need to include behavioral criteria -- where (anatomic site), when (age), and in whom (sex, race, and population). Identification of any distinctive characteristic for the lesion will provide a useful marker, considerable insight into the processes involved, and perhaps a clue regarding the cause of its progression. The marker may be a particular cell type, a special lipid, a distinctive connective tissue alteration, or some other component.

The importance of the transitional lesion is difficult to overestimate. This lesion signals the conversion of an initially innocuous process of lipid accumulation in the arterial intima to a progressive and clinically serious process that eventually will result in high risk of arterial occlusion. The age at and conditions under which transitional lesions occur will determine when and how clinically significant progression can be prevented or retarded. Intervention at later ages already has been shown to be helpful, but intervention at this early stage may be more nearly definitive.

The question is important, but the difficulties in obtaining answers are great. Animal models already have suggested that prolonged hyperlipidemia results in the progression of fatty streaks into fibrous plaques by continued lipid deposition and other tissue changes. These lesions include many that resemble the hypothetical transitional lesion. It appears that little more information is to be gained from animal models on this issue unless the same sequence can be demonstrated in humans. The difficulties center around the problem of reconstructing a dynamic process by capturing enough still frames from the motion picture so that the proper sequence of changes can be deciphered. This is a classical problem of both experimental and observational pathology when dealing with a process that cannot be observed continuously *in situ*. We must obtain enough tissue samples from humans in the appropriate age range to reconstruct a convincing motion picture.

In our society, deaths in the 20 to 30 year old age group are very low, even in men, and moth of the deaths are traumatic and result from suicide, homocide, or accidents. These deaths most certainly are not representative of the population in which they occur, but they are the best we have. Autopsies on such deaths usually are performed in medical examiners' or coroners' laboratories, and the needs of the forensic pathologist sometimes take precedence over the needs of the investigator who seeks his cooperation. Consequently, special efforts are necessary to obtain the large numbers of cases required from young men in the early 20's.

The second major difficulty in studying lesions in young men dying under these conditions is that of measuring the risk factors that we suspect may be involved in the progression of atherogenesis. The probability that any ever have had serum lipid or blood pressure measurements is very low, and the effort required to locate the values, if any have been recorded, is great. Smoking habits must be reconstructed from interviews of surviving family members or associates. Family histories are also difficult to obtain.

Some progress has been made in measuring these risk factor variables in deceased persons by analyzing post-mortem blood for serum lipids and apolipoproteins, estimating blood pressure by examining renal arterioles, and measuring plasma thiocyanate as marker for recent smoking. Considerable efforts have been devoted to validating these methods, and they offer some promise in answering these questions about the conditions associated with the progression of atherosclerosis in young persons.

In summary, the transitional lesion is important, and the answer will make a difference in our concept of pathogenesis and also in our strategies for prevention of atherosclerotic disease. The questions are difficult to answer, but are not impossible.

The Fatty Streak

Juvenile fatty streaks remain one of the great mysteries of atherosclerosis. They appear in the aorta shortly after birth, and increase rapidly in extent in the aorta during the second decade. They occur in children of all populations, regardless of environment or disposition to advanced lesions later in life.

The major question about juvenile fatty streaks is whether they progress to more advanced lesions, as hypothesized previously in the discussion of transitional lesions and fibrous plaques; and, if they do, what are the conditions that lead to such progression. Clearly, not all fatty streaks undergo such progression, and this discrepancy has led to much of the skepticism about the relationships of fatty streaks to fibrous plaques.

The second important set of questions about fatty streaks is why they form and whether they are associated with the risk factors for clinical events. A recent report described a remarkable positive correlation of juvenile fatty streaks with plasma low density lipoprotein levels (4). Nevertheless, a substantial extent of aortic fatty streaks can be found in children from populations that have very low serum cholesterol and lipoprotein levels. It is difficult, therefore, to imagine that they are due entirely to hyperlipidemia. We would like to know much more about their associations with the risk factors, but the problems of collecting tissue and risk factor data are even greater than those for the transitional lesions discussed previously because death rates are lower in the first and second decades.

In summary, the origin and fate of the fatty streak are important, but answers beyond those that we already have are quite difficult to obtain.

Current Efforts to Answer Questions about Pathogenesis

A group of investigators, under the leadership of Robert Wissler of the University of Chicago, has organized a cooperative research project designed to answer some of the difficult questions about the atherosclerotic lesions of childhood and young adulthood. This project, titled

"Pathobiological Determinants of Atherosclerosis in Youth",
focuses on coronary artery and aortic lesions in 15-34 year
old victims of traumatic death autopsied in 10 medical
examiner's laboratories about the U.S. Blood and other
materials are collected along with the arteries, and standardized samples are sent to central laboratories for uniform
processing and analysis. The left coronary artery is perfused with fixative under pressure at the autopsy site.
Standardized histologic sections are made through the
proximal portion of the left anterior descending coronary
artery, the site well known to be disposed to early and
frequent occlusive lesions. The right coronary artery and
right half of the aorta are stained with Sudan IV for
grading by conventional visual estimation and by computerized
image analysis. Post-mortem blood is analyzed for cholesterol concentration and distribution among the major lipoprotein classes, and a subset of blood samples is assayed
for apolipoprotein distribution among lipoproteins. Smoking
exposure is estimated from serum thiocyanate concentrations.
Blood pressure is estimated by measurement of the wall thicknesses of renal arterioles. A variety of supplementary
studies of platelets, connective tissues, arterial proteins,
and viruses are conducted on selected samples. The data are
collected in a central laboratory for quality control and
eventual statistical analysis.

We hope that, about 5 years from now, we will begin to
see some answers to these difficult questions about fatty
streaks and fibrous plaques in young persons, and perhaps
about the elusive transitional lesions.

The Initial Event

The initial lesion is the Holy Grail of atherosclerosis
research, and it has been pursued with zeal equal to that of
King Arthur's knights -- and perhaps with equal success.
Almost every conceivable possibility has been proposed and
examined. Endothelial injury permitting the influx of lipoproteins or platelets, smooth muscle cell proliferation and
degeneration, connective tissue alteration, monocyte infiltration -- some evidence has been accumulated for each of
these. Much of the evidence supporting one or the other of

these processes as the initial stage of atherogenesis has been derived from cell cultures or animal models in which interesting and important processes can be isolated and studied, but the relevance of these processes to what takes place in the human artery remains uncertain. A new generation of observational studies is needed to assist in bridging the gap between cell biology and human pathophysiology.

The ongoing cooperative research project described in connection with the fatty streak may provide some partial or preliminary answers to this question, but its primary focus is on the hypothesized progression of lesions between 15 and 34 years, and not on the initiation of the fatty streak, which we know is well established in the aorta and is beginning in the coronary arteries by age 15. The difficulties of such research are even greater than those of studying fatty streaks and transitional lesions described previously. We are looking for a change that predicts the future occurrence of clinically significant atherosclerosis. Unless one accepts the idea that fatty streaks progress to fibrous plaques, this means that we are looking for a change that predicts a lesion that will develop, 10 to 20 years later. If one is looking for the precursor of the fatty streak, one must deal with the reservation that the earliest and most frequent site of intimal lipid deposition is the thoracic aorta, which is least likely to develop fibrous plaques.

One promising approach to answering this question is to examine systematically a site in the arteries of young children known to have high predisposition to develop fatty streaks and subsequently fibrous plaques and more advanced occlusive lesions. Such a site is the proximal portion of the left anterior descending coronary artery. Herbert Stary has conducted such a study of children and young adults from birth to 29 years of age, and reports selected observations later in this workshop to supplement those already published (5,6). The most striking feature of Stary's findings is the presence of isolated macrophage foam cells deep within the coronary artery intima in even the youngest infants. By about 10 years of age, macrophage foam cells began to appear in clusters and often are associated with lipid in smooth muscle cells. These microscopic lipid deposits are not visible as gross fatty streaks on the intimal surface because of the thickness of the overlying intima. Endothelium, connective tissue, and smooth muscle show no morphologic abnormalities in these sites. One, of course, must simultaneously acknowledge the limits of even the best light and electron microscopy to detect subtle functional changes, but the presence of lipid-filled macrophages and smooth muscle cells appears to support strongly the primary roles of abnormal lipid and lipoprotein metabolism and of the tissue monocyte-macrophage in the earliest stages of atherogenesis.

The resolution of questions about the initial event is important because it will give us a better guide to the importance of the risk factors, initially identified for adult disease, in childhood, and where to expend preventive efforts. One of the major controversial topics in the overall diet-heart issue is whether to recommend diet modification for children. The present case for making such a recommendation is based almost exclusively on extrapolation backward from observations on middle-aged adults. Pediatricians have good reason to be conservative regarding changing childrens' diets which have been associated with the virtual disappearance of scourges such as rheumatic fever and tuberculosis. A stronger case must be made for avoiding the potential long deferred effects of diet-induced hyperlipidemia in children. A close relationship between high plasma lipoproteins and intimal lipid deposition in a vulnerable portion of the coronary arteries of children would close another gap in the evidence linking childhood hyperlipidemia to adult atherosclerotic disease.

In summary, the nature of the initial event is important, because the answer makes a big difference in many ways. Obtaining an answer is difficult and tedious, but perhaps not impossible. Study of human tissues is an essential part of the spectrum of research effort.

REFERENCES

1. DeBakey ME, Gotto AM Jr (1983) Factors Influencing
    the Course of Myocardial Ischemia. Amsterdam:
    Elsevier Science Publishers B.V.
2. Pinckard RN, McManus LM, Crawford MH, et al. (1983)
    The role of the acute inflammatory process in the
    pathogenesis of ischemic myocardial tissue injury.
    In: Factors Influencing the Course of Myocardial
    Ischemia. Amsterdam: Elsevier Science Publishers
    B.V., pp 173-189.
3. Wilhelmsen L, Svardsudd K, Korsen-Bengtsen K,
    Larsson B, Welin L, Tibblin G (1984) Fibrinogen as
    a risk factor for stroke and myocardial infarction.
    N Engl J Med 311:501-505.
4. Newman WP III, Voors AW, Freedman DS, et al. (1986)
    Relation of serum lipoprotein levels and systolic blood
    pressure to early atherosclerosis: The Bogalusa Heart
    Study. N Engl J Med 314:138-144.
5. Stary HC (1987) Evolution and progression of athero-
    sclerosis in the coronary arteries of children and
    adults. In: Bates RS, Gangloff EC (eds) Atherogenesis
    and Aging. New York: Springer-Verlag, pp. 20-36.
6. Stary HC (1987) Macrophages, macrophage foam cells,
    and eccentric intimal thickening in the coronary
    arteries of young children. Atherosclerosis 64:91-108.

Cellular Contents

2
Arterial Endothelial Structure and Permeability as It Relates to Susceptibility to Atherogenesis

Ross G. Gerrity

INTRODUCTION

Over the past decade, the arterial endothelium has been the subject of intense scrutiny, both *in vivo* and *in vitro*. This interest stems primarily from the belief that since this cellular lining provides the first level of interaction between the blood and the arterial wall, and presents to the blood a non-thrombogenic and selectively permeable surface, it may play a decisive role in the processes leading to atherogenesis. Once considered little more than a passive barrier to diffusion, the vascular endothelium has, in recent years, been shown to exhibit a wide range of tissue-specific structural and functional characteristics which demonstrate this cell type to be highly differentiated and specialized. Vascular endothelium clearly exhibits the ability to regenerate when injured, both *in vivo* and *in vitro*, in order to maintain its functional state (1-9), and when intact, selectively controls the transport and permeability of both large and small molecules into the vessel wall (10-14). Endothelial cells contain contractile protein (15-17), plasminogen activator (18), fibrinolysins and tissue thrombospondins (20,21), and synthesize factor VIII (22) and connective tissue components, including collagens type III (23) and IV (24) and heparin and heparitin sulfate (25). More recently (26), the vascular endothelium

has been shown to actively synthesize PGI_2 (a potent vasodilator and antiaggregatory substance for platelets),
endothelial cell-derived growth factor (EDGF), a smooth
muscle cell mitogen resembling platelet-derived growth
factor (27-29), and lipoprotein lipase (30). The presence
of PGI_2 and EDGF in arterial endothelium has obvious implications relating to control of vascular spasm, thrombosis,
and proliferative responses of the arterial wall, whereas
lipoprotein lipase activity on the endothelial surface
could have important implications not only in the conversion
of very low density lipoprotein (VLDL), but also in the
initial degradation of chylomicrons, with resultant release
of small cholesterol-rich particles (30). All these mechanisms have potential relevance to vascular injury and
atherogenesis. Endothelial cells also exhibit surface
receptors for a wide variety of molecules, including low
density lipoprotein (LDL), which is modified by the endothelial cell to a form recognized by the scavenger receptor
of macrophages (31).

In other words, as our understanding of the structural-
functional relationships of the vascular endothelium has
become more precise due to improved *in vivo* perfusion
fixation techniques and the broad range of *in vitro* approaches
now available, it has become obvious that the endothelial
lining is a dynamic cellular layer whose functions are largely
specific to a particular vessel and tissue site. However, it
is also clear that most of our understanding of arterial endothelial function is derived from studies of animal cells in
tissue culture, and that *in vivo* structural-functional
relationships have resulted from studies on animal models
which approximate, to varying degrees, the human condition.
This is particularly true of studies relating the function
of arterial endothelium to the cellular biology of atherosclerosis. Our knowledge of endothelial cell structure in
development and aging, altered hemodynamics, or in conditions of hyperlipidemia leading to atherogenesis is derived
almost solely from studies in animal models. Certain
parallels exist, however, particularly those relating to the

focal nature of atherosclerosis in man, which can be
reproduced and studied in certain animal models. The
existence of focal, lesion-susceptible sites in human
arteries (32) suggests that such areas may have inherent
structural-functional properties which render them prone
to atherogenic stimuli. Studies on similar sites in animal
models (33-43) would support this concept. This chapter is
intended to review our knowledge of arterial endothelial
cell structure as it may relate to lesion susceptibility
in experimental models, in the absence of similar knowledge
in human disease.

Normal Arterial Endothelial Structure

The arterial endothelium, when viewed in sections of
perfusion-fixed arteries at either the light (Figure 1a)
or electron (Figure 1b) microscopy level, can be seen to
consist of a thin cellular layer on the luminal surface,
ranging in thickness from 0.1 μ at the tapering edges of
the cells to 3-4 μ in the central portion containing the
nuclei. Even at the ultrastructural level, endothelial
cells show a sparse complement of organelles when viewed
in cross-, or longitudinal section, probably due to the
laminar orientation of organellar structures within the
flattened cytoplasm of this cell type, together with the
small cytoplasmic area visible in cross-section. As a
result, early ultrastructural studies on arteiral endothelium (44-49) reported very little development of cytoplasmic organelles. In fact, French (49), commenting on
the paucity of organelles in arterial endothelium, stated
"apart from their primary requirements, endothelial cells
are not engaged at a high level in specialized metabolic
activities." Subsequent studies (referred to above) have
shown this not to be true, and the use of "en face"
sections, in which the endothelium is sectioned parallel
to the flattened surface of the cell, have shown not only
that arterial endothelium is rich in organelles, but also
that the organellar component varies with development and
aging (50).

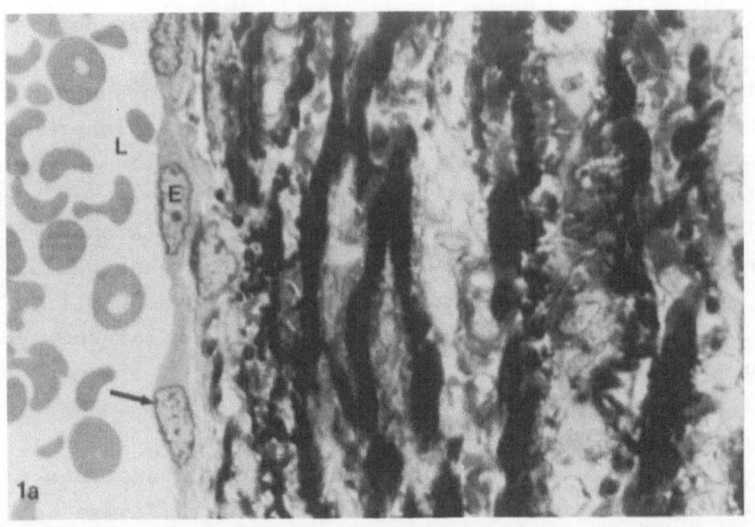

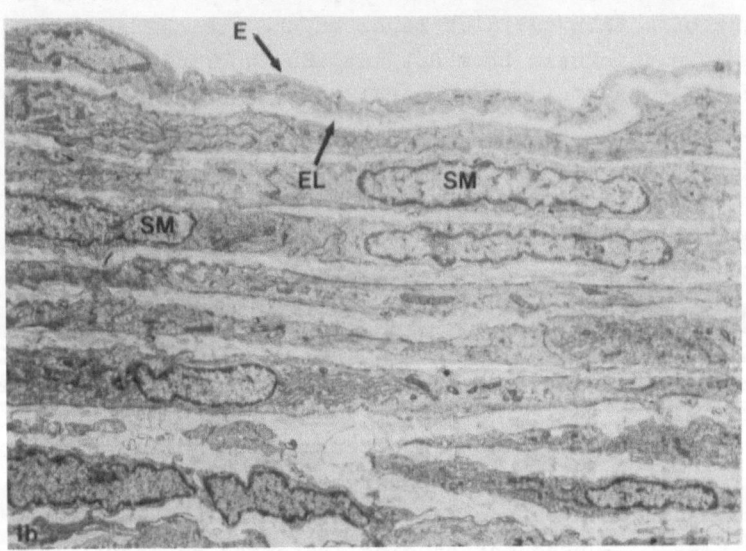

Figure 1.   (A)   Light photomicrograph of 1μ-thick section through intima and inner media of perfusion-fixed monkey
thoracic aorta.   Endothelium (E) appears as a thin monolayer
separating the arterial wall from the lumen (L).   Endothelial
cells bulge slightly into lumen in area around nuclei (arrow).
Methylene blue-azure II-basic fuchsin (x 780).   (B)   Transmission electron micrograph of cross-section through the
thoracic aorta of 1 week old rat.   Endothelium (E) rests
directly on developing internal elastic lamina (EL).
Organelles appear sparse in cross-sections through endothelial
cells compared to underlying smooth muscle (SM) rich in endoplasmic reticulum and Golgi (x 7,200).

The aortic endothelium of the young, both in animals and man, when seen in "en face" sections, is characterized by its extraordinary development of cellular organelles (Figure 2). The Golgi complex is very prominent, as is the endoplasmic reticulum (ER), the cisternae of which are often swollen and contain granular material (Figure 2). Coated vesicles and large numbers of free ribosomes, which do not form ergosomal clusters, are seen. Mitochondria are numerous. Centrioles and multivesicular bodies can be found at all ages. However, as maturity is reached, organellar development declines. In particular, the amounts of Golgi and ER diminish, and there are fewer free ribosomes, although ergosomes are present at these stages. During maturity, but prior to old age, or disease in humans, the appearance of the cells is relatively constant (Figure 3). The Golgi zone remains small in size, and the ER is fragmented so that only short profiles are observed. Coated vesicles are present in small numbers beyond two months of age (50) in the rat. In contrast, the endothelial cytoplasm of 2- and 3-year-old rats (Figure 4) and other aged animals is almost as active morphologically as that of the newborn (Figure 2). The Golgi apparatus is hypertrophied, and membrane-bound inclusions containing both osmiophilic and nonosmiophilic lipid are associated with it (Figure 4). ER is more prominent than in the middle aged groups, and free ribosomes are numerous. Mitochondria are larger and less electron-dense than in younger rats, and coated vesicles and multivesicular bodies are present in moderate numbers.

Endothelial cells are flat to ovoid in cross-section in the young (Figure 1B) and subsequently flatten with age. When viewed in cross-section, the cell is more irregular on the luminal side at all ages, and with increasing age develops numerous microvillus projections (Figure 5), which are also more frequently seen overlying atherosclerotic lesions (34). Cytoplasmic flaps, extending into the lumen from the surfaces of endothelial cells near junctions are seen at all ages and are often very complex. On the abluminal surface, peg-like extensions of endothelial cells project into and through the

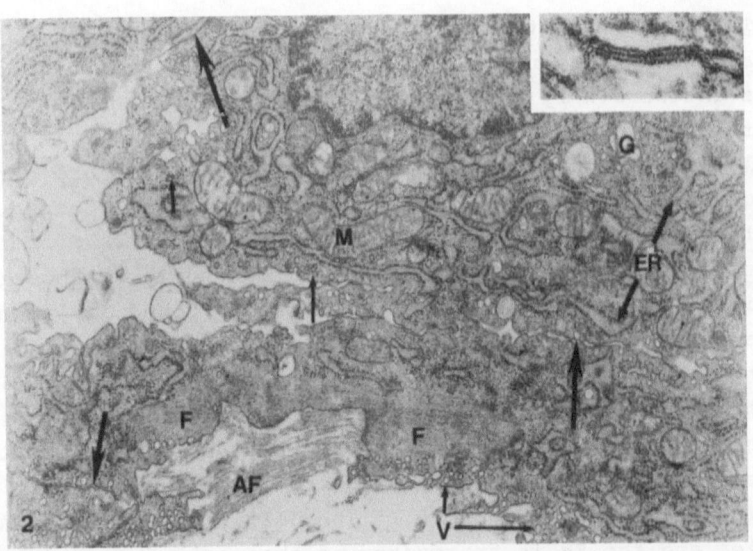

Figure 2. Transmission electron micrograph of section through endothelium cut parallel to endothelial layer (*en face*). Same specimen as in Figure 1B. Well-developed dilated endoplasmic reticulum (ER), Golgi (G), cytoplasmic filament bundles (F), numerous mitochondria (M), vesicles (V), and free ribosomes (small arrows) are visible in *en face* view which are not seen in cross-section. Elongate, complex junctions (large arrows) are visualized, as is proximity of anchoring filaments (AF) to cytoplasmic filaments (F) on basal aspect of cell (x 31,000). Inset. Transmission electron micrograph of punctate tight junction between endothelial cells common to all ages (x 120,000). Reprinted from Exp. Molec. Pathol. 16:382-402, 1972, by permission of Academic Press.

subendothelial space in the neonate. Such projections often extend between patches of developing elastin and come into close contact with medial smooth muscle cells (Figure 6). After the formation of an intact internal elastic lamina, endothelial projections are rarely seen in contact with medial smooth muscle, although they may extend into the internal elastic lamina. The endothelial nuclei at all ages are granular with dense peripheral chromatin, and contain nucleoli. In both young animals and humans, their profiles are smooth with few indentations (Figure 1B, 2), whereas with

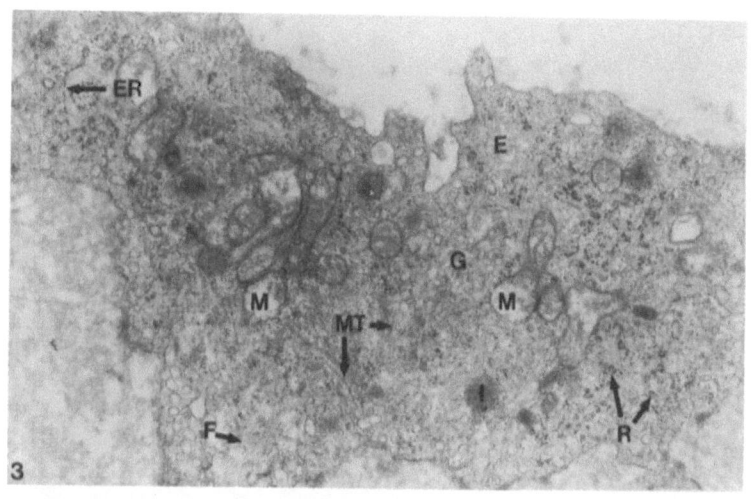

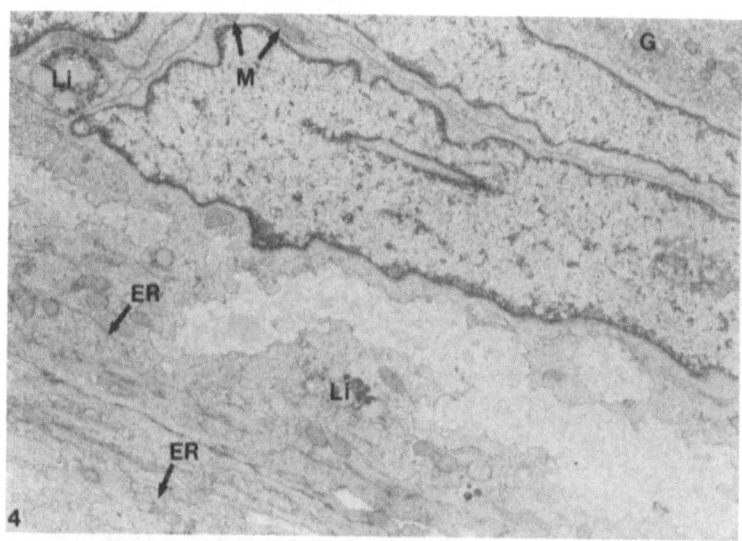

Figure 3.   Transmission electron micrograph of endothelium (E)
from a twenty-year-old human cut slightly *en face*.   Short profiles of endoplasmic reticulum (ER), a small Golgi (G), numerous
ribosomal clusters or ergosomes (R), membrane-bound inclusions
(I), microtubules (MT) and filaments (F) are visible.   Partial
degeneration of mitochondria (M) is a post-mortem artefact
(x 27,000).
Figure 4.   Transmission electron micrograph of *en face* section
of aortic endothelium of two-year-old rat.   Golgi apparatus
(G) is extremely well-developed, frequently associated with
lipid inclusions (Li).   Endoplasmic reticulum (ER) shows
elongate profiles, and mitochondria (M) are large and electron-
translucent (x 23,000).   Reprinted from Exp. Molec. Pathol.
16:382-402, 1972, by permission of Academic Press.

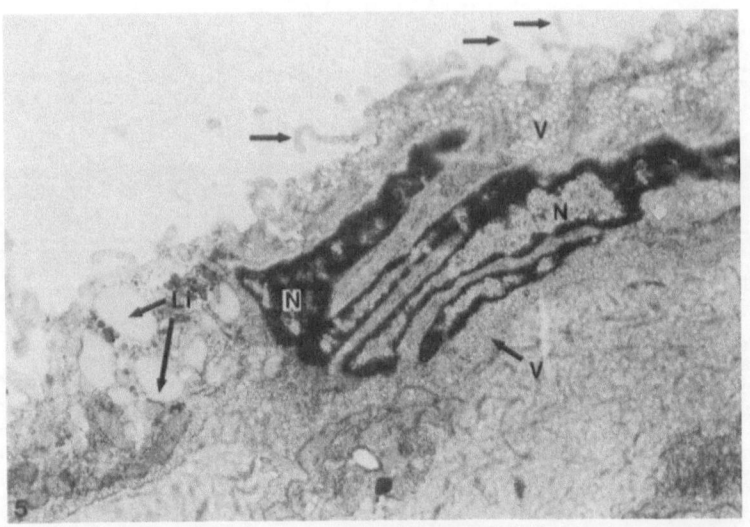

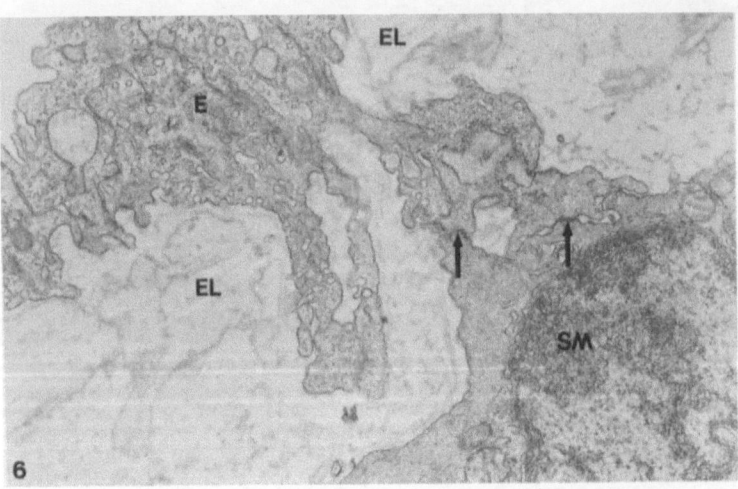

Figure 5. Transmission electron micrograph of slightly
oblique section through aortic endothelial cell of three-year-
old rat. Numerous microvilli (arrows) extend from the luminal
surface, and lipid inclusions (Li) are associated with Golgi
apparatus. Nucleus (N) is extremely tortuous with dense
peripheral chromatin. Large numbers of plasmalemmal vesicles
(V) can be seen on both luminal and abluminal aspects of
the cell (x 21,600).

Figure 6. Transmission electron micrograph of cross-section
through aortic intima of one-week-old rat. Projections of
endothelium (E) extend through developing internal elastic
lamina (EL) and come into close contact (arrows) with medial
smooth muscle cells (SM) (x 31,000). Reprinted from Exp.
Molec. Pathol. 16:382-402, 1972, by permission of Academic
Press.

advanced age, they frequently become very thin, with tortuous, folded contours (Figure 5), even in perfusion-fixed vessels. Peripheral chromatin is frequently more densely stained in older than in younger animals (Figure 5). Occasional mitoses can be identified in the endothelium of the neonate, but are seldom seen after maturity in experimental animals.

The endothelium of all species examined, including humans, contains tubular structures and filaments. Numerous microtubules 20-24 nm in diameter and of indefinite length occur free in the cytoplasm (Figures 3,7,8A,8B). These do not appear to have any specific orientation. Rod-shaped bundles of fine tubules (Weibel-Palade bodies) enveloped by tightly-fitted membranes are routinely found at all ages. In rodents, large clusters of these organelles are frequently observed near the nucleus, generally on the luminal side of the cell (Figure 7). These bodies are about 0.1 μ in diameter and 0.5-1.0 μ in length, and of variable density. The microtubules within them are similar in appearance and diameter to those found free in the cytoplasm. The frequency of Weibel-Palade bodies (51) appears to be species-dependent. In our experience, they are numerous in the arterial endothelium of rodents, rarely seen in swine, and present in moderate numbers in dogs, primates and humans.

Bundles of fine cytoplasmic filaments of about 9 nm diameter are present at intermittent intervals related to the abluminal surface of arterial endothelial cells. These filaments often merge into dense bodies on the internal surface of the plasma membrane (Figures 2,8). There is generally no obvious orientation of the filament bundles within endothelial cells, and the angle of their meeting with the plasma membrane is random. In some cases these filament bundles exhibit a cross-striated appearance (Figure 8). There is an apparent relationship between these cytoplasmic filaments and other filaments in the subendothelial space, described below. Cytoplasmic filaments also occasionally occur along junctional surfaces, but are not associated with specialized membrane complexes. In lesion-susceptible areas in swine, however, such filaments are often arranged in a circular pattern around the nuclei (Figure 8B).

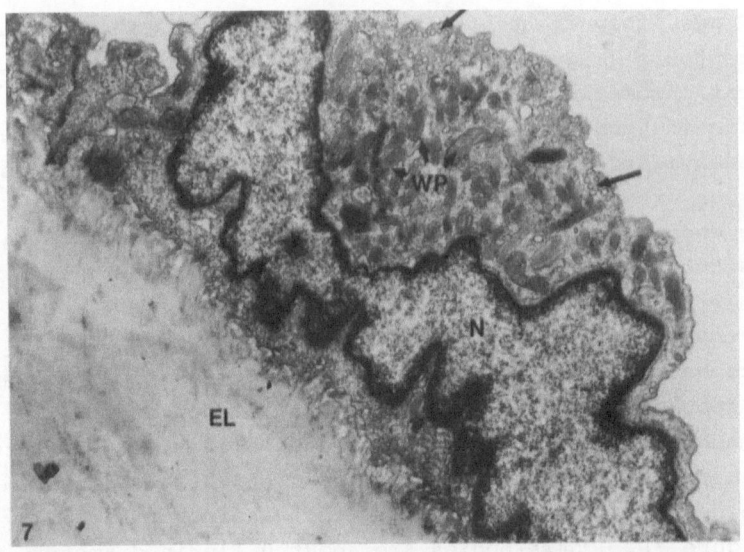

Figure 7. Transmission electron micrograph of cross-section
of aortic endothelium from a two month old rat showing large
cluster of Weibel-Palade bodies (WP) on luminal side of
nucleus (N). Numerous vesicles (arrows) are also visible.
Endothelial cell rests directly on internal elastic lamina
(EL) (x 24,700).

Junctional surfaces between endothelial cells are
complex, especially when observed in "en face" sections. In
this orientation, junctional regions several microns in length
can be seen in one plane. In these areas the peripheral cytoplasm of the cells is thrown into folds which interdigitate
with those of adjacent cells (Figures 2,4). A space of 3-8 nm
generally separates the two plasma membranes. Membrane fusions
between arterial endothelial cells are seldom observed in
cross- or longitudinal sections of the aorta. In the "en
face" orientation, however, localized, punctate areas of
membrane fusion are encountered frequently at all ages
(Figure 2, inset). Serial sections through such areas reveal
that their long axes are approximately parallel to the luminal
and abluminal surfaces of the cell, but they extend for only
very short distances in the luminal-abluminal axis of the
junctions.

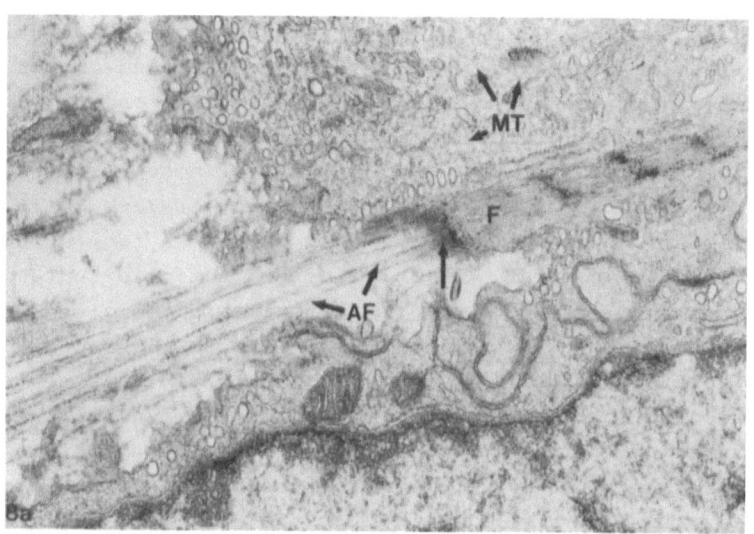

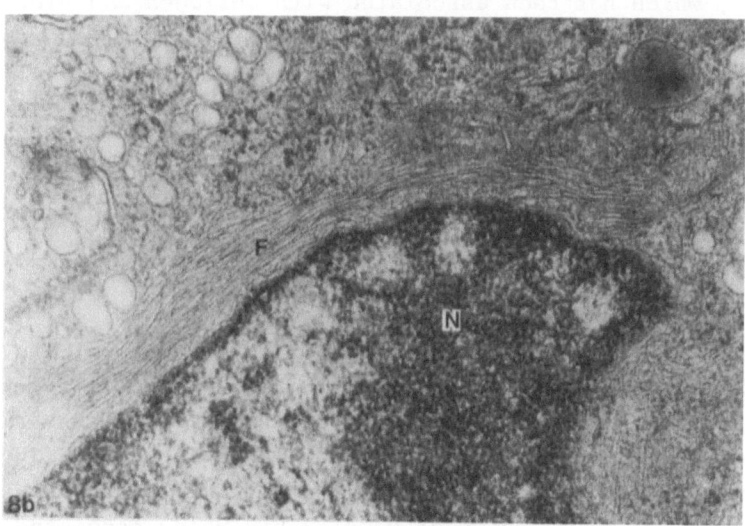

Figure 8. (A) Transmission electron micrograph *en face*
section through abluminal aspect of aortic endothelial cell
of a rat, showing striated intracytoplasmic filament
bundles (F) merging with dense body (arrow) at plasma membrane.
Subendothelial anchoring filaments (AF) merge with dense body
on extracellular surface and are aligned with intracellular
filaments. Numerous microtubules (MT) are present in the
cytoplasm (x 50,200). (B) Transmission electron micrograph
through endothelium of lesion-susceptible area in swine
aorta showing cytoplasmic filaments (F) arranged in circular
pattern around nucleus (N) (x 64,600). Reprinted from Exp.
Molec. Pathol. 16:382-402, 1972, by permission of Academic
Press.

By sectioning the endothelium in an en face orientation, large areas of plasma membrane on both luminal and abluminal surfaces can be viewed. Large numbers of vesicles or "caveolae intracellulares" cover these areas in all age groups, regardless of species (Figures 2,4,7,8A). These vesicles vary in diameter between 34 and 68 nm and there are 34 to 140 vesicles/μ^2 when cells are viewed in the en face orientation. Studies in swine, described below, indicate that age-related changes in the density of cytoplasmic vesicles exist.

The presence of a well-developed ER and Golgi apparatus in the aortic endothelium of the young probably represents its metabolic involvement in the rapid development of the cardiovascular system occurring at that time. Medial smooth muscle cells at this age also exhibit more organelles than at later stages, presenting a fibroblast-like appearance (52-53), which has been associated with collagen and elastin synthesis (53). With maturity and homeostasis, it is probable that less-active synthesis is required, and these organellar components are reduced to a minimum. The return of the system to a highly active state in old age may well represent hypertrophic response to changing conditions in the extra-cellular environment due to breakdown in the general homeo-static mechanisms. Buck (54) and Daoud, Jones and Scott (55) have reported an increase in endothelial organelles in dietary-induced atherosclerosis, and Huttner, More and Rona (56) have shown similar results in hypertensive rats.

Although the arterial endothelium, as previously stated, has been shown to be capable of active synthesis of a variety of biologically-active molecules, little is known relating the structure of the synthetic apparatus to specialized synthetic function. The rough ER-Golgi complex has been associated in general with protein synthesis, transport, and secretion (57-60), and Golgi with production and secretion of nonproteinaceous materials (61-62). A possible product of this system in aortic endothelial cells are the rod-shaped bodies identified in the cytoplasm. These tubular structures were first described by Weibel and Palade (51) and Majno (63), and have since been linked with the release of thromboplastic and fibrinolytic

substances by blood vessel endothelium (64-66); which may
occur after administration of epinephrine (67-68). Sengel
and Stoebner (69) have shown that the rod-shaped bodies
are assembled and possibly synthesized in the Golgi complex.
Other proteinaceous molecules (15-17,23-24,27-30) are
obviously produced and secreted by the ER-Golgi complex, but
the mechanisms governing the relative synthesis of each are
relatively unexplored.

There is no apparent connection between the tubular
bodies and the microtubules found free in the cytoplasm. The
functional significance of the latter has been uncertain since
Sanborn et al. (70) initially reported their existence in a
wide variety of tissues fixed with aldehydes. It is generally
accepted that they provide an inner support mechanism or
cytoskeleton which prevents deformation of the endothelial
cells due to physical forces. Similarly, there is no apparent
structural connection between the microtubules and the cytoplasmic filaments found within these cells. Bierring and
Kobayasi (46) initially suggested that these filaments may
be elastin precursors, but other workers have maintained that
they perform a structural function, and have connections with
the subendothelial space (71-73). Leak and Burke (72) found
similar filaments in endothelial cells of lymphatics, in areas
where elastin was not present. All of the above workers
reported the presence of extracellular "microfibrils" in close
apposition to the endothelial plasma membrane in areas where
intracellular filaments were found, and Leak and Burke
termed the former "anchoring filaments." The long axis of
the anchoring filaments are aligned with that of the cytoplasmic filaments, suggesting a common alignment along lines
of stress. No continuity through the plasma membrane is
observed. Giacomelli, Wiener and Spiro (74) observed cross-
striated bundles of filaments in the endothelium of cerebral
cortical arteries similar to those described in the aorta by
Gerrity and Cliff (50). They suggested a contractile function
in relation to increased permeability in hypertension. It is
thus likely that the filament system serves at least to anchor
the endothelium to the wall at various points, preventing

deformation and mechanical detachment, and aiding in the
distribution of shearing forces caused by pulsatile blood
flow in the lumen. Supporting this view is the fact that
anchoring filaments apparently merge with the internal
elastic lamina in many areas. Stresses on the endothelium
may therefore be transferred along the anchoring filaments to
the underlying elastin, which acts to distribute the forces
evenly (75).

Endothelial Structure in Lesion-Susceptible Areas

The focal nature of atherosclerosis in man has recently
led to studies which have quantitatively demonstrated the
existence of focal sites with high probability of developing
atherosclerotic lesions (32). Similar lesion-susceptible
areas have been studied extensively in the swine (33-37),
dog (38) and non-human primate (41-42). Recently, Cornhill
et al. (43) have generated probability-of-occurrence maps of
lesion development in swine. These sites of lesion susceptibility correlate well with earlier qualitative studies demonstrating focal areas of altered intimal structure and function
(33-37) which have been demonstrated to be lesion-prone in
hyperlipidemic swine. The presence of such focal sites of
lesion susceptibility in both man and animal models has led
to studies in the latter to determine whether such areas
exhibit inherent structural-functional differences which
account for, or contribute to preferential lesion development.
The most extensively-studied model in this respect is the
Evans blue model in swine, in which areas of spontaneously-
occurring enhanced accumulation of blood macromolecules (33-37)
can be demarcated, even in normal swine, by their uptake of
intravenously-injected Evans blue. Such "blue" areas are
located at branch sites and inflow tracts of ostia in the
arterial tree. In the thoracic aorta, these blue areas are
the sites of earliest foam cell lesions in hyperlipidemic
swine (34,76,77), a process associated with active recruitment
of monocytes (76,78). In the abdominal aorta blue areas have
been associated with sites of intimal cushions containing
smooth muscle cells, which are considered to form the initial

proliferative cell population in the genesis of fibrous plaques (79-82).

The arterial endothelium and intima of lesion-susceptible (blue) areas, differs structurally from that overlying adjacent areas which are devoid of dye uptake and which are not susceptible to early lesion formation (white areas). In the latter, endothelial cells are consistently elongated, flattened, and oriented in the direction of blood flow (Figures 9A and 9B). In contrast, blue area endothelium exhibits an almost cuboidal structure in both surface (Figure 10A) and sectional (Figure 10B) view. Although early light microscopic studies (33) were unable to detect, quantitatively, differences in cell shape and size between the two areas, subsequent ultrastructural quantitative studies (34,83) using perfusion-fixed vessels showed that endothelial cells in lesion-susceptible (blue) areas are larger and more rounded than those in white areas (surface area $741 \pm \mu m^2$ vs $545 \pm 38 \mu m^2$; length: width ratio $1.39 \pm .03$ vs $3.30 \pm .09$, respectively). Moreover, these parameters in white areas can be made to duplicate those in blue areas by altering hemodynamic and flow conditions through partial coarctation of the vessel distal to the area (83). These differences in cell size in lesion-susceptible areas are of particular interest with respect to human vessels, in that Repin et al. (84) have reported that the arterial endothelium of infants exhibits smaller cells and greater cell density than that of uninvolved adult endothelium. Moreover, they demonstrated that the size of endothelial cells over fatty streaks and plaques, like that of swine aortic susceptible areas, is greater than that of uninvolved areas or infant vessels, with a corresponding decrease in cell density. Giant and large cells covered up to 41% of plaque surfaces, and small cells occupied only 24% of the entire surface. In contrast, in normal infant vessels, 75% of the surface is covered by small cells.

Endothelial Cell Organelles

On a qualitative basis, both the structure and frequency of a number of cellular organelles - including mitochondria,

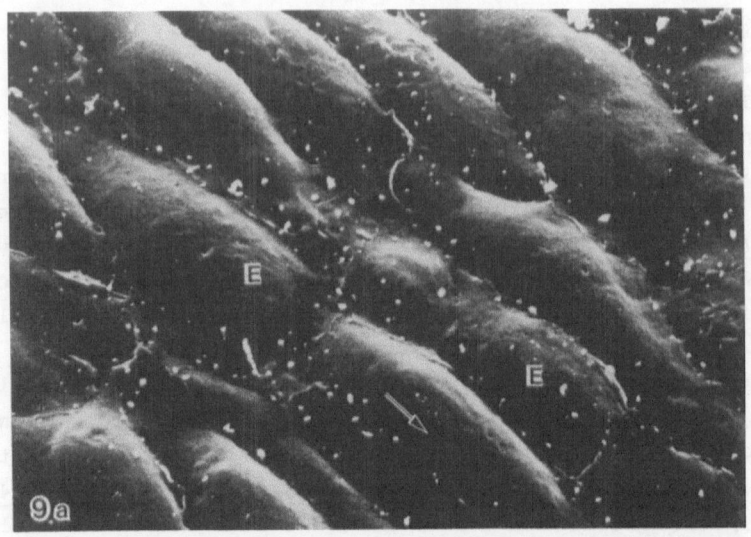

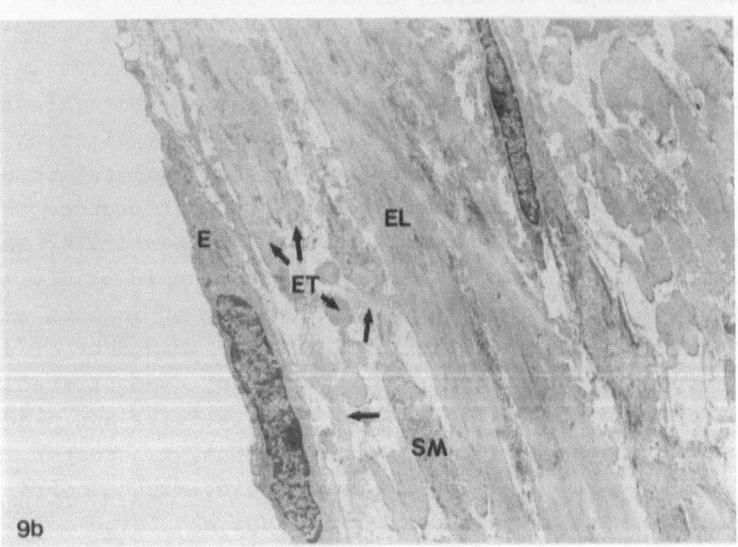

Figure 9. (A) Scanning electron micrograph of endothelial
surface from a non-susceptible (white) area of normal swine
aorta. Endothelial cells (E) are elongate, and aligned in
direction of blood flow (arrow). Compare size, shape and
orientation with cells in Figure 10A (x 5,600). (B) Transmission electron micrograph of section through endothelium
(E) and intima of non-susceptible (white) area adjacent to
that in Figure 9A. Intima is delineated on medial side by
internal elastic lamina (EL), and contains fragments of
elastic tissue (ET), collagen (arrows) and portions of smooth
muscle cells (SM). Endothelial cells are flat and elongate
(x 6,500).

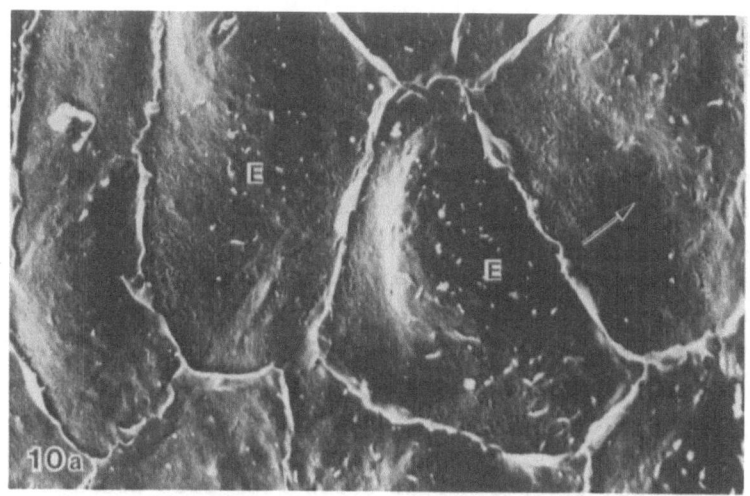

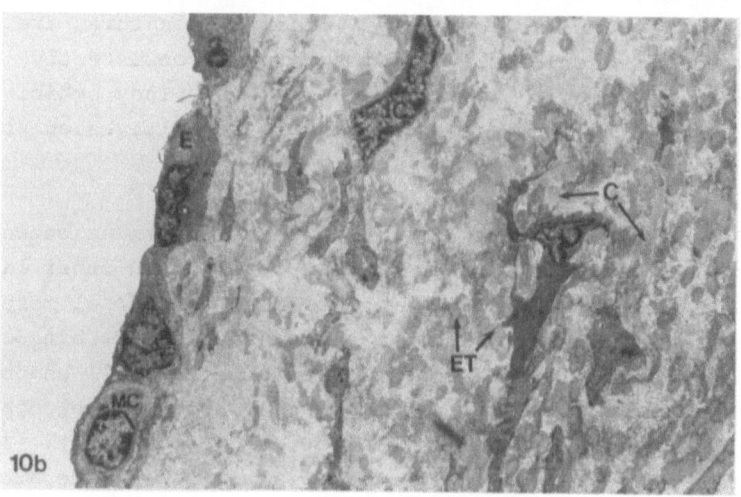

Figure 10. (A) Scanning electron micrograph of endothelial
surface from a lesion-susceptible (blue) area of normal swine
aorta. Endothelial cells (E) are large, cuboidal in shape,
and not aligned in direction of blood flow (arrow). Compare
with Figure 9A at approximately same magnification (x 5,200).
(B) Transmission electron micrograph of section through endothelium (E) and greatly expanded intima of lesion-susceptible
(blue) area adjacent to that seen in Figure 10A. Internal
elastic lamina is not visible. Compare depth of intima with
that of non-susceptible area in Figure 9B shown at approximately twice the magnification. Intima contains elastic
tissue fragments (ET), collagen (C), elongate undifferentiated
intimal cells (IC) and occasional mononuclear cells (MC).
Endothelial cells are cuboidal with simple end-to-end junctions.
Compare with Figure 9B (x 3,700).

nucleoli, free ribosomes, pinocytotic vesicles, cytoplasmic filaments, and microtubules - appear similar in endothelial cells from susceptible and non-susceptible areas. In contrast, however, definite differences in the prominence and development of the rough endoplasmic reticulum (ER), Golgi apparatus, and lysosomal bodies have been noted between lesion-susceptible (blue) and non-susceptible (white) areas in swine. The ER is more prominent in endothelial cells of blue areas (Figure 10B, 11A), although it generally exhibits shorter profiles than in white areas (Figure 11B). Of particular interest is the observation that the Golgi apparatus is consistently well developed in the endothelium of white areas (Figure 11B), whereas it is poorly developed and seldom seen in endothelial cells from blue areas (Figure 11A), despite their larger cross-sectional areas. A variety of inclusions, probably lysosomal in nature, are observed in the endothelium of both areas, consistently occurring in greater numbers in the latter. They exhibit variable density and in some instances are multivesicular.

Junctions

Although the general architecture of junctions between endothelial cells is similar to that observed in other large arteries, considerable focal variation in junctional morphology is observed between endothelial cells of blue and white areas. Associated with the differences in endothelial cell shape described above, most junctions in white areas are elongate and tortuous, with many interdigitations (Figure 12A). In contrast, the more cuboidal endothelial cells of blue areas form shorter, less complex, end-to-end junctions, with little or no interdigitation or cellular overlap (Figure 12B). Such junctions frequently exhibit a marked segmental dilatation or vacuolation (Figure 11A). Tight junctions are sometimes observed adjoining dilated segments and are frequently observed between endothelial cells in both blue and white areas.

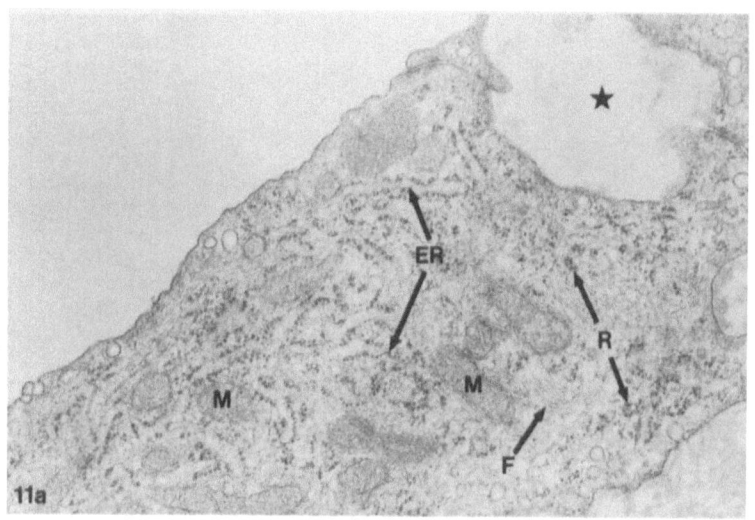

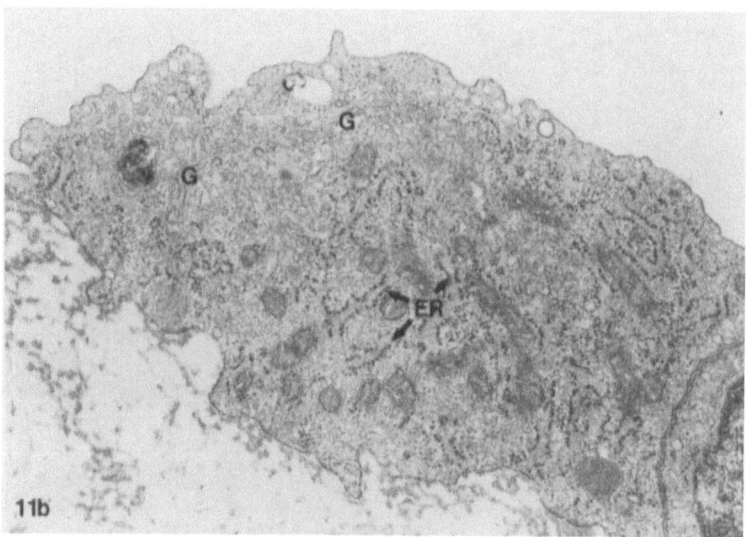

Figure 11.   (A) Transmission electron micrograph showing
cytoplasmic details of endothelial cell from lesion-susceptible
(blue) area of swine aorta.   Numerous short profiles of endoplasmic reticulum (ER), ribosomal clusters (R), filaments (F)
and mitochondria (M) are visible.   Note segmental dilation
(*) of junctional region common to these areas (x 39,400).
(B) Transmission electron micrograph showing cytoplasmic
details of endothelial cells from non-susceptible (white)
area of swine aorta.   Endoplasmic reticulum (ER) profiles
are generally longer, but less extensive than in blue areas.
Golgi (G) is well developed (x 39,400).   Reprinted from Exp.
Molec. Pathol. 16:382-402, 1972, by permission of Academic
Press.

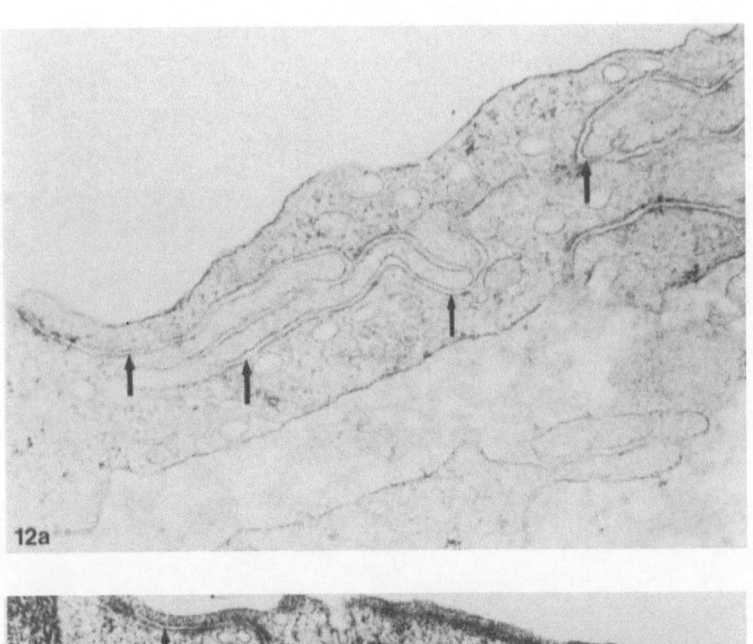

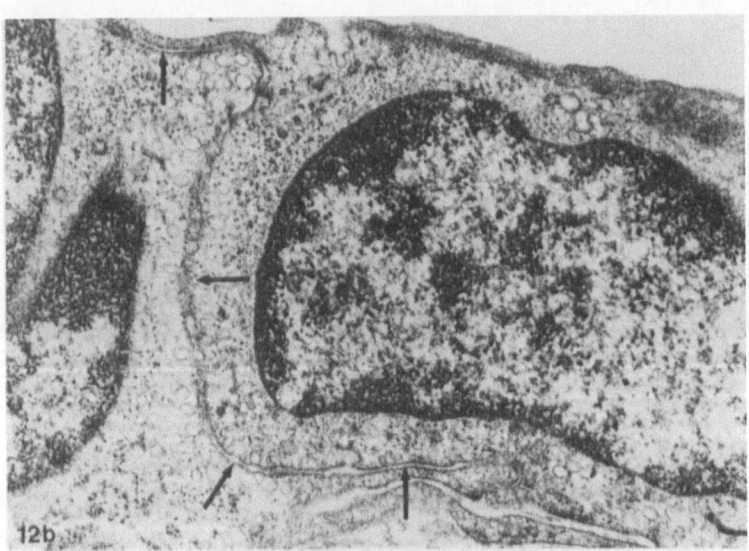

Figure 12. (A) Transmission electron micrograph showing
complex interdigitating junction (arrows) common to elongated
endothelial cells of non-susceptible (white) areas (x 65,000).
(B) Transmission electron micrograph showing end-to-end
junction (arrows) common to cuboidal endothelial cells of
lesion-susceptible (blue) areas. Such junctions frequently
show dilatation, as in Figure 11A (x 36,800).

Subendothelial Space

The subendothelial space, although variable, is consistently and strikingly thicker in lesion-susceptible
(Figure 10B) than in non-susceptible (Figure 9B) areas. In
Figure 9B (from a non-susceptible white area), the internal
elastic lamina is clearly evident, delineating the subendothelial space some 7-8 μ below the endothelium. Figure 10B
(from a lesion-susceptible blue area) is shown an approximately half the magnification of Figure 9B. The internal
elastic lamina is not visible at a depth of 30-35 μ below
the endothelium. In non-susceptible (white) areas, the
endothelium is closely applied either to the developing
internal elastic lamina or to modified smooth muscle cells
which lie parallel to the endothelial layer (Figure 9B). In
blue areas, the subendothelial space appears markedly
edematous, with variable amounts of collagen, elastic tissue,
and microfibrils scattered in a background of floccular
material of low electron density (Figure 10B). Intima cells
in blue areas are seldom in close proximity to the endothelium and are either very elongate with numerous cytoplasmic
processes or ovoid in shape (Figure 10B). In the former, the
presence of myofilaments and dense bodies suggest a smooth
muscle cell origin, while the latter more closely resemble
blood-derived mononuclear cells. Both the above cell types
contain frequent lysosome-like inclusions.

Endothelial Glycocalyx

In sections stained with uranium and lead salts, a
definite, though lightly-staining, glycocalyx can often be
observed on the luminal surface of endothelial cells from
white areas. In contrast, this layer is barely perceptible
or apparently absent over endothelial cells in blue areas.
With ruthenium red staining, this difference in the thickness
of the glycocalyx is accentuated. The glycocalyx in both
areas has two components; a dense lamina closely applied to,
or continuous with, the plasmalemmal membrane, and superficially, a layer of decreasing density exhibiting a finely
fibrillar meshwork (Figure 13A and B). Both components - the

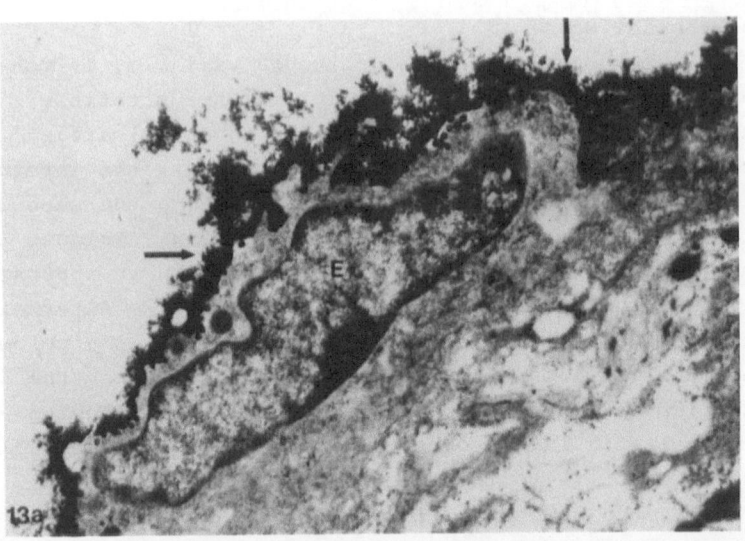

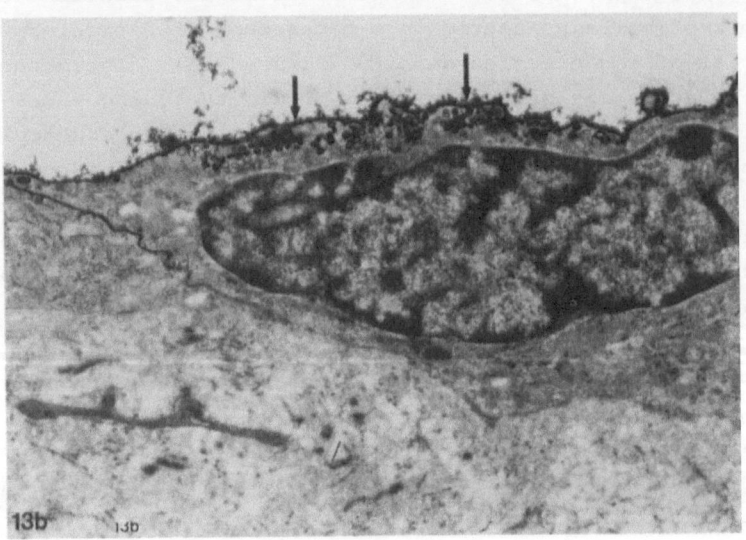

Figure 13. (A) Transmission electron micrograph of endothelial cell (E) from non-susceptible (white) area of swine
aorta stained with ruthenium red to demonstrate glycocalyx
(arrow) consisting of dense layer closely applied to endothelial plasma membrane, and flocculent material extending
from this into lumen. Compare glycocalyx thickness with
that in Figure 13B at same magnification (x 22,700).
(B) As in Figure 13A, but from a lesion-susceptible area.
Compare thickness of glycocalyx (arrow) and absence of
flocculent material with that of non-susceptible area in
Figure 13A (x 22,700).

inner dense lamina and the superficial fibrillar meshwork -
are each much thicker in white (Figure 13A) than in blue
(Figure 13B) areas. Additionally, circular or oval structures
of densely-stained material are conspicuous in the surface
coat from white (Figure 13A), but not from blue areas
(Figure 13B). The mean glycocalyx thickness in blue areas
has been found to be 13 nm, as compared to 44 nm in white
areas, a statistically significant difference. Additionally,
the amount of ruthenium present in the glycocalyx as measured
using energy dispersive analysis of x-rays was found to be
threefold greater in white than in blue areas, a finding consistent with the thickness measurements (34).

A spectrum of changes consonant with endothelial cell
structural alteration can be observed in lesion-susceptible
areas which may be of relevance to atherogenesis. Of particular importance may be endothelial cell shape and short, non-
convoluted junctions. However, the more overt forms of endothelial cell injury in swine blue areas described in early
works on this model by ourselves (33,34) and others (39)
have not manifested themselves in subsequent studies. It is
now our belief that these severe structural abnormalities,
such as mitochondrial disruption, cytoplasmic vacuolation,
and endothelial cell sloughing are at least partially due to
poor fixation and mechanical trauma in early attempts at
large animal perfusion fixation. However, in silver-stained
Hautchen preparations of endothelium, in which injured or
dead cells show intense silver staining, such cells were
found to occur with significantly greater frequency in
blue (2.91%) than in white (0.71%) areas. This finding is
consistent with other studies in swine (35), which demonstrate
enhanced ^{3}H-thymidine uptake by endothelial cells in blue
areas, and those in dogs (38) which show increased susceptibility to endotoxin-induced endothelial injury in such areas.
Thus, although more recent studies have not been able to
demonstrate frequent overt endothelial structural damage and
denudation, even in hyperlipidemia, there is little doubt
that the endothelium and intima in such areas are structurally
altered; the frequency of endothelial cell death is 2-3 times

that of other areas; and the endothelium in these areas
is more susceptible to induced injury. It has been suggested
by Fry (40) that the altered characteristics of these areas
may be due to altered hemodynamic stress.

Endothelial Transport and Intimal Accumulation

Whereas receptor-mediated endocytosis is considered to
be the chief mechanism by which specific macromolecules are
taken up for metabolism by that cell, it is primarily non-
receptor mediated bulk-phase pinocytosis by the endothelium
which results in the passage of blood macromolecules through
the intact endothelial layer into the vessel wall (13,14).
This process is thus of considerable interest with respect
to the transport and accumulation of plaque lipids, particularly cholesterol, from the lipoproteins of the blood into
lesion-susceptible sites. Studies using intravenously-
injected labelled molecules (36,37) or electron-dense probes
such as ferritin (85) have provided considerable insight into
this problem, and have demonstrated that lesion-susceptible
areas exhibit enhanced intimal accumulation of blood macromolecules (36,37,85).

Such studies in young, normal swine (85) have also
shown that the numbers of endothelial pinocytotic vesicles
are similar in lesion-susceptible and non-susceptible areas,
and that the carrying capacity of vesicles for electron-dense
probes such as ferritin is likewise the same. In older swine,
white area endothelial cells exhibit more vesicles per unit
sectional area that adjacent blue areas. Despite this age-
related change, which would favor greater intimal accumulation
in white areas, approximately two to three times as many
vesicles take up intravenously-injected ferritin in blue
compared to white areas (Table). As a result, more ferritin
accumulates in the intima of such areas in normal animals,
and such accumulation is further enhanced under conditions of
hyperlipidemia (Table). In addition, intimal accumulation
is greatly enhanced by intracellular uptake of the probe by
macrophages (Table). Our previous studies demonstrated that
a further characteristic of lesion-susceptible areas is the

Table. Bulk-Phase Endothelial Vesicular Transport and Intimal Accumulation of Ferritin in Swine Aorta

Diet Group/Aortic Site [a]	Vesicles/Endo Area	% Vesicles Labelled	Grains/SES Area	Grains/Macrophage Area
1 Min Circulation				
Control White	21 ± 2	20 ± 3	3 ± 0.4	3 ± 0.7
Atherogenic White	27 ± 1	18 ± 2	3 ± 0.2	2 ± 0.6
Control Blue	12 ± 1[b]	38 ± 4[b]	6 ± 0.3[b]	7 ± 2[b]
Atherogenic Blue	15 ± 1[b]	34 ± 3[b]	6 ± 0.4[b]	8 ± 1[b]
15 Min Circulation				
Control White	21 ± 1	17 ± 4	3 ± 0.7	1 ± 0.2
Atherogenic White	21 ± 2	15 ± 3	2 ± 0.2	2 ± 0.4
Control Blue	13 ± 2[b]	46 ± 4[b]	9 ± 0.5[b]	26 ± 8.0[b]
Atherogenic Blue	10 ± 1[b]	38 ± 2[b]	18 ± 1.0[b,c]	58 ± 9.0[b,c]

a Swine were fed an atherogenic diet or control diet for 15 weeks. Blue = lesion-susceptible area, White = non-susceptible area.

b Significantly different ($p < 0.05$) from corresponding white area.

c Significantly different ($p < 0.05$) from blue area in control swine.

specific chemotatic recruitment (78) of blood monocytes, which provide the major source of foam cells in early lesions. Thus the expanded intima of lesion-susceptible areas may provide a "sink" for enhanced accumulation of molecules taken up by bulk-phase vesicular transport. It is of considerable importance to note that hyperlipidemia does not increase the percentage of vesicles carrying ferritin, which is 2-3 times greater in lesion-susceptible (blue) areas compared to non-susceptible (white) areas. However, intimal accumulation is increased by hyperlipidemia both extracellularly, and to an even greater extent, within macrophages (Table). Lesion-susceptible areas demonstrate increased accumulation of albumin (36), fibrinogen (37), cholesterol (86) and lipoprotein (87,88) in addition to ferritin, supporting the hypothesis that this property is due to non-specific bulk-phase vesicular transport across the endothelium.

Of interest in these studies is that ferritin was never observed in the shorter, sometimes vacuolated junctional regions of lesion-susceptible endothelium, and secondly, in those rare cases in which focal endothelial denudation was observed, almost no ferritin accumulation was observed in the exposed intima. These findings are consistent with those of Minick et al. (89), who showed that intimal lipoprotein accumulation occurred subsequent to reendothelialization in ballooned arteries, but did not occur in exposed intima. More recent studies in swine have demonstrated, both structurally (88) and biochemically (87) that lesion-susceptible areas preferentially accumulate apo B-containing lipoproteins even in normal animals, a condition exaggerated by hyperlipidemia. With prolonged hyperlipidemia, however, even non-susceptible areas accumulate lipoprotein. Since these lipoproteins are of a molecular size necessitating vesicular transport, it is highly likely that the preferential lipoprotein accumulation in susceptible areas is a result of the greater bulk-phase vesicular transport and enhanced accumulation in the thickened intima demonstrated by the ferritin studies. Hoff, in a series of papers, has

demonstrated the presence of apo B-containing lipoproteins
in a wide variety of human arteries (90-95). Although this
accumulation has not been linked to specific predilection
sites, it is significant that he has demonstrated the
presence of apo B-containing lipoproteins even in grossly-
normal vessels (95). If, as suggested by studies of ferritin
and lipoprotein accumulation in swine, lesion-susceptible
areas preferentially accumulate lipoprotein through inherent
differences in bulk-phase transport, coupled with enhanced
intimal "trapping", then the concept of endothelial injury
as an initiating factor in atherogenesis must be re-examined.
Enhanced bulk-phase transport, as well as increased accumulation of a wide variety of large blood macromolecules (36,37,
85-87) occurs in these areas even in normal swine. Thus the
preferential accumulation of atherogenic lipoproteins in such
regions is not the result of endothelial injury, but rather,
the superimposition of altered blood composition on areas of
normally-altered structural and functional characteristics
which are independent of induced injury. The resultant focal
accumulation of atherogenic macromolecules may then trigger
the events leading to lesion formation. The focal nature
of lesion formation in human atherosclerosis (32) would
suggest the existence of areas analagous to blue areas in
swine. The possibility therefore exists that human lesions
may also initiate through a similar mechanism. Certainly, at
the very least, the results of animal studies would suggest
that we must look for more subtle forms of endothelial
"injury" in the form of altered function as an initiating
factor in atherogenesis.

REFERENCES

1. Blose SH, Chacko S (1975) *In vitro* behaviour of guinea pig arterial venous endothelial cells. Dev Growth Diff 17:153-165.
2. Caplan BA, Schwartz CJ (1973) Increased endothelial turnover in areas of *in vivo* Evans Blue uptake in the pig aorta. Arteriosclerosis 17:401-417.
3. Gimbrone MA, Cotran RS, Folkman J (1974) Human vascular endothelial cells in culture. J Cell Biol 60:673-684.
4. Jaffe EA, Nachman RL, Becker CG, Minick CR (1973) Culture of human endothelial cells derived from umbilical veins. J Clin Invest 52:2745-2756.

5. Lewis LJ, Hoak JC, Maca RD, Fry GL (1973) Replication
    of human endothelial cells in culture. Science 181:
    453-454.
6. Poole JCF, Sanders AG, Florey HW (1958) The regenera-
    tion of aortic endothelium. J Pathol Bacteriol 75:133-144.
7. Schwartz SM, Stemerman MB, Benditt EP (1975) The aortic
    intima: II. Repair of the aortic lining after mechanical
    denudation. Am J Pathol 81:15-31.
8. Stehbens WE (1965) Endothelial cell mitosis and perme-
    ability. J Exp Physiol 50:90-92.
9. Wright HP (1971) Mitosis patterns in aortic endothelium.
    Atherosclerosis 15:93-100.
10. Cotran RS, Karnovsky MJ (1968) Ultrastructural studies
    on the permeability of the mesothelium to horseradish
    peroxidase. J Cell Biol 37:123-137.
11. Karnovsky MJ (1967) The ultrastructural basis of
    capillary permeability studied with peroxidase as a
    tracer. J Cell Biol 35:213-236.
12. Majno G (1965) Ultrastructure of the vascular membrane.
    In: Hamilton WF, Dow P (eds) Handbook of Physiology,
    Section 2. Washington, DC: American Physiological
    Society, pp. 2293-2375.
13. Simionescu N, Simionescu M, Palade GE (1973) Perme-
    ability of muscle capillaries to exogenous myoglobin.
    J Cell Biol 57:424-452.
14. Simionescu N, Simionescu M, Palade GE (1975) Perme-
    ability of muscle capillaries to small heme-peptides.
    Evidence for the existence of patent transendothelial
    channels. J Cell Biol 64:586-607.
15. Becker CG, Murphy GE (1969) Demonstration of contractile
    protein in endothelium and cells of the heart valves,
    endocardium, intima, arteriosclerotic plaques, and
    Aschoff bodies of rheumatic heart disease. Am J Pathol
    55:1-37.
16. Joris I, Magno G, Ryan GB (1972) Endothelial contraction
    in vivo: A study of the rat mesentery. Virchows Arch
    (Zellpathol) 12:73-83.
17. Magno G, Shea SM, Leventhal M (1969) Endothelial con-
    traction induced by histamine-type mediators. An
    electron microscopic study. J Cell Biol 42:647-672.
18. Pugatch EMJ, Foster EA, MacFarlane GE, Poole JCF (1970)
    The extraction and separation of activators and inhibi-
    tors of fibrinolysis from bovine endothelium and meso-
    thelium. Br J Haematol 18:669-681.
19. Todd AS (1959) The Histological localization of fibrino-
    lysin activator. J Pathol Bacteriol 78:281-285.
20. Nemerson Y, Maynard J, Pitlich FA (1975) Activation of
    blood coagulation by tissue factor. New York: New York
    Heart Association Symposium on the Intima.
21. Zeldis SM, Nemerson Y, Pitlich FA, Lentz TK (1972)
    Tissue factor (thromboplastin) localization to plasma
    membranes by peroxidase-conjugated antibodies. Science
    175:766-768.
22. Jaffe EA, Hoyer LW, Nachman RL (1973) Synthesis of
    antihemophilic factor antigen by cultured human endo-
    thelial cells. J Clin Invest 52:2757-2764.

23. Sage H, Crouch E, Bornstein P (1979) Collagen synthesis by bovine aortic endothelial cells in culture. Biochemistry 24:5433-5449.

24. Jaffe EA, Adelman B, Minick CR (1975) Synthesis of basement membrane by cultured endothelial cells. Circulation 51:11-17.

25. Buonassisi V, Root M (1975) Enzymatic degradation of heparin-related mucopolysaccharides from the surface of endothelial cell cultures. Biochim Biophys Acta 383:1-10.

26. Moncada S, Higgs EA, Vane Jr (1977) Human arterial and venous tissue generate prostacyclin, a potent inhibitor of platelet aggregation. Lancet 2:18.

27. Gajdusek CM, DiCorleto P, Ross R, Schwartz SM (1980) An endothelial cell derived frowth factor. J Cell Biol 85:467-472.

28. DiCorleto PE, Gajdusek CM, Schwartz SM, Ross R (1983) Biochemical properties of the endothelium-derived growth factor: Comparison to other growth factors. J Cell Physiol 114:339-345.

29. DiCorleto PE, Bowen-Pope DF (1983) Cultured endothelial cells produce a platelet-derived growth factor-like protein. Proc Natl Acad Sci USA 80:1919-1923.

30. Zilversmit DB (1973) A proposal linking atherogenesis to the interaction of endothelial lipoprotein lipase with triglyceride-rich lipoproteins. Circ Res 33:633-638.

31. Steinberg D (1983) Lipoproteins and atherosclerosis: A look back and a look ahead. Arteriosclerosis 3:283-301.

32. Cornhill JF (1986) Topographic probability mapping of atherosclerosis. Report 763813/715703, The Ohio State University Research Foundation (NHLBI, N01-HV-38019).

33. Caplan BA, Gerrity RG, Schwartz CJ (1974) Endothelial cell morphology in focal areas of *in vivo* Evans Blue uptake in the young pig aorta. I. Quantitative light microscope findings. Exp Mol Pathol 21:102-117.

34. Gerrity RG, Richardson M, Bell FP, Somer JB, Schwartz CJ (1977) Endothelial cell morphology in areas of *in vivo* Evans Blue uptake in the young pig aorta. II. Ultrastructure of the intima in areas of differing permeability to proteins. Am J Pathol 89:313-334.

35. Caplan BA, Schwartz CJ (1973) Increased endothelial cell turnover in areas of *in vivo* Evans Blue uptake in the pig aorta. Atherosclerosis 17:401-417.

36. Bell FP, Adamson IL, Schwartz CJ (1974) Aortic endothelial permeability to albumin: Focal and regional patterns of uptake and transmoral distribution of ^{131}I-albumin in the young pig. Exp Mol Pathol 20:57-68.

37. Bell FP, Gallus AS, Schwartz CJ (1974) Focal and regional patterns of uptake and the transmural distribution of ^{131}I-fibrinogen in the pig aorta *in vivo*. Exp Mol Pathol 20:281-292.

38. Gerrity RG, Richardson M, Caplan BA, Cade JF, Hirsh J, Schwartz CJ (1976) Endotoxin-induced vascular endothelial injury and repair. II. Focal injury, en face morphology [^{3}H] thymidine uptake and circulating endothelial cells in the dog. Exp Mol Pathol 24:59-69.

39. Packham MA, Rowsell HC, Jorgensen L, Mustard JF (1967) Localized protein accumulation in the wall of the aorta. Exp Mol Pathol 7:214-232.

40. Fry DL (1973) Responses of the arterial wall to certain physical factors. In: Atherogenesis: Initiating Factors. Ciba Foundation Symposium, No. 12. New York: Excerpta Medica Foundation, pp. 93-125.

41. Faggiotto A, Ross R, Harker L (1984) Studies of hyper-cholesterolemia in the nonhuman primate. I. Changes that lead to fatty streak formation. Arteriosclerosis 4:323-340.

42. Faggiotto A, Ross R (1984) Studies of hypercholesterol-emia in the nonhuman primate. II. Fatty streak conversion to fibrous plaque. Arteriosclerosis 4:341-356.

43. Cornhill JF, Barrett WA, Herderick EE, Mahley RW, Fry DL (1985) Topographic study of sudanophilic lesions in cholesterol-fed minipigs by image analysis. Arterio-sclerosis 5:415-426.

44. Buck RC (1958) The fine structure of endothelium of large arteries. J Biophys Biochem Cytol 4:187-190.

45. Rhodin JAG (1962) Fine structure of vascular walls of mammals, with special reference to smooth muscle component. Physiol Rev 42:5-48.

46. Bierring F, Kobayasi T (1963) Electron microscopy of the normal rabbit aorta. Acta Pathol Microbiol Scand 57:154-168.

47. Karrer HE (1961) An electron microscope study of the aorta in the young and in aging mice. J Ultrastruct Res 5:1-27.

48. Pease DC, Paule WJ (1960) Electron microscopy of elastic arteries; the thoracic aorta of the rat. J Ultrastruct Res 3:469-483.

49. French JE (1963) Endothelial structure and function. In: Jones RJ (ed) Evolution of the Atherosclerotic Plaque. Chicago: University of Chicago Press, pp. 15-28.

50. Gerrity RG, Cliff WJ (1972) The aortic tunica intima in young and aging rats. Exp Mol Pathol 16:382-402.

51. Weibel ER, Palade GE (1964) New cytoplasmic components in arterial endothelia. J Cell Biol 23:101-112.

52. Cliff WJ (1967) The aortic tunica media in growing rats studied with the electron microscope. Lab Invest 17(6):599-615.

53. Gerrity RG, Adams EP, Cliff WJ (1975) The aortic tunica media of the developing rat. II. Incorporation by medial cells of ^{3}H-proline into collagen and elastin. Autoradiographic and chemical studies. Lab Invest 32:601-612.

54. Buck RC (1962) Lesions in the rabbit aorta produced by feeding a high cholesterol diet. Brit J Exp Pathol 43:236-240.

55. Daoud AS, Jones R, Scott RF (1968) Dietary induced atherosclerosis in miniature swine. Exp Mol Pathol 8:277-289.

56. Huttner I, More RH, Rona G (1970) Fine structural evidence of specific mechanism for increased endothelial permeability in experimental hypertension. Am J Pathol 61(3):395-403.

57. Ziegel RF, Dalton AJ (1962) Speculations based on the morphology of the Golgi systems in several types of protein-secreting cells. J Cell Biol 15:45-54.

58. Warshawsky H, LeBlond CO, Droz B (1963) Synthesis and migration of proteins in the cells of the exocrine pancreas as revealed by specific activity determination from radioautographs. J Cell Biol 16:1-23.

59. Caro LG, Palade GE (1964) Protein synthesis, storage and discharge in the pancreatic exocrine cell. An autoradiographic study. J Cell Biol 20:473-495.

60. Jamieson JD, Palade GE (1967) Intracellular transport of secretory proteins of the pancreatic exocrine cell. J Cell Biol 34:577-615.

61. Wissig SL (1963) The anatomy of secretion in the follicular cells of the thyroid gland. J Cell Biol 16:93-118.

62. Neutra M, LeBlond CP (1966) Synthesis of the carbohydrate of mucus in the Golgi complex as shown by electron microscope radioautography of goblet cells from rats injected with glucose-^{3}H. J Cell Biol 30:119-136.

63. Majno G (1965) Ultrastructure of the vascular membrane. In: Hamilton WJ, Dow P (eds) Handbook of Physiology, Section 2, Volume 3. Washington, DC: American Phyiol Soc, pp. 2293-2375.

64. Astrup T, Buluk K (1963) Thromboplastic and fibrinolytic activities in vessels of animals. Circ Res 13:252-260.

65. LaTaillada JN, Gutstein WH, Lazzarini-Robertson (1964) A study of experimental vasodilation of rabbit abdominal aorta and its relationship to arterio-atherosclerosis. J Atheroscler Res 4:81-95.

66. Warren BA (1963) Fibrinolytic properties of vascular endothelium. Brit J Exp Pathol 44:365-372.

67. Schimamoto T, Ishioka T (1963) Release of a thromboplastic substance from arterial walls by epinephrine. Circ Res 12:138-144.

68. Burri PH, Weibel ER (1968) Beeinflussung einer spezifischen cytoplasmatischen organelle von endothelzellen durch adrenalin. Z Zellforsch Mikrosk Anat 88:426-440.

69. Sengal A, Stoebner P (1969) Golgi origin of tubular inclusions in endothelial cells. J Cell Biol 44:223-226.

70. Sandborn E, Koen PF, McNabb JD, Moore G (1964) Cytoplasmic microtubules in mammalian cells. J Ultrastruct Res 11:123-138.

71. Stehbens WE (1966) The basal attachment of endothelial cells. J Ultrastruct Res 15:389-399.

72. Leak LU, Burke JF (1968) Ultrastructural studies on the lymphatic anchoring filaments. J Cell Biol 36:129-149.

73. Tsao C, Glagov S (1970) Basal endothelial attachment. Tenacity at cytoplasmic zones in the rabbit aorta. Lab Invest 23(5):510-516.

74. Giacomella F, Weiner J, Spiro D (1970) Cross-striated arrays of filaments in endothelium. J Cell Biol 45:188-192.

75. Glagov S, Wolinsky H (1963) Aortic wall as a two phase material. Nature (London) 199:606-608.

76. Gerrity RG (1981) The role of the monocyte in athero-
    genesis. I. Transition of blood-bone monocytes into
    foam cells in fatty lesions. Am J Pathol 103:181-190.
77. Gerrity RG (1981) The role of the monocyte in athero-
    genesis. II. Migration of foam cells from athero-
    sclerotic lesions. Am J Pathol 103:191-200.
78. Gerrity RG, Goss JA, Soby L (1985) Control of monocyte
    recruitment by chemotactic factor(s) in lesion-prone
    areas of swine aorta. Arteriosclerosis 5:55-66.
79. Scott RF, Thomas WA, Lee WM, Reiner JM, Florentin RA
    (1979a) Distribution of intimal smooth muscle cell
    masses and their relationship to early atherosclerosis
    in the abdominal aortas of young swine. Atherosclerosis
    34:291-301.
80. Thomas WA, Florentin RA, Nam SC, Reiner JM, Lee KT (1971)
    Alterations in population dynamics of arterial smooth
    muscle cells during atherogenesis. I. Activation of
    interphase cells in cholesterol-fed swine prior to gross
    atherosclerosis demonstrated by "postpulse salvage"
    labeling. Exp Mol Pathol 15:245-267.
81. Thomas WA, Florentin RA, Reiner JM, Lee WM, Lee KT (1976)
    Alterations in population dynamics of arterial smooth
    muscle cells during atherogenesis. IV. Evidence for
    a polyclonal origin of hypercholesterolemic diet-induced
    atherosclerotic lesions in young swine. Exp Mol Pathol
    24:244-260.
82. Thomas WA, Reiner JM, Florentin RA, Lee KT, Lee WM (1976b)
    Population dynamics of arterial smooth muscle cells. V.
    Cell proliferation and cell death during initial 3 months
    in atherosclerotic lesions induced in swine by hyper-
    cholesterolemic diet and intimal trauma. Exp Mol Pathol
    24:360-374.
83. Gerrity RG, Naito KH (1980) Alteration of endothelial
    cell surface morphology after experimental aortic
    coarctation. Artery 8:267-274.
84. Repin VS, Dolgov VV, Zaikina OE, Novikov ID, Antonov AS,
    Nikolaeva MA, Smirnov VN (1984) Heterogeneity of endo-
    thelium in human aorta. A quantitative analysis by
    scanning electron microscopy. Atherosclerosis 50:35-52.
85. Gerrity RG, Schwartz CJ (1977) Structural correlates of
    arterial endothelial permeability in the Evans blue
    model. In: Sinzinger H, Averswald WA, Jellinek H,
    Feigl W (eds) Prog Biochem Pharmacol, Volume 13. Basil:
    S. Karger, pp. 134-137.
86. Somer JB, Schwartz CJ (1972) Focal [^{3}H]-cholesterol
    uptake in the pig aorta. II. Distribution of [^{3}H]-
    cholesterol across the aortic wall in areas of high
    and low uptake in vivo. Atherosclerosis 16:377-388.
87. Hoff HF, Gerrity RG, Naito HK, Dusek D (1983) Quanti-
    tation of apolipoprotein B in aortas of hypercholesterol-
    emic swine. Lab Invest 48:492-504.
88. Feldman DL, Hoff HF, Gerrity RG (1984) Immunohisto-
    chemical localization of Aprprotein B in aortas from
    hyperlipemic swine. Preferential accumulation in
    lesion-prone areas. Arch Pathol Lab Med 108:817-822.

89. Minick CG, Stemmerman MB, Insul W (1979)   Role of endo-
    thelium and hypercholesterolemia in intimal thickening
    and lipid accumulation.   Am J Pathol 95:131-142.
90. Hoff HF (1976)   Apolipoprotein localization in human
    cranial arteries, coronary arteries and the aorta.
    Stroke 7:390-393.
91. Hoff HF, Ruggles BM, Bond MG (1980)   A technique for
    localizing LDL by immunofluorescence in formalin-fixed
    and paraffin-embedded atherosclerotic lesions.   Artery
    6:328-339.
92. Hoff HF, Heideman CI, Gaubatz JW (1975)   Apo-low density
    lipoprotein localization in intracranial and extra-
    cranial atherosclerotic lesions from human normolipo-
    proteinemics and hyperlipoproteinemics.   Arch Neurol
    32:600-605.
93. Hoff HF, Heideman CI, Noon JP, Meyer JS (1975)
    Localization of apolipoproteins in human carotid artery
    plaques.   Stroke 6:531-534.
94. Hoff HF, Jackson RI, Mao JT, Gotto AM (1974)   Locali-
    zation of low density lipoproteins in arterial lesions
    from normolipemics employing a purified fluorescent
    labeled antibody.   Biochim Biophys Acta 351:407-415.
95. Hoff HF, Lie JT, Titus JL, Jackson RL, DeBakey ME,
    Bayardo R, Gotto AM (1975)   Lipoproteins in athero-
    sclerotic lesions.   Localization by immunofluorescence
    of apo- low density lipoproteins in human atherosclerotic
    arteries from normal and hyperlipoproteinemics.   Arch
    Pathol 99:253-258.

3

Second Messengers in Human Vascular Endothelial Cells: Regulation of Endothelial Monolayer Formation and Repair

Vladimir N. Smirnov, Alexander S. Antonov, Matvey E. Lukashev,
Yuri A. Romanov, J. Frederic Cornhill, and Ross G. Gerrity

INTRODUCTION

The endothelial lining of blood vessels comprises a pivotal
interface between flowing blood and vessel wall, performing
a variety of specific functions to maintain normal functioning
of vessel wall and normal blood flow. It is widely accepted
now that injury of vascular endothelium may be the initial
step in development of some pathologies, i.e., thrombosis,
atherosclerosis, etc. Studies have indicated that endothelial
functions are closely related to morphological organization
of endothelial monolayer, the latter reflecting changes in
circulatory system and vessel wall.

In this paper the attempt was made to understand some
of the mechanisms which may control organization of endothelial monolayer and its changes in atherosclerosis.

It is known that the morphology of endothelial cells (EC)
is affected by such factors as hemodynamic forces (1,2); blood
pressure (3); vasoactive amines (4,5); the products of lipid
metabolism (6); and other physiologically active substances
(7,8). Of special interest are the mechanisms which mediate
the effects of these factors on endothelial morphology.

It is well known that the action of a majority of hormones, neuromediators, growth factors and other endocrine and
paracrine regulators is mediated by the systems of second
messengers, which include cyclic nucleotides (cAMP and cGMP),
Ca^{2+} ions and the products of phosphoinositide metabolism,
namely, triphosphoinositol and diacylglycerol (DAG).

Convenient tools to study processes controlled by the systems of second messengers are the substances capable of selectively activating certain steps in each of these metabolic pathways. To study the effects of cAMP, we used forskolin, an activator of adenylate cyclase, the enzyme which catalyzes cAMP formation. To study the role of the products of phosphoinositide metabolism, Phorbol-12-myristate-13-acetate (PMA) was used which has a physiological analogue, namely, diacylglycerol. Both forskolin and PMA were used in experiments on primary cultures of endothelial cells from human aorta and umbilical vein and in experiments with short-term organ cultures of human aorta.

Regulation of Endothelial Cell Morphology in Monolayer
    The addition of forskolin (10^{-5}M) to a confluent primary culture of human umbilical vein endothelium caused rapid (40-80 min) and well expressed changes in the cell shape (Figure 1). These changes did not result in the loss of the integrity of the monolayer (Figure 1C). Colchicine (10^{-6}M) completely abolished the effects of forskolin. Similar morphological changes were induced by dibutyryl-cAMP (10^{-5}M) and by the inhibitor of cyclic nucleotide phosphodiesterase, isobutylmethylxanthine (10^{-4}M). Morphological changes caused by forskolin were maximal in 60-80 min which was followed by the restoration of the original shape (Figure 2).

    PMA (10^{-7}M) also caused changes in the morphology of human umbilical vein endothelium, but these changes were less pronounced compared to the effects of forskolin (Figure 2). Forskolin and PMA at the concentration 10^{-6}M and 10^{-8}M, respectively, did not affect cell morphology. At the same time, simultaneous addition to the cells of forskolin and PMA at these concentrations resulted in very rapid and well-expressed changes in the cell morphology (Figure 2). Morphological changes induced by the substances which elevate intracellular level of cAMP and protein kinase C were completely reversible: 30-60 min after removal of the agents from culture medium, the cells restored initial morphology.

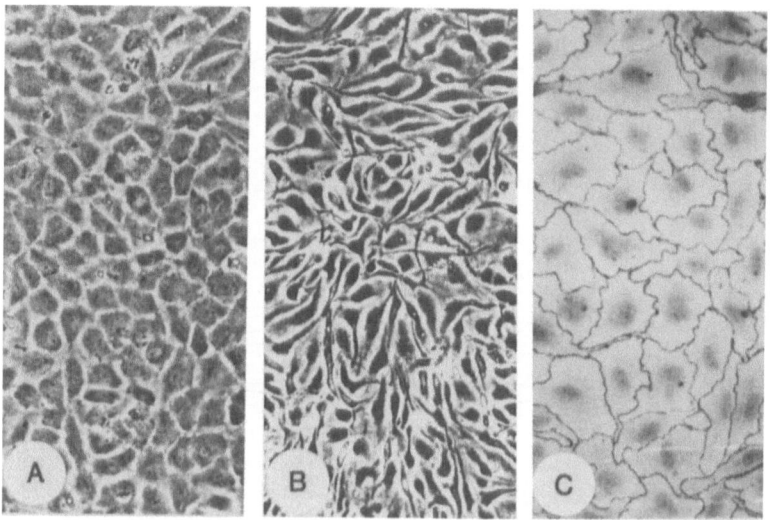

Figure 1. Effect of forskolin on morphological features of human umbilical vein EC in primary culture. (A) Control, cells were incubated in medium 199 with 0.5% BSA. (B,C) Cell culture after 1 h incubation with forskolin (10^{-5}M). (A,B) Phase contrast (x 200), (C) Silver nitrate stain (x 350).

In human aortic EC forskolin and PMA caused morphological changes which were similar to the changes in human umbilical endothelium (Figure 3). The most pronounced effect was registered with small and medium size cells. The changes in large multinucleated cells were less prominent.

In the experiments with short-term tissue cultures of adult human aortic segments the shape changes in the presence of forskolin were also noticed (Figure 4A,B). In these experiments after addition of forskolin cells acquired the morphology characteristic of endothelium in the regions of expected altered hemodynamic stress (Figure 4C). The most pronounced effect after addition of forskolin was found in homogeneous small size EC from child aortae (Figure 4D,E).

In our experiments the most pronounced effects of PMA were seen in the presence of agents which essentially increase the intracellular concentration of cAMP (forskolin, isobutyl-methylxanthine and dibutyryl-cAMP). It has been recently

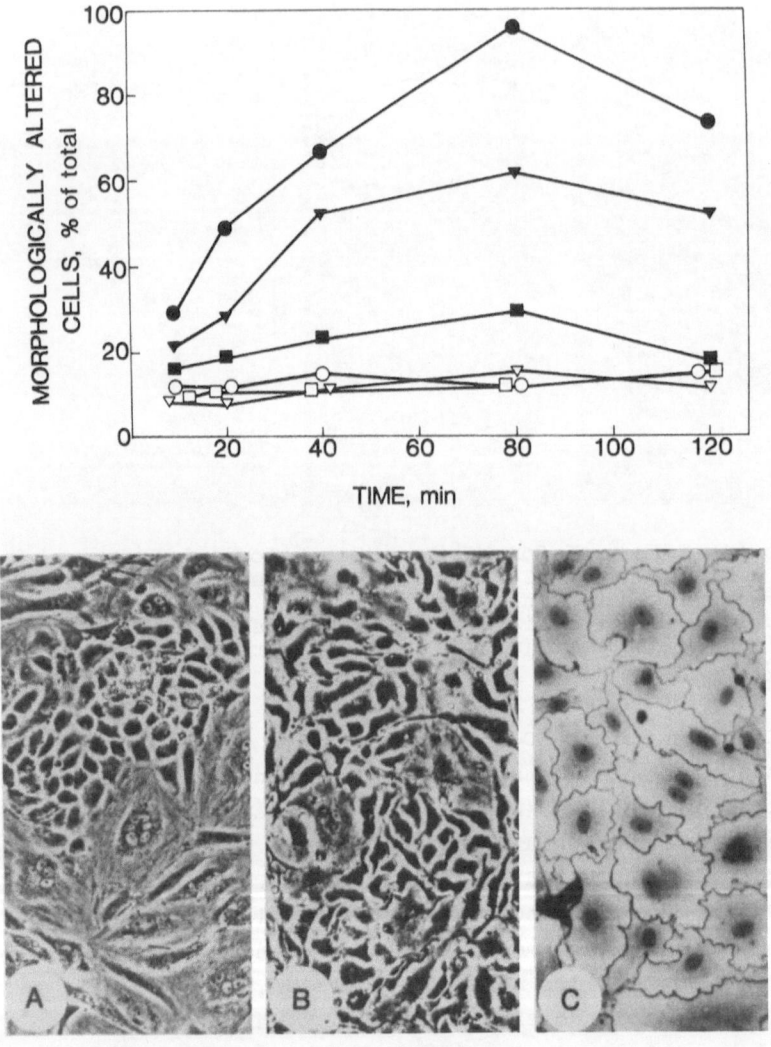

Figure 2. Synergistic effects of PMA and forskolin on the
morphology of human umbilical vein EC. Cultures were incubated in medium 199 with 0.5% BSA ($\bigcirc$) or in medium 199 with
0.5% BSA supplemented with effectors: 10^{-5}M forskolin($\blacktriangledown$);
10^{-7}M PMA ($\blacksquare$); 10^{-6}M forskolin ($\triangledown$); 10^{-8}M PMA ($\square$); 10^{-6}M
forskolin with 10^{-8}M PMA ($\bullet$). After the incubation cultures
were stained with silver nitrate and shape index of EC was
determined, EC of shape index $\leq$ 0.5 were regarded as altered.
Figure 3. Effect of forskolin on the morphological features
of human aortic EC in primary culture. (A) Control, cells
were incubated in medium 199 with 0.5% BSA. (B,C) Cell
culture after 1 h incubation with forskolin (10^{-5}M).
(A,B) Phase contrast (x 200), (C) Silver nitrate stain
(x 350).

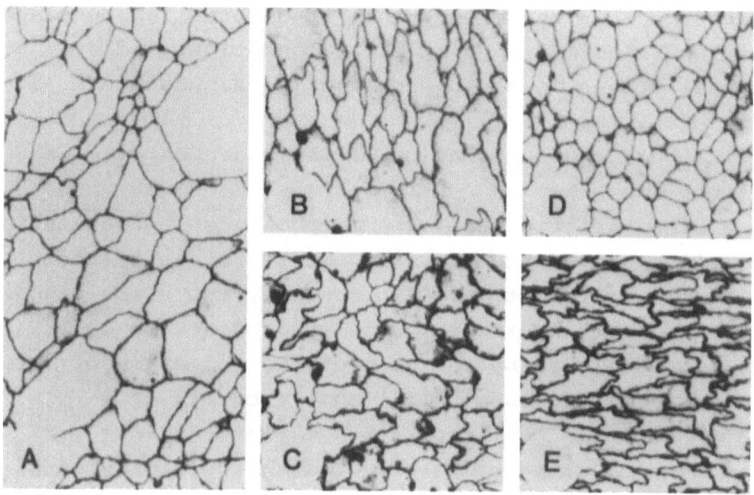

Figure 4. Effect of forskolin on EC from adult human (A,B) and child (D,E) aortae in short-term organ culture. Explants were incubated in medium 199 with 0.5 BSA (A,D) or in medium containing forskolin (10^{-5}M) (B,E) for 1 h; (C) endothelium in the zone of hemodynamic stress (ostia of arteria carotis). Silver nitrate stain (x 350).

shown that PMA, as well as phosphoinositide turnover activating hormones, potentiates cAMP accumulation induced by adenylate cyclase activators in various cell types (9-11). Thus, the synergism of forskolin and PMA may be due either to potentiation by PMA of the forskolin-induced cAMP synthesis, or to simultaneous phosphorylation of cytoskeletal proteins by cAMP-dependent protein kinases and protein kinase C. The polymorphous response pattern of adult human aortic EC may be due either to differences in cAMP metabolism and protein phosphorylation systems or to differences in the cytoskeleton organization of the large, multinuclear endothelial cells.

The exact physiological relevance of morphological alterations induced by activation of second messenger systems in endothelial cells still remains to be ascertained and may be somewhat different in different physiological conditions. We propose that such or similar changes in endothelial cell morphology in both normal and diseased arteries may be of

great importance in the maintenance of endothelial monolayer
integrity under normal physiological conditions and in
pathological states involving endothelial denudation.

Proliferation and Formation of Cellular Contacts in Culture

To a significant degree, the morphological organization
of endothelium can be predetermined at the stage of endothelial monolayer formation. Arbitrarily, two steps can be
distinguished in this process: the step of active cellular
proliferation followed by the step of the formation of intercellular contacts and endothelial monolayer per se.

Using selective activators of adenylate cyclase and
protein kinase C, we have investigated the role of second
messenger systems in the regulation of proliferation of EC
and the formation of intercellular contacts in culture.

PMA at the concentrations of 10^{-7}-10^{-9}M markedly stimulated both the proliferation of EC and the incorporation of
^{3}H-thymidine in DNA (Figure 5). In the presence of PMA (10^{-8}M),
the average time of the cell population doubling was shortened
from 72-76 h to 16-18 h. Confluent monolayers were formed at
seeding densities from 2×10^2 to 2×10^4 cells/cm^2. The
final density of the monolayer and the cell size in the monolayer correlated with initial seeding density. At low seeding
densities in PMA-containing medium, the monolayers with the
density of 2-3×10^4 cells/cm^2 were formed containing large
and giant, often multinucleated cells (Figure 6A,B). High
seeding density resulted in the formation of dense monolayers
(8×10^4-10^5 cells/cm^2) were elongated and mutually oriented
cells were predominant (Figure 6C,D). PMA did not suppress
contact inhibition of endothelial cell growth. We never
observed the growth and migration of cells over each other,
or the formation of multilayer culture even after prolonged
treatment of endothelium with PMA. This fact, in addition
to the observation on the reversibility of PMA effects, led
to the conclusion that mitogenic effect of PMA on EC may not
be related to cell transformation. It is thought that PMA

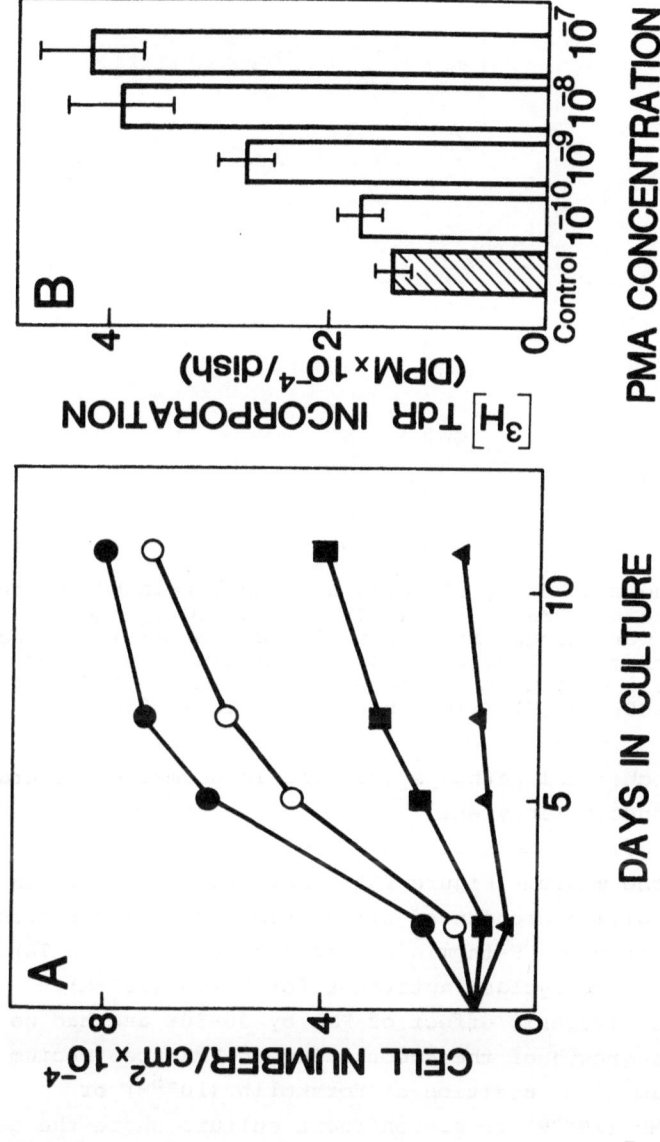

Figure 5. Effect of PMA on human umbilical vein EC. (A) Dose-dependent effect of PMA on EC growth rate: Control (▲), 10^{-10}M PMA (■), 10^{-9}M PMA (○), 10^{-8}M PMA (●); (B) Effect of PMA on [3H] thymidine incorporation in DNA.

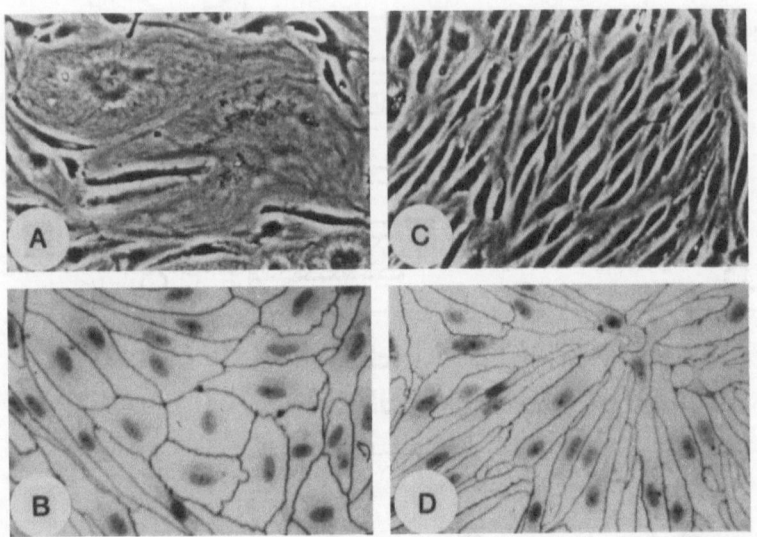

Figure 6. The morphology of human umbilical vein EC, cultured in the presence of PMA at low (A,B) or high (C,D) seeding density. EC were seeded at density 10^3 cells/cm^2 (A,B) and 5×10^4 cells/cm^2 (C,D) and cultured in medium containing 10^{-8}M PMA until confluent monolayer was formed. (A,C) Phase contrast (x 200), (B,D) Silver nitrate stain (x 350).

activates biochemical pathways involved in normal proliferative response of endotheliocytes.

The mitogenic effect of PMA depended on the concentration of serum in the medium (Figure 7A). Nevertheless, even in serum-free medium a pronounced stimulation of proliferation and incorporation of ^{3}H-thymidine was observed (Figure 7B).

The adenylate cyclase activator forskolin (10^{-5}M) inhibited the mitogenic effect of PMA by 30-50% and had no effect on the growth of the endothelium in PMA-free medium with 10% serum. The addition of forskolin (10^{-5}M) or dibutyryl-cAMP (10^{-5}M) to preconfluent culture where the cell junctions were not yet stained with silver nitrate, resulted in a fast (1-4 hours) reorganization of the monolayer, and cell boundaries became easily stained with silver nitrate (Figure 8). These changes were accompanied by the accumulation

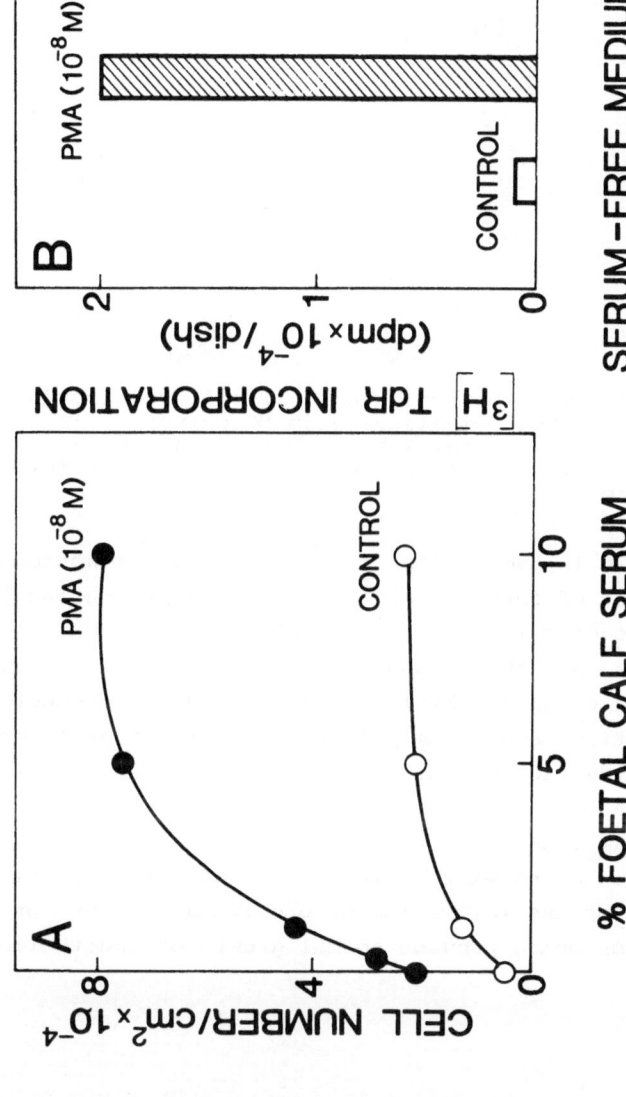

Figure 7. Effect of serum on the mitogenic action of PMA on EC from human umbilical vein (A) and effect of PMA on DNA synthesis in serum-free medium (B).

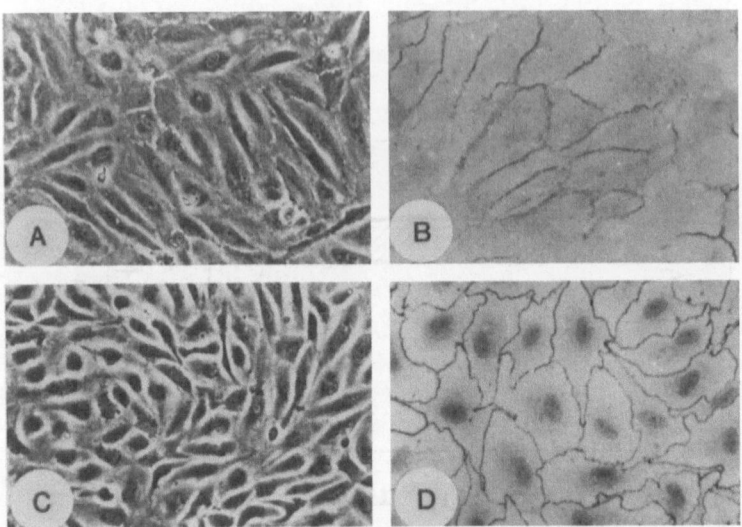

Figure 8. Effect of forskolin of cell-cell contact formation in preconfluent human umbilical vein EC culture. (A,B) Control culture; (C,D) After 1 h incubation in the presence of forskolin (10^{-5}M). (A,C) Phase contrast (x 200); (B,D) Silver nitrate stain (x 350).

of fibronectin in the regions of intercellular junctions. A similar effect of forskolin was observed in preconfluent cultures of endothelium grown in the presence of PMA. These findings show that the second messengers are able to regulate the formation of endothelial monolayer, and the products of phosphoinositide metabolism primarily stimulate proliferation of EC; the elevation of intracellular cAMP is important for the formation of intercellular contacts and the organization of endothelial monolayer.

It should be noted that in EC PMA activates systems responsible for the initiation of proliferation but not all the mechanisms which provide normal growth of endotheliocytes.

This idea is supported by the fact that the mitogenic effect of PMA is potentiated by serum components. Growth factors in a number of cell types are known to activate both phosphoinositide metabolism and the synthesis of cGMP. At the same time, PMA is able to imitate the effect of only one of the products of phosphoinositide metabolism, namely, DAG. It is thought that for normal proliferation of EC it is necessary to switch on the system of cGMP metabolism, and, in parallel, to imitate the effect of the second product of phosphoinositide metabolism, triphosphoinositol. Selective activation of the systems which are affected by PMA is likely to result in the formation of certain morphotypes of EC (elongated, mutually oriented and giant multinucleated cells).

Repair and Protection of Endothelium

It is commonly accepted that the injury of endothelium plays an important role in atherogenesis (12), and morphological criteria of endothelial injury were described by many authors (13-15). Of special interest is the understanding of the intracellular mechanisms mediating the effects of physiologically active substances involved in the regulation of homeostasis of EC, and the maintenance of their viability and stability against those effects of external factors which produce cell damage.

In the previous section it was shown that the behavior of EC in monolayer, the proliferation of endothelium and the formation of contacts between cells may be controlled by the systems of second messengers which mediate the external signals. The question arises, whether these systems are also involved in the control of endothelium homeostasis and its stability against external damaging effects.

An important role in atherogenesis is ascribed now to the products of cholesterol metabolism, particularly to cholesterol oxidized derivatives which exert powerful cytotoxic effect on various cells. The addition to confluent endothelial cells of one of the product of cholesterol oxidation, 1,3,5-cholestantriol, results in a death of endothelium within 35 hours (Figure 9A). The same derivative

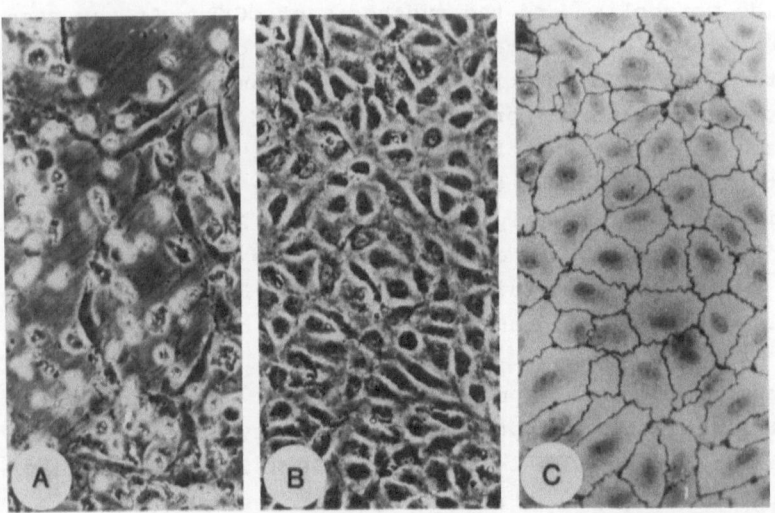

Figure 9. Chemical injury of cultured EC, protective effect
of forskolin. (A) EC monolayer was incubated for 24 h in
the presence of cholestantriol (5 µg/mL); (B,C) Cholestantriol with forskolin (10^{-5}M). (A,B) Phase contrast (x 200);
(C) Silver nitrate stain (x 350).

of cholesterol has no toxic effect on similar cultures when
the level of cAMP is elevated by activation of its synthesis,
or by the addition of cAMP analogues capable of penetrating
into cells (Figure 9B). Under these conditions the endothelium is completely preserved, and even minimal deteriorations
of cellular contacts are absent (Figure 9C). These data
demonstrate that the system of cAMP metabolism is closely
involved in the regulation of the ability of endothelium to
sustain chemical damage.

However, this is not the only way by which the protective
effect of cAMP is exerted. The same system may play an important role in the restoration of the integrity of endothelial
monolayer. We have found that the elevation of cAMP in EC can
significantly accelerate the repair of endothelium after mechanical injury of an endothelial sheet. In Figure 10A, an
endothelial monolayer after mechanical assault is shown.
After addition of forskolin (10^{-5}M) the integrity of the

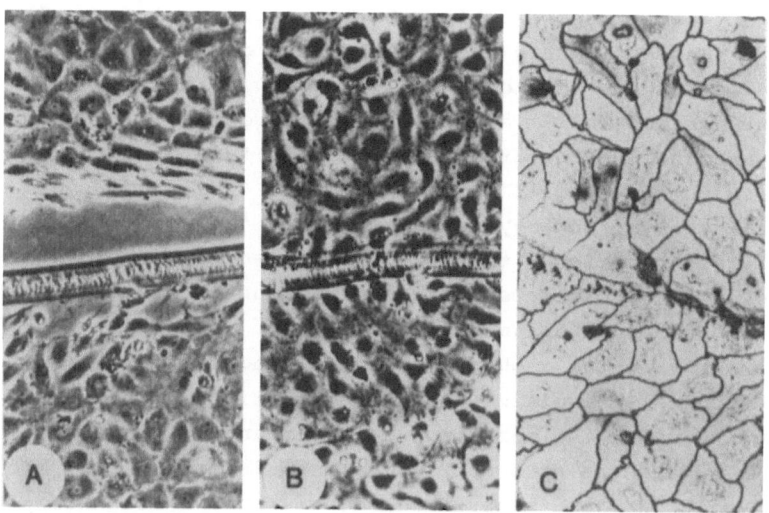

Figure 10. Effect of forskolin on EC monolayer reparation
after mechanical damage. (A) EC culture after mechanical
damage (a scrape). (B,C) Repair of the monolayer after 2 h
incubation in the presence of forskolin (10^{-5}M). (A,B) Phase
contrast (x 200); (C) Silver nitrate stain (x 350).

monolayer is completely restored within 1-2 hours (Figure 10B),
whereas in its absence the repair of endothelium after
similar damage requires from 1-3 days. The effect of forskolin
can not be explained by the increase in the cell number;
earlier in this paper it was mentioned that cAMP does not
stimulate, but rather inhibits endothelial growth. The repair
of the endothelial monolayer in this case is due to the
stimulation of migration and spreading of endothelial cells.
The cells migrate into the zone of injury and form a continuous monolayer with completely formed intercellular contacts.
This is well seen after staining of the culture with silver
nitrate (Figure 10C).

CONCLUSION
For many years the viewpoint has been commonly shared
that the decisive role in atherosclerotic transformation of
vessel wall belongs to the subendothelial layers of intima.

In animal experiments it was demonstrated that the accumulation of cells, lipids and extracellular matrix is the consequence of the activation of proliferation, metabolic and synthetic activity of smooth muscle cells. On the other hand, according to the "response-to-injury" hypothesis, the damage or partial loss of EC plays the role of a trigger which activates the subsequent development of atherosclerotic process. The primary event in endothelium-mediated initiation of this process may be the changes in endothelial morphology (12). The studies of endothelial cell morphology in "normal" and "atherosclerotic" human arteries have shown that the development of atherosclerotic lesions correlates with alterations in morphological organization of endothelium (16).

To understand the mechanisms controlling the formation and morphological reorganization of endothelium, we have made an attempt to model the morphological rearrangements of endothelium in culture using specific chemical interventions. It was shown that fast and reversible changes in the morphology of EC are effectively controlled by the change in the concentrations of second messengers, cAMP and DAG. These substances are formed by activation of adenylate cyclase and via the cascade of the enzymes of phosphoinositide metabolism caused by such compounds as catecholamines, angiotensin, histamine, prostaglandins, leukotrienes, etc.

According to our findings, hormones and vasoactive compounds which act by the increasing concentration of cAMP may affect mostly the morphology of cells and the state of intercellular contacts. Hormones, which stimulate phosphoinositide metabolism, are capable of triggering or accellerating the proliferation of EC. Both systems of second messengers function not in an isolated fashion, but are complementary. The activators of cAMP basically act on the population of nonproliferating EC, increasing their viability and the resistance to a number of cytotoxins and unfavorable mileau factors. In the zones of injury these agents may accelerate repair processes due to faster cell migration and intensive spreading of EC. Simultaneously, the formation of dense intercellular contacts is stimulated by the cAMP system.

Phosphoinositide metabolism activators restore and support the morphological integrity or the monolayer in a different way, acting by the activation of proliferation and by the increase in the number of cells in the monolayer. Both mechanisms are essential for normal morphological integrity of the endothelial lining. The role of second messengers in the control of morphology and the viability of endothelium allow one to predict the likely changes in the vascular wall at different combinations of endocrine factors and stress mediators and to suggest a way to look for potential drugs which protect endothelium from damage by the selective effects on receptors or on the systems of second messengers.

REFERENCES

1. Langille BL, Adamson SL (1981) Relationship between blood flow direction and endothelial cell orientation at arterial branch sites in rabbit and mice. Circ Res 48:481-485.
2. Levesque MJ, Liepsch D, Moravec S, Nerem RM (1986) Correlation in endothelial cell shape and wall sheer stress in a stenosed dog aorta. Arteriosclerosis 6:220-229.
3. De Chastonay C, Gabbiani G, Elemer G, Huttner I (1983) Remodeling of the rat aortic endothelial layer during experimental hypertensia: Changes in replication rate, cell density, and surface morphology. Lab Invest 48:45:52.
4. Shepro D, Welles SL, Hecjtman HB (1984) Vasoactive agonists prevent erythrocyte extravasation in thrombocytopenic hamsters. Thromb Res 45:421-427.
5. Welles SL, Shepro D, Heichtman HB (1985) Vasoactive amines modulate actin calbes (stress fibres) and surface area in cultured bovine endothelium. J Cell Physiol 123:337-342.
6. Sandra A, Bar RS, Dolash S, Marshall SJ, Kaduce TL, Spector AA (1985) Morphological alterations in cultured endothelial cells induced by arachidonic acid. Exp Cell Res 158:484-492.
7. Galdal KS, Evensen SA, Brosstad F (1981) Effects of divalent cations and various vasoactive and haemostatically active agents on the integrity of monolayers of cultured human endothelial cells. Thromb Res 21:273-284.
8. Galdal KS, Evensen SA, Nilsen E (1983) Thrombin-induded shape changes of cultured endothelial cells: Metabolic and functional observations. Thromb Res 32:57-66.
9. Nabika T, Nara Y, Yamori Y, Lovenberg W, Endo J (1985) Angiotensin II and phorbol ester enhance isoproterenol- and vasoactive intestinal peptide (VIP)-induced cyclic AMP accumulation in vascular smooth muscle cells. Biochem Biophys Res Communs 131:30-36.

10. Vanecek I, Sugden D, Weller J, Klein D (1985) Atypical synergistic $alpha_1$- and beta-adrenergic regulation of adenosine 3',5'-monophosphate and guanosine 3',5'-monophosphate in rat pinealocytes. Endocrinology 116:2167-2173.

11. Sibley DR, Jeffs RA, Daniel K, Nambi P, Lefkowitz RJ (1986) Phorbol diester treatment promotes enhanced adenylate cyclase activity in frog erythrocytes. Arch Biochem Biophys 244:373-381.

12. Reidy MA (1985) Biology of disease. A reassessment of endothelial injury and arterial lesion formation. Lab Invest 53:513-520.

13. Christensen BC (1974) Repair of arterial tissue. A scanning electron microscopic (SEM) and light microscopic study on the endothelium of rabbit thoracic aorta following noradrenaline in toxic doses. Virchows Arch [A] 363: 33-38.

14. Repin VS, Dolgov VV, Zaikina OE, Novikov ID, Antonov AS, Nikolaeva MA, Smirnov VN (1984) Heterogeneity of endothelium in human aorta - A quantitative analysis by scanning electron microscopy. Atherosclerosis 50:35-52.

15. Zimmerman M, McGeachie J (1986) Quantitation of the relationship between aortic endothelial intercellular morphology and peameability to albumin. Atherosclerosis 59:277-282.

16. Antonov AS, Nikolaeva MA, Klueva TS, Romanov YuA, Babaev VR, Bystrevskaya VB, Perov NA, Repis VS, Smirnov VN (1986) Primary culture of endothelial cells from atherosclerotic human aorta. Part I. Identification, morphological and ultrastructural characteristics of two endothelial cell subpopulations. Atherosclerosis 59:1-19.

4

Cytoskeletal Characterization of Smooth Muscle Cells of Human and Experimental Atherosclerotic Plaques

G. Gabbiani

It is presently well accepted that smooth muscle
cells (SMC) are the major contributor to the formation of
atheromatous plaque (1-4). However, little is known
about morphologic and/or biochemical differences between
SMC of the media and atheromatous SMC (1,2,5). The cytoskeletal features of SMC in the arterial wall have been
clarified only recently (6-10). Practically all SMC contain intermediate filaments (IF) composed of vimentin, and
in addition, many (more than 50%) contain IF composed of
desmin. Moreover, vascular SMC are characterized by the
prevalence of a special α-actin isotype (7,9). It has been
shown that the large majority of rat aortic SMC located in
intimal thickening after endothelial injury (the most
commonly used model for the atheromatous plaque) contain
IF composed only of vimentin (8). This suggests that
changes in cytoskeletal elements may represent useful
markers of SMC adaptation during experimental and possibly
human atheromatosis. Recent studies of human atheromatous
plaques have shown that fibrous plaques contain SMC with
"dedifferentiated" cytoskeletal features similar to those
of the experimental early aortic intimal thickening, while
complicated plaques contain SMC which have reacquired cytoskeletal features similar to those of the quiescent media
(11).

We have compared the cytoskeletal features of rat
aortic SMC during normal conditions, experimental intimal

thickening and *in vitro* culture (12, 13). Our results show that the modification of cytoskeletal elements during intimal thickening or tissue culture furnish new useful information on SMC reaction to stimuli inducing their replication and movement.

Normal Conditions and Isolated Cells

Total tissues were treated as previsouly described (13). Cells were isolated by means of enzymatic digestion (14). Vimentin and desmin positive cells were identified by means of indirect immunofluorescent staining using affinity purified polyclonal antibodies against vimentin purified from eye lens and desmin purified from chicken gizzard (13). For the biochemical evaluation of total actin we first determined the quantities of DNA and protein per mg of tissue in the different specimens (13); then, we evaluated actin as percentage of total protein by densiometric analysis of sodium dodecyl-sulfate polyacrylamide gels. These data, correlated with the estimations of DNA and total proteins per mg of tissue, allowed us to calculate the quantities of actin per cell (13). The proportion of actin isoforms was calculated in two-dimensional gels according to Quitschke and Schechter (15). The values were obtained as a percentage of total actin in the same gel.

Results using total tissues or isolated cells were similar and hence will be reported together. The percentage of vimentin-positive and vimentin plus desmin cells was 30 and 70 respectively. The content of actin per cell was about 20 pg and the proportions of α-, β- and γ-actin isoforms were 58%, 29% and 13% respectively.

Intimal Thickening After Endothelial Injury

Fifteen days after balloon-induced endothelial injury, the percentage of vimentin-positive cells in the intimal thickening was 79 and the percentage of vimentin plus desmin-positive cells was 21. Total actin per cell decreased to 13.62 pg and the proportions of actin isoforms was 35% for α, 45% for β and 20% for γ. Seventy-five days after endothelial injury, when the lesion was reendothelialized and SMC were not replicating, the percentage of vimentin-positive cells was 48 and the percentage of vimentin plus desmin-positive cells 58. The content of actin per cell was 18 pg and the proportions of different actin isoforms were 55% for α, 30% for β and 15% for γ, practically the same as that of normal cells.

Primary Confluent Cells

SMC cultured in 10% FCS reached confluence about 7 days after seeding. At that time the percentage of vimentin-positive cells was about 52 and the percentage of vimentin plus desmin-positive cells about 48. The content of actin per cell was about 15 pg and the proportions of actin isoform were 34% for α, 43% for β and 23% for γ.

DISCUSSION

Our results, summarized in Table I, show that in experimental intimal thickening observed in the rat aorta 15 days after balloon-induced endothelial injury, distinct cytoskeletal changes appear in SMC compared with normal media SMC. These consist of: a) increased amount of cells containing only vimentin and decreased amount of cells containing in addition desmin; b) decreased actin content per cell, and c) a switch in pattern of actin isoform expression from a predominant α-smooth muscle type to a predominant β-type and an increased γ-type. These changes are present also in primary cultures of SMC in the presence of 10% FCS and are similar to those previously reported in human aortic atheromatous plaques (12). All the described intimal changes regress by 75 days after injury when endothelial repair is complete; thus, at least in our experimental conditions, it appears that: a) absence of endothelium is important in order to maintain SMC cytoskeletal changes, and b) after proliferation and migration into the intima, SMC can evolve *in situ* toward a mature type of cell morphologically and biochemically similar to the SMC of the normal media. The finding of a molecular switch of actin expression in rat SMC during intimal thickening and primary cultures provides a new biochemical marker allowing a better definition of the phenotype of these cells and suggests that cultured SMC may represent a useful experimental model for atheromatous SMC.

Table 1. Cytoskeletal Features of Rat Aortic SMC During Normal and Experimental Conditions

	Vimentin positive %	Vimentin + desmin positive %	Total actin (pg/cell)	Proportions of actin isoforms (% of total actin in gels)		
				α	β	γ
Normal conditions or isolation after enzymatic digestion	30	70	20.79	58	29	13
Experimental intimal thickening 15 days after injury	79	21	13.62	35	45	20
Experimental intimal thickening 75 days after injury	48	52	18.06	55	30	15
Primary culture at confluence	52	48	15.45	34	43	23

In conclusion, it appears that evaluation of cytoskeletal changes of SMC under various conditions furnishes useful information as to the expression of SMC phenotype during experimental and human atheromatosis. It is conceivable that a better understanding of the mechanisms leading to the described cytoskeletal alterations will help in the clarification of the molecular phenomena resulting in the production of experimental and human atheromatous plaques.

REFERENCES

1. Benditt EP, Gown AM (1980) Atheroma: The artery wall and the environment. Int Rev Exp Pathol 21:55-118
2. Haust MD (1974) Reaction patterns of intimal mesenchyme to injury and repair in atherosclerosis. Adv exp Med Biol 43:35-57
3. Ross R, Glomset JA (1976) The pathogenesis of atherosclerosis (first of two parts) N Eng J Med 295:369-377
4. Ross R, Glomset JA (1976) The pathogenesis of atherosclerosis (second of two parts) N Eng J Med 295: 420-425
5. Chamley-Campbell J, Campbell GR, Ross R (1979) The smooth muscle cell in culture. Physiol Rev 59: 1-61
6. Frank ED, Warren L (1981) Aortic smooth muscle cells contain vimentin instead of desmin. Proc Natl Acad Sci USA 78:3020-3024
7. Gabbiani G, Schmid E, Winter S, Chaponnier C, de Chastonay C, Vandekerckhove J, Weber K, Franke WW (1981) Vascular smooth muscle cells differ from other smooth muscle cells:Predominance of vimetin filaments and a specific α-type actin. Proc Natl Acad Sci USA 78:298-302
8. Gabbiani G, Rungger-Brändle E, de Chastonay C, Franke WW (1982) Vimentin-containing smooth muscle cells in aortic intimal thickening after endothelial injury. Lab Invest 47:265-269
9. Schmid E, Osborn M, Rungger-Brändle E, Gabbiani G, Weber K, Franke WW (1982) Distribution of vimentin and desmin filaments in smooth muscle tissue of mammalian and avian aorta. Exp Cell Res 137:329-340
10. Travo P, Weber K, Osborn M (1982) Co-existence of vimentin and desmin type intermediate filaments in a subpopulation of adult rat vascular smooth muscle cells growing in primary culture. Exp Cell Res 139:87-94
11. Kocher O, Gabbiani G (1986)   Cytoskeletal features of normal and atheromatous human arterial smooth muscle cells. Hum Pathol 17:875-880
12. Gabbiani G, Kocher O, Bloom WS, Vandekerckhove J, Weber K (1984) Actin expression in smooth muscle cells of rat aortic intimal thickening and human atheromatous plaque. J Clin Invest 73: 148-152

13. Kocher O, Skalli O, Bloom WS, Gabbiani G (1984)
    Cytoskeleton of rat aortic smooth muscle cells.
    Normal conditions and experimental intimal thickening.
    Lab Invest 50:645-652
14. Ives HE, Schultz GS, Galardy RE, Jamieson JD (1978)
    Preparation of fractional smooth muscle cells from the
    rabbit aorta. J Exp Med 148: 1400-1413
15. Quitschke W, Schechter N (1982) A noncomputerized
    scanning method for determining relative protein
    quantities and synthesis rates on two-dimensional
    electrophoretic gels. Anal Biochem 124: 231-238

5

Phenotypic Changes in Smooth Muscle Cells of Human Atherosclerotic Plaques

G.R. Campbell, J.H. Campbell, A.H. Ang, I.L. Campbell, S. Horrigan, J.A. Manderson, P.R.L. Mosse, and R.E. Rennick

Smooth Muscle Cells of the Media of Normal Arteries

General Morphology

The smooth muscle cell is usually the only cell type present in the media of mammalian arteries and occupies 40-50% of the volume of the media in large elastic arteries and 80-85% in smaller muscular arteries (Gabella, 1984); the rest of the media is composed of extracellular matrix components such as elastin, collagen and proteoglycans.

In the normal young adult, myofilaments occupy the major volume density of the smooth muscle cytoplasm (60-70%) and tend to be located towards the peripheral regions of the cell. Other organelles such as rough and smooth endoplasmic reticulum (ER) which together occupies 5-10% of volume, mitochondira (about 8%), Golgi, free ribosomes, lysosomes and inclusions (such as glycogen and lipid droplets) are usually found in the central region of the cell extending from the nuclear poles (1).

Three distinct types of filaments are found in smooth muscle: thin, thick and intermediate filaments. By far the largest number of filaments are thin, 50-80$\overset{o}{A}$ in diameter and are composed predominantly of actin. Three different isotypes of actin can be distinguished by isoelectric focusing and chemical analysis of the amino-terminal peptides; these have been termed the α, β and γ isoforms (2). Smooth muscle cells

of the human aortic media contain more than 60% of actin
in the α isoform, 31% in the β isoform and negligible amounts
of the γ isoform. Mammalian nonmuscle cells, including
fibroblasts, contain only the β- and γ-isoforms (3,4).

Thick filaments are 102-180Å in diameter and contain
myosin. They differ biochemically from those of striated
muscle, as well, their preservation for electron microscopy
is variable. Limited data suggests that smooth muscle
myosin, like that of cardiac muscle myosin, expresses some
heterogeneity (5,6). Cardiac muscle myosin exists in three
different isoforms, each with a different ATPase activity
which affects shortening velocity of the cells (7).

There are two major classes of intermediate filament
proteins presently recognized in smooth muscle: vimentin
and desmin. Mature visceral smooth muscle contains predominantly desmin, but vascular smooth muscle expresses
various ratios of desmin and vimentin. In the rat aortic
media 51% of the smooth muscle cells contain only vimentin,
48% contain both vimentin and desmin, and 1% of cells have
only desmin. By comparison, fibroblasts contain only
vimentin filaments (8).

Function
The smooth muscle cell is responsible for maintaining
tension (tone) via contraction-relaxation as well as vessel
integrity by proliferation and synthesis of extracellular
matrix (9).

Structure/Function Changes

Concept of modulation of phenotype
In recent years a number of studies have shown that
various cell types can alter their character when the
environment changes. These alterations in character are
called modulations of the differentiated state and involve
reversible interconversions between different phenotypes
(from Greek, phän -show). Modulations in cell phenotype
may occur as a result of cell interactions, alterations to
the extracellular matrix, or in response to other signals
such as hormones (10,11).

In keeping with the multiplicity of functions required of it, the arterial medial smooth muscle cell is capable of expressing a range of phenotypes (i.e., modulating its differentiated state). At one end of the spectrum of phenotypes is the smooth muscle cell whose function is almost exclusively contraction. The cytoplasm of the "contractile-state" cell contains numerous myofilament bundles. Organelles such as rough ER, Golgi and free ribosomes are few in number and located in the perinuclear region. In the media of normal adult arteries the majority of cells are towards this "contractile-state". At the opposite end of the spectrum of phenotypic expression is the muscle cell whose function is almost exclusively synthesis ("synthetic-state") (10). In line with the other cell types actively engaged in production of extracellular matrix, the cytoplasm of the synthetic state cell contains few filament bundles but large amounts of rough ER, Golgi and free ribosomes.

Smooth Muscle Cells of the Intima of Arteries

Diffuse intimal thickenings (DITs) in human arteries are sites of predilection for atheromatous plaque formation, but do not invariably develop into lesions (12-14). The vast majority of cells in these intimal thickenings are smooth muscle (12,15) and it is their nodular proliferation together with the accumulation of foam cells and extracellular lipid which results in the reorganization of the intima seen in atheroma (13,14).

In an attempt to gain a better understanding of the role of SMC in atherogenesis, we have recently been examining the phenotypic expression of smooth muscle cells of DIT's of human carotid arteries. Cells from regions of DIT adjacent to atheromatous plaques (16) and those from regions of DIT in vessels free from atheroma (17) have been compared with cells of the underlying media.

An ultrastructural analysis of the cell types present in DIT's near lesions showed that 87% were smooth muscle. The remaining 13% included monocyte/macrophages, lymphocytes, mast cells, plasma cells and those which were not readily identified. The smooth muscle cells in the DIT expressed a range of phenotypes, from those whose cytoplasm was filled with myofilaments (Figure 1) to cells whose cytoplasm contained few myofilaments and was largely filled with synthetic organelles such as rough ER, free ribosomes, and Golgi apparatus (Figure 2). As an indication of their phenotypic state, the volume density of myofilaments in these cells was estimated using morphometry (16,17). In regions free from atheroma there was no significant difference in the volume density of myofilaments between smooth muscle cells of the intima and media (75% intima versus 79% media, V_v myo expressed as a percentage of the cytoplasmic volume) (Figure 3). However, when regions adjacent to atheromatous plaques (but not involved directly in the lesion) were examined there was a significant difference in the volume density of myofilaments between muscle cells of the intima and those of the media (52% intima versus 77% media) (Figure 3).

Thus, while there are no significant differences between intimal smooth muscle cells of regions free from atheroma and medial cells both from the same region and from regions adjacent to atheromatous plaques, smooth muscle cells in DIT's adjacent to atheromatous plaques express a different phenotype - one in which there is a lowered volume fraction of myofilaments and a concomitant increase (of approximately 100%) in synthetic organelles. Consistent with this finding is recent data that smooth muscle cells in the human diffuse intimal thickening contain 15% of their actin in the α-isoform, 70% in the β-isoform and 15% in the γ-isoform, unlike the aortic media which shows a predominance of actin in the α-isoform (4). The presence of phenotypically altered cells in the DIT's adjacent to atheromatous plaques raises two questions:

1. Do these alterations in smooth muscle phenotypic expression play a part in the development of the atheromatous plaque?
2. What causes these changes in phenotypic expression?

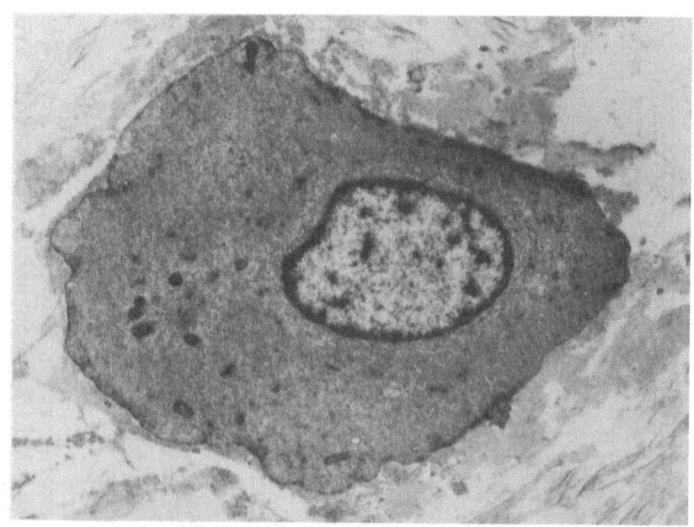

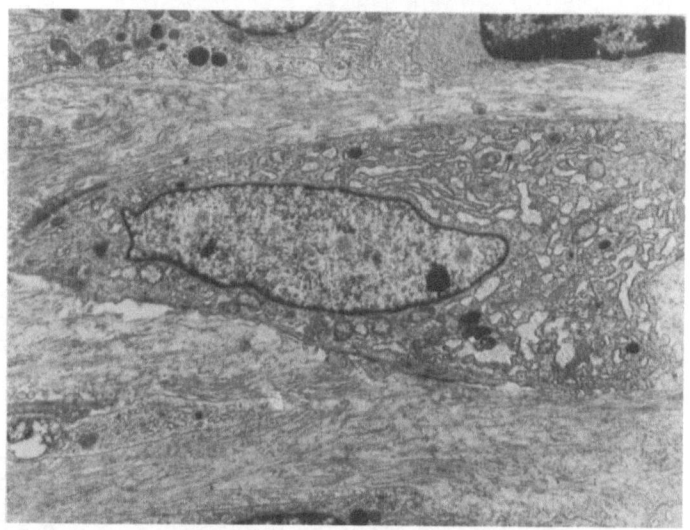

Figure 1. Smooth muscle cell from a diffuse intimal thickening of human carotid artery showing the range of phenotypes
expressed. Cell with high volume density of myofilaments
(V_V myo) and only a few synthetic organelles in the perinuclear region. (x 16,000). (From Mosse et al., 1985,
Laboratory Investigation 53:556-562.)
Figure 2. Smooth muscle cell from a diffuse intimal thickening of human carotid artery showing the range of phenotypes
expressed. Cell with low volume density of myofilaments
(V_V myo), most of the cytoplasm being filled with synthetic
organelles. (x 20,000).

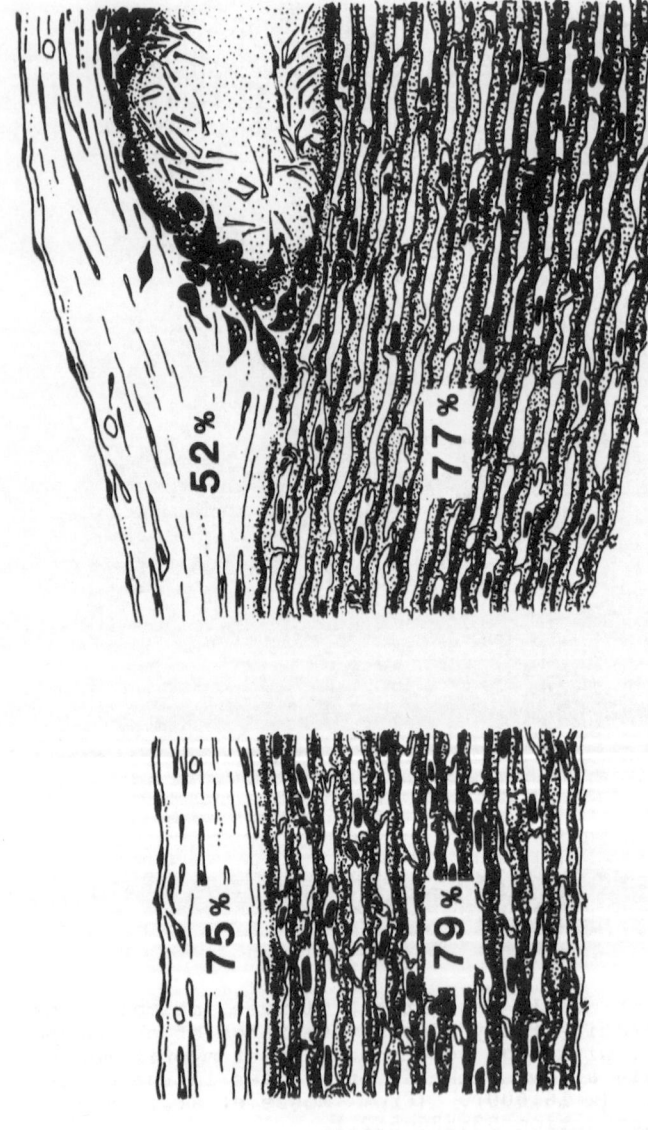

Figure 3. The volume densities of myofilaments (V_V myo), expressed as a percentage of cyto-plasmic volume, in smooth muscle cells of diffuse intimal thickenings and underlying media from human carotid arteries. The two regions compared are areas free from atherosclerosis versus areas adjacent to, but not involved with, atherosclerotic plaques.

Our studies on primary cultured smooth muscle cells suggest some answers to these important questions.

Vascular Smooth Muscle Cells in Primary Cell Culture

Smooth Muscle Phenotypic Modulation in Primary Culture

When smooth muscle cells from the aortic media are enzymatically dispersed into single cells and seeded into primary culture the cells are functionally contractile (18). Ultrastructurally these cells closely resemble "contractile state" smooth muscle cells in the intact aortic media. If the cells are seeded at 10^6 cells/mL in primary culture such that a confluent monolayer is present from day zero, then the cells remain indefinitely in the contractile state. However, if the isolated cells are seeded at less than 10^6 cells/mL, then after a variable number of days (dependent on species, donor age and organ), they spontaneously undergo a change in phenotype whereby there is a gradual decrease in V_v myo and a concomitant increase in synthetic organelles (the synthetic state). This has been verified by Thyberg et al. (19).

Proliferation

As a population, the smooth muscle cells from adult animals in culture do not begin to proliferate until their V_v myo has decreased over a variable number of days from the original 60-70% to 30-40%. The V_v myo then plateaus and the cells proliferate logarithmically until confluence.

Reversibility of Phenotypic Change

Smooth muscle cells which have modulated from the contractile to synthetic phenotype in primary culture can spontaneously revert to the contractile state (i.e., with an increase in V_v myo) upon achieving confluence. This may occur if the cells are seeded sufficiently densely (5×10^4 - 1×10^5/mL) that a confluent monolayer of cells is reached within five cell doublings and within 5-7 days of the original change in phenotype ("reversible synthetic" state cells). If the cells are seeded sparsely (1×10^3 - 5×10^3/mL) such that 3 weeks

of proliferation and more than five cell doublings is
necessary for confluence to be achieved, then the cells
remain permanently in the synthetic phenotype. These cells
are immediately responsive to serum mitogens upon subculture
("irreversible synthetic" cells) (20).

Lipid Accumulation

Morphological examination of rabbit aortic smooth muscle
cells incubated for 24 hours in 75 µg/mL cholesteryl ester-rich
very low density lipoprotein (β-VLDL) from the serum of
cholesterol-fed rabbits, shows few lipid droplets in "contractile"
state cells. Some increase in lipid is observed in "reversible
synthetic" state cells, but there are substantial numbers of
lipid droplets in "irreversible synthetic" state cells. This
pattern of differential cholesteryl ester accumulation has
been confirmed by gas chromatography and by incorporation of
[3]H-sodium oleate into cholesteryl oleate. Furthermore,
"irreversible synthetic" state cells have a considerably
greater capacity to bind and degrade β-VLDL than "reversible
synthetic" state cells. With all phenotypes the binding is
receptor-mediated, of high affinity and saturable (Figures 4
and 5) (21,22).

When macrophages and endothelial cells are coincubated
with SMC's of different phenotype they influence the binding
and uptake of lipoproteins by the SMC's. In the presence of
macrophages (Figure 4) and endothelial cells (Figure 5) there
is greater specific binding to the muscle cells than in their
absence for all three phenotypes. Whether this is due to an
alteration in the lipoprotein itself or a change in function
of the smooth muscle induced by the macrophages and/or endothelial cells (23) is currently under investigation.

Synthesis of Extracellular Matrix

Pulse-labelling cultures with tritiated proline and
measuring the collagenase-susceptible protein by the method
of Peterkofsky and Diegelmann (24) reveals that reversible and
irreversible synthetic state smooth muscle cells have twice

SPECIFIC BINDING OF β-VLDL TO SMC IN THE

PRESENCE AND ABSENCE OF MACROPHAGES

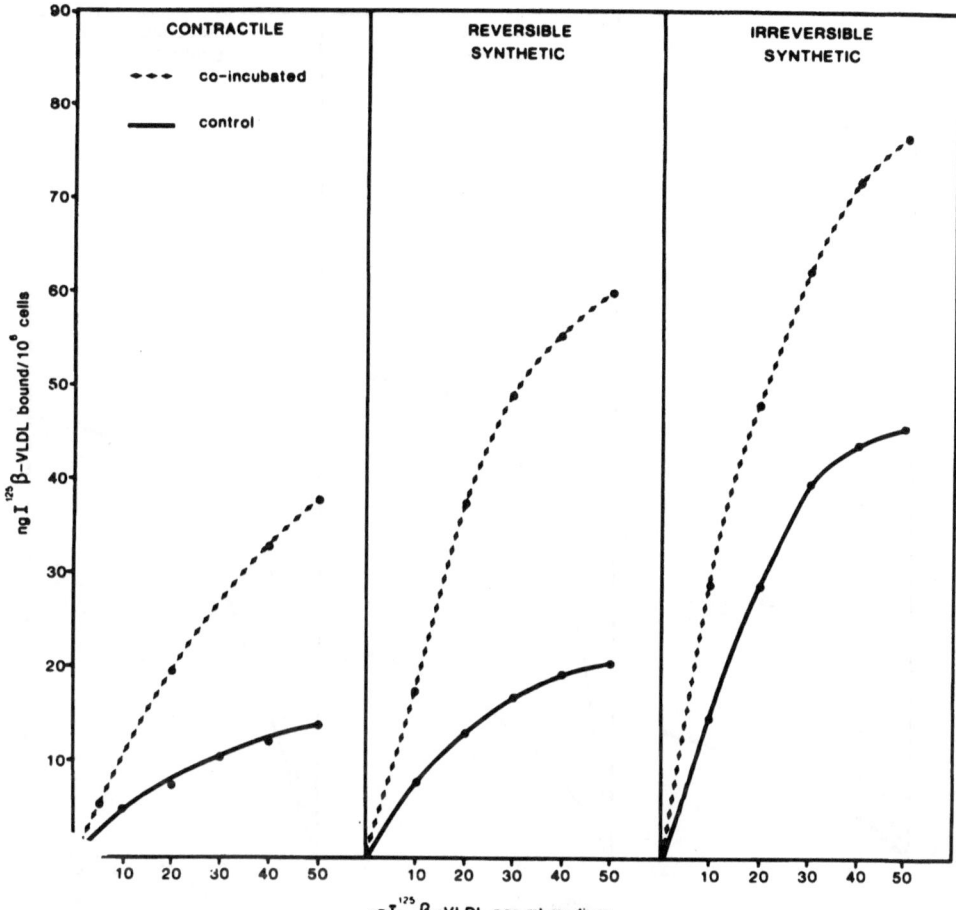

Figure 4. Specific binding of β-VLDL to smooth muscle cells in the contractile, reversible synthetic and irreversible synthetic phenotypes in the presence and absence of macrophages in culture.

SPECIFIC BINDING OF β-VLDL TO SMC IN THE

PRESENCE AND ABSENCE OF ENDOTHELIUM

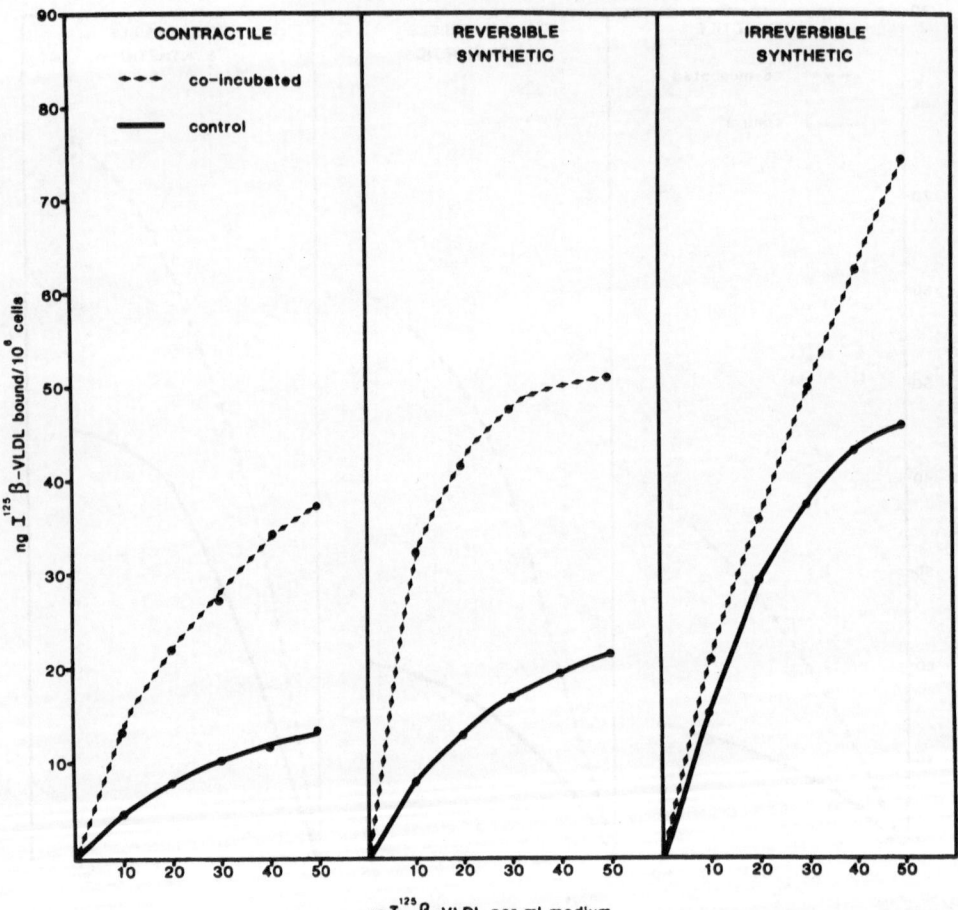

Figure 5. Specific binding of β-VLDL to smooth muscle cells in the contractile, reversible synthetic and irreversible synthetic phenotypes in the presence and absence of endo-thelium in culture.

the rate of synthesis of collagen as contractile state
cells (Table 1). There is no significant difference (p > 0.05)
in the rate of collagen synthesis between reversible and
irreversible synthetic state cells. The increase in collagen
production is specific since non-collagenous protein synthesis
is not significantly altered (p > 0.05) between the three cell
phenotypes (Table 1).

To determine the types of collagen produced, analysis
of pepsin-resistant radiolabelled proteins in 5% polyacrylamide gel electrophoresis in the presence of SDS has also
been made. The collagen distribution in both the medium and
cell layer fractions have been analyzed separately and the
combined synthesis of types I, III and V collagens taken to
be 100%. In the medium fraction, there is a small but significant change in the distribution of types I and III collagens
between contractile and synthetic cells (Table 2). Contractile
SMC synthesize approximately 84% type I and 14% type III
whereas synthetic SMC synthesize 92% type I, 6% type III;
type V synthesis remains essentially unaltered (2-3%). A
similar pattern is observed in the cell layer fraction. As
with rate of collagen synthesis, reversible and irreversible
synthetic cells do not show differences in the relative
distribution of types I, III and V collagens they produce.

Factors Which Affect the Spontaneous Change in Phenotype
of Primary Cultured Smooth Muscle

Cell Seeding Density
As mentioned previously, smooth muscle cells in primary
culture remain in the contractile phenotype if they are seeded
sufficiently dense that they are confluent on day zero. If
they are seeded less densely they spontaneously undergo a
change in phenotype which is reversible or irreversible
depending on the number of doublings the cells undergo before
achieving a confluent monolayer (20,25).

Table 1. Rates of Collagen, Non-Collagenous Protein (NCP) and Total Protein Synthesis by Contractile, Reversible and Irreversible Synthetic Pig Aortic SMC

	Collagen Synthesis[a,b]	NCP Synthesis[a,c]	Total Protein Synthesis[a,d]
Contractile SMC	13,639 ± 2,454	320,559 ± 32,365	334,237 ± 33,339
Reversible-Synthetic SMC	32,449 ± 4,053	294,053 ± 42,537	326,502 ± 44,495
Irreversible Synthetic SMC	26,515 ± 2,415	215,180 ± 22,835	241,695 ± 25,031

a   mean ± SEM (n = 10), expressed as dpm/10^6 cells/h

b   dpm in collagenase-susceptible protein

c   dpm in collagenase-insusceptible protein x 5.4

d   collagen synthesis + NCP synthesis

Table 2. Distribution of Collagens Synthesized by Phenotypically Different Pig Aortic SMC in the Medium and Cell Layer Fractions

	Contractile SMC			Reversible-Synthetic SMC			Irreversible-Synthetic SMC		
	Collagen percentages[a]			Collagen percentages[a]			Collagen percentages[a]		
	%I	%III	%V	%I	%III	%V	%I	%III	%V
Medium fraction[b]	83.8 ± 4.6	14.1 ± 3.5	2.2 ± 1.7	92.5 ± 3.8	5.2 ± 3.6	2.4 ± 1.4	91.5 ± 2.9	5.8 ± 2.8	2.7 ± 0.9
Cell layer fraction[b]	74.7 ± 3.4	13.1 ± 3.5	12.3 ± 2.8	82.3 ± 5.0	5.8 ± 2.7	11.9 ± 3.8	81.7 ± 4.8	4.7 ± 3.4	13.6 ± 3.7

[a] I + III + V = 100%

[b] mean ± SD; n = 8, 11 and 9 for contractile, reversible- and irreversible-synthetic cells respectively

Co-Culture with Endothelium or Smooth Muscle

Spontaneous phenotypic modulation of sparsely seeded smooth muscle from the contractile to synthetic phenotype in primary cell culture is prevented if the cells are grown in co-culture with a confluent monolayer of endothelial cells (20,25,26). The two cell layers do not have to be in contact, just bathed by the same nutrient medium. This occurs in modified Rose chambers where the test and feeder cell layers are grown on opposite coverslips. A feeder layer of confluent, contractile smooth muscle cells (which is above the critical cell density and does not undergo the spontaneous phenotypic change) also prevents the test, sparsely-seeded contractile smooth muscle cells from spontaneously modulating their phenotype. Co-culture with confluent adventitial fibroblasts, confluent subcultured synthetic state smooth muscle cells, or sub-confluent proliferating endothelial cells, does not prevent the spontaneous phenotypic change of contractile smooth muscle (20).

The studies suggest that confluent smooth muscle cells or endothelial cells release an inhibitory substance for smooth muscle phenotypic modulation. The approximate MW of this inhibitory substance or substances produced by confluent endothelial cells and contractile smooth muscle cells is 10,000-15,000 daltons (25). These results agree with our earlier study showing that glycosaminoglycan extract of about 12,000 MW from the artery wall inhibits smooth muscle phenotypic change (20). Treatment of the aortic glycosaminoglycan extract with 4 units/mL heparinase from *Flavobacterium heparinum* for 6 hours at 37°C destroys the active factor. Addition of sodium heparin to culture medium also inhibits smooth muscle phenotypic change (20).

Co-Culture of Smooth Muscle with Peritoneal Macrophages

When smooth muscle cells are grown in co-culture with peritoneal macrophages such that the two cell layers are not in contact but bathed by the same medium, the smooth muscle cells spontaneously modulate to the synthetic phenotype earlier than smooth muscle cells in the absence of the macrophages (Table 3) (28). We are currently carrying out studies to characterize the substance which has this effect.

Hypothesis

On the basis of the above results we have suggested that a heparin-like glycosaminoglycan in the basal lamina of smooth muscle cells maintains the cells in the contractile phenotype. Any factor which removes this substance (i.e., enzyme dispersion in primary culture, or substances released from cells such as monocyte/macrophages *in vivo*), will allow the cells to undergo a change in phenotype to the synthetic state (28).

Relevance of Changes in Smooth Muscle Phenotype to Athero-genesis

Atherosclerotic plaques are superimposed on pre-existing DIT's in arteries and are composed mainly of smooth muscle cells, with smaller numbers of macrophages and T-lymphocytes (29). Proliferation of smooth muscle cells in focal regions of DIT, their synthesis of extracellular matrix and accumu-lation of lipid are well established events in atherogenesis (30). In primary cell culture before smooth muscle cells proliferate as a general population there is a decrease in their V_v myo, i.e., the cells modulate their phenotype from a contractile state towards a synthetic state; change towards the synthetic phenotype is accompanied by an increase in rate of collagen synthesis; and change towards the synthetic pheno-type is accompanied by an alteration in the capacity to bind atherogenic lipoproteins, with subsequent accumulation of lipid. These findings, if they can be extrapolated to the artery wall, suggest that change in smooth muscle phenotype towards a synthetic state may play a central role in atherogenesis.

Why is There an Accumulation of Smooth Muscle Cells with an Altered Phenotypic Expression in DIT's Near Atheromatous Plaques?

It is possible that atherosclerotic plaques develop in regions of DIT where there are already accumulations of

Table 3. Volume Density of Myofilaments in Smooth Muscle
Cells Cultured with and without Macrophages

	Control	Coincubated
Day 3	54.1 + 0.7	51.0 + 2.1
Day 4	52.6 + 1.2	38.8 + 1.5
Day 5	28.1 + 1.7	35.8 + 1.3

Using a two way Analysis of Variance the effect of coincubation
of macrophages with smooth muscle cells over time has a significant effect on the phenotype which the smooth muscle cell
expresses (p < 0.005).

synthetic state cells. That is, in forming the DIT cells in
certain areas going through more than 5 cell doublings, the
cells remain in the synthetic state and form a focal site for
the development of the lesion.

However, in our studies of DIT's unaffected by atheroma
in human carotid arteries, synthetic state smooth muscle
appeared to be randomly distributed and showed no preferential
localization (17). This argues against the above proposition.
However, the question can only be resolved by further studies
in which specific sites of predilection of atheroma are
examined in a range of age groups from young adults to 70-
year-olds.

The second possibility is that all smooth muscle cells
of DIT (except for those involved in normal turnover) are in
an essentially contractile state before the onset of atherogenesis, and change in phenotype is influenced by local
factors during the pathogenesis of the disease, for instance,
by damage to the vessel wall.

Damage to the Vessel Wall

Injury to the endothelium can be caused experimentally
by a variety of traumata such as balloon catheterization (31)
and air drying (32,33). If the damage is of sufficient size,
smooth muscle cells from the media migrate to the intima

where they subsequently proliferate forming a neo-intima of longitudinally oriented smooth muscle cells.

We have recently quantified the volume density of myo-filaments (V_v myo) in smooth muscle cells in the neo-intima of a rabbit carotid artery formed after endothelial denudation (for methods see Mosse et al. 1985). Two weeks after denudation the V_v myo (37%) (expressed as a percentage of cytoplasmic volume) was significantly less than for control medial smooth muscle (68%). Six weeks after injury the volume density had risen to 54% and by 26 weeks after injury had returned to levels (70%) equivalent to that of the control media (Figure 6).

Recent studies have shown a different filamentous expression in smooth muscle cells of a neo-intima formed 2-3 weeks after endothelial injury from that of the media. Fifteen days after injury, cells in the intima contain decreased amounts of actin and desmin and increased amounts of vimentin. Moreover, β-actin is the predominant actin isotype in these cells and significant amounts of γ-actin appear, whereas α-actin decreases. Seventy-five days after injury when the endothelium has completely regenerated the cytoskeletal elements of the neo-intimal smooth muscle cells are similar to those of the media (3,4,34).

This indicates that phenotypic modulation from the contractile to synthetic state can occur in the vessel wall in response to an injury, and that the change in phenotype, as in culture, can be reversible.

Influence of Leukocytes

Macrophages

As well as the established role in atherogenesis of macrophages accumulating lipid to become "foam" cells (35,36), macrophages secrete a growth-promoting activity that acts on several non-lymphoid mesenchymal cell types including smooth muscle (37,38).

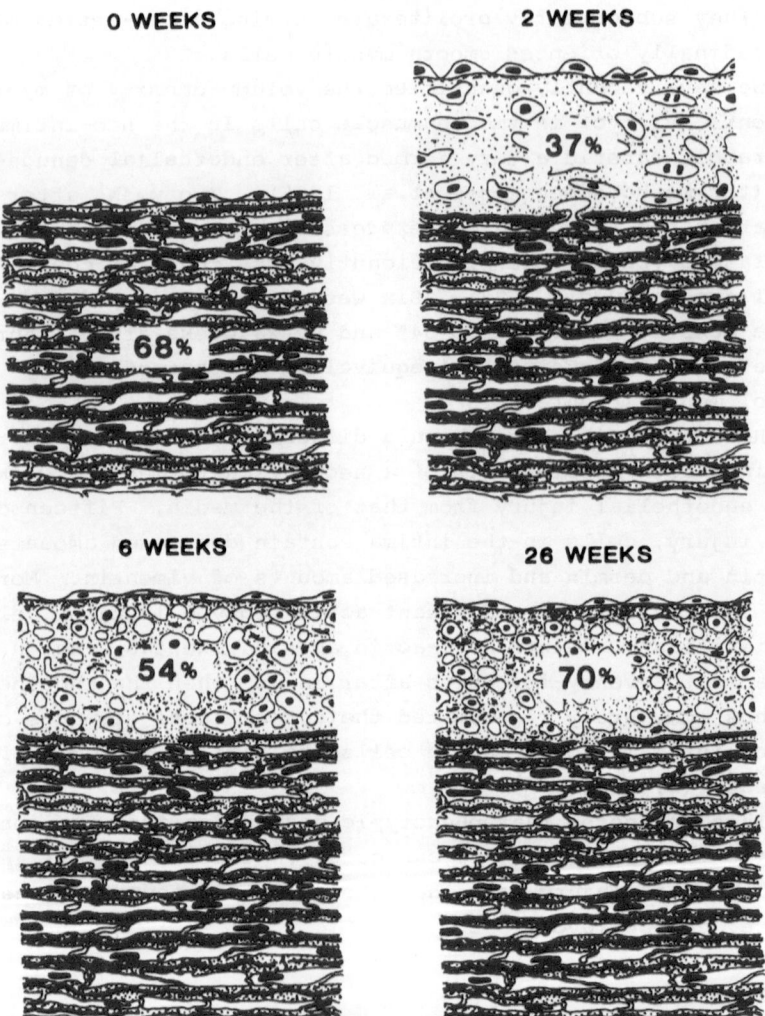

Figure 6. The volume densities of myofilaments (V_V myo), expressed as a percentage of cytoplasmic volumes, in smooth muscle cells in the neo-intima and media of control (0 weeks) and experimental arteries, 2,6 and 26 weeks following balloon catheter injury.

Our results show that macrophages can also stimulate SMC phenotypic change from the contractile to synthetic state, and influence SMC interactions with an atherogenic lipoprotein, β-VLDL.

T-Lymphocytes

The class II transplantation antigen HLA-DR is expressed in immunocompetent cells such as monocytes, macrophages, B-cells and certain T-cells (39). It may, however, also be expressed in several different types of epithelial cell (40,41), dermal fibroblasts (42) and endothelium (40,42,43). Cultured endothelial cells start to express HLA-DR when stimulated by recombinant immune interferon (IFN-γ) or conditioned medium from activated T-lymphocytes (42,43).

The presence of T-lymphocytes in atherosclerotic plaques (29) therefore raises the possibility of their interaction with neighboring cells. The same group (44,45) showed that smooth muscle cells adjacent to atheromatous plaques express HLA-DR. Very few DR-positive cells were found in the DIT of normal human arteries. Since both synthetic state smooth muscle cells and smooth muscle which express HLA-DR antigens are found in the same location adjacent to atheromatous plaques, the possibility exists that they are the same population of cells.

We have recently verified the presence of DR-positive smooth muscle cells in and adjacent to atheromatous plaques. These cells still express HLA-DR when enzymatically isolated and grown in culture for up to one week (Figure 7). DR expression can be induced in some human saphenous vein smooth muscle cells by growing them in the presence of recombinant IFN-γ (200 units for 4 days) (Figure 8). This suggests that DR expression in the smooth muscle cells adjacent to athero-matous plaques may be due to IFN-γ release from other cells within the plaque, such as T-lymphocytes.

CONCLUSIONS

Culture studies indicate that smooth muscle cells with a low V_v myo (synthetic phenotype) have a different biology

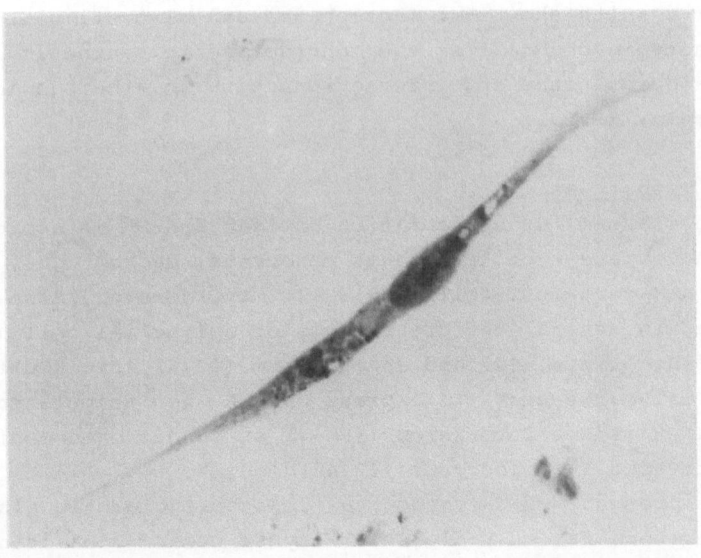

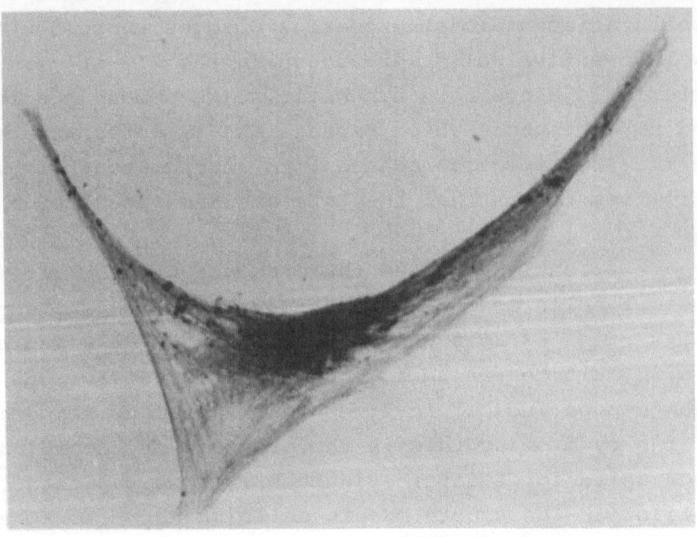

Figure 7. Smooth muscle cells enzymatically isolated from
human carotid artery adjacent to atherosclerotic plaques and
grown in cell culture for 7 days. The cells stain positively
with peroxidase labelled anti HLA-DR. (x 1,200)
Figure 8. Smooth muscle cells enzymatically isolated from
human saphenous vein and grown in the presence of recombinant
γ-interferon (200 units) for 4 days. These cells stain positively with peroxidase labelled anti HLA-DR. (x 1,200)

from cells with a high V_v myo (contractile phenotype) in
that they more readily proliferate, synthesize collagen and
accumulate lipid. These three features are important in the
formation of atheromatous plaques.

Consistent with the hypothesis that an altered smooth
muscle cell phenotype may play an important role in atherogenesis, we have shown that the smooth muscle cells in DIT's
adjacent to atherosclerotic plaques exhibit a low V_v myo
(synthetic phenotype).

Why these cells express a different phenotype in this
location is not known. However, a number of factors could be
involved such as injury to the vessel wall of the influence
of macrophages and T-lymphocytes.

The expression of HLA-DR by smooth muscle cells in DIT's
adjacent to atherosclerotic plaques suggests an additional
change in properties of the SMC from those of the normal
media.

REFERENCES

1. Gabella G (1984) Structural apparatus for force transmission in smooth muscles. Physiol Rev 64:455-477.
2. Vanderkerckhove J, Weber K (1981) Actin typing on total
   cellular extracts: A highly sensitive protein-chemical
   procedure able to distinguish different actins. Eur J
   Biochem 113:595-603.
3. Kocher O, Skalli O, Bloom WS, Gabbiani G (1984) Cytoskeleton of rat aortic smooth muscle cells. Normal
   conditions and experimental intimal thickening. Lab
   Invest 50:645-652.
4. Gabbiani G, Kocher O, Bloom WS, Vanderkerckhove J,
   Weber K (1984) Actin expression in smooth muscle cells
   of rat aortic intimal thickening, human atheromatous
   plaque, and cultured rat aortic media. J Clin Invest
   73:148-152.
5. Larson DM, Fujiwara K, Alexander RW, Gimbrone MAJr (1984)
   Heterogeneity of myosin antigenic expression in vascular
   smooth muscle *in vivo*. Lab Invest 50:401-407.
6. Larson DM, Fujiwara K, Alexander RW, Gimbrone MAJr (1984)
   Myosin in cultured vascular smooth muscle cells: Immunofluorescence and immunochemical studies of alterations
   in antigenic expression. J Cell Biol 99:1582-1589.
7. Hoh JFY, McGrath PA, Hale PT (1977) Electrophoretic
   analysis of multiple forms of rat cardiac myosin:
   Effects of hypophysectomy and thyroxine replacement.
   J Mol Cell Cardiol 10:1053-1076.

8. Gabbiani G, Schmid E, Winter S, et al. (1981) Vascular smooth muscle cells differ from other smooth muscle cells: Predominance of vimentin filaments and a specific alpha-type actin. Proc Natl Acad Sci USA 78:298-302.

9. Chamley-Campbell JH, Campbell GR, Ross R (1979) The smooth muscle cell in culture. Physiol Rev 59:1-61.

10. Campbell GR, Chamley-Campbell JH, Burnstock G (1981) Differentiation and phenotypic modulation of arterial smooth muscle. In: Schwartz CJ, Werthessen NT, Wolf S (eds) Structure and Function of the Circulation, Vol 3. New York: Plenum Press, pp. 357-399.

11. Campbell JH, Campbell GR (1986) Chemical stimuli of the hypertrophic response in smooth muscle. In: Seidel CL, Weisbrodt N (eds) Hypertrophic Response of Smooth Muscle. Boca Raton: CRC Press.

12. Geer JC, Haust MD (1972) Smooth muscle cells in athero-sclerosis. In: Pollack OJ, Simms HS, Kirk SE (eds) Monographs on Atherosclerosis, Vol. 2. Basel: S Karger, pp. 1-140.

13. Velican C, Velican D (1976) Intimal thickening in developing coronary arteries and its relevance to athero-sclerotic involvement. Atherosclerosis 23:345-355.

14. Velican C, Velican D (1980) The precursors of coronary atherosclerotic plaques in subjects up to 40 years old. Atherosclerosis 37:33-46.

15. Haust MD (1983) Atherosclerosis and smooth muscle cells. In: Stephens NL (ed) Biochemistry of Smooth Muscle, Vol. II. Boca Raton: CRC Press, pp. 189-250.

16. Mosse PRL, Campbell GR, Wang Z-L, Campbell JH (1985) Smooth muscle phenotypic expression in human carotid arteries. I. Comparison of cells from diffuse intimal thickenings adjacent to atheromatous plaques with those of the media. Lab Invest 53:556-562.

17. Mosse PRL, Campbell GR, Campbell JH (1986) Smooth muscle phenotypic expression in human carotid arteries. II. Atherosclerosis-free diffuse intimal thickenings compared with the media. Arteriosclerosis 6:664-669.

18. Chamley JH, Campbell GR, McConnell JD, Gröschel-Stewart U (1977) Comparison of vascular smooth muscle cells from adult human, monkey and rabbit in primary culture and in subculture. Cell Tiss Res 177:503-522.

19. Thyberg J, Palmberg L, Nilsson J, Ksiazek T, Sjölund M (1983) Phenotype modulation in primary cultures of arterial smooth muscle cells. On the role of platelet-derived growth factor. Differentiation 25:156-167.

20. Chamley-Campbell JH, Campbell GR (1981) What controls smooth muscle phenotype? Atherosclerosis 40:347-357.

21. Campbell JH, Popadynec L, Nestel PJ, Campbell GR (1983) Lipid accumulation in arterial smooth muscle cells. Influence of phenotype. Atherosclerosis 47:279-295.

22. Campbell JH, Reardon MF, Campbell GR, Nestel PJ (1985) Metabolism of atherogenic lipoproteins by smooth muscle cells of different phenotype in culture. Arterio-sclerosis 5:318-328.

23. Campbell JH, Reardon MF, Koudounas S, Poapdynec L, Nestel PJ, Campbell GR (1986) Influence of smooth muscle phenotype on lipid accumulation. Athero-sclerosis VII:399-402.

24. Peterkofsky B, Diegelmann R (1971) Use of a mixture of proteinase-free collagenase for the specific assay of radioactive collagen in the presence of other proteins. Biochemistry 10:988-999.

25. Campbell JH, Campbell GR (1984) Cellular interactions in the artery wall. In: Hunyor S, Lundbrook J, McGrath M, Shaw J (eds) The Peripheral Circulation. New York: Elsevier, North Holland, pp. 33-39.

26. Chamley JH, Campbell GR, Burnstock G (1974) Dedifferentiation, redifferentiation and bundle formation of smooth muscle cells in tissue culture: The influence of cell number and nerve fibres. J Embryol and Exp Morph 32: 297-323.

27. Campbell GR, Campbell JH, Rennick R, Wang Z-L (1986) The influence of endothelial cells and macrophages on smooth muscle phenotype and proliferation. Atheroscleorsis VII:389-393.

28. Campbell GR, Campbell JH (1985) Smooth muscle phenotypic changes in arterial wall Homeostasis: Implications for the pathogenesis of atherosclerosis. Exp Mol Pathol 42: 139-162.

29. Jonasson L, Holm J, Skalli O, Bondjers G, Hansson GK (1986) Regional accumulations of T cells, macrophages, and smooth muscle cells in the human atherosclerotic plaque. Arteriosclerosis 6:131-138.

30. Ross R (1981) Atherosclerosis: A problem of the biology of the arterial wall cells and their interactions with blood components. Arteriosclerosis 1:293-311.

31. Baumgartner HR, Studer A (1966) Consequences of vessel catheterization in normo- and hypercholesterolemic rabbits (German). Pathology Microbiology 29:393-405.

32. Fishman JA, Ryan GB, Karnovsky MJ (1975) Endothelial regeneration in the rat carotid artery and the significance of endothelial denudation in the pathogenesis of myointimal thickening. Lab Invest 32:339-351.

33. Manderson JA, Campbell GR (1986) Venous response to endothelial denudation. Pathology 18:77-87.

34. Gabbiani G, Rungger-Brändle E, DeChastonay C, Franke WW (1982) Vimentin-containing smooth muscle cells in aortic intimal thickening after endothelial injury. Lab Invest 47:265-269.

35. Gerrity RG (1981) The role of the monocyte in atherogenesis. I. Transition of blood-borne monocytes into foam cells in fatty lesions. Am J Pathol 103:181-190.

36. Faggioto A, Ross R, Harker L (1984) Studies of hypercholesterolemia in the nonhuman primate. I. Changes that lead to fatty streak formation. Arteriosclerosis 4:323-340.

37. Calderon J. Unanue ER (1975) Two biological activities regulation cell proliferation found in cultures of peritoneal exudate cells. Nature 253:359-361.

38. Martin BM, Gimbrone MA, Unanue ER, Cotran RS (1981) Simulation of non-lymphoid mesenchymal cell proliferation by a macrophage-derived growth factor. J Immunol 126: 1510-1515.

39. Kaufman JF, Auffay C, Korman AJ, Shackelford DA, Strominger J (1984) The class II molecules of the human and murine major histocompatibility complex. Cell 36:1-13.

40. Hirschberg H, Braathen LR, Thorsby E (1982) Antigen presentation by vascular endothelial cells and epidermal Langerhans cells: The role of HLA-DR. Immunol Rev 66: 57-77.

41. Barclay AN, Mason DW (1982) Induction of Ia antigen in rat epidermal cells and gut epithelium by immunological stimuli. J Exp Med 156:1665-1685.

42. Pober JS, Collins T, Gimbrone MA et al. (1983) Lymphocytes recognize human vascular endothelial and dermal fibroblast Ia antigens induced by recombinant immune interferon. Nature 305:726-729.

43. Pober JS, Gimbrone MA, Cotran RS et al. (1983) Ia expression by vascular endothelium is inducible by activated T cells and by human interferon. J Exp Med 157:1339-1354.

44. Jonasson L, Holm J, Skalli O, Gabbiani G, Hansson GK (1985) Expression of class II transplantation antigen on vascular smooth muscle cells in human atherosclerosis. J Clin Invest 76:125-131.

45. Hansson GK, Jonasson L, Holm J, Claesson-Welsh L (1986) Class II MHC antigen expression in the atherosclerotic plaque: Smooth muscle cells express HLA-DR, HLA-DQ and the invariant gamma chain. Clin Exp Immunol 64: 261-268.

6

Changes in the Cells of Atherosclerotic Lesions as Advanced Lesions Evolve in Coronary Arteries of Children and Young Adults

H.C. Stary

INTRODUCTION

As early as 1913 Anitschkow (1) described the cells of the aortic intimal lesions of rabbits that had been eating food rich in cholesterol. In his drawings of lesions, Anitschkow pictured both smooth muscle cells and macrophages. Some of the macrophage foam cells are pictured in mitosis, and lesion smooth muscle cells are described as modified (equivalent to the terms RER-rich or synthetic). His observations, although limited by the methods of his time, remain nevertheless valid not only for experimental atherosclerotic lesions, but also for human lesions.

With the availability of new techniques a great effort is underway to understand the range, origins, and functions of intimal and lesion cells. This work includes characterization and quantitation of the contractile and structural proteins of intimal and lesion smooth muscle cells (2), and a search for macrophage chemoattractants (3). The topics are considered elsewhere in this volume.

My task is to summarize some findings in a study on the evolution and progression of atherosclerotic lesions in children and young adults. We began this study in 1979 and it is still continuing. I will emphasize our data on

This work was financially supported by the National Institutes of Health, Grant HL-22739.

changes in the cellular composition of the intima as lesions
develop and changes in lesion cells as lesions enter progressively more complex stages. Specifically, I will
describe the changing spectrum of several smooth muscle
cell phenotypes and their locations in normal intima and in
intimal lesions. I will also summarize our observations
on the numbers and locations of intimal and lesion macrophages and macrophage foam cells.

METHODS

The work reported here is part of a continuing study
of the coronary arteries and aortas of human subjects that
die between fullterm birth and 29 years. In the period
from 1979 to 1986 we obtained the arteries of 1140 subjects
autopsied in New Orleans within this age range. In 560
of these cases, we fixed the coronary arteries by perfusing
them under pressure because the relatively short interval
between death and autopsy of these cases (the mean interval
was about 9 hours) lead us to expect that the tissue would
be well enough preserved to be studied by high-resolution
light microscopy and electron microscopy. These 560 pressure-perfusion fixed cases were used to obtain the data
outlined in this paper. In cases in which coronary arteries were not fixed by pressure-perfusion, they were
removed from the heart, opened along their full length,
flattened, fixed in formalin, and stained with Sudan-IV.
Data from these coronary arteries are not being reported
here. Most subjects were victims of accidents and homocides.
Serum lipid levels were not determined in these individuals while they were alive, but we determined the serum
cholesterol from postmortem blood in many of these subjects.

Our microscopic observations were made on a segment of
the left coronary artery that extended from the beginning
of the left main branch through the first 15-25 mm of the
left anterior descending branch. This segment usually contained the origins of diagonal and septal branches. We
used this segment because clinically important atherosclerotic lesions, if they occur in the coronary arteries
at all, occur in this location with predictable regularity.
This coronary segment is therefore ideally suited for

sequential studies of lesions from their inception to stages of great complexity.

We perfused the coronary arteries with 3% phosphate-buffered glutaraldehyde, which was allowed to run into the coronary artery system through the ascending aorta by the force of gravity. The pressure was about 100 mm Hg. After perfusion, we removed the unopened and rigid left coronary artery from the heart. We then cut the proximal part, including the main branch, the main bifurcation, and the proximal left anterior descending branch, into a minimum of five consecutive tubelike portions, each measuring from 3 to 5 mm in length. Length depended on age (*i.e.* heart size). We marked the anterior wall and the flow divider wall of each tubelike portion with small incisions. In the subsequent histological sections these cuts determined the precise location of intimal structures and the location of lesions. The portions were then immersed in the fixative used for perfusion (1 1/2 hours), washed in buffer, post-fixed in osmium, dehydrated, and embedded upright in Beem capsules containing Maraglas. From each tubelike portion, we cut multiple 1-micron thick cross-sections with glass knives. In many cases, we made semiserial cross-sections. We stained sections with toluidine blue, basic fuchsin, and sodium borate.

We identified and counted macrophages, smooth muscle cells, and other intima and lesion components in the 1-micron cross-sections by light microscopy with Nikon NCG 60x and 100x (dry) objectives. We used electron microscopy to check light microscopic quantitations and to identify different smooth muscle phenotypes and other vascular or lesion components. For electron microscopy we chose parts of the tissue that were of interest as determined by microscopy of 1-micron cross-sections. The 65-nm sections were obtained with a diamond knife, stained with uranyl acetate and lead citrate, and photographed in a Philips 201 or 300 electron microscope. We could not classify some intimal cells by light or by electron microscopy. We believe, however, that we correctly identified the majority. We also obtained some data on sizes and areas by projecting 1-micron cross-sections on a horizontal digitizer board, and by digitizing the structures we wished to measure.

RESULTS

Classification and Composition of Normal Intima

We found two intimal patterns in coronary arteries.
Both patterns were always present from birth (4). They
were continuous and complemented each other. We applied
the terms eccentric thickening and diffuse thickening to
them.

Eccentric intimal thickening (eccentric thickening)
was related to bifurcations, and generally restricted to
the half of the coronary circumference that was opposite
the flow divider wall. In pressure-perfusion fixed arteries
eccentric thickening appeared as a crescent-shaped increase
in intima thickness which at its midpoint could attain
several times the thickness of the media. It is also known
as cushion, pad, or bolster, but it resembles all of these
only in an artery that has been fixed after it has collapsed.
Some have used the term fibromuscular plaque. I have avoided the word plaque for these structures because the term has
the connotation of a lesion. In coronary arteries, the most
prominent eccentric thickening was that associated with the
left main bifurcation. It varied in length but it often
extended from the main branch through the proximal 5-10 mm
of the anterior descending branch.

Diffuse intimal thickening (diffuse thickening)
extended wherever eccentric thickening was not present.
Here the intima was of relatively uniform thickness, less
thick than, or just equaling the media. At and near a
bifurcation, diffuse thickening was continuous with eccentric thickening, involving the half of the coronary circumference without eccentric thickening. Away from bifurcations it encompassed the entire circumference. In the literature, the terms diffuse intimal thickening, and fibromuscular or musculoelastic thickening are used. Some
authors may not distinguish between the diffuse and the
eccentric patterns, applying one of the terms I listed here
and further above to both.

Both eccentric and diffuse thickening were composed of
two main layers which differed in density and nature of
smooth muscle cells, and in denisity and nature of extra-

cellular matrix. The inner (luminal) layer was rich in proteoglycan (GAG) matrix and poor in elastic fibers. Here, smooth muscle cells were widely spaced and more often of a myofilament-poor, RER-rich (synthetic) phenotype. The GAG-rich intima that was immediately subendothelial contained isolated macrophages. The thicker, underlying (musculo-elastic) layer was poor in GAG, and rich in elastic fibers. Smooth muscle cells were densely packed, in an orderly arrangement, and of the myofilament-rich (contractile) phenotype. Eccentric thickening differed from diffuse thickening only by a greater thickness of each layer and by a several fold larger number of macrophages.

Classification of Atherosclerotic Lesions

I have categorized the morphological spectrum of lesions we found in the first three decades of life into five stages or types (5). The composition of each type is described under the subsequent headings. A uniformly accepted terminology of atherosclerotic lesions does not exist and the classification that I use differs from that proposed by the World Health Organization (6) or the one used in the International Atherosclerosis Project (7). I have used familiar terms whenever appropriate.

Isolated Macrophage Foam Cells (Type-I Lesion)

The earliest evidence of an oversupply of lipid in the intima occurred in some infants and consisted of macro-phages overloaded with lipid droplet inclusions (macrophage foam cells). Type-I lesions were macroscopically invisible in Sudan-IV stained coronary arteries. Macrophages without inclusions were increased over the number normally present. Macrophage foam cells usually occurred as isolated cells and sometimes as small clusters of cells. Macrophage foam cells and macrophages were more numerous in eccentric thick-ening than in coronary locations with only diffuse thicken-ing. While macrophages remained in the immediately sub-endothelial region, macrophage foam cells were frequent in the deep part of the GAG-rich intima layer. Macrophage foam cells occurred in 45% of infants in the first eight months of life (4). Over the next four years of life the

number of cases with macrophage foam cells was only 17%.
Macrophage foam cells reappeared in greater number at
puberty as a component of the type-II lesion.

Lipid-laden smooth muscle cells were not a component
of type-I lesions and the phenotypic range of intimal smooth
muscle cells did not differ from normal. Nor did we see
extracellular lipid particles by electron microscopy.

Fatty Streak - Superficial or Submerged (Type II Lesion)

The lesion we classified microscopically as a fatty
streak appeared at puberty. It was present in 43% of
children 10-14 years old. Fatty streaks were composed of
multiple layers of cells overloaded with lipid droplet
inclusions. Cells with inclusions were intimal smooth
muscle cells of the two main phenotypes and macrophages.
RER-rich smooth muscle cells with inclusions had more RER
than usual for their phenotype in human intima. Myofilament-rich smooth muscle cells with inclusions now also had
RER. The number of macrophages and macrophage foam cells
was greater than it had been in infants with foam cells.
Sometimes smooth muscle cells with inclusions predominated
and at other times macrophage foam cells predominated.
Occasionally, the proportions of the two cell types that
contained droplets were about equal. Particles of electron
microscopically visible extracellular lipid were part of
the matrix.

Superficial fatty streak: Because the GAG layer of the
intima was narrow in diffuse thickening and at the shoulders
of eccentric thickening, lipid-laden cells, particularly
the more lipid-laden macrophage foam cells, occupied the
full thickness of the GAG layer. Therefore, since the lipid-
laden cells were located superficially they were macroscopically visible as fatty streaks.

Submerged fatty streak: The GAG layer was wide at the
thick center of eccentric thickening, the lipid-laden macrophages aggregated in its deepest part. Thus, these foam
cells occupying the center of eccentric thickening were
concealed some distance below the endothelial surface, and

macroscopically less obvious, even after staining with
Sudan-IV.

Preatheroma (Type-III Lesion)

This is the lesion that is transitional or intermediate
(8) between the fatty streak and the atheroma (type-IV). In
young people only the fatty streaks located in eccentric
thickening were disposed to this type of transformation. In
addition to the components that make up fatty streaks, such
intimal lesions now contained many separate pool-like
aggregates of extracellular lipid particles. The pools of
lipid particles were below the foam cell layer, that is,
they were in the musculoelastic intima layer of eccentric
thickening. By increasing the volume of the intercellular
space, they disrupted the coherence of structural smooth
muscle cells in the affected regions, and somewhat dispersed
them. This was associated with a phenotypic change in these
normally myofilament-rich cells. The cells were now thin,
long, very rich in RER and encased in gigantic basement membranes. The thickness of the basement membranes was in no
relation to the diameter of the cells, sometimes exceeding
this several fold. Myofilaments often were entirely
absent.

Atheroma (Type-IV Lesion)

The feature that distinguished atheroma was a single
and massive expanse of extracellular lipid particles (the
lipid core) that was grossly visible. Lipid cores occupied
the musculoelastic layer of eccentric thickening. Thus, the
location was the same as that of the separate pools of extracellular lipid particles that we found in other cases, and
classified as preatheroma. The lipid core separated the
musculoelastic intima layer into a luminal (inner) and a
medial (outer) part, and it greatly thickened the intima.
However, a similtaneous mild dilatation of the arterial wall
forestalled a significant loss of arterial lumen.

Our sequential electron microscopic observations indicate that lipid cores are the result of progression and
coalescence of smaller, separate pools of extracellular
lipid particles. The lipid particles that constituted

cores were identical in their fine structure to the more or
less degraded lipid droplets within the cytoplasm of macrophage foam cells and smooth muscle cells. Macrophage foam
cells did not occur within lipid cores. Instead, macrophage foam cells, some dead and decomposing, bordered the
core along its inner periphery, that is, along the aspect
that was towards the lumen. The preexisting structural
intimal smooth muscle cells that were trapped within the
region of the lipid core were widely separated and scattered.
They were thinner and more elongated still than those trapped
within the multiple smaller lipid pools of preatheroma.
Their basement membranes were equally massive.

Fibroatheroma (Type-V Lesion)

The feature that distinguished fibroatheroma was a more
or less thick "cap" of RER-filled smooth muscle cells embedded in a matrix of collagen. This cap formed the uppermost
part of the lesion. Caps replaced and thickened the GAG-
rich intima layer which, except for accumulation of macrophages, had remained relatively unchanged right into the
atheroma stage. Thus, caps were located just above the
foam cell layer and above the lipid core.

The smooth muscle cells of caps were stratified in
parallel layers, and longitudinally arranged around the
artery circumference. The fine structure of cap smooth muscle cells varied somewhat. Some differed from the smooth
muscle cell phenotypes described earlier. Their cytoplasm
was completely packed with cisternae of RER, and basement
membranes were not massive. However, in some regions of the
caps RER-rich smooth muscle cells resembled those in the
lipid cores in their basement membrane gigantism. Lipid
droplet inclusions in cap smooth muscle cells were small
and often infrequent or absent.

DISCUSSION AND CONCLUSIONS
Eccentric Intimal Thickening is Not an Atherosclerotic
Lesion but a Normal Structure in Man

Eccentric thickening, composed of at least two smooth
muscle cell phenotypes and of infrequent macrophages and

located opposite flow divider walls of bifurcations, was
present in coronary arteries from birth. Since we found
eccentric thickening in the coronary arteries of all
subjects, we consider it to be a normal, not a pathological
structure. Our observations support the view that eccentric
thickening is a physiologic adaptation to hemodynamic forces
to which parts of the vasculature are exposed from the very
development of the vascular system(9).

The Macrophage Is the First Cell in the Intima to Accumulate
Lipid Droplets and Most Important in Lipoprotein Uptake and
Degradation

In the youngest children, the macrophage was the one
cell type to accumulate intracytoplasmic lipid droplets.
While the macrophage foam cells of infants may not be the
first stage of atherosclerosis, their presence indicates
that macrophages are intended as the first line of defense
in the intima. When the fatty streak, the lesion which
lead into advanced atherosclerosis, developed at puberty,
the preexisting intimal smooth muscle cells also contained
lipid droplet inclusions. But in the majority of pubertal
children, the greater portion of the lipid that was stored
intracellularly was still stored in macrophages. As fatty
streaks become larger (older), the number of smooth muscle
cells that contained droplet inclusions increased and they
began to outnumber macrophage foam cells. Smooth muscle
cells have a longer life span than macrophages and they may
resist injury better. In any case, we saw fewer dead smooth
muscle cells than dead macrophage foam cells. It is probably for this reason that smooth muscle cells become the
predominant cell type that stores lipid.

While at any one time the proportion of macrophage foam
cells may be smaller than that of muscle cells with droplets,
the total number of macrophage foam cells that was present
over the lifetime of a lesion clearly is enormously greater
than that of smooth muscle cells. This is documented by
radioautographic and electron-microscopic evidence of rapid
macrophage turnover in lesions. Thus, most of the lipoprotein uptake and degradation clearly occurs in macrophages.

Fatty Streaks Located in Eccentric Thickenings Are the
Fatty Streaks That Are Subject to Progression to Atheroma

In the youngest children eccentric thickenings was the
preferred location of macrophage foam cells (4). This con-
currence between the locations of greatest lipid accumulation
and eccentric thickening continued when fatty streaks
emerged at puberty. Lipid deposits having the microscopic
configuration of fatty streaks were greatest in eccentric
thickening although their locations ranged beyond eccentric
thickenings. When subsequently we encountered preatheroma
and atheroma in older children and young adults, the spacial
coincidence with eccentric thickening was again present.
Lipid cores, the expression of particularly heavy lipid
accumulation, did not occur outside eccentric thickenings.
The predilection of eccentric thickening for the larger lipid
deposits was present whether eccentric thickening was particularly thick or not. This is evidence that eccentric thickening and lipid deposition are independently produced by,
as yet, poorly understood hemodynamic forces.

Lipid Cores Are Accumulations of Macrophage Foam Cells
That Have Died

At present, there is disagreement both on the mechanism
of evolution and on the nature of lipid cores. In perhaps
the most widely held view, cores represent a more or less
extensive region of arterial wall necrosis, being composed
primarily of smooth muscle cells that had died (10). In
this view, at least some of the macrophage foam cells at the
periphery of cores are there to phagocytize the cores (11).
In another view, lipid cores consist largely of plasma lipoproteins (12). Here too, the view seems to be that macrophage foam cells respond to the lipid core rather than being
the cause of it.

Our own evidence points to another mechanism of evolution,
although it does not exclude that, to some extent, both of the
above mechanisms coexist. The data indicate that a greater influx of lipoprotein into the intima at locations with eccentric
thickenings is accompanied by a greater influx of macrophages
and generation of macrophage foam cells. In the presence of
continued excessive influx of lipoprotein, many macrophage
foam cells are created over the span of years. Because

of their short life they do not accumulate as intact cells.
As they die, their smaller remnants shift to deep parts of
eccentric thickening. Here they accumulate. In the rapid
generation and death of macrophages the situation in hyperlipidemic intima resembles the situation in the lungs (13,
14). But while the remnants of dead alveolar macrophages
are readily eliminated through the tracheobronchial tree,
those of intimal macrophages are subject to complete extracellular degradation, a slow process that does not keep
pace with rapid forms of accumulation.

Past experiments with rhesus monkeys provide supportive
evidence that lipid cores are the graveyards of macrophage
foam cells. When we reduced high serum cholesterol levels
in monkeys, proliferation of intimal lesion macrophages
ceased and the number of macrophages and macrophage foam
cells declined (15). While macrophage foam cells were
dying, the size of extracellular lipid pools did not decrease
much. Their size decreased only after cells recognizable
as macrophage foam cells had disappeared. We take this as
evidence that the remnants of dead macrophage foam cells
rather than lipoproteins from the blood are the main component of cores.

Lesion Smooth Muscle Cells Are Indigenous Intimal Smooth
Muscle Cells and Their Descendants

We have evidence that the smooth muscle cells that com-
pose intimal lesions in man and in some experimental species
are indigenous intimal smooth muscle cells and their progeny.
Many layers of smooth muscle cells are present in the human
arterial intima from birth at points at which advanced atherosclerotic lesions develop. At every age many are present,
particularly in the upper intima layer, that contain RER and
few myofilaments. We do not see these cells in the media.
There is also increasing evidence of differences with respect
to their contractile and structural proteins (2). Radioautography shows that the preexisting intimal smooth muscle
cells can label with tritiated thymidine, an indication of
cell division (16).

There is no evidence in our present studies in young
people that medial smooth muscle cells contribute to the
smooth muscle cells of intimal lesions by migrating into them

or by being in other ways incorporated into them. A central
role for medial smooth muscle cells in atherogenesis had been
proposed 20 years ago in an editorial in Circulation (17). In
this view, medial smooth muscle cells migrate to become components of intimal lesions. The hypothesis of a medial origin
of intimal lesion cells received support from investigators
who noted medial smooth muscle cells or their cell processes
at the intima-media junction within fenestrations or gaps of
the internal elastic lamina, and who accept this observation
as evidence of cell transmigration. In my view, the presence
of cells of this location does not represent migration.

A Cap of Stratified Smooth Muscle Cells and Collagen is
Added to Lesions After a Lipid Core Has Formed
    We began to encounter lesions consisting of both a
lipid core and of a cap of collagen-producing smooth muscle
cells in persons who were in the third decade of their life,
nearly a decade after lesions with a core but without a cap
appeared. Clearly, establishment of collagenous caps trailed
the establishment of lipid cores. Caps formed by two mechanisms. They formed slowly as a reaction to the underlying
lipid core. Those caps remained relatively thin. Or they
formed when thrombotic surface deposits were incorporated
into the intima. Such caps were thick.
    Caps were present only when a lesion with a lipid core
was also present. However, caps, particularly those caused
by mural thrombi, extended for a variable distance beyond
the limits of a lipid core, and cross-sections made through
the artery at such points would simulate a lesion with a
collagenous cap but lacking a lipid core.
    In the atheroma stage, the increase in intimal thick-
ness had been generated mainly by the formation of the lipid
core deep within eccentric thickening. The GAG-rich layer
that was above the core had only been moderately modified
and thickened by the presence of lipid-laden cells. In the
subsequent fibroatheroma stage, the character of the GAG-
rich layer changed completely. It became a dense and thick
layer composed of new layers of smooth muscle cells and
collagen. That there is a difference between the upper
layer of atheroma and the collagenous cap of fibroatheroma
can be recognized by microscopy of 65 nm or 1-micron sections.

It can not be resolved in conventional 6-micron sections.

RER-rich smooth muscle cells with basement membrane gigantism were the residual cells of lipid cores and, when collagenous caps developed, they were present in some parts of these. Ross and his coworkers (18) who studied lesions in the superficial femoral arteries of old adult subjects described identical cells as characteristic for the cap of lesions. Most of their lesions did not have a lipid core and may represent organized thrombi which in arteries of the lower extremities extend far beyond the primary atheroma. In our material, change of smooth muscle cells into the RER-rich phenotype with basement membrane gigantism occurred when smooth muscle cells became widely separated by an increase in unstructured extracellular material. Massive basement membranes were closely associated with collagen fibers, and may represent a step in collagen synthesis.

While macrophages clearly play a role in the evolution and progression of the lipid core, the role of macrophages, if any, in the formation of a collagenous cap is not clear to us. Some investigators have suggested that, in the presence of thrombosis, monocytes might redifferentiate into collagen-producing cells (19).

REFERENCES

1. Anitschkow N (1913) Uber die veranderungen der kanin-chenaorta bei experimenteller cholesterinsteatose. Beit path Anat Allgem Pathol 56:379-404
2. Kocher O, Gabbiani G (1986) Cytoskeletal features of normal and atheromatous human arterial smooth muscle cells. Hum Pathol 17:875-880
3. Gerrity RG, Goss JA, Soby L (1985) Control of mono-cyte recruitment by chemotactic factor(s) in lesion-prone areas of swine aorta. Arteriosclerosis 5:55-66
4. Stary HC (1987) Macrophages, macrophage foam cells, and eccentric intimal thickening in the coronary artery intima of young children. Atherosclerosis 64:91-108
5. Stary HC (1987) Evolution and progression of athero-sclerosis in the coronary arteries of children and adults. In: Bates RS, Gangloff EC (eds) Atherogenesis and Aging, Springer-Verlag, New York, pp 20-36
6. World Health Organization (1958) Classification of atherosclerotic lesions. Report of a study group. WHO Techn Rep Ser 143, pp 1-20
7. Guzman MA, McMahan CA, McGill HC Jr, Strong JP, Tejada C, Restrepo C, Eggen DA, Robertson WB, Solberg LA (1968) Selected methodologic aspects of the international atherosclerosis project. Lab Invest 18:479-497

8. Katz SS, Shipley GG, Small DM (1976) Physical
    chemistry of the lipids of human atherosclerotic les-
    ions. Demonstration of a lesion intermediate
    between fatty streaks and advanced plaques. J Clin
    Invest 58:200-211
9. Naumann A, Schmid-Schonbein H (1983) A fluid-
    dynamicist's and a physiologist's look at arterial
    flow and arteriosclerosis. In: Schettler G *et al*
    (eds) Fluid dynamics as a localizing factor for
    atherosclerosis. Springer-Verlag, Berlin Heidelberg,
    pp 9-25
10. Constantinides P (1984) Ultrastructural pathobiology.
    Elsevier, Amsterdam, p 110
11. Daoud AS, Jormolych J, Augustyn JM, Fritz KE (1981)
    Sequential morphologic studies of regression of
    advanced atherosclerosis. Arch Pathol Lab Med
    105:233-239
12. Bocan TMA, Schifani TA, Guyton JR (1986) Ultrastructure
    of the human aortic fibrolipid lesion. Formation of
    the atherosclerotic lipid-rich core. Am J Pathol
    123:413-424
13. Bowden DH (1983) Cell turnover in the lung. Am Rev
    Respir Dis 128:S46-S48
14. van Furth R (1985) Cellular biology of pulmonary
    macrophages. Int Archs Allergy Appl Immun 76 (suppl
    1):21-27
15. Stary HC (1979) Regression of atherosclerosis in
    primates. Virchows Arch A (Path Anat) 383:117-134
16. Stary HC (1974) Proliferation of arterial cells in
    atherosclerosis. In: Wagner WD, Clarkson TB (eds)
    Arterial Mesenchyme and Arteriosclerosis. Adv Exp
    Med Biol 43:59-81, Plenum Press, New York
17. Wissler RW (1967) The arterial medial cell, smooth
    muscle, or multifunctional mesenchyme? Circulation
    36:1-4
18. Ross R, Wight TN, Strandness E, Thiele B (1984) Human
    Atherosclerosis. I. Cell constitution and character-
    istics of advanced lesions of the superficial femoral
    artery. Am J Pathol 114:79-93
19. Feigl W, Susani M, Ulrich W, Matejka M, Losert U,
    Sinzinger H (1985) Organisation of experimental
    thrombosis by blood cells. Virchows Arch A (Path
    Anat) 406:133-148

7

Inflammatory Components of the Human Atherosclerotic Plaque

Colin J. Schwartz, Eugene A. Sprague, Anthony J. Valente, Jim L. Kelley, Ellen H. Edwards, and C. Alan Suenram

INTRODUCTION

For many years atheroma, or atherosclerosis as it is more commonly denoted, has been regarded as a disease exclusively affecting the tunica intima. In later years this misconception has been slowly eroded, and it is now generally recognized that this disorder affects all three coats of the arterial wall. Apart from the prominent medial thinning, advanced disease typically exhibits a triad of changes in the adventitia, namely fibrosis, increased vascularity, and a prominent cellular infiltrate which is predominantly lymphocytic. The frequent granulomatous foci of advanced human plaques, together with the lymphocytic infiltration (1-3) are but two overt histologic manifestations of the inflammatory nature of human atherosclerosis. Additionally, in both human and experimental atherosclerosis, and in experimentally-induced hypercholesterolemia, an enhanced monocyte macrophage recruitment to the arterial intima has been observed (4-16). If, then, we accept the contemporary criteria defining inflammation as a process characterized by the focal tissue accumulation of blood constituents including plasma proteins, and the interstitial or extravascular accumulation of the formed elements of blood, then the atherosclerotic plaque adequately fulfills these criteria.

Inflammation as a component of atherogenesis is by no means a new concept, for it was recognized by Rudolf Virchow

(17) in 1862. Elsewhere in this volume, the participation
of the monocyte macrophage in human atherogenesis is described in some detail. In this brief review our primary
purpose is to describe the lymphocytic infiltrates which
characterize advanced human disease, emphasizing but one of
the inflammatory manifestations of this complex disease
process.

Historical Background

Aggregates of inflammatory cells in the tunica adventitia
have been the subject of a number of reports over the years.
As seen in Table 1, they received but a passing mention by
Clifford Allbutt in 1915, and Ophuls in 1933. A more
definitive statement emerged in 1940 when Horn and Finkelstein
reported lymphocytic cellular changes in the adventitia of
human coronary arteries, noting that they were particularly
frequent in "sclerotic vessels". Von Hausammann confirmed
these observations, emphasizing their prevalence in diseased
coronary arteries from patients aged 40 years and older.

Table 1. Inflammatory Cells in the Human Arterial Tunica
Adventitia: An Historical Perspective

Year	Author(s)	Reference
1915	Allbutt	18
1933	Ophuls	19
1941	Horn & Finkelstein	20
1941	Nelson	21
1949	von Hausammann	22
1956	Gerlis	23
1956	Morgan	24
1962	Schwartz & Mitchell	3

It was in 1956 that Gerlis described the histologic features
of the inflammatory cellular aggregates in the adventitia of
coronary arteries, concluding erroneously, however, that they
were unrelated to the degree of coronary artery disease. He
went on to suggest that they might reflect the mode of death,
particularly anoxia. Lymphocytic adventitial aggregates were

also described by Morgan in 1956 who suggested that the
process represents "a low grade reaction to the atherosclerosis, possibly concerned in the scavenging of the
degenerate material".

It was in 1962, as part of a study undertaken by Mitchell
and Schwartz at the Radcliffe Infirmary, Oxford, over the
years 1959-1961, that the following data on the relationship
of lymphocytic infiltration of the tunica adventitia and
atheromatous plaque severity was assembled. These authors
concluded in their initial report (2,3), that the lymphocytic infiltrates might reflect an auto-immune component
in plaque pathogenesis.

Histologic Assessment of Adventitial Lymphocytosis

In order to correlate plaque severity and the degree of
adventitial lymphocytic infiltration, three arbitrary
histologic grades of plaque severity were employed, namely
(a) free, i.e. no evidence of disease or only a minor degree
of diffuse intimal thickening; (b) severe disease, i.e.,
massive plaques with a thickness greater than the original
arterial wall, or in smaller arteries, plaques reducing the
lumen on cross-section to less than half the original diameter, and (c) present, plaques less severe than in category
(b).

Additionally, three grades of adventitial cellularity
were recognized, namely (a) absent; (b) slight, i.e., several
foci of less than 20 cells or a single focus of less than 100
cells; (c) marked, i.e., numerous foci or 20 or more cells or
a single focus of 100 cells or more. In all instances both
plaque severity, and the degree of adventitial lymphocytic
infiltration were assessed jointly by two observers.
Microscopic Features of the Adventitial Cellular Infiltrates

In approximately 80% of blocks showing atheroma of a
severe histologic grade, adventitial cellular aggregates can
be observed. These occur as discrete foci, within the
fibrotic adventitia, the smallest comprising only some 10-20
cells and the largest many hundreds or thousands of cells.
The aggregates are remarkably homogenous, consisting predominantly of small round cells morphologically identifiable
as small lymphocytes. Only occasional plasma cells are

present within these infiltrates. These lymphocytes are often seen encircling adventitial vasa vasorum. Sometimes they have a perineural distribution, and frequently they occur as attenuated ellipsoid bands within the adventitial fibrous stroma. Histologically they are similar in composition and distribution irrespective of the arterial bed examined. Examples of the adventitial lymphocytic infiltration are illustrated in Figures 1-6, which are derived from coronary artery, carotid, and aortic lesions.

Although lymphocytic infiltrates are most prominent within the adventitial coat, scattered lymphocytes are not infrequent within the intima and plaque, and may also be seen in relatively large numbers within plaque granulomata (Figure 7). It is of some importance to note that adventitial lymphocytes are not a feature of human fatty streaks, and further that they have been described in experimental lesions in nonhuman primates receiving dietary coconut oil supplements (25), and also in advanced rabbit lesions produced by intermittent hyperlipidemia.

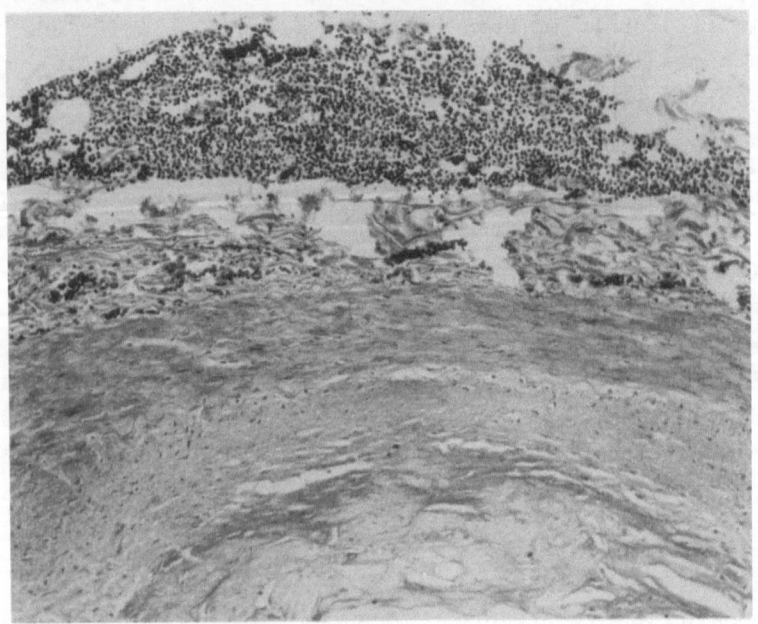

Figure 1. Segment of severely diseased coronary artery showing ellipsoid adventitial lymphocytic infiltrate of a marked degree. (Trichrome X 220)

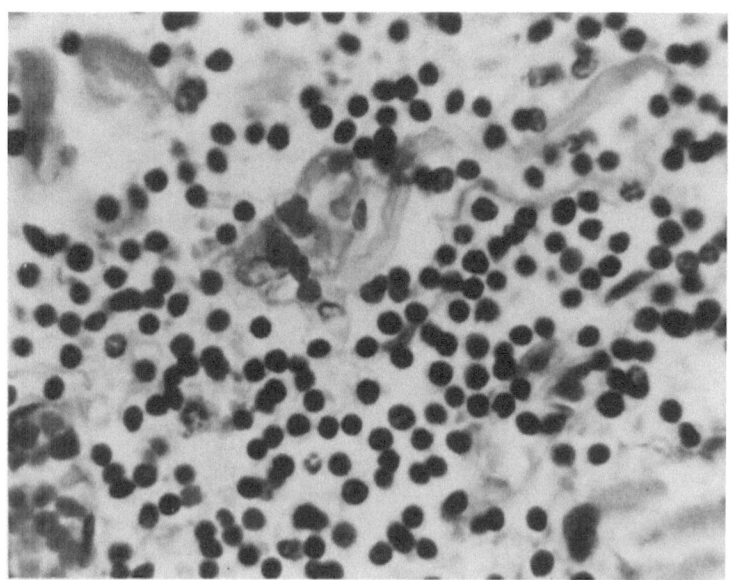

Figure 2. Adventitial lymphocytic infiltrate, showing the relatively homogenous nature of the cells morphologically identifiable as small lymphocytes. (Trichrome x 870)

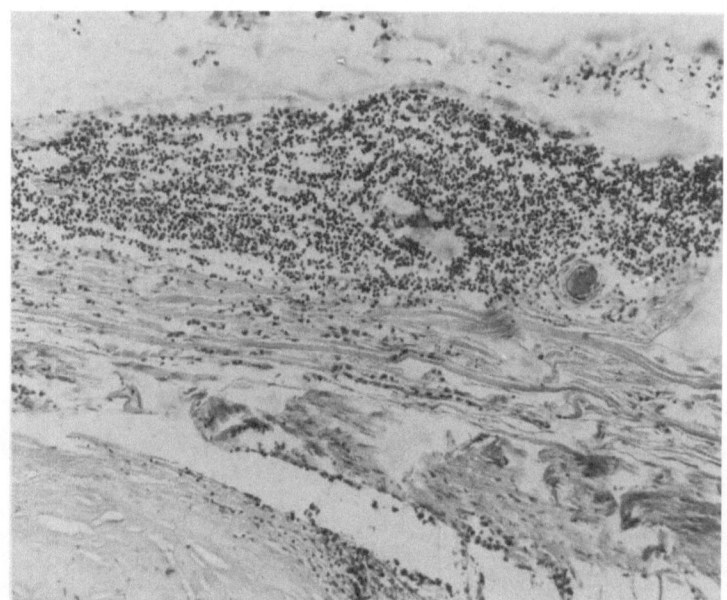

Figure 3. Adventitia of severely diseased coronary artery showing both prominent fibrosis and a marked grade of lymphocytic infiltration (H & E x 220)

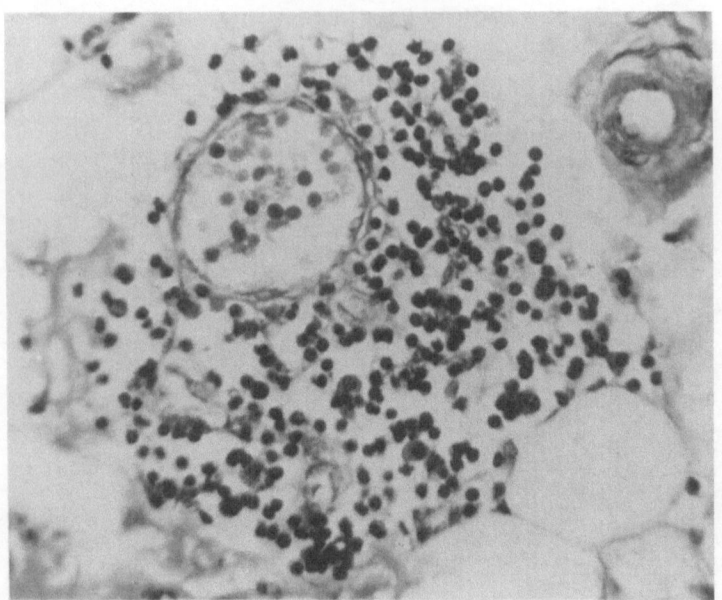

Figure 4. Adventitial lymphocytic aggregate in the common carotid artery. (Trichrome X 810)

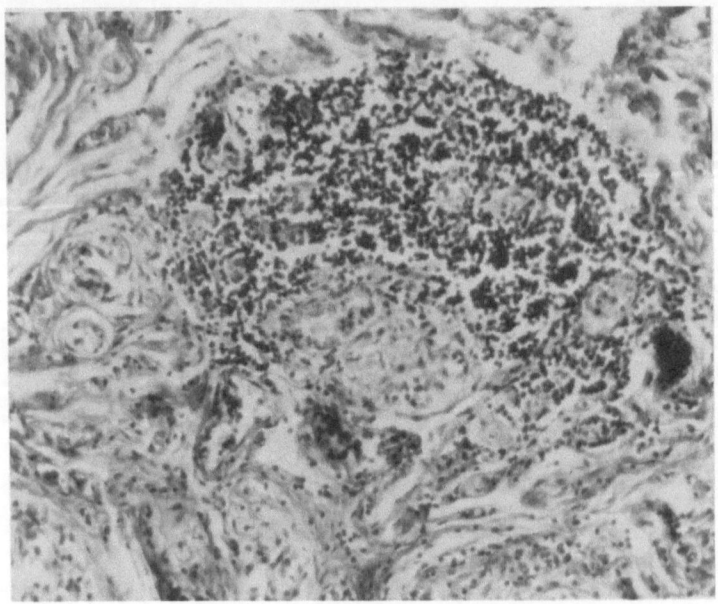

Figure 5. Adventitial lymphocytic infiltration within the carotid body, associated with severe atherosclerotic disease. (Trichrome X 320)

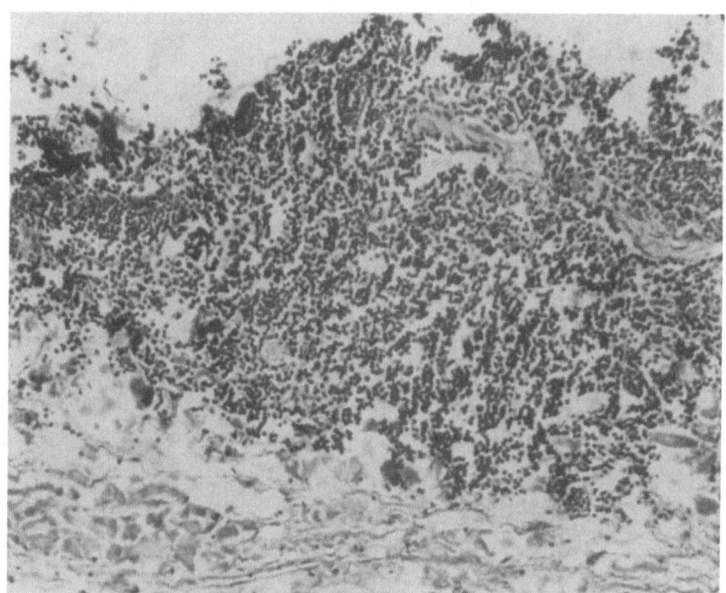

Figure 6. Aortic adventitial lymphocytic infiltration of a marked degree associated with severe atherosclerosis. (Trichrome X 260)

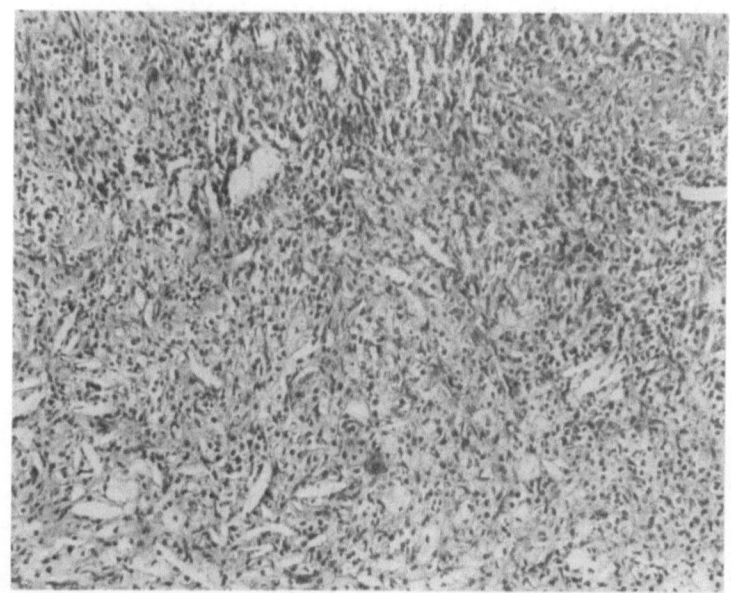

Figure 7. Atherosclerotic plaque granuloma, containing cholesterol clefts, macrophages, and copious small round cells morphologically identifiable as lymphocytes. (Trichrome X 160)

Relationship Between Plaque Severity and Adventitial
Lymphocytic Infiltration

Table 2 summarizes the overall relationship between
plaque severity and the degree of adventitial lymphocytic
infiltration in the aortas, and cervical and iliac arteries
of men and women derived from an unselected necropsy sample
obtained at the Radcliffe Infirmary, Oxford, during the
years 1959-1962 (2). It is apparent that arteries microscopically free of disease exhibit no adventitial lymphocytic infiltration. With some disease present an infiltrate
is present in 17% of the blocks examined, while in severely
diseased arteries some 80% of the blocks exhibit lymphocytic
aggregates, of which 20% are of a marked degree. So-called
fatty streaks, identified macroscopically and microscopically
are not associated with any adventitial lymphocytic aggregates, an observation which suggests a potentially important
difference in pathogenesis between these lesions and
advanced atherosclerotic plaques.

As illustrated in Table 3, a remarkably similar
relationship between plaque severity and the degree of
adventitial lymphocytic infiltration also holds for the
coronary arteries derived from an unselected necropsy sample
(2). It should be noted that these relationships are not
age-dependent, nor are there any consistent differences
between men and women.

Table 2. Prevalence and Degree of Adventitial Lymphocytic
          Infiltration in Aortic, Cervical, and Iliac
          Arteries

Plaque Severity	(% of blocks examined)		
	Cellularity Grade		
	Absent	Slight	Marked
Free n = 94	100	0	0
Present n = 124	83	17	0
Severe n = 128	21	60	19

(Unselected necropsy sample, 1959-1961, Radcliffe Infirmary,
Oxford) (2)

Table 3.   Prevalence and Degree of Adventitial Lymphocytic
           Infiltration

Coronary Plaque Severity	(% of blocks examined)		
	Cellularity Grade		
	Absent	Slight	Marked
Free n = 223	100	0	0
Present n = 149	82	15	3
Severe n = 65	25	52	23

(Unselected necropsy sample, 1959-1961, Radcliffe Infirmary, Oxford) (2)

Reprinted from Mitchell and Schwartz, Arterial Disease, 1965 by permission of Blackwell Scientific Publishers, Oxford, UK.

From the above, it would appear that there is no consistent influence of arterial site on the relationship of plaque severity and adventitial lymphocytic infiltration. This question is explored in Table 4, where, for simplification, the prevalence and degree of lymphocytic infiltration is compared for 4 arterial sites, each having microscopically severe disease. These data were also derived from an unselected necropsy sample (2). It can be seen, that with the possible exception of the cervical arteries, the prevalence and degree of lymphocytic infiltration appears to be determined by plaque severity, irrespective of the arterial site affected.

Relationship Between Plaque Severity and Adventitial Lymphocytic Infiltration in Males and Females with Transmural Myocardial Infarction

It is particularly important to determine if the presence of myocardial ischemia or ischemic necrosis has any influence on the prevalence or degree of coronary artery adventitial lymphocytic infiltration. Table 5 addresses this question, and illustrates the prevalence and degree of lymphocytic infiltration in both men and women with transmural myocardial infarction. Several conclusions can be drawn from Table 5. First, it is readily apparent that adventitial lymphycytic aggregates are not observed in the absence of atherosclerotic disease,

in spite of the presence of myocardial necrosis. In other
words, myocardial ischemia and ischemic necrosis are not
per se the determinants of lymphocytic infiltration. Second,
in men the presence of transmural infarction does not significantly alter the relationship between plaque severity and
the prevalence and degree of adventitial lymphocytic infiltration. In women, however, some differences can be seen.
Although the total prevalence of lymphocytic aggregates (62%)
in association with severe disease is less than is seen in
other sites, the number of blocks showing a marked degree
of lymphocytic infiltration is somewhat greater. The reasons
for this apparent discrepancy are elusive, but may reflect,
among other things, the greater frequency of diabetes mellitus
in women dying from myocardial infarction, a possibility
certainly worth exploring.

Table 4. Prevalence and Degree of Adventitial Lymphocytic
Infiltration in the Presence of Severe Disease

Arterial Site Examined	(% of blocks examined		
	Absent	Slight	Marked
Aorta n = 44	20	57	23
Cervical n = 51	22	67	11
Iliac n = 33	21	55	24
Coronary n = 75	25	52	23

(Unselected necropsy sample, 1959-1961, Radcliffe Infirmary,
Oxford) (2)

Reprinted from Mitchell and Schwartz, Arterial Disease, 1965
by permission of Blackwell Scientific Publishers, Oxford, UK.

Because of the frequency and importance of occlusive
thrombosis in the genesis of transmural myocardial infarction, Table 6 summarizes the relationship between adventitial lymphocytic infiltration and plaque severity in men
with transmural myocardial infarction, according to the
presence and nature of occluding thrombi. In coronary

Table 5.   Prevalence and Degree of Adventitial Lymphocytic
           Infiltration in Coronary Arteries of Patients
           with Transmural Myocardial Infarction

Plaque Severity	(% of blocks examined)					
	Cellularity Grade					
	Males			Females		
	Absent	Slight	Marked	Absent	Slight	Marked
Free n = 126M 15 F	100	0	0	100	0	0
Present n = 138M 44F	73	22	5	75	21	4
Severe n = 226M, 61F	28	46	26	38	28	34

arteries without histologic evidence of thrombosis, the
relationship between the prevalence and degree of lymphocytic
infiltration is similar to that seen in men without myocardial infarction.   In the presence of acute or recent thrombus,
however, the prevalence and degree of lymphocytic aggregates
are significantly greater than that observed in patients
from an unselected necropsy sample with comparble degrees
of plaque severity, or in patients with transmural infarction
with no histologic evidence of recent thrombosis.   Clearly,
there is an association between the presence of recent
thrombus, but not recanalizing thrombus, and the prevalence
and degree of adventitial lymphocytic cellularity.   This
association is of considerable interest and potential importance.   It is possible that thrombosis is more likely to
develop in diseased arteries in which there is an underlying
inflammatory process, of which the adventitial lymphocytosis
is but one overt manifestation.   On the other hand, it could
be that the lymphocytic cellular aggregates are the end
result of an inflammatory process invoked by the thrombus
itself.   This latter possibility is unlikely for several
reasons.   First, adventitial lymphocytic infiltrates are not
seen in the presence of recent thrombus in the absence of

Table 6. Prevalence and Degree of Adventitial Lymphocytic Infiltration in Males with Transmural Myocardial Infarction (% of blocks examined)

Plaque Severity	Blocks without Thrombus			Blocks with Recent Thrombus			Blocks with Recanalizing Thrombus		
	Absent	Slight	Marked	Absent	Slight	Marked	Absent	Slight	Marked
Free n = 101	100	0	0	–	–	–	–	–	–
Present n = 142	77	19	4	31	50	19	–	–	–
Severe n = 227	35	41	24	5	65	30	30	48	22

(Column group header: Cellularity Grade)

From Schwartz CJ, and Mitchell JRA, 1962 (3)

Reprinted from Schwartz and Mitchell, Circ., 26; 73-78, 1962 by permission of the American Heart Association.

a severe degree of atherosclerosis. Secondly, adventitial
lymphocytosis is not enhanced in frequency or degree in
the presence of old or recanalizing thrombus.

SUMMARY AND CONCLUSIONS

In this brief review we have illustrated the morphology,
and prevalence data relating to the adventitial lymphocytic
infiltration associated with atherosclerotic disease. Lymphocytic aggregates are present in some 80% of severely diseased
arteries in the presence of recent but not recanalizing
thrombus. As in our earlier reports (2,3), we continue to
believe that these adventitial lymphocytic infiltrates
represent an auto-immune inflammatory component in atherogenesis, which may reflect the antigenicity of lipid peroxidation products such as ceroid (27). It is possibly also
that this immune inflammatory process may participate in
thrombogenesis.

REFERENCES
1. Schwartz CJ, Mitchell JRA (1962) The morphology,
    terminology and pathogenesis of arterial plaques.
    Postgrad Med J 38:25-34
2. Mitchell JRA, Schwartz CJ (1965) Arterial Disease.
    Oxford: Blackwell Scientific Publications
3. Schwartz CJ, Mitchell JRA (1962) Cellular infiltration
    of the human arterial adventitial associated with
    atheromatous plaques. Circulation 26:73-78
4. Stary HC (1980) The intimal macrophage in atherosclero-
    sis. Artery 8:205-207
5. Schaffner T, Taylor K, Bartucci EJ, et al (1980)
    Arterial foam cells with distinctive immunomorphologic
    and histochemical features of macrophages. Am J Pathol
    100:57-80
6. Gerrity RG, Naito HK, Richardson M, Schwartz CJ (1979)
    Dietary induced atherogenesis in swine. Am J Pathol
    95:775-792
7. Gerrity RG (1981) The role of the monocyte in athero-
    genesis: 1. Transition of blood-borne monocytes into
    foam cells in fatty lesions. Am J Pathol
8. Still WJS, O'Neal RM (1962) Electron microscopic
    study of experimental atherosclerosis in the rat. Am
    J Pathol 40:21-35
9. Joris I, Zand T, Nunnari JJ, et al (1983) Studies on the
    pathogenesis of atherosclerosis: 1. Adhesion and emigra-
    tion of mononuclear cells in the aorta of hypercholester-
    olemic rats. Am J Pathol 113:341-358
10. Lewis JC, Taylor RG, Jones ND, et al (1982) Endothelial
    surface characteristics in pigeon coronary artery athero-
    sclerosis: 1. Cellular alterations during the initial
    stages of dietary cholesterol challenge. Lab Invest
    46:123-138

11. Duff GL, McMillan GC, Ritchie AC (1957) The morphology of early atherosclerotic lesions of the aorta demonstrated by the surface technique in rabbits fed cholesterol. Am J Pathol 33:845-873

12. Barbolini G, Scilabra GA, Botticelli A, Botticelli S (1969) On the origin of foam cells in cholesterol-induced atherosclerosis of the rabbit. Virchows Arch (Cell Pathol) 3:24-32

13. Schwartz CJ, Sprague EA, Kelley JL, et al (1985) Aortic intimal monocyte recruitment in the normo- and hyper-cholesterolemic baboon (Papio cynocephalus): An ultra-structural study. Implications in atherogenesis. Virchows Arch (A) 405:175-191

14. Kelley JL, Sprague EA, Carey KD, et al (1986) Athero-sclerosis in vervet monkeys (Cercopithecus aethiops) after a seven-year dietary challenge. Unpublished data

15. Schwartz CJ, Gerrity RG (1978) Initial events in athero-genesis. Excerpta Med 435:47-55

16. Schwartz CJ, Valente AJ, Sprague, et al (1986) Monocyte-macrophage participation in atherogenesis: Inflammatory components of pathogenesis. Seminars in Thrombosis and Hemostasis 12:79-86

17. Virchow R (1862) Gesammelte Abhandlungen z. wissenschaft-lichen Medizin. In: Phalogose und Thrombose Gefässystem. Berlin: Max Hirsch

18. Albutt C (1915) Diseases of the arteries including angina pectoris. London: McMillan Co., Vol I, p 468.

19. Ophulus W (1933) The pathogenesis of arteriosclerosis. In: Cowdrey EV, ed, Arteriosclerosis: A survey of the problem. New York: McMillan Co., p 249

20. Horn H, Finkelstein LE (1940) Arteriosclerosis of the coronary arteries and the mechanism of their occlusion. Am Heart J 19:655-682

21. Nelson MG (1941) Intimal coronary artery haemorrhage as a factor in the causation of coronary occlusion. J Path Bact 53:105-116

22. von Hausammann E (1949) Die Koronarsklerose im höheren Alter in ihrer Beziehung zur Koronarsklerose der Jugendlichen. Cardiologia 14:225-242

23. Gerlis LM (1956) The significance of adventitial infiltra-tions in coronary atherosclerosis. Brit Heart J 18:166-172

24. Morgan AD (1956) The pathogenesis of coronary occlusion. Oxford: Blackwell Scientific Publications, pp 60-67.

25. Wissler RW (1974) The development of atherosclerotic plaque. In: Braunwald E, ed, The myocardium: Failure and infarction. New York: HP Publishing Co. Inc, p 155.

26. Constantinides P (1965) Experimental atherosclerosis. Amsterdam, London, and New York: Elsiever, pp 27-39.

27. Parums DV, Chadwick DR, Mitchinson MJ (1985) The local-ization of immunoglobulin G in chronic periaortitis. Atherosclerosis 61:117-123.

8

The Role of Macrophages in Human Atherosclerosis

Malcolm J. Mitchinson, Keri L.H. Carpenter, and Richard Y. Ball

INTRODUCTION

Lipid-laden foam cells are characteristic features of small human and experimental arterial lesions (fatty streaks) and are also found in most advanced lesions, especially at the periphery. The nature of these cells, however, has been a matter of controversy for many years. In the 1930's, Anitschkow and others regarded the foam cells of experimental lesions as monocyte-derived macrophages. In the 1960's, the recognition by electron microscopy of smooth muscle cells in the lesions led to the assumption by many that the foam cells were also smooth muscle cells. This view gained credence when platelet-derived growth factor (PDGF) was discovered. A popular view of the origin of atherosclerosis then was that focal loss of endothelium led to platelet adhesion, PDGF release and therefore smooth muscle cell replication.

In recent years, a good deal of evidence from electron microscopy (EM), scanning EM and studies with various cell-markers has led to a revival of the view that, at any rate in experimental atherosclerosis, the foam cells are monocyte-derived. Evidence on human foam cells is harder to come by,

Acknowledgements: The monoclonal antibody studies were carried out with the collaboration of Dr. N.M. Aqel, Dr. H. Waldmann, and Dr. E.S. Lennox. We gratefully acknowledge the expert technical help of B. Potter, J.H. Enright, and J. King. The work was supported by the Elmore and John Lucas Walker Funds of Cambridge University, by the East Anglian Regional Health Authority and by the British Heart Foundation.

but Fowler and others have provided evidence for a monocytic origin in man (1,2). We have studied a large number of fresh human arterial lesions by immunohistochemistry, using certain monoclonal antibodies that distinguish between macrophages and smooth muscle cells (Table 1). The results are clear-cut and consistent in a variety of lesions from over 20 subjects, some of which have been described elsewhere (3,4).

Table 1. Monoclonal Antibodies Used to Identify Macrophages and Smooth Muscle Cells (3,4)

Code No.	Reacts with
YAML 501.4	"Leukocyte-common" (T200) antigen
YTH 8.18	Macrophage cytoplasm
YAML 555.6	P28,33 complex (HLA Class II)
YPC 1/3.12	Smooth muscle cell cytoplasm

Findings in Human Arteries

The cells in diffuse intimal thickening react as smooth muscle cells, but a very occasional isolated cell reacting as a macrophage is found in an immediately subendothelial position (Figure 1), just as Stary described on EM (5).

Focal lesions examined in the same way show several different patterns. The smallest focal lesion we have found is a collection of subendothelial macrophages too small to make a raised lesion (Figure 2). Sometimes these are lipid-laden, sometimes not, suggesting that lipid uptake occurs within the intima.

The smallest raised lesions (fatty streaks) consist of a larger collection of foam cells, reacting as macrophages, raised above the level of the diffuse intimal thickening populated by smooth muscle cells (Figure 3).

Exactly similar lesions may be found with the additional feature of a fibrous cap (Figure 4). This cap contains smooth muscle cells and, because few macrophages are found within it, suggests that it hinders further monocyte recruitment. Sometimes areas of early necrosis may be found among

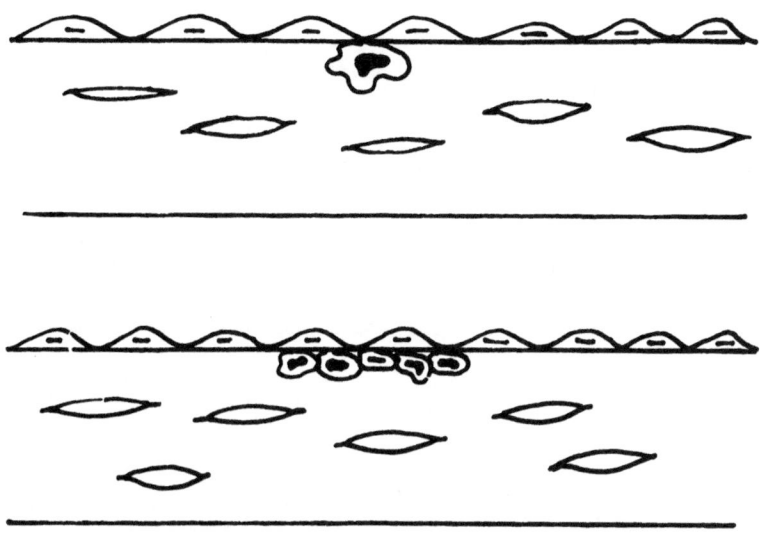

Figure 1. Intima, showing diffuse intimal thickening.
Almost all the cells react as smooth muscle cells, but
solitary subendothelial macrophages are found.
Figure 2. A very small, flat focal lesion, consisting of
a group of subendothelial macrophages.

the macrophages in such lesions. The other feature found
in such plaques is that the underlying smooth muscle cells
(but not those in the fibrous cap, nor in nearby diffuse
intimal thickening) often contain modest amounts of stainable
lipid.

The largest plaques always have a fibrous cap covering
a substantial area of basal necrosis. In such lesions macrophages are found, in very variable numbers, mainly at the
periphery of the plaque. Sometimes they extend as a continuous band from the endothelium to the borders of the necrosis,

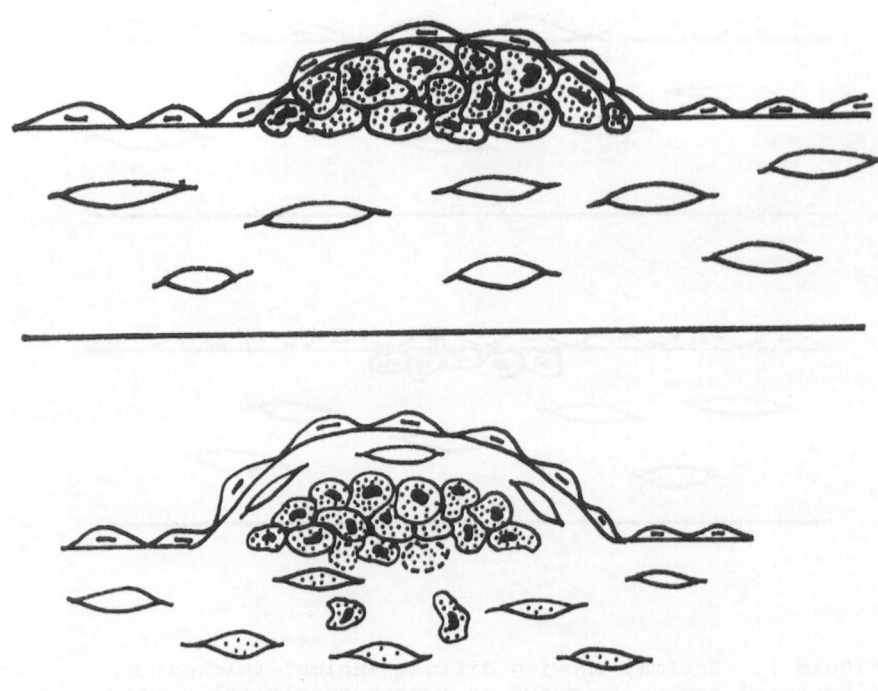

Figure 3. A fatty streak. The raised lesion consists
predominantly of lipid-filled macrophages, overlying the
diffuse intimal thickening.
Figure 4. A larger fatty lesion, with a fibrous cap
composed predominantly of smooth muscle cells and fibers.
Sometimes such lesions show early necrosis, scattered macrophages deeper in the intima and small numbers of lipid
droplets in the local deep smooth muscle cells.

where they appear to be dying and spilling their contents into
the gruel (Figure 5). In such areas, smooth muscle cells
appear to be rare. Occasionally, however, macrophages are
virtually absent from the shoulders of a lesion.

In our view, the appearances suggest a possible mode of
progression of small lesions into large ones. Of course,
some small lesions might regress and leave little or no
trace. Occasionally we find raised lesions composed
principally of smooth muscle cells, with few macrophages

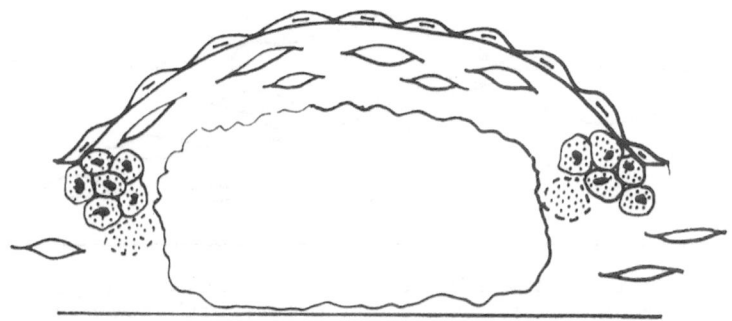

Figure 5. Advanced plaque, showing fibrous cap, basal
necrosis and macrophage foam cells at the shoulders
(periphery) of the lesion.

and no necrosis (Figure 6). Perhaps these might result
from regression.

It is therefore possible to interpret atherosclerosis
as an essentially inflammatory lesion, as Virchow did.
There are reasons to suppose that macrophage activity might
be harmful and tend to enlarge the lesion, whereas the
smooth muscle cell has an essentially reparative role. Thus
the relative proportions of the two cell types might be an
indication of the activity or rate of progression of a lesion.

Possible Functions of Macrophages in Atherosclerosis
The significance of macrophages in the plaque hinges
on their characteristic activities which might be important
in plaque development. Space does not allow more than a
brief indication of some of the possibilities.

1. Avid uptake of lipid, including modified low-
density lipoprotein (LDL) by scavenger receptors, allowing
foam cell formation and intracellular modification of lipids.

2. Death of macrophages, for unknown reasons, providing
some at least of the necrotic base.

3. Re-entry into the bloodstream, as an alternative
outcome, is a possible means of plaque regression.

4. Secretion of molecules that are chemotactic for
monocytes and perhaps for smooth muscle cells.

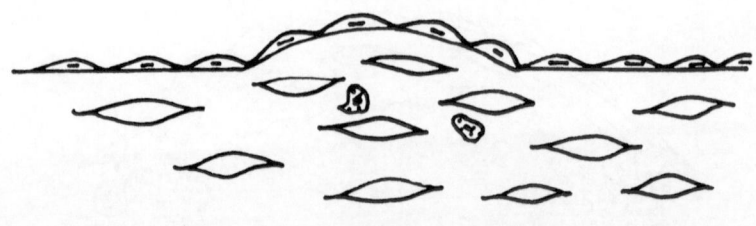

Figure 6. Raised predominantly fibrous lesion, composed mainly of smooth muscle cells and fibers with few macrophages.

5. Secretion of factors enhancing cell division in smooth muscle cells and perhaps endothelial cells.

6. Secretion of factors increasing LDL transport through endothelial cells and increasing LDL uptake by smooth muscle cells.

7. Leakage of enzymes affecting intercellular matrix and fibers.

8. Leakage of oxygen radicals causing cellular damage, e.g., to endothelial cells.

9. Oxidation of intracellular lipids and secretion of the oxidation products.

10. In the advanced lesion, phagocytosis of peripheral contents of the necrotic zone.

11. Antigen presentation.

All the above activities are presumably influenced by local and systemic factors affecting macrophage function, e.g., activating factors, anti-inflammatory drugs.

Lipid Oxidation by Macrophages

One aspect of macrophage function which is of particular interest to us is their known capacity for lipid oxidation (6) which is supported by their tendency to accumulate ceroid. Ceroid is insoluble material produced when various lipid-protein mixtures (including human LDL) are artificially oxidized. It can therefore be stained with oil red 0 in paraffin sections of tissue. It is present as granules in the cytoplasm of most macrophages in the earliest human lesions, sometimes as "rings" representing an insoluble skin around intracellular lipid droplets and, again as granules and rings, in the necrotic base of advanced plaques (7). There is evidence that it is antigenic and may be responsible for the inflammatory reaction to advanced plaques (8); it might incarcerate the lipid droplets and prevent their dispersal *in vivo* (7); most important, it may indicate the sites at which diffusible lipid oxidation products are produced in the macrophage. Among the possible oxidation products are some that are cytotoxic and others, such as prostaglandins and leukotrienes, with important effects on the behavior of nearby cells.

Lipid may of course be oxidized to an unknown extent before being taken up by the foam cells - in the diet, in the blood, by endothelial cells or ectracellularly in the intima - and ceroid production by macrophages is enhanced by preoxidation of LDL (9). Ceroid itself, however, only seems to develop in macrophages, which suggests they at least contribute to the process of oxidation.

In vitro, macrophages take up lipid avidly from serum-containing medium and produce ceroid rings within 24 hours (10). Emulsions of bovine serum albumin with defined content of cholesterol esters or triglycerides are also rapidly phagocytosed. Those containing arachidonate or linoleate lead to ceroid production. Those containing oleate, with only one double bond, do not. The ceroid production is inhibited by butylated hydroxytoluene, a free radical scavenger (10). It is therefore possible that among the many functions of macrophages in human atherosclerosis, they may oxidize unsaturated lipids to produce molecules of central importance in the progression of the disease. We are investigating this possibility in more detail.

The recognition of foam cells as macrophages raises many such new questions for investigators. We must hope it will usher in a period of rapid increase in understanding of this deadly disease.

128

REFERENCES

1. Fowler SD (1983) Role of macrophage foam cells in
    arterial lesions. In: Schettler G, Gotto AM et al.
    (eds) Atherosclerosis VI. New York: Springer-Verlag,
    pp 452-456.
2. Vedeler CA, Nyland H, Matre R (1984) *In situ*
    characterization of the foam cells in early human
    atherosclerotic lesions. Acta Pathol Microbiol
    Immunol Scand, Sect C 92:133-137.
3. Aqel N, Ball RY, Waldmann H, Mitchinson MJ (1984)
    Monocytic origin of foam cells in human atherosclerotic
    plaques. Atherosclerosis 53:265-271.
4. Aqel N, Ball RY, Waldmann H, Mitchinson MJ (1985)
    Identification of macrophages and smooth muscle cells
    in human atherosclerosis using monoclonal antibodies.
    J Pathol 146:197-204.
5. Stary HC (1983) Macrophages in coronary artery and
    aortic intima and in atherosclerotic lesions of children
    and young adults up to age 29. In: Schettler G,
    Gotto AM, et al. (eds) Atherosclerosis IV. New York:
    Springer-Verlag, pp 462-466.
6. Cathcart MK, Morel DW, Chisolm GM (1985) Monocytes
    and neutrophils oxidize low density lipoprotein making
    it cytotoxic. J Leukocyte Biol 38:341-350.
7. Mitchinson MJ, Hothersall DC, Brooks PN, de Burbure CY
    (1985) The distribution of ceroid in human athero-
    sclerosis. J Pathol 145:177-183.
8. Parums DV, Chadwick DR, Mitchinson MJ (1985) The
    localization of immunoglobulin G in chronoc peri-
    aortitis. Atherosclerosis 61:117-123.
9. Ball RY, Bindman JP, Carpenter KLH, Mitchinson MJ (1986)
    Oxidized low density lipoprotein induces ceroid accumu-
    lation by murine peritoneal macrophages *in vitro*.
    Atherosclerosis 60:173-181.
10. Ball RY, Brodley H, Brooks PN, Mitchinson MJ (1984)
    The production of ceroid by mouse peritoneal macro-
    phages *in vitro*. Brit J Exp Pathol 65:719-724.

9

Recent Observations on Human Atherosclerotic Lesions, and their Possible Significance

M. Daria Haust

INTRODUCTION

In 1984 cilia were observed in the smooth muscle cells of experimental atherosclerosis in rabbits (1). These cilia were not of the classical type characteristically present in the epithelia lining the upper respiratory tract, certain segments of the female reproductive system and some other tissues (2-4), but were of the unusual variety; these latter have been variously named "single", "solitary", rudimentary", "primary" or "oligo"-cilia, and reported to occur in cells of diverse nature in normal and pathological tissues of man and other living organisms (5,6). However, these organelles have not been reported to occur in mural cells of either normal or pathological arteries of man.

To test whether in analogy to these observations in rabbits, ciliated smooth muscle cells may be also present in human atherosclerotic lesions, these lesions were scrutinized with appropriate controls (normal intima) by electron microscopy for that purpose.

It was surprising to find that these unusual cilia occurred not only in the smooth muscle cells but also were present in the endothelial cells. A preliminary report on this subject was published recently (7), and detailed accounts are in press (8,9).

The author wishes to thank Ms Irena Wojewodzka for her expert technical assistance and Mrs. Sheila Collard and Mrs. Betty Gardiner for efficient typing of the manuscript.

The purpose of this presentation is to summarize the
recent findings on the occurrence of ciliated smooth muscle
cells (7,8) and endothelium (9) in human atherosclerotic
lesions, and to discuss briefly the possible significance
of these observations.

MATERIALS AND METHODS

Tissues obtained from 48 fatty dots and streaks removed
at necropsy of 15 patients (whose age ranged from 8 to 40
years) were utilized for these studies; the appropriate
controls were removed at various aortic levels, and processed for light and transmission electron microscopy (TEM) as
described previously (8-10). All the tissues served as the
basis of a broader study designed for another purpose (10).

Thin sections for TEM were picked up on 300-mesh
copper grids, stained doubly with uranyl acetate and lead
citrate, and examined in a Philips-300 electron microscope.
Electron micrographs of lesions and control intima were
selected from the randomly photographed sections by criteria as outlined elsewhere (8,9).

The recently reported studies or the present account
were not designed to assess the incidence of ciliated cells
in atherosclerotic lesions or the normal intima.

RESULTS

Normal Intima

A pair of centrioles was identified easily in a number
of both the endothelial and smooth muscle cells (SMCs).
The axes of the centrioles were almost invariably perpendicular or slightly tangential to each other. In most
instances the centrioles were short and stubby; they were
associated with a prominent Golgi complex and a variable
number of cytoplasmic microtubules. In most centrioles the
moderately electron-lucid core and the tubular nature of
the periphery was apparent. On rare occasion a couple or
three electron-opaque ladder-like arrangements were present
between the two centrioles of the endothelial cells. The
rungs of the ladder showed a variability in thickness and
width. Thin filaments connected the rungs to each other
and to the centrioles (Figure 1).

Atherosclerotic Lesions

Endothelial Cells. Whereas with respect to their
general cytoplasmic features the endothelial cells varied
from one area of the same lesion to another, and from lesion
to lesion, the observations relating to the centrioles and
cilia were similar.

When both centrioles were visualized, each was present
at the opposite pole of the nucleus and directed with its
longitudinal axis towards the luminal plasma membrane.
Occasionally, one of the centrioles gave rise to a "primary"
cilium; its shaft and the apex of the enclosing vacuole were
pointing to the endothelial surface (Figures 1 and 2). At
times, a structure with features of an elongated centriole
was situated close to the surface and was on either side
surrounded by a large (separate) vacuole. Transitional
fibers, extending from the distal end of this structure to
the base of the vacuoles suggested that it actually represented a cilium, the distal end being the basal body. Semi-
serial sectioning disclosed that the two vacuoles fused with
each other and ultimately "opened" into the lumen; thus, the
short ciliary shaft assumed a luminal position (Figures 3
and 3-inset). The lateral foot process of the (now) basal
body became readily visible.

In view of the shortness of the shaft and non-availabil-
ity of its transverse section for study, it was not possible
to assess the internal structure of this ciliary segment;
there is not reason to doubt, however, that this internal
configuration was similar or identical to that of the cilia
in the SMCs observed in the same lesions (vide infra).

Since the cilia were accompanied by or were enclosed
in vacuoles within the cytoplasm, they qualify in the endothelial cells as "primary" cilia of Sorokin (11,12). Of
interest was that the endothelial ciliary shafts were always
short in the tissues examined, but it is not possible to
state whether this is a true feature.

Smooth Muscle Cells. As was observed in the endothelial cells, the centrioles and cilia varied in appearance
in the SMCs not only from one to the other, but even within
the same lesion. Nevertheless the basic structure was
similar (Figures 4 and 5).

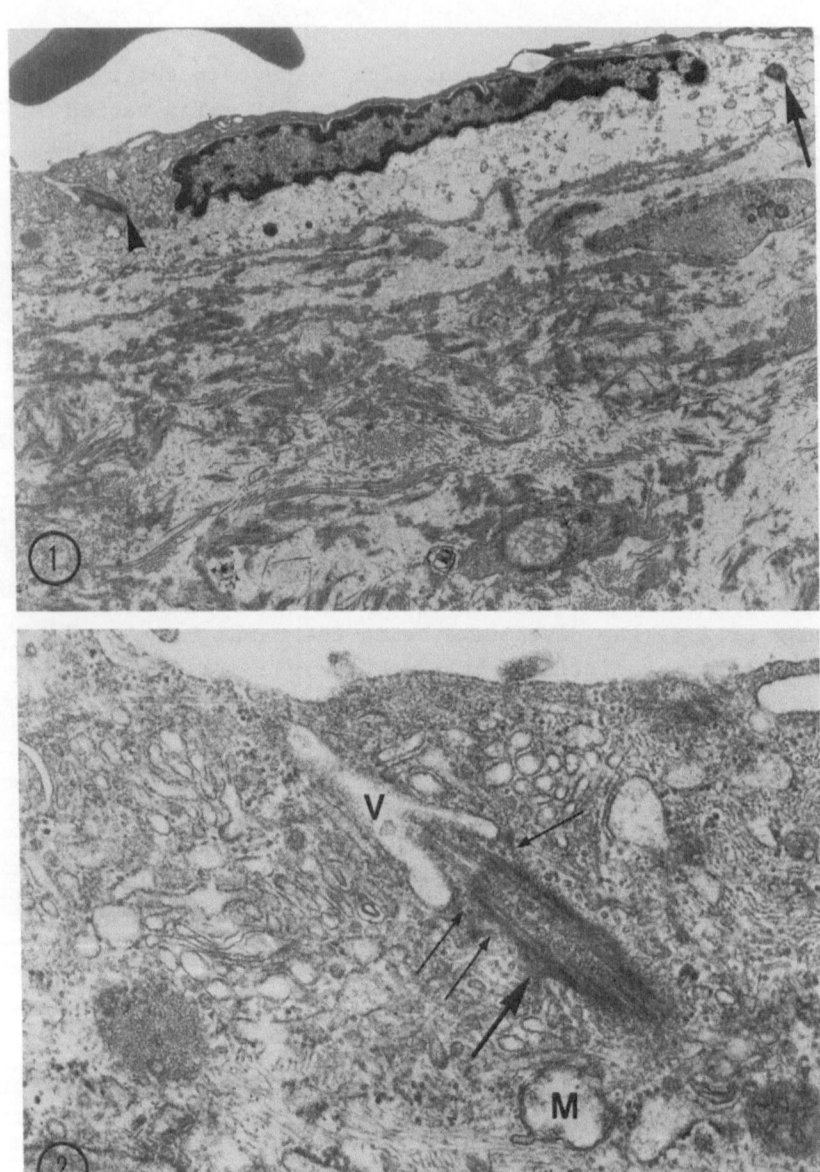

The pair of centrioles was often placed in close proximity to the plasma membrane. Their longitudinal axes were usually not perpendicular to each other, and at times were almost parallel. On occasion, one of the centrioles was in apposition to the plasma membrane displaying some or all features of a ciliary basal body (*vide infra*), and in other instances only a single centriole was observed.

Each fully visualized cilium consisted of two segments: a cytoplasmic basal body and a shaft projecting into the extracellular space (Figures 4 and 4-inset). The shaft varied from a considerable length (Figures 4 and 4-inset; Figure 1 in: 8) to a stubby short form (Figure 5 and 5-inset). The ciliary shafts emerged from the cytoplasmic surface in a surrounding recess (Figure 4 and 4-inset), that at times was unilateral (Figure 5 and 5-inset). In the cytoplasm of the SMCs cilia or their segments (i.e. the basal body) were not seen to be associated with or be enclosed within vacuolar formations as were those observed in the endothelium (Figure 2).

On several occasions both centrioles gave rise to cilia (8), although in a given section one was indicated only in part, *i.e.* by the presence of the basal body only (Figures 5 and 5-inset).

Figure 1. Electronmicrograph of a lesion shows an endothelial cell with one centriole to the right of the nucleus (arrow) and the other, giving rise to a primary cilium, on the left (arrowhead). Magnification = X 7,500.

Figure from: Haust MD. Endothelial cilia in human aortic atherosclerotic lesions. Virchows Arch A. Pathological Anatomy and Histopathology 410:317-326, 1986. Reproduced with permission of the Editor and Publisher.

Figure 2. Details of the primary cilium indicated by an arrowhead in Figure 1. A lateral foot process projects from the mid-portion of the basal body (large arrow). The microtubular nature of the basal body and ciliary shaft (in vacuole = V) is evident. Small arrows indicate transitional fibers. Mitochondria (M) are not well preserved. Magnification = X 45,000.

Figure from: Haust MD. Endothelial cilia in human aortic atherosclerotic lesions. Virchows Arch A. Pathological Anatomy and Histopathology 410:317-326, 1986. Reproduced with permission of the Editor and Publisher.

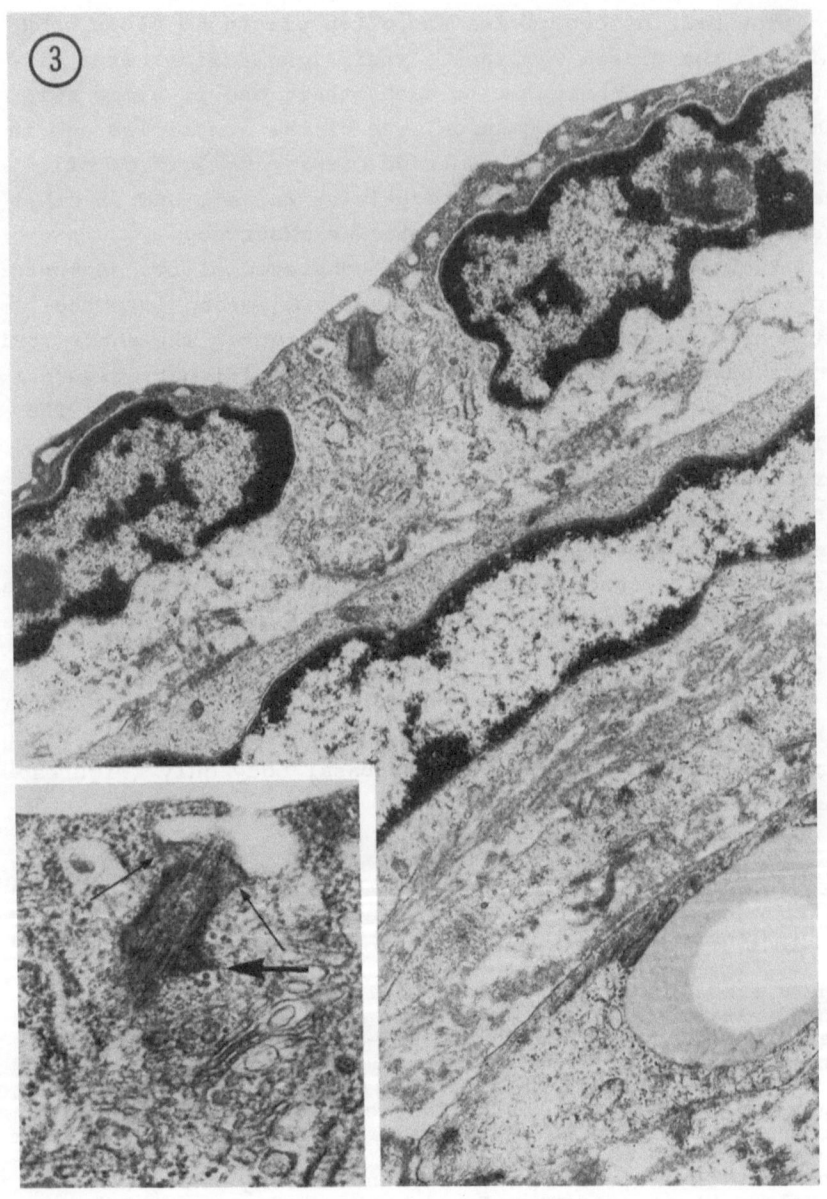

The internal structure of the ciliary shaft varied somewhat in longitudinal cuts, reflecting probably the plane of sectioning. In most, microtubules could be identified at either side of the periphery and parallel to the longitudinal axis of the shaft (Figures 4 and 4-inset). Short segments of centrally placed microtubules were visualized on occasion (1,8), but they probably represented an image termed the "median longitudinal section" (13). The peripheral microtubules seemed to be in continuity with similarly placed tubules of the basal body (Figures 4 and 4-inset).

The transverse section of the shaft of the non-classical cilium has reportedly "9 + 0" axonemal configuration (5,6). Thus, it consists of peripherally arranged 9 pairs (doublets) of hollow microtubules, but the central microtubules and the linkage structures that in addition are present in the classical ciliary shafts (Figure 6), are missing. No suitable transverse section was available in our material for evaluation.

The ciliary basal body was more electron-dense than the shaft, and had a thick limiting membrane (Figures 4 and 5). The constituent microtubules were at the periphery in continuity with those of the shaft (*vide supra*). The basal body showed a lateral "spur" or foot process (14) of triangular shape that gradually tapered off in the cytoplasm (Figure 5 in: 8). On occasion, structures resembling rootlets extended from the proximal end of the basal body (Figure 1 in:8), into the surrounding cytoplasm.

Figure 3. Electronmicrograph representing a semi-serial section of that depicted elsewhere (not shown). The two lateral vacuoles seen previously on either side of the forming primary cilium are here fused with each other and with the plasma membrane of which only a thin discontinuous

Figure 3-inset. Details of the primary cilium illustrated in Figure 3. Note the slight transverse periodicity of the short shaft; the lateral foot process (large arrow) and transitional fibers (small arrows) originate from the basal body. Magnification = X 47,000.

Figure from: Haust MD. Endothelial cilia in human aortic atherosclerotic lesions. Virchows Arch A. Pathological Anatomy and Histopathology 410:317-326, 1986. Reproduced with permission of the Editor and Publisher.

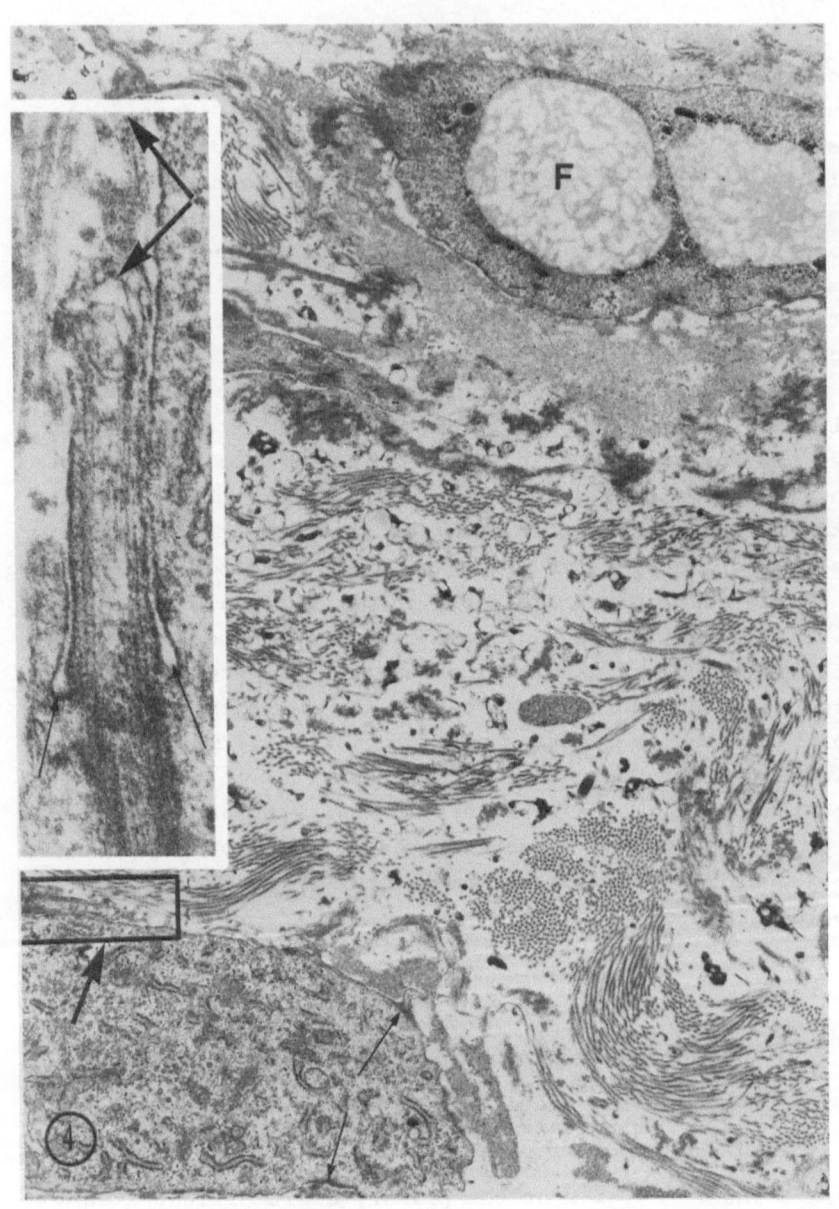

The internal structure of the basal body was basically that of a centriole, i.e., it consisted of peripherally arranged 9 triplets of fused microtubules embedded in a moderately electron-opaque amorphous substance. Spokes of alar sheets (15) attached to the triplets could be demonstrated on occasion when the cut was made in close proximity to the plasma membrane (Figure 6-inset in:8).

The basal bodies of the cilia in the SMCs often were not accompanied by a nearby-situated centriole, - a feature different than that observed in the SMCs in lesions of experimental atherosclerosis (1).

DISCUSSION

There is only a small number of reports on ciliated endothelium (16-23) and none related to its occurrence in human normal or pathological arteries. At other sites they were observed rarely in man (5,17,23). Thus, the finding of ciliated endothelium in atherosclerotic lesions in human aorta (9) was the first such observation on several accounts.

Figure 4. Moderately large fatty streak. Two smooth muscle cells (top) contain fat droplets (F). The fat-free cell (bottom, left) contains a cilium whose longitudinal axis is parallel and in close apposition to the main cell body. Note that this smooth muscle cell has numerous but narrow profiles of rough surface endoplasmic reticulum, and prominent Golgi and other vesicles, but few myofilaments and triangular densities (small arrows); it is enveloped by a discontinuous, thickened basement membrane material. The arrowed square indicates the position of the cilium. Magnification = X 10,500.

Figure 4-inset. Higher magnification of the square indicated in Figure 4. The base of the shaft of the cilium is surrounded by a circular recess (small arrows) which results from a moderate dilatation of an invagination of the cellular membrane enveloping the shaft. The shaft, extending into the intercellular space, contains microtubular structures which are parallel to its longitudinal axis and in continuity with similar tubules of the basal body. These microtubules are present in either side of the cilium (shaft + basal body); in addition, centrally placed similar structures are visualized with difficulty and only in short segments of both parts of the cilium. It is also difficult to determine where the cilium terminates as its tip may be folded and/or cut tangentially (large arrows). Note that the basal body is more electron-opaque than the shaft. Magnification = X 55,000.

Figure and inset from: Haust MD. Ciliated smooth muscle cells in atherosclerotic lesions of human aorta. Am J Cardiovasc Pathol 1:115-129,1987. Reproduced with the permission of the Editor and Publisher.

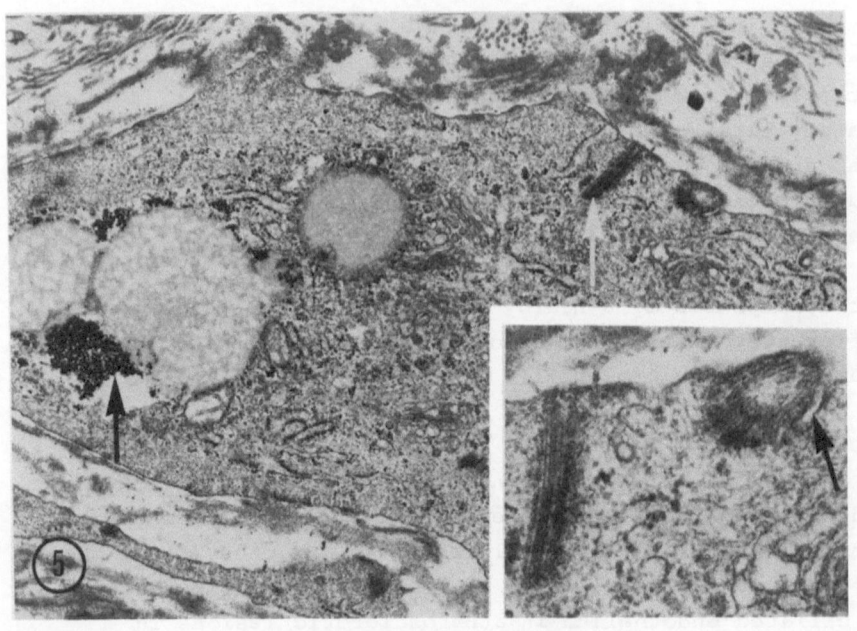

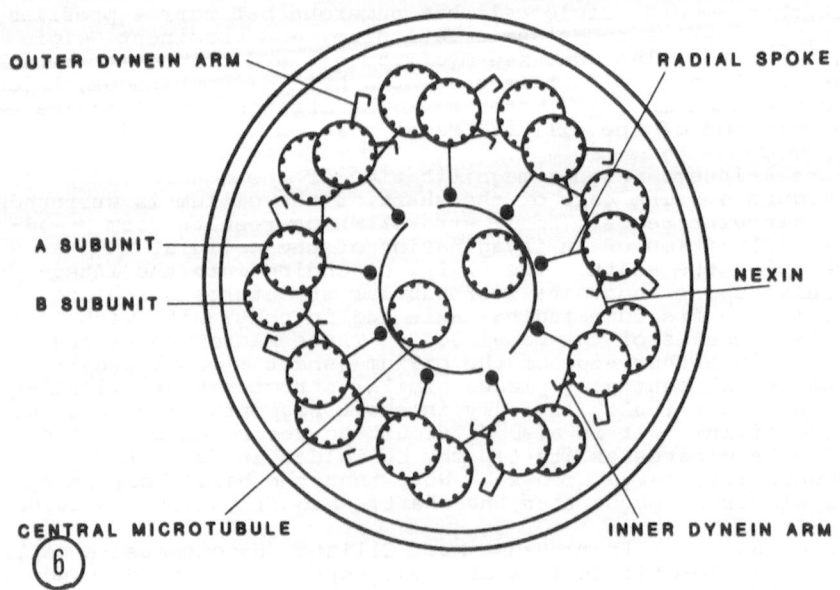

Prior to 1984 (1) ciliated smooth muscle cells (SMCs) were reported in four publications; all of these cells were observed in extra-arterial sites and none in human tissues (11,24-26). Recent studies showed that ciliated SMCs occur not only in experimental atherosclerosis (1), but also in similar lesions of man (7,8).

Whereas cilia were not observed in either the endothelium or SMCs of control tissues, this does not preclude their possible occurrence in normal intima. However, should they be present in the latter, their incidence must be considerably lower in the normal intima than in the lesions where they were observed with relative ease.

Figure 5. Fat droplets associated with localized aggregates of glycogen (arrow) are present in a smooth muscle cell (left half). The cell also contains one long basal body (white arrow) and, to its right, another but shorter similar body in continuity with a stubby ciliary shaft. Since basal bodies are parts of cilia, it may be stated that this cell contains two rudimentary cilia. No accompanying centrioles are seen. Magnification = X 19,000.

Figure 5-inset. Higher magnification of the two ciliary structures shows the presence of microtubules in the basal bodies and in the shaft. The shaft emerges from the cell with only one-sided invagination of the cellular membrane (arrow). Note the difference in electron-opacity of the basal body and that of the shaft. Magnification = x 40,000.

Figure and inset from: Haust MD. Ciliated smooth muscle cells in atherosclerotic lesions of human aorta. Am J Cardiovasc Pathol 1:115-129, 1987. Reproduced with permission of the Editor and Publisher.

Figure 6. Schematic representation of a transverse section of a shaft of a classical cilium. The outer two circles represent the trilaminar cytoplasmic envelopment. For details see Refs 2-6, 8 and 9. The axonemal complex is enlarged approximately X 400,000 but the relative measurements of the microtubules and the associated structures were not taken into consideration.

Figure, at reduced magnification from: Haust MD. Ciliated smooth muscle cells in atherosclerotic lesions of human aorta. Am J Cardiovasc Pathol 1:115-129, 1987. Reproduced with permission of the Editor and Publisher.

It is of interest to consider the possible significance of the presence of these non-classical cilia in
atherosclerotic lesions in the light of the ongoing uncertainty regarding the genesis and function of these unusual
organelles in general.

Ciliogenesis was proposed to proceed under normal
circumstances by at least three different mechanisms (11,12,
27); the role of centrioles has been considered to be crucial
in this process. Our studies indicate that the ciliogenesis
in the endothelial cells in lesions resembles the process
described by Sorokin (11,12), $i.e.$, the formation of the
"primary" cilium in association with, or within cytoplasmic
vacuolar configurations (Figures 2 and 3). However, in no
instance were vacuoles observed to be associated with cilia
in the SMCs. In these cells, it appeared that one centriole
(at a time) "migrated" toward the plasma membrane, where it
assumed the position of a ciliary basal body, (presumably
always?) giving rise to a ciliary shaft. Moreover, in some
circumstances both centrioles (successively) "converted" to
cilia (8).

For the above reasons the terminologies such as: "primary", "single", "solitary" or "oligo" cilia do not apply
to these organelles in the SMCs, the most suited term being
"rudimentary" cilia.

Several theories have been proposed with respect to
the function, and the implications of the presence of the
rudimentary cilia. Since the two central tubules [of their
"9 + 0" rather than "9 + 2" - axonemal configuration (Figure
6)] are absent, and these are believed to be involved in
ciliary motion, rudimentary cilia are generally considered
to lack motility. In fact, in only one instance (in
$vitro$), were the rudimentary cilia observed to be motile
(28).

It has been variously proposed that the non-classical
cilia have a chemoreceptor (29) or sensory (30) function,
or represent remnants of an evolutionary stage of cells (31).
It has been shown that in certain cell types many centrioles
form cilia during rapid division (32) and in quiescent cells
arrested in Gl (33).

Mulhaud and Pappas proposed that the ciliary formation follows a stimulation of centriolar reproduction without subsequent mitosis (34). The last concept was expanded by suggesting that the sudden transformation from mitotic replicative to non-mitotic structuring tissue could be correlated with the disappearance of centrioles and with ciliary formation (35).

In the context of our present-day-knowledge in atherosclerosis, the theory linking the appearance of the non-classical cilia to mitotic activity of both the endothelial and SMCs of lesions, would be more attractive. In the course of their development, the early atherosclerotic lesions may pass the boundary of potential reversibility, and progress to the common form of advanced lesion, $i.e.$, the atherosclerotic plaque (36). This progress is characterized by proliferation of intimal SMCs (37,38). The endothelial cells overlying these intimal SMCs-foci also multiply, either in response to the same injurious factor "evoking" the proliferation of the SMCs, or as a secondary phenomenon, $i.e.$, in order to accommodate the growing lesion. This process of cellular multiplication, once in progress, may not be easily "switched-off". Whereas much has been learned about the stimuli capable of inducing cellular proliferation in the course of injury and repair operating as the pathogenetic mechanism in atherosclerosis (39,40), little is known of factors capable of limiting this proliferative process once this useful reparative phase has been achieved. It is of interest to speculate that at least the SMC-mitosis may be blocked under the above circumstances by agents that redirect one or both of the centrioles for ciliary formation. In $vitro$, colcemid was shown to be capable of blocking mitosis by such "redirection" (28) while other agents may exert their antimitotic action by different mechanisms. For example, diazepam inhibits mitosis by preventing the separation of centrioles in man (41) and the separation of the two basal bodies (42) in a green flagellate alga (Dunaliella).

If in fact the non-classical rudimentary cilia reflect or are the consequence of aborted mitoses of SMCs (and endothelia?), they may be useful in the testing of various substances for their ability to arrest or reduce the multiplication of these cells in atherosclerosis. They may become, thus, an indicator of a "switch-off" mechanism so desirable for arresting the progression of lesions in this disease.

REFERENCES

1. Haust MD (1984) Ciliated smooth muscle cells in aortic atherosclerotic lesions of rabbit. Atherosclerosis 50:283-293
2. Gibbons IR (1981) Cilia and flagella of Eukaryotes. J Cell Biol 91:107s-124s
3. Laschi R, Baccetti B (1983) (eds) International Conference on Development and Function in Cilia and Sperm Flagella. J Submicrosc Cytol 15(1):1-374
4. Stephens RE (1983) Reconstitution of ciliary membranes containing tubulin. J Cell Biol 96:68-75
5. Wheatley DN (1982) (ed) The Centriole: A Central Enigma of Cell Biology. New York: Elsevier Biomedical Press pp 147-184
6. Pysher TJ, Neustein HB (1984) Ciliary dysmorphology. Perspect Pediatr Pathol 8:101-131
7. Haust MD (1986) Myohistiocytes and ciliated smooth muscle cells in human atherosclerotic lesions. In: Fidge NH, Nestel PJ (eds), Atherosclerosis VII. Amsterdam-New York-Oxford:Elsevier Exerpta Medica pp 377-380
8. Haust MD (1987) Ciliated smooth muscle cells in atherosclerotic lesions of human aorta. Am J Cardiovasc Pathol 1:115-129
9. Haust MD (1986) Endothelial cilia in human aortic atherosclerotic lesions. Virchows Arch A Pathol Anat Histopathol 410:317-326
10. Haust MD (1980) The nature of bi- and trinuclear cells in atherosclerotic lesions in man. Atherosclerosis 36:365-377
11. Sorokin S (1962) Centrioles and the formation of rudimentary cilia by fibroblasts and smooth muscle cells. J Cell Biol 15:363-377
12. Sorokin SP (1968) Reconstructions of centriole formation and ciliogenesis in mammalian lungs. J Cell Sci 3:207-230
13. Dingle AD, Funton C (1966) Development of the flagellar apparatus of Naegleria. J Cell Biol 31:43-54
14. Greiner JV, Weidman TA, Bodley HD, Greiner CAM (1981) Ciliogenesis in photoreceptor cells of the retina. Exp Eye Res 33:433-446
15. Anderson RGW (1972) The three-dimensional structure of the basal body from the rhesus monkey oviduct. J Cell Biol 54:246-265
16. Corbett WEN (1961) The fine structure of the intima of muscular and elastic arteries. M.Sc. Thesis. Queen's University, Kingston, Ontario, Canada
17. Vegge T (1963) Ultrastructure of normal human trabecular endothelium. Acta Ophthal 41:193-199
18. Hogan MJ, Alvarado JA, Weddell JE (1971) (eds) Histology of the Human Eye. An Atlas and Textbook. Philadelphia: WB Saunders Co
19. Edanaga M (1974) A scanning electron microscope study on the endothelium of the vessels. I. Fine structure

of the endothelial surface of aorta and some other arteries in normal rabbits. Arch Histol Jap 37(1): 1-14

20. Edanaga M (1975) A scanning electron microscope study on the endothelium of vessels. II. Fine surface structure of the endocardium in normal rabbits and rats. Arch Histol Jap 37(4):301-312

21. Renard G, Hirsch M, Galle P, Pouliquen Y (1976) Ciliated cells of corneal endothelium. Functional and morphological aspects compared to cilia of other organs. Arch Ophthalmol 36(1):59-72

22. Gallagher BC (1980) Primary cilia of the corneal endothelium. Am J Anat 159:475-484

23. Yamamoto K and Fujimoto S (1980) Endothelial cilium in the capillaries of the human fetal pineal gland. J Electron Microsc 29:256-258

24. Laguens R (1964) Ciliated smooth muscle cells in the uterus of the rat. Experientia (Basal) 20:322-323

25. Fussell EN, Roberts JA (1979) Ciliated smooth muscle cells in the monkey ureter. Vet Pathol 16:619-622

26. Gardiner SL, Rieger RM (1980) Rudimentary cilia in muscle cells of Annelids and Echinoderms. Cell Tissue Res 213:247-252

27. Pitelka DR (1974) Basal bodies and root structures. In: Sleigh MA (ed) Cilia and Flagella. New York: Academic Press

28. Stubblefield E, Brinkley BR (1966) Cilia formation in Chinese hamster fibroblasts *in vitro* as a response to colcemid treatment. J Cell Biol 30:645-652

29. Munger BL (1958) A light and electron microscopic study of cellular differentiation in the pancreatic islets of the mouse. Am J Anat 103:275-311

30. Barnes BG (1961) Ciliated secretory cells in the pars distalis of the mouse hypophysis. J Ultrastruct Res 5:453-467

31. Latta H, Maunsbach AB, Madden SC (1961) Cilia in different segments of the rat nephron. J Biophys Biochem Cytol 11:248-252

32. Fonte VG, Searls RL, Hilfer SR (1971) The relationship of cilia with cell division and differentiation. J Cell Biol 49:226-229

33. Tucker RW, Pardee AB (1979) Centriole ciliation is related to quiescence and DNA synthesis in 3T3 cells. Cell 17:527-537

34. Milhaud M, Pappas GD (1968) Cilia formation in the adult cat brain after pargline treatment. J Cell Biol 37:599-609

35. Rush JE, Shay JW, Biesele JJ (1969) Cilia in cardiac differentiation. J Ultrastruct Res 29:470-484

36. Haust MD (1971) The morphogenesis and fate of potential and early atherosclerotic lesions in man. Human Pathol 2:1-29

37. Haust MD, More RH, Movat HZ (1960) The role of smooth muscle cells in the fibrogenesis of arteriosclerosis. Am J Pathol 37:377-389

38. Geer JC, Haust MD (1972) .Smooth Muscle Cells in Atherosclerosis In: Pollack OJ, Simms HS, Kirk JE (eds) Monographs on Atherosclerosis, Vol 2, Basel-London, New York: S Karger

39. Haust MD (1970) Injury and repair in the pathogenesis of atherosclerotic lesions. In: Jones RJ (ed) Atherosclerosis: Proceedings of the Second International Symposium, New York-Heidelberg-Berlin, Springer Verlag, pp 12-20

40. Haust MD, More RH (1972) Development of modern theories on the pathogenesis of atherosclerosis. In: Wissler RW, Geer JC (eds) The Pathogenesis of Atherosclerosis. Baltimore: The Williams and Wilkins Company, pp 1-19.

41. Anderson LC, Lehto V-P, Stenman S, Badley RA, Virtanen I (1981) Diazepam induces mitotic arrest at prometaphase by inhibiting centriolar separation. Nature 291:247-248

42. Marano F, Santa-Maria A, Fries W (1984) Effects of Diazepam on mitosis and basal body duplication of synchronously dividing flagellate cells. Biol Cell 50:163-172

Tissue Organization and Architecture

10
Intimal Lipids and Associated Changes in Intimal Composition

Elspeth B. Smith

"Insoluble" lipid accumulates in normal intima with aging, and in some (but not all) atherosclerotic lesions. In this paper I want to raise some questions about the source of this lipid, and the factors involved in its deposition.

Normal Intima

From about age 15 upwards intimal esterified cholesterol increases at a rate of approximately 0.6 mg/100 mg defatted dry tissue/decade (1). This parallels the accumulation of fine lipid droplets, mainly less than 200 nm in diameter, which are particularly associated with elastin, but also occur adjacent to and within collagen bundles (2,3). The close similarity of chemical composition suggests that these droplets are derived directly from plasma low density lipoprotein (LDL) (1,2), and they still appear to contain some apoprotein B (4).

Early Fibrous Plaques

The problem with human lesions is their enormous diversity, and the fact that we can only speculate about their sequence of development. Some of the changes that occur can be highlighted by description of three specific lesions.

Acknowledgments: The author's work was supported by grants from the British Heart Foundation and the Medical Research Council. The names of the author's coworkers are cited in the references.

The first is a large gelatinous lesion from a woman aged 60 who died following a pulmonary embolism. We found massive focal proliferation of smooth muscle cells and collagen, maximum thickness 1600 μm, virtually no stainable lipid apart from a faint diffuse sudanophilia, but quite a large deposit of fibrin right in the center of the plaque, just above the internal elastic lamina (IEL). A striking feature of this representative lesion is its water content, which, compared with the patient's normal intima, has increased three-fold in the upper (luminal) layer and five-fold in the deeper layers. However, the proportion of water which is in the interstitial fluid space is unchanged (Table 1). LDL content is increased five- to six-fold, but in the interstitial fluid its concentration is only increased by about 40%, so that the environment of the cells is not particularly abnormal. Immobilized cholesterol is slightly lower than normal intima in the upper layers of the lesion, and slightly higher in the deep layers. In normal intima free LDL accounts for less than 10% of total cholesterol but in the lesion it makes a significant contribution of 33% and 25% in the upper and lower layers, respectively.

The second lesion is from a woman aged 58 who died following a subarachnoid hemorrhage. This was classified as being slightly more advanced - a "transitional" lesion - grayish rather than translucent pink, and even thicker. There appeared to be a pool of insudation adjacent to a patch of fibrin that was partially invaded by collagen. The only lipid staining was in wide collagen bundles in close proximity to the insudation pool, which showed a uniform, diffuse sudanophilia.

This plaque has been analyzed in a different way and the results are compared with the lipid-rich center of an adjacent white fibrous plaque. There is actually less cholesterol in this lesion than in the normal intima (Table 2), and more than half of it is accounted for by LDL. This is in marked contrast to the plaque center where cholesterol has increased more than twenty-fold, and only 2% of it is accounted for by LDL.

What is the mechanism of this localized lipid accumulation? One possibility is increased "tight binding" of LDL.

Table 1. Large Gelatinous Plaque[a]

	Normal Intima	Lesion Upper	Lesion Lower
Tissue hydration:			
mg water/100 mg dry tissue	376	1004	1811
% of tissue water as interstitial fluid (IF)	62	65	61
LDL			
Dry tissue: μl/100 mg	606	3114	3597
IF: % of plasma concentration	265	376	360
Residual cholesterol:			
mg/100 mg dry tissue	11.5	9.0	16.0
Maximum thickness: μm	110	1600	

[a] From a woman aged 60 with pulmonary embolism

Table 2. LDL Cholesterol in Normal Intima and Lesions from a Single Aorta[a]

	Concentration in Intima: mg/100 mg dry tissue		
	Semi-Normal	Transitional Lesion	"Early Amorphous" Lipid Center of Small Plaque
LDL cholesterol[b]			
Mobile	1.0	1.3	0.8
Released by crude collagenase	0.2	0.6	1.4
Residual cholesterol	3.2	1.6	117.6
Maximum thickness	220 μm	2500 μm	1120 μm total 700 μm fatty center

[a] Woman aged 58 with subarachnoid hemorrhage
[b] Calculated from immunoelectrophoretic apo-B

Tightly bound LDL is released by incubation with crude
collagenase, but equally effectively, by the fibronolytic
enzyme, plasmin. It is not released by chondroitinase ABC.
Purified collagenase is much less effective than plasmin in
releasing bound LDL (5,6) and plasmin appears to cause
simultaneous release of a large fibrin fragment (Smith and
Keen, unpublished). There was no quantitative relationship
between the massive release of fibronectin by pure collagenase, and release of LDL (6). The implication of these
findings is that in some way fibrin is involved in the
tight-binding of LDL. Plasmin-releasable LDL is high in
plaques that have accumulated large amounts of extracellular
lipid (Table 3). This is true both for mature fibrous
plaques with white collagen caps, and for apparently younger
soft, translucent gelatinous plaques.

Relation Between Extracellular and Intracellular Lipid

Unlike most experimental models, human lesions cover an
enormous morphological range, and although there is a
tendency for one type to predominate in an individual patient, most types can be found in most patients. At one
end of the spectrum is the pure fatty streak, with virtually
all the lipid in large droplets within cells. Fatty streaks
seem to progress by increase in fat-filled cells, accumulation of some extracellular lipid, and moderate proliferation
of collagen to give a raised fatty plaque with fat-filled
cells at all levels. At the other end of the spectrum, the
early gelatinous lesion is a focal proliferation of smooth
muscle cells and collagen with virtually no increase in
intra- or extracellular lipid. These lesions continue to
grow into large space-occupying plaques, about half of which
do not accumulate any lipid whereas the remaining half
accumulate extracellular lipid in the form of fine perifibrous droplets in the central deep layer of the lesion.

I have no doubt that these are two independent processes. The chemical composition of the intracellular lipid
is quite different from perifibrous lipid (1,2); the composition of perifibrous lipid closely resembles LDL except that,
with increasing lipid accumulation there is a disproportionate
increase in free cholesterol.

Table 3. Plasma-Releasable LDL in Atherosclerotic Lesions

| | Concentration: mg/100 mg Lipid-Extracted Dry Tissue | | | | |
| | LDL | | Soluble FRA | Insoluble Fibrin | Residual Cholesterol |
	Free	Released by Plasmin			
Normal intima (n = 12)	5.2	0.8	2.2	2.0	3.2
Gelatinous lesions: low lipid (n = 15)	15.7	1.5	6.6	5.1	5.3
Gelatinous plaques: low lipid cap and sides (n = 10)	12.3	2.9	8.0	10.3	9.4
lipid-rich centers (n = 22)	8.5	16.5	9.2	28.3	106.1
White fibrous plaques: lipid-rich centers (n = 13)	4.3	7.4	3.5	19.8	108.5

In addition to these two ends of the spectrum, there is a third group comprised of proliferative lesions that also contain numerous fat-filled cells scattered through the fibrous cap, and at the shoulders of the plaque. It is not clear if the two processes described above have occurred independently at the same location, or if one has stimulated the other. Chemical analysis of layers through plaques isolated by microdissection suggested that the characteristic cholesterol oleate-rich lipid in fat-filled cells did undergo change when the cells disintegrated, that extracellular accumulation of LDL-type lipid occurred even in lesions rich in fat-filled cells, and that preferential hydrolysis of cholesterol linoleate was a possible source of free cholesterol (7). In a recent ultrastructural study of early lesions, Bocan et al (8) also concluded that the extracellular lipid did not arise via foam cell necrosis, and that lipid deposition in association with extracellular matrix constituents is an early event in development of the lipid-rich core. Thus there is strong evidence to support the idea of direct extracellular deposition of LDL lipid in fibrous plaques, but we do not know the mechanism involved, or why plaques in the same aorta, exposed to the same concentration of LDL, may differ markedly in the amount of lipid deposited. Whether the excess of free cholesterol results from hydrolysis of cholesterol ester or some form of preferential uptake is not clear. Kruth (9) has described subendothelial deposition of free cholesterol at a very early stage in cholesterol fed rabbits, before the appearance of foam cells, and in the same model Simionescu et al. (10) observed accumulation of extracellular phospholipid liposomes rich in unesterified cholesterol. In human tendon xanthoma, free cholesterol deposition was separate from cholesterol ester (11).

Intracellular Lipid

There is a general agreement that the large intracellular lipid droplets contain a high proportion of cholesterol ester in which oleic acid is the major fatty acid (1,2, 3,8,12), but the source or sources of this lipid in fat-filled cells of human lesions is not clear.

The very extensive studies on lipid accumulation in
cultured smooth muscle cells and macrophages are reviewed
in Part 1 of this volume, but direct evidence from lesions
is minimal. In intimal homogenates Clevidence et al. (13)
found an apo B-containing fraction with increased net
negative charge that was taken up by macrophages. In interstitial fluid, which is the cells' immediate environment,
Smith and Ashall (14) found no consistent differences in net
negative charge of the LDL from normal intima or intima
containing fat-filled cells. Some fat-filled cells seem
capable of degrading LDL with enormous avidity. In samples
of interstitial fluid from fatty streaks containing very
numerous fat-filled cells we detected only trace amounts of
LDL although the concentrations of other plasma proteins
were normal (Table 4). This seems to imply that either the
cells have become abnormal, with unregulated uptake of
normal LDL, or they themselves modify the LDL in their
immediate vicinity. The behavior of the cells in early
fatty streaks is not really compatible with the concept that
they are scavenging deposited lipid. In advanced plaques,
by contrast, they are often adjacent to deposits of fibrin and
extracellular lipid and thus may have a scavenging function.

Table 4. Macromolecule Concentrations in Interstitial Fluid
from Lesions Containing Fat-Filled Cells

	Percent of Concentration in Adjacent Normal Intima		
	LDL	α_2-M	Albumin
Fatty streaks: numerous fat-filled cells (n = 4)	tr	77 ± 28[a]	91 ± 19
Extracellular lipid and scattered fat-filled cells (n = 4)	35 ± 6	123 ± 41	137 ± 36

[a] Standard deviation

Formation of foam cells is not unique to the artery wall; they develop in, for example, experimental carrageenan granulomas in both normal and hyperlipidemic rabbits, but in this model the proportion of the cholesterol that is esterified is much lower (15).

We now have a large amount of information on the chemistry, physical chemistry and morphology of lipid in plaques, but the vital question of how and why it accumulates is still not answered.

REFERENCES

1. Smith EB (1974) The relationship between plasma and tissue lipids in human atherosclerosis. Advances in Lipid Research 12:1-49.
2. Smith EB, Evans PH, Downham MD (1967) Lipid in the aortic intima; the correlation of morphological and chemical characteristics. J Atheroscler Res 7:171-186.
3. Guyton JR, Bocan TMA, Schifani TA (1985) Quantitative ultrastructural analysis of perifibrous lipid and its association with elastin in nonatherosclerotic human aorta. Arteriosclerosis 5:644-652.
4. Walton KW, Williamson N (1968) Histological and immunofluorescent studies on the evolution of the human atheromatous plaque. J Atheroscler Res 8:599-624.
5. Smith EB, Massie IB, Alexander KM (1976) The release of an immobilized lipoprotein fraction from atherosclerotic lesions by incubation with plasmin. Atherosclerosis 25:71-84.
6. Smith EB, Ashall C (1986) Fibronectin distribution in human aortic intima and atherosclerotic lesions: Concentration of soluble and collagenase-releasable fractions. Biochim Biophys Acta 880:10-15.
7. Smith EB, Slater RS (1972) The microdissection of large atherosclerotic plaques to give morphologically and topographically defined fractions for analysis. Part 1. The lipids in the isolated fractions. Atherosclerosis 15:37-56.
8. Bocan TMA, Schifani TA, Guyton JR (1986) Ultrastructure of the human aortic fibrolipid lesion. Formation of the atherosclerotic lipid-rich core. Am J Pathol 123:413-424.
9. Kruth HS (1985) Subendothelial accumulation of unesterified cholesterol. An early event in atherosclerotic lesion development. Atherosclerosis 57:337-341.
10. Simionescu N, Vasile E, Lupu F, Popescu G, Simionescu M (1986) Accumulation of extracellular cholesterol-rich liposomes in the arterial intima and cardiac valves of the hyperlipidaemic rabbit. Am J Pathol 123:109-125.
11. Kruth HS (1985) Lipid deposition in human tendon xanthoma. Am J Pathol 121:311-315.
12. Small DM (1977) Cellular mechanisms for lipid deposition in atherosclerosis. N Engl J Med 297:873-877.

13. Clevidence BA, Morton RE, West G, Dusek DM, Hoff HF
    (1984) Cholesterol esterification in macrophages.
    Stimulation by lipoproteins containing apo B isolated
    from human aortas. Arteriosclerosis 4:196-207.
14. Smith EB, Ashall C (1983) Variability of the electro-
    phoretic mobility of low density lipoprotein - Compari-
    son of interstitial fluid from human aortic intima,
    and serum. Atherosclerosis 49:89-98.
15. Kelley JL, Suenram CA, Valenta AJ, Sprague EA, Rozek MM,
    Schwartz CJ (1985) Evolution of foam cells in sub-
    cutaneous rabbit carrageenan granulomas. II Tissue
    and macrophage lipid composition. Am J Pathol 120:
    391-401.

11
Evolution of the Atherosclerotic Plaque—A Physicochemical Approach to Lipid Deposition

Donald M. Small

The pathogenesis of atherosclerosis involves the development of a space occupying lesion in the intima of major arteries. The lesion appears to start in an area of slightly thickened intima with very low lipid concentration. It progresses first into a fatty streak lesion and later into a plaque with a necrotic core. A major fraction of the volume of the atherosclerotic plaque is made up of lipid. While the normal intima contains less than 5% of the dry weight as lipid about 25% of fatty streaks and 60% of an atheromatous plaque dry weight is lipid (1,2).

There are three main classes of lipids which accumulate in atherosclerotic lesions: free sterols (almost exclusively cholesterol), cholesterol esters (mainly cholesteryl linoleate, oleate and palmitate), and phospholipids (mainly phosphatidylcholines and sphingomyelins). These lipids make up about 95% of the total lipids in the normal intima and atheromas. Minor lipids present in small amounts include triglycerides, fatty acids and lysophospholipids (3). The three major classes of lipids are virtually insoluble in water (4,5,6). Free cholesterol forms crystals of cholesterol monohydrate with melting point of 85° C (4), phospholipids such as lecithin (5) and sphingomyelin (6) swell in water to form bilayered or membrane-like structures

This research was supported by research grant HL-26335 and training grant HL-07291 from the National Institutes of Health. We thank Irene Miller for the preparation of the manuscript.

and cholesterol esters separate from water as an oil above
their melting points, and, as liquid crystalline structures
below their melting points (4). If a cholesterol ester mixture is particularly high in saturated and mono-unsaturated
esters the melting point will be above 37° and the state of
esters will be liquid crystalline. On the otherhand if the
cholesterol esters are rich in linoleic acid or other polyunsaturates or are contaminated with triglycerides (7), the
melting point will be below body temperature and the esters
will be present as an unstructured oil (4).

These three classes of lipids have been shown not to
be completely miscible especially in the presence of water
(8). The phospholipids can incorporate appreciable amounts
of free cholesterol up to a molar ratio of 1 cholesterol to
1 phospholipid in the bilayered-membrane-like phase (9),
but very little cholesterol ester (2 mol% or less) can be
incorporated (10,11). Cholesterol esters on the otherhand
cannot incorporate any phospholipid and only small amounts
of free cholesterol, about 4 wt.% (4,12). Thus, when equal
amounts of phospholipids and cholesterol esters are present
they separate into the phospholipid bilayer phase and an
oily (or liquid crystalline) cholesterol ester phase (8).
Because the cholesterol ester phase is less dense it may be
separated by centrifugation. Further, if large amounts of
free cholesterol are added to the system it will precipitate
as cholesterol monohydrate (8). Thus, depending upon the
relative composition of lipids in the arterial intima, lipids
may be present in at least 3 separate phases, 1) phospholipid bilayer phases containing cholesterol up to 1:1 molar
ratio with phospholipid, 2) cholesterol ester phases containing small amounts of cholesterol, and 3) cholesterol monohydrate crystals (8).

In fresh unfixed tissue these different phases may be
identified under a polarizing microscope with a heating
stage according to the criteria presented in Figure 1 (13).

Normal Intima

Composition of the normal intima becomes enriched with
cholesterol ester as a function of age (2,14). Katz (2)
studied the chemical composition and physical state of
normal appearing intima from birth to old age. The intima

Identification of Tissue Lipids by Hot Stage Polarizing Microscope

Lipid	State at Body Temperature	Morphology	Thermal Behavior	Neutral Lipid Staining
Cholesterol Monohydrate	Crystal		melt > 85℃	No
Cholesterol Esters rich in Oleate and Palmitate	Liquid Crystal	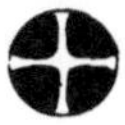	melt to liquid at 40-55℃, reversible	Yes
rich in Linoleate	Oil		form on cooling to 37-20°C	Yes
Triglycerides more saturated	Crystal	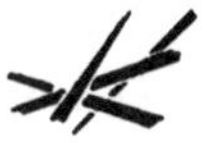	melt on heating crystallize after undercooling >20°C	No
more unsaturated	Oil		crystallize after undercooling <20°C	Yes
Phospholipids and Complex Membrane Lipids	Liquid Crystal multilamellar liposomes vesicles membranes	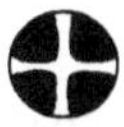	melt > 85°C	No

Figure 1. Identification of tissue lipids by hot stage
polarizing microscope. The major lipids of biological
importance can be identified in fresh, unfixed, unstained,
hydrated tissue samples by hot stage polarizing microscope
(6,13).   Cholesterol monohydrate crystals such as occur in
gallstones and atherosclerosis and other necrotic deposits
have typical plate-like morphology with acute edge angles
of 79°.   They melt to a liquid crystalline form at about
85° (4).   Mixtures of cholesterol esters rich in saturated
and mono-unsaturated acyl moeties tend to be liquid crystalline at body temperature and melt between 40 and 55 °C.   The
liquid crystals are present as maltese crosses under crossed
polars.   When mixtures of esters are rich in polyunsaturates
such as cholesteryl linoleate they are liquid at body temperature and form maltese crosses at lower temperatures.
Triglycerides do not form liquid crystals but rather needle-
like crystalline structures.   While most triglyceride deposits
are in the liquid state *in vivo* they can become crystalline
when cooled well below their melting point.   The undercooling
and lack of liquid crystalline phases is characteristic of
triglycerides.   The more saturated the triglyceride the
higher the melting point (4).   Mixtures of phospholipids or
complex membrane lipids generally form a variety of bilayered
structures which are strictly liquid crystalline but may be
present as multi-lamellar liposomes, uni-lamellar vesicles
or membrane-fragments.   Multi-lamellar liposomes appear as
spherical or tubular-like processes (myelin figures).   The
spherical particles exhibit a maltese cross under crossed
polars and are indistinguishable from cholesterol ester droplets except that their melting points are much higher than
85°C (Modified from ref. 13).

of newborns contains only phospholipid and free cholesterol.
Thus, these lipids are situated in a bilayered phospholipid
phase, presumably the membranes of the cells in the intima.
As age increases a substantial increase in the quantity of
cholesterol ester occurs, so that by age 50 at least half
of the lipid in the normal arterial intima is cholesterol
ester. Cholesterol ester forms a separate largely extracellular phase consisting of small VLDL-LDL sized particles
(15,16) whose lipid composition is similar to LDL (2). The
relation of this age-related increase in LDL-like lipids to
the development of atherosclerotic lesions is not yet clearly understood. It is quite possible that the small extracellular particles having a lipid composition similar to
LDL are denatured, modified or oxidized particles derived
from plasma lipoproteins which can be taken up and metabolized by intimal smooth muscle cells or macrophages (17).
It has been recognized that certain anatomic regions in
normal arteries are thickened (18) even at birth (19,20),
and, that these eccentric thickenings may be sites of
future lesions (21,22). To my knowledge the lipids of these
eccentric thickenings, or endothelial cushions have not been
compared to adjacent intima.

Atherosclerotic Lesions
    Fatty Streaks
    The earliest intimal lesions visible to the naked eye
or low power dissecting microscope which contain an abun-
dance of lipid are fatty streaks. These are flat or
slightly raised, fairly discrete, pale yellow lesions present just beneath the glistening surface of the endothelium.
They appear to develop in regions in which the intima was
thickened (18,21,22,23) and begin around puberty (22,23).
They increase in frequency in the early decades of life and
then decrease later in life (22,24). These lesions contain
a very large amount of cholesterol ester and a varying
amount of free cholesterol (3,25). Those lesions which
contain an amount of cholesterol which would not be expected to precipitate and form cholesterol crystals have been
called ordinary fatty streaks (3). Their cholesterol esters
are high in oleate and they contain little sphingomyelin,
lysolecithin or fatty acid and most of the cholesterol

esters are contained in cytoplasmic droplets within foam cells. These foam cells appear to be derived principally from macrophages (26).

Intermediate, Transitional, or Pre-Atheromatous Lesions

A subset of fatty streak lesions indistinguishable grossly from ordinary fatty streaks, contain an increased amount of free cholesterol, enough that they should contain cholesterol crystals. These fatty streaks not only contain more free cholesterol but more fatty acid, sphingomyelin, lysolecithin and triglyceride, and have an intermediate composition between that of an ordinary fatty streak and an atheromatous plaque (3). These fatty streaks have been called intermediate lesions (3). Only about 1 in 4 of these contain microscopically observable sparse and small crystals (3) and necrosis is minimal. These lesions appear to be analagous to what McGill has termed a "transitional" lesion (27) and Stary has called a "pre-atheroma" (22). We have called them intermediate because they are intermediate or transitional between a fatty streak and an atheromatous plaque. On a physical-chemical basis they are cholesterol-supersaturated fatty streaks whose potential metastability renders them poised to nucleate and grow cholesterol crystals and thus become necrotic and develop into an atheroma.

Atheroma

The atheromatous plaque or atheroma contains an increased amount of free cholesterol and microscopically observable cholesterol monohydrate crystals (3,8). In fact, cholesterol monohydrate crystals are the hallmark of the atheroma. They also contain higher quantities of unsaturated cholesterol esters, fatty acid, lysolecithin, sphingo-myelin and triglyceride (3). Deep in the lesion they harbor a nearly acellular, necrotic core consisting of cholesterol crystals, extracellular cholesterol esters, phospholipids, connective tissue, cellular debris, calcium apatite, gly-coproteins and other poorly described materials.

The Progression from Thickened Intima to Atheroma

The evolution of the atherosclerotic plaque requires progression from thickened intima to a foam cell lesion (that is a fatty streak), to an intermediate or transitional lesion and finally to an atheromatous plaque.

The development of the foam cell lesion has been the subject of much work over the past several years. Whether the first foam cells are of macrophage (26) or smooth muscle cell origin or both is not entirely clear and may depend upon the animal species and the nature of the factors inducing atherosclerosis (e.g., dietary, immunologic, hereditary, etc.). Certainly either macrophages or smooth muscle cells must go into positive cholesterol balance, that is, they must take up more cholesterol from lipoproteins or lipid particles then they metabolize or secrete (28). Thus, a positive cholesterol balance occurs in the cell producing a cholesterol ester loaded foam cell. The nature of the lipoprotein or lipid particle leading to foam cells has been avidly discussed and putative candidates could be native LDL, β-VLDL, large LDL, chemically or physically modified LDL or VLDL, or even remnants of triglyceride-rich lipoproteins. Even lipid particles disgorged by dying cells might be an aggravating factor in producing smooth muscle-derived foam cells (29).

The transition from fatty streak to intermediate lesion, that is the supersaturation of fatty streak lesions, has not been carefully explored. It is probable that the free cholesterol content increases in the lesion either because there is an increased cholesterol esterase activity within the cell releasing free cholesterol over and above that which ACAT can esterify or a decreased esterification of cholesterol secondary to an inhibition of ACAT (28). The former could occur if particle cholesterol ester uptake continued to increase and lysosomal degradation of cholesterol ester to cholesterol proceeded more rapidly than normal ACAT could re-esterify the liberated cholesterol. On the other hand a damaged or inhibited ACAT might lead to an increase in free cholesterol. Alternatively an abnormal transport of cholesterol from lysosomes to endoplasmic reticulum could account for an increase in lysosomal free cholesterol. Such defects appear to account for decreased cholesterol esterification in a strain of BALB/C mice (30) and in a variant of Neimann-Pick disease in humans (31). If crystallization took place in lysosomes these bodies might rupture and release their destructive enzymes into the cytoplasm. The mechanism by which free cholesterol leads to necrosis is not understood, but it is quite possible that when free cholesterol reaches a certain level of supersaturation it nucleates, grows into crystals, disrupts the lysosome, liberating lytic enzymes into the cell. Such a sequence of events could lead to necrosis, further cholesterol esterase activity and the production of increased quantities of free cholesterol. This chain reaction would lead to a necrotic atheromatous core and the production of an atheroma.

The Turnover of Cholesterol in Atheroma

The different phases of plaque lipid, that is, the phospholipid membrane phase, the cholesterol ester phase, and cholesterol crystals have been isolated in relatively pure form from human atherosclerotic plaques by density gradient centrifugation (32). Using this isolation procedure we have been able to estimate the turnover of cholesterol and cholesterol ester in the different lipid phases of human atherosclerotic plaques isolated at surgery (33). Many years ago several groups including Chobanian and Hollander (34) and Jagannathan and associates (35) measured the specific activity of cholesterol from plaques excised from patients who were given radioactive cholesterol to measure cholesterol pool sizes. The cholesterol specific activity was low when compared to plasma and they concluded that the turnover rate of cholesterol in atheroma was slow. In plasma and liver the cholesterol turns over very rapidly. It turns over more slowly in muscle, even more slowly in skin, and extremely slowly in tendon (36). The turnover of cholesterol ester in the different physical phases (e.g., phospholipid membranes, oily cholesterol esters) of the atherosclerotic plaque is similar to that in tendons (33). However, free cholesterol showed marked differences in turnover depending upon the physical state. It was most rapid from the oily cholesterol ester phase, somewhat slower from the membrane phase, and so slow as to be unmeasurable from the crystalline phase (33). Thus, once the cholesterol has entered the crystalline phase its turnover appears to be exceptionally slow. This finding has relevance to the problem of reversal and removal of lipids from atherosclerotic plaques. In fact cholesterol crystals appear to be removed much more slowly than cholesterol ester from plaques (37).

The Stratification of Lipid Deposits in Atheroma

Accepting the consensus that some fatty streaks become intermediate or transitional lesions and some of these become atheromatous plaques it becomes important to understand how a lesion grows from a nearly flat innocuous lesion with a total volume of a few thousandths of a cubic centimeter to one which has a volume approaching a few tenths of a cubic centimeter and is capable of impinging on luminal blood flow. Using a technique which preserves the normal anatomical relationships of structures in tissues while also preserving the lipids in their *in vivo* physical state (13) we were able to study the plaques of a familial homozygote patient who had been given several doses of radioactivity over the years to follow cholesterol pool sizes (38). We found layers deep in the atheroma which contained no cholesterol radioactivity and layers closer to the surface which contained a large amount of radioactivity in the foam cell region of the lesions (39,40). From the sequence of the radioactive cholesterol doses given and the radioactive and nonradioactive layers in the plaques of this individual, I would like to suggest that atherosclerotic lesions grow by deposition of cholesterol at the luminal edge of the lesion (Figure 2). First, starting with a thickened intima, a high level of atherogenic lipoprotein enters the vessel wall, cells are recruited from both blood media and these cells take up the lipoproteins (either normal or altered) to become foam cells. A cluster of these foam cells becomes a fatty streak. With time the lesion grows and the cells towards the bottom, that is those which are nearest the internal elastic lamina,

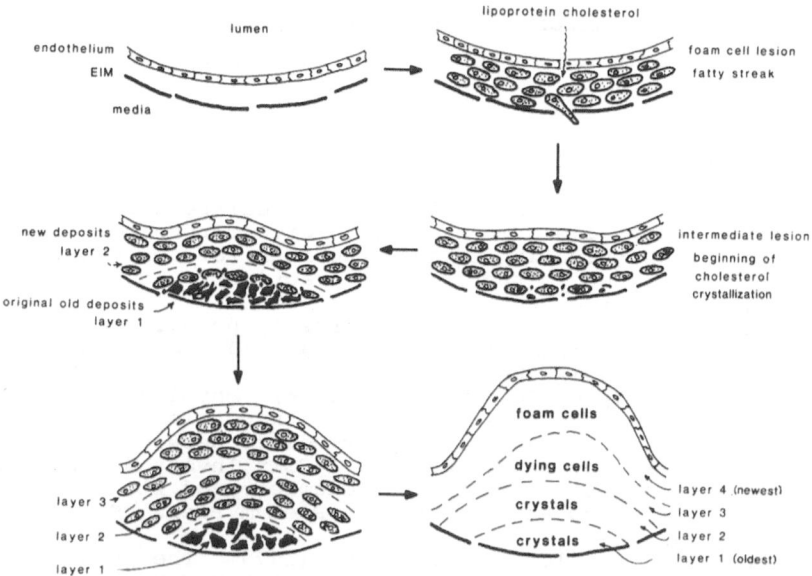

Proposed Sequential Lipid Deposition During Progression

Figure 2. <u>Proposed stratification of sequential lipid deposits during progression</u>. This sequence suggests that the normal intima, upper left, progresses through a series of stages (fatty streak, intermediate lesion) to an atheroma, bottom. Cholesterol appears to come from the luminal side with the newest deposits being just beneath the intima and the older deposits being deeper in the lesion. For further discussion see text.

become supersaturated with cholesterol possibly because the intracellular hydrolysis of cholesterol ester exceeds re-esterification by ACAT. In this region of the intermediate or transitional lesion, crystals then nucleate and grow to cause cellular death and impending necrosis in the base of the lesion. Coincident with the crystal deposition and necrosis at the base of the lesion new cell layers form below the endothelium and above the necrotic base. This process continues enlarging the lesion. As the lesion becomes thicker further crystal formation and necrosis occur enlarging the core. Thus, the atheroma consists of mainly new cells at the luminal edge and the crystallized tombstones of the older deposits at the base. Atheroma may thus be stratified with respect to their deposits with the oldest being at the base and the most recent being at

the surface. Simple atheroma may then become complicated
with thrombofibrous cap formation and calcium apatite
crystallization leading to the more complicated advanced
atheroma.

REFERENCES

1. Smith EB, Slater RS (1972) The microdissection of
   large atherosclerotic plaques to give morphologically
   and topographically defined fractions for analysis.
   I. The lipids in the isolated fractions. Atherosclerosis 15:37-56
2. Katz SS (1981) The lipids of grossly normal human
   aortic intima from birth to old age. J Biol Chem
   256(23):12275-12280
3. Katz SS, Shipley GG, Small DM (1976) Physical
   chemistry of the lipids of human atherosclerotic lesions.
   Demonstration of a lesion intermediate between fatty
   streaks and advanced plaques. J Clin Invest 58:200-211
4. Small DM (1986) The Physical Chemistry of Lipids
   from Alkanes to Phospholipids. Plenum Press, New York,
   pp 1-672
5. Loomis CR, Shipley, GG, Small DM (1979) The phase of
   behavior of hydrated cholesterol. J Lipid Res 20:525-
   535
6. Shipley GG, Avecilla L, Small DM (1974) Phase behavior
   and structure of aqueous dispersions of sphingomyelin.
   J Lipid Res 15:124-131
7. Croll DH, Small DM, Hamilton JA (1985) Molecular
   motions and thermotropic phase behavior of cholesteryl
   esters with triolein. Biochemistry 24:7971-7980
8. Small DM, Shipley GG (1974) Physical-chemical basis
   of lipid desposition in atherosclerosis. Science
   185:222-229
9. Bourges M, Small DM, Devichian DG (1967) Biophysics
   of lipid associations. II. The ternary systems.
   Cholesterol-lecithin-water. Biochim et Biophys Acta
   137:157-167
10. Janiak JM, Loomis CR, Shipley GG, Small DM (1974) The
    ternary phase diagram of lecithin, cholesteryl lino-
    lenate and water. J Molec Biol 86:325-339
11. Hamilton JA, Small DM (1982) Solubilization and local-
    ization of cholesteryl oleate in egg phosphatidylcho-
    line vesicles: A carbon-13 NMR study. J Biol Chem
    257:7318-7321
12. North BE, Katz SS, Small DM (1978) The dissolution of
    cholesterol monohydrate crystals in atherosclerotic
    plaque lipids. Atherosclerosis 30:211-217
13. Waugh DA, Small DM (1984) Methods in Laboratory
    Investigation. Identification and detection of *in situ*
    cellular and regional differences of lipid composition
    and class in lipid-rich tissue using hot stage polariz-
    ing light microscopy. Laboratory Investigation
    51(6):702-714
14. Smith EB, Evans PH, Downham MD (1967) Lipid in the
    aortic intima. The correlation of morphological and
    chemical characteristics. J Atheroscler Res 7:171-186

15. Hollander W, Paddok J, Colombo M (1979) Lipoproteins in human atherosclerotic vessels. Exp Mol Path 30: 144-171

16. Hoff HF, Heideman CL, Gaubatz JW (1980) Low density lipoproteins in the aorta: Relation to atherosclerosis. In: Atherosclerosis V. Gotto Jr AM, Smith LC, Allen B (eds) Springer-Verlag, New York, pp 533-536

17. Parathasarathy S, Printz, DJ, Boyd D, Joy L, Steinberg D (1986) Macrophage oxidation of low density lipoprotein generates a modified form recognized by the scavenger receptor. Atherosclerosis 6(5):505-510

18. Dock W (1946) The prediction of atherosclerosis for the coronary arteries. J Am Med Assoc 131:875-878

19. Fangman RJ, Hellwig CA (1947) Histology of coronary arteries in newborn infants. Am J Path 23:901-902

20. Minkowski W (1947) The coronary arteries of infants. Amer J Med Sci 214:623-629

21. McMillan GC (1965) The onset of plaque formation in arteriosclerosis. Acta Cardiol (suppl XI):43-62

22. Stary HC (1987) Evolution and progression of atherosclerosis in the coronary arteries of children and adults. In:Atherogenesis and Aging, Springer-Verlag, New York, Chapter 3, pp 20-36

23. Greer JC, McGill Jr, HC, Robertson WB, Strong JP (1968) Histologic characteristics of coronary artery fatty streaks. Lab Invest 18(5):565-570

24. Velican C, Velican D (1980) The precursors of coronary atherosclerotic plaques in subjects up to 40 years old. Atherosclerosis 37:33-46

25. Lang PD, Insul Jr W (1970) Lipid droplets in atherosclerotic fatty streaks of human aorta. J Clin Invest 49:1479-1488

26. Aqel NM, Ball RY, Waldmann H, Mitchinson MJ (1985) Identification of macrophages and smooth muscle cells in human atherosclerosis using monoclonal antibodies. J Pathol 146:197-204

27. McGill Jr HC (1986) Questions about the natural history of human atherosclerosis. Prepared for the workshop of the Evolution of Human Atherosclerotic Plaque, Rockville, Maryland, September 20-27, 1986

28. Small DM (1977) Cellular mechanisms for lipid deposition in atherosclerosis. N Eng J Med (Seminars in Physiology) 297:873-877 and 924-929

29. Wolfbauer G, Glick JM, Minor LK, Rothblat GH (1986) Development of the smooth muscle foam cell: Uptake of macrophage lipid inclusions. Proc Natl Acad Sci USA 83:7760-7764

30. Pentchev PG, Boothe AD, Kruth HS, Weintroub H, Stivers J, Brady RO (1984) A genetic storage disorder in BLAB/C mice with a metabolic block in esterification of exogenous cholesterol. J Biol Chem 259(9):5784-5791

31. Pentchev PG, Comly ME, Kruth HS, Vanier MT, Wenger DA, Patel S, Brady RO (1985) A defect in cholesterol esterification in Niemann-Pick disease (type C) patients. Proc Natl Acad Sci USA 82:8247-8251

32. Katz SS, Small DM (1980) Isolation and partial characterization of the lipid phases of human atherosclerotic plaques. J Biol Chem 1255:9753-9759

33. Katz SS, Small DM, Smith FR, Dell RB, Goodman D-WS (1982) Cholesterol turnover in lipid phases of human atherosclerotic plaque. J Lipid Res 23:733-737

34. Chobanian AV, Hollander W (1962) Body cholesterol metabolism in man. I. The equilibration of serum and tissue cholesterol. J Clin Invest 41:1732-1737

35. Jagannathan SN, Connor WE, Baker WH, Bhattacharyya AK (1974) The turnover of cholesterol in human athero-sclerotic arteries. J Clin Invest 54:366-377

36. Ramakrishnan R, Dell RB, Goodman DS (1981) On deter-mining the extent of side-pool synthesis in a three-pool model for whole body cholesterol kinetics. J Lipid Res 2:1174-1180

37. Small DM, Bond MG, Waugh D, Prack M, Sawyer JK (1984) Physicochemical and histological changes in the arter-ial wall of non-human primates during progression and regression of atherosclerosis. J Clin Invest 73:1580-1605

38. McNamara DJ, Aherns Jr EH, Kolb R, Brown C, Parker TS, Davidson NO, Samuel P, McVie RM (1983) Treatment of familial hypercholesterolemia by portacaval anasto-mosis: Effect on cholesterol metabolism and pool sizes. Proc Natl Acad Sci USA 80(2):564-568

39. Small DM, Tercyak AM, Fonferko E, McCormack C, Hudgins LC and Aherns Jr EH (1984) Properties and sequential deposition of cholesterol in aortic lesions of a familial hypercholesterolemic homozygote (FHH). Arteriosclerosis 4:567a

40. Small DM (1985) Some speculations on the deposition of cholesterol in aortic lesions of familial hyper-cholesterolemia. Saratoga Springs Conference, New York. Annals NY Acad Sci, Vol 464, Atherosclerosis, pp 207-208

12

Modification of Collagen and Elastin in the Human Atherosclerotic Plaque

William D. Wagner

Collagen

The collagen-rich fibromuscular cap is the hallmark
of the advanced human atherosclerotic plaque. Collagen is
the major extracellular product representing one-third
of the dry weight and up to 60% of the total protein content of the plaque (1-3). In the normal human intima,
collagen increases with increasing age (Table 1). With
atherosclerosis there is significantly more collagen with
increases of up to 57% (Table 2). Important functions of
collagen may be altered in atherosclerotic tissue.

Normally, collagen plays a role in the attachment of
endothelial cells to the subendothelial matrix, thus contributing to endothelial cell integrity. Any modification
in this structure may render the endothelial cells more
susceptible to damage or loss. Collagen may play a role
in the activation of platelets during early or late states
of lesion formation or it may contribute to the occlusive
nature of the lesion. At later stages of atherosclerosis,
collagen may serve as a thrombogenic agent.

Collagen Structure

Collagen molecules in general contain a triple helical region characterized by the presence of a basic repeat
triplet unit of amino acids where glycine occupies every
third amino acid position. The basic triplet unit is gly-
X-Y and a variety of amino acids can occupy the X and Y

Table 1. Changes in Human Aortic Collagen with Age

Age in Years	Number of Cases	Youngest - Oldest	
1 - 80	20	30.2 - 53.0*	Bertelsen (3)
11 - 90	58	16.0 - 26.1**	Levene & Poole (2)
11 - 75	23	23.1 - 27.0***	Smith (1)

* Mg hydroxyproline/gm dry delipidated decalcified artery.

** Mg collagen/100 mg dry weight.

*** Mg collagen mg protein.

Table modified from Table 8 (4).

Table 2. Changes in Human Aortic Collagen with
          Atherosclerosis

Age in Years	Number of Cases	Youngest - Oldest	
43 - 80	11	47 - 74*	Bertelsen (3)
41 - 90	42	30 - 34**	Levene & Poole (2)
10 - 80	70	32 - 45*	Wagner & Clarkson (5)

* Mg hydroxyproline/gm dry delipidated decalcified artery.

** Mg collagen/100 mg dry weight.

Table 3. Genetically Distinct Collagen Types

Collagen Type	Constituent α Chains	Chain Association	Major Tissue Distribution
I	$\alpha1(I)$ $\alpha2(I)$	$[\alpha1(I)]_2\alpha2(I)$	Skin, tendon, bone, placenta, arteries
I trimer	$\alpha1(I)$	$[\alpha1(I)]_3$	Skin, tendon, liver, dentine, cultured skin, fibroblasts, tumours
II	$\alpha1(II)$	$[\alpha1(II)]_3$	Cartilage, vitreous humour, chondrosarcoma, intervertebral disc
III	$\alpha1(III)$	$[\alpha1(III)]_3$	Skin, lung, arteries, uterus, chorioamnion liver, stroma and connective tissue of organs
IV	$\alpha1(IV)$ $\alpha2(IV)$	$[\alpha1(IV)]_2, 2(IV)$	Basement membranes
V	$\alpha1(V)$ $\alpha2(V)$ $\alpha3(V)$	$[\alpha1(V)\ 2\alpha(V)]$ $\alpha1(V)\ 2(V)\alpha3(V)$ $[\alpha1(V)]_3$	Placenta, skin chorioamnion pericullular stromal in most connective tissue, rhabdomyosarcoma
VI	$\alpha1(VI)$ $\alpha2(VI)$	Unknown	Blood vessels, uterus, ligament, skin, lung, kidney
VII	$\alpha1(VII)$	$[\alpha1(VII]_3$	Chorioamniotic membranes, skin, esophagus
VIII	$\alpha1(VIII)$	Uncertain: structure composed of collagenous peptides proposed	Culture medium from endothelial astrocytoma and other cells from normal and malignant tissues
IX	$\alpha1(IX)$ $\alpha2(IX)$ $\alpha3(IX)$	$[\alpha1(IX)\alpha2(IX)\alpha3(IX)]$	Cartilage, vitreous humour, intervertebral disc
X	$\alpha1(X)$	$[\alpha1(IX)]_3$	Cartilage
XI	1α 2α 3α	$(1\alpha2\alpha3\alpha)$	Cartilage, vitreous humour, intervertebral disc

Modified from Table 1 (9)

positions, but most often, the position is occupied by
proline and hydroxyproline. The triplet unit is essential
for the formation of a semi-rigid triple helical molecule
composed of three polypeptide chains. The variation in
length, primary structure, and the presence, extent and
location of either noncollagenous domains or interchain
disulfide bonding all form the basis for characterizing the
different collagen types.

Collagen Types

The family of collagen consists of at least 10 or
more genetically distinct protein types (Table 3). Based
on current studies, there are at least 18 genes to code
for the constituent α chains. In different tissues there
are specific types, quantities or molecular compositions
of collagen. Several reviews have been published on the
collagen types and collagen genes, including those of
Bornstein and Sage (6), Miller and Gay (7), Burgeson (8),
and Cheah (9).

The classification of the different collagen types
can be grouped according to the type of fiber formed.
Types I, II and III have been classified as interstitial
collagens where they form a fibrillar structure. Of the
non-fibrillar collagens, Type IV, which is a major component of the basement membranes, is the best understood.
The remaining types of collagens are usually present in
tissue in very small amounts and those such as VI and VIII
are less well characterized.

Each collagen type has unique properties and functions.
As one example, Type IX collagen is thought to bridge
collagen Type I fibers. A chondroitin sulfate/dermatan
sulfate glycosaminoglycan has been described as a component of the fourth noncollagenous domain of this molecule (10).

Collagen Types in the Artery Wall - Types I and III

It is now well established that there are a number of
genetically different collagen types in the artery wall.
The major types are the two interstitial collagens -
Types I and III. Information on the alteration of these

collagens is relevant to the pathogenesis of early atherosclerotic lesions since it is linked to the proliferation
of the cells in the intima and the ensuing fibrotic changes.

Collagen Types in the Normal Human Artery

In the normal intima, Gay (11,12) demonstrated
immunologically in the aorta of a 4-year-old that Type III
collagen was localized in the subendothelial space between
the endothelium and the internal elastic lamina. No Type
I collagen was detected in this location. McCullagh *et al*
(13) reported, following immunolocalization, studies, that
artery intimas of older humans ranging in age from 45-65
years had increased amounts of Type III and Type I collagen.
When Morton and Barnes (14) chemically analyzed the collagen
types present in thickened aortic intimas of aged humans a
greater amount of Type I was detected. It appears, therefore, that as the normal intima thickens with age, there
is predominantely a change in ratio of I and III collagen
to favor Type I. It is assumed that the Type III collagen
localized in the subendothelial space of arteries of young
individuals is synthesized by the endothelium since endothelial cells in culture can synthesize this collagen
type (15-19).

In the thickened intima, increased amounts of Type I
may reflect the metabolic property of an increased number
of smooth muscle cells present in the tissue since these
cells in culture synthesize both Types I and III collagen.

In the media of the aorta, both Gay (11,12) and
McCullagh (13) have demonstrated by using immunofluorescent
techniques that both Types I and III are localized throughout the tissue. There is a close association of these two
collagen types in the space between the smooth muscle cells
and elastic fibers. Type III localizes preferentially
near the elastic fibers, whereas Type I is found adjacent
to smooth muscle cells.

One of the first attempts to quantitate the collagen
types biochemically in the normal human aorta was the work
of McCullagh and Balian (20). Low extraction with pepsin
led to the conclusion that there was a preponderance of
Type III collagen in the media. However, other studies

of human aorta including the arch, thoracic and abdominal
aorta and the carotid artery (14,21-25) have consistently
indicated that Type I collagen and not Type III is the
major type. Based upon extractions of about 65 to 75% of
the total artery collagen, all of these studies have demonstrated that Type I collagen represents about 50 to 75% of
the total collagen of the normal media. Of note is the
work by Ooshima (22) who analyzed individually 28 samples
of human aorta. In every sample, Type I collagen was the
major collagen type. Within the entire artery there
appears to be a concentration gradient in the ratio of
Type I collagen to total collagen. Based upon the studies
of Murata (25), Type I is greater in the adventitia,
compared to the media.

Collagen Types in the Artery Wall - Types IV, V and VI

The presence of other collagen types has been described
in human arteries but in relatively smaller amounts compared to Types I and III. These include Types IV, V, and VI
which collectively comprise only about 0.5 to 1% of the
total arterial collagen.

Chung et al (26) first isolated Type V from human
aorta. Later studies by Morton and Barnes (14), as well
as by Ooshima (22) showed the presence of the α2(V) as well
as the α1(V) chains in both the media and the intima. More
recently, Murata (25) demonstrated α3(V) chains in the
human aorta. Type V collagen is a pericellular collagen
and may function to bind interstitial collagen to cells or
to basal lamina. This collagen has been localized immunologically in close association with the endothelial cells
and the basal lamina of the smooth muscle cell and in the
subendothelial basement membrane (13,27-29). Several
studies have demonstrated that both arterial smooth muscle
cells and endothelial cells synthesized Type V collagen
(15,16,18,19,28,30,31).

Type IV collagen, the collagen characteristic of
basement membrane, has been isolated from human aorta
(25,32) and immunolocalization studies by Madri et al (28)
and Gay et al (27) have demonstrated its presence in the
subendothelial basement membrane and the basal lamina of

the smooth muscle cell. Cultures of smooth muscle cells
(19) and endothelial cells (15,17,28,33,34) have been
shown to synthesize Type IV collagen.

Chung *et al* (26) was also the first to isolate Type
VI collagen or "short chain" collagen from human aortic
intima. This type of collagen has been suggested by Gay
and Miller (35) to serve as a link between collagenous
and non-collagenous structures. Its precise function is
still unclear.

Collagen Types in Atherosclerotic Plaque - Types I and III

Biochemical analyses have consistently demonstrated
that the major type of collagen present in the human atherosclerotic plaque is Type I (Table 4). It represents an
average of 70% of the total collagen which is very similar
to the 65% levels of Type I collagen in grossly normal artery.

Table 4. Level of Type I in the Human Atherosclerotic
Plaque

McCullagh and Balian (20)	65%
Ooshima (22)	66%
Morton and Barnes (14)	76%
Murata *et al* (25)	77%
Hanson and Bentley (24)	88%

No consistent shifts in the ratios of the major collagen
Types I and III in atherosclerosis have been established.
Morton and Barnes (14) did not see any significant shift
in the composition of the plaque collagen to favor Type I,
whereas Ooshima (22) found an enrichment of Type III collagen in the plaque in only a few samples. An interesting
observation was made by Murata (25) that the ratio of $\alpha 1$
(I) to $\alpha 2(I)$ chains in the atherosclerotic plaque was less
than 2 which is the expected ratio of Type I collagen
chains with the structure $[\alpha 1(I)]_2 \alpha 2(I)$. This implies that
there is a possibility for a modified Type I chain in the
atherosclerotic artery, possibly with the structure $\alpha 1(I)_3$.

When the synthesis of collagen types in the normal human aorta has been examined, Type I synthesis is favored over Type III. This ratio is similar to that seen for synthesis by segments of intact rabbit aorta or by smooth muscle cells in culture (Table 5).

Collagen Types in the Atheroslcerotic Plaque - Types IV, V and VI

One significant and consistent change in the minor collagen types of the atherosclerotic plaque is the increase in Type V collagen (14,22,25). Based on the studies of Ooshima (22) and Murata (25), Type V collagen is very prominent in intimal plaques and it increases with advancing fibrosis of the lesion.

Table 5. Synthesis of Collagen Types in Aorta and Aorta Derived Smooth Muscle Cells

				I/III	
Smooth muscle cells of chick aorta	I	III	V	1:1 2:1	Morton and Barnes (14)
Smooth muscle cells of rabbit aorta	I	III		1.5:1 2:1	Holderbaum and Ehrhart (36)
Aortic tissue of rabbits	I	III	V	2:1 3:1	Barnes (37)
Human thoracic aorta	I	III		2.3:1	Krieg and Muller (38)

Synthesis of Types IV and VI below detection limit.

There appears to be a difference in the Type V chains that are present in the different parts of the aorta. Murata showed that the $\alpha 3(V)$ chain was detected only in the intima and the subintima. Type V collagen has been reported to play a role in cell migration (39) and also appears to reduce the thrombogenic properties of the sub-endothelium (28). Although the exact role of Type V collagen remains to be determined, the increase of Type V may

simply reflect smooth muscle cell hyperplasia in the subendothelial space. As mentioned, the synthesis of Type V
collagen by smooth muscle cells has been reported (19,30).
In a recent study by Murata *et al* (25), Type V collagen in
the internal layer of the human atherosclerotic plaque
increased with the advancement of atherosclerosis and
$a3(V)$ collagen was detected in the aortas.

Based on the findings of Murata (25), it appears as
if Type IV collagen increases with the increasing atherosclerosis. As mentioned in that study, the short chain or
basement membrane collagens Types IV and V were also seen
to increase. Type VI collagen was also detected in the
intima and subintima of the human aorta.

The relative ratios of the synthesis of Types III, I
and V collagen by atherosclerotic tissue has been investigated (Table 6). Barnes (37) found that the atherosclerotic arteries of rabbits that were fed a beef tallow diet for
12 months synthesized sixfold greater levels of collagen
compared to controls. There was a significantly elevated
level of collagen Type I compared to collagen Type III.

Table 6. Collagen Synthesis by Rabbit Aorta

Study		III	I	V	III:I:V
1	Control	18	34	7	31:57:2
1	Atherogenic Diet, 12 mos 20% beef tallow-- no cholesterol	68	258	26	19:73:8
2	Intimal injury	117	556	56	16:76:8
2	Intimal injury + cholesterol diet	53	188	23	20:71:9

Numbers represent incorporation of ^3H proline (cpm x 10^{-2}
gm wet aorta).
Data modified from Tables 1 and 2, Barnes (37).

Barnes also studied collagen synthesis in rabbit aortas
after endothelial denudation by balloon catheter (Study 2,
Table 5). Removal of the endothelium again caused an

increased synthesis of collagen and the ratios of collagen types synthesized were similar to those seen with cholesterol feeding alone. Therefore, although there may be minor change in ratios of III, I, and V compared to the control, there was an increased synthesis of all three collagen types. In another species, McCullagh and Ehrhart (40) examined the synthesis of collagen in dogs fed an atherogenic diet for one year. In these animals, Type I collagen was exclusively synthesized.

The change in synthesis of the relative types of collagens reported in atherosclerosis therefore does not appear to be very markedly different. It appears that there may be some enrichment of Type I, but still the ratio of Types III, I and V remains fairly constant. The increased production of collagen in the atherosclerotic plaque is probably a result of the smooth muscle cells of the lesion assuming a synthetic rather than a contractile state. It appears therefore that evaluation of the role of collagen in atherosclerosis should be concerned principally with the increase in the total amount of the collagen synthesized.

Hyperlipemia and Collagen Synthesis

The stimulus for the increase in collagen production by the smooth muscle cells of the atherosclerotic artery is of major interest. It appears as if the effect of hyperlipemia *per se* is not sufficient to cause increased collagen synthesis. When Holderbaum *et al* (41) and St. Clair (42) studied the effects of hyperlipemia on collagen synthesis by arterial tissue or smooth muscle cells, both reported the lack of any stimulatory effect. In fact, some investigations have demonstrated that there is a reduction in synthesis in response to hyperlipemic serum. In studies done by Holderbaum and Ehrhart (43) where the hyperlipemic effect on collagen synthesis by cultured smooth muscle cells was examined, a stimulation of collagen synthesis per cell by hyperlipemic serum was noted only when there was an actual decline in the overall cell population. It appears therefore that when an increased collagen synthesis is reported, it is related to a

cytotoxic effect of the serum. Holderbaum and Ehrhart (43)
showed that when the proliferative effect of the serum was
taken into consideration, there was an increased cell population and the actual level of collagen per cell showed a
decline. Thus, convincing evidence is lacking that hyperlipemic serum specifically stimulates collagen synthesis.
Rather, any reported effect appears to be secondary as
the result of factors causing alterations in cells or cell
number.

In summary, the exact stimulus for increased collagen
accumulation in atherosclerosis is unknown. The control
presumably lies in some regulatory gene or regulatory protein affecting the different collagen genes of smooth
muscle cells which may be modified in the hyperplastic
state.

Elastin

With increasing age there is a decrease in the
elastin content in the grossly normal human aorta (44).
Parallel with this change there is increased collagen.
These changes in the collagen to elastin ratio result in
less vessel elasticity with increasing age.

In the human atherosclerotic plaque with increasing
atherosclerosis, there is a reduction in the total mass of
elastin. At the base of the lesion the elastic fibers are
split or frayed and histologically can be demonstrated to
contain lipid and calcium deposits.

Elastic Fiber Structure

In large arteries, elastin may comprise more than 50%
of the dry weight of the vessel. At the light microscopic
level, the elastic fibers are highly refractive and are
identified by their characteristic staining reactions with
Orcein or Resorcin-Fuchsin. By electron microscopy (45-47),
the elastic fibers can be seen to be comprised of two
distinguishable components: 1) an amorphous component,
elastin, which does not possess any regular repeating
structure or banding pattern and 2) a microfibrillar component. The amorphous elastin is the major part of the
fiber and comprises about 90% of a mature fiber. The

microfibrillar component is found as small fibrils of about
10-12 nm in diameter located primarily around the periphery
of the amorphous elastin. These components differ both
morphologically and chemically. In the formation of an
elastic fiber it is thought that the microfibrillar protein
serves as a nidus or a scaffold for the amorphous elastin
released from the cell following synthesis. Several
reports review the amorphous elastin (48-50), the microfibrillar protein (51), and the intact elastic fibers (52).
Elastin which appears amorphous in electron micrographs is
a very apolar and an extremely insoluble protein. The
specific amino acid sequences in the protein render the
molecule resistant to mild hydrolysis. Quantitation of
elastin involves either gravimetric methods which are easily
interpreted when the amount of elastin as a percentage of
total tissue protein is high or quantitation of crosslinking amino acids, a method more suitable when the tissue
concentration of elastin is low.

The precursor to the elastin component of the elastic
fiber is tropoelastin (48,52) which is secreted from cells
as a 72,000 molecular weight protein (48,49,52-54). Studies
suggest that tropoelastin is a modification of an earlier
precursor, proelastin, with a molecular weight of 76,000 to
78,000 daltons (49,53-57). When cell-free translations of
aortic mRNA preparations were performed, the major elastin-
like translation product appeared to resemble tropoelastin
with perhaps a short extension peptide.

It is unclear whether different cell types synthesize
different types of elastin. According to the work of
Foster (57), mRNA from embryonic chick aorta and lung translate elastin-like polypeptides that differ in size and
composition. Other studies suggest that chick aorta (49)
and avian lung (57,58) tropoelastin have very nearly
identical chemical properties and molecular weights. There
are several cell types in arteries that are capable of
synthesizing tropoelastin and the microfibrillar protein.
Both smooth muscle cells (59-61) and endothelial cells (62-
63) and in addition, fibroblasts (64) such as those that
exist in the adventitia all have been reported to synthesize
elastin. It appears therefore that a variety of mesenchymal
cells are capable of elastin synthesis.

The general view of the elastic fiber synthesis indicates that the elastic fibers first appear as bundles of microfibrils close to smooth muscle cells. Later these fibrils appear as an amorphous core of elastin and a peripheral microfibrillar component (51). Once elastin is synthesized it is stabilized by crosslinking amino acids and undergoes extremely slow turnover rates estimated in normal human beings to be measured in years (48). Harel (75) showed that in man the excretion of desmosine was 40 to 50 mg per day which would suggest a turnover of less than 1% of the total body pool of elastin per year.

Elastin Structure

The elastic recoil property of the elastic fiber is attributed largely to the elastin moiety. Postranslational modification of lysine residues results in extensive crosslinking of elastin which influences the biophysical properties of the protein. The major crosslinks of elastin were largely defined based on the work of Partridge (65-68) who first recognized that isomers of desmosine were the major crosslinking components. Further work on crosslinking amino acids (69,70) has resulted in the identification of desmosine, isodesmosine, lysinorleucine and merodesmosine as the major crosslinking amino acids of elastin.

The crosslinks restrict the elastic fiber so that upon stretching the individual polypeptide chains are constrained. Therefore, realignment and organization occurs upon the release of tension. In blood vessels, elastic fibers are crosslinked in a three-dimensional network but have a lamellar arrangement in the form of concentric sheets. The elastic fibers are parallel to the direction of stress and are therefore necessary for mechanical recoil during pulsatile blood flow.

With aging, shifts in the distribution of crosslinks of elastin result in a more chemically stable crosslink. The enzyme lysyl oxidase that catalyzes the oxidative deamination of specific lysine residues has been characterized from artery (71). Lysyl oxidase is a copper dependent enzyme (72) and in states of reduced lysyl oxidase activity, such as in nutritional copper deficiency or zinc intoxication there is reduced crosslinking of elastin in arteries, thus rendering animals susceptible to aneurysms.

Elastin is a very apolar protein. It contains very high concentrations of valine-proline sequences. About one-third of the total residues is glycine. The alanine and lysine residues in tropoelastin are clustered together to comprise the cross-linking amino acids (69,70). Between the crosslinking regions are amino acid sequences that are rich in valine, glycine and proline. Sequence data from chick tropoelastin suggest that certain sequences such as gly-gly-val-pro, pro-gly-val-gly-val, and pro-gly-val-gly-val-ala appear to repeat (52,69). In tropoelastin of chicks, a series of collagen-like repeats, gly-val-pro has been described (73). These amino acid sequences have been useful in determining elastin structure and have resulted in several proposed models for elastin (Reviewed by Sandberg, 74).

Elastin and Lipid Deposition

In atherosclerosis the arterial elastic fibers are fragmented, deranged and altered. Many morphologic studies have documented these changes to be progressive with the development of atherosclerosis. Since the elastin is very hydrophobic in nature, one would expect that the elastin could bind lipid. Such binding of plasma low density lipoprotein (LDL) by elastin has been demonstrated to occur in studies of human aortas (76). In addition, *in vitro* studies have demonstrated a transfer of cholesterol and cholesteryl esters of LDL to amorphous elastin (77). Such transfer did not occur with high density lipoproteins (HDL) although it has been demonstrated by others (78) that both LDL and HDL bind to elastin *in vitro*. One report by Tokita (79) suggested that portions of elastin that are enriched in the polar amino acids preferentially bind cholesterol. This binding of lipid is important because the lipid may diminish the elasticity of the tissue by altering the conformation of the elastin through hydrophobic interactions. Binding may also increase the sensitivity of elastin to proteolytic degradation (80), an effect that has been observed in an *in vitro* system (81). In addition, degradation of elastin may produce peptides which are chemotactic to macrophages (82). Therefore, cholesterol binding to elastin may be a contributory factor in the progression of atherosclerosis through enhanced recruitment of monocyte-derived macrophages.

Early reports by Kramsch (76) described the relationship of the cholesterol deposits in human aorta to the amount of elastin present and to the degree of severity of atherosclerosis. Elastin from the intimal plaque areas of the aorta contained increasing amounts of lipid and polar amino acids and decreasing amounts of crosslinking amino acids. These changes were also seen in normal-appearing areas adjacent to complicated lesions but not in normal artery. Kramsch originally believed that a prerequisite for the transfer of cholesterol to plaque elastin was an altered amino acid composition of the plaque elastin protein. Later studies by Keeley and Partridge (83) were unable to confirm that there was a change in the polar amino acids and suggested that contaminating micro-fibrillar protein and collagen in samples that were not decalcified properly was the reason for an altered amino acid composition. In addition, it has been suggested that the presence of calcium and lipid in an atherosclerotic lesion might be expected to cause changes in composition as a result of selective cleavage of elastin peptides upon alkali extraction (84,85).

Elastin and Calcification of Atherosclerotic Plaque

An important site of calcification in atherosclerosis appears to be associated with elastic fibers. Yu (86) reported that a carbonate apatite is the predominant mineral form in calcified plaque. Although carboxyl groups have been suggested to serve as nucleation sites for calcification of elastin, the apolar nature of the protein does not favor calcium binding. Urry (87) proposed that elastin can act as a calcifying protein even in the absence of ionic interactions which would arise from charged amino acids. The results of those *in vitro* studies by Urry suggest that calcium binds at neutral binding sites that involve complexes arising from the orientation of acyl oxygens in the elastin polypeptide. There is evidence (88) that matrix vesicles in the aorta may be a route of plaque calcification. Therefore, it is possible that, although elastin can bind calcium and act as a calcifying matrix, the matrix vesicles may be of primary importance in calcification of the artery. Certainly, when elastin is partially hydrolyzed or cleaved, calcium can bind to elastin, Rucker (89) showed that in solutions of low ionic strength elastin bound calcium (1 μmole calcium per 250-350 μmole of amino residues). This degree of binding is sufficient for hydroxyapatite nucleation and growth. An additional consequence of calcification of elastin is an enhancement of the binding of cholesterol and other lipids by elastin (90).

Elastolysis

Several proteases have been shown to attack elastic fibers. These proteases have been described in neutrophils (91), platelets, macrophages (92), and smooth muscle cells (93). For reviews, see 94,95). In a recent report, Robert (93) summarized studies of an elastase-type protease isolated from smooth muscle cells of the aorta. In cultures of smooth muscle cells derived from rat and pig aorta, this protease was localized on the cell membrane. This protease was inhibited by the usual serine protease inhibitors. In other studies enzyme activity was shown to increase with subsequent passage of smooth muscle cells and also as a result of added LDL to the culture media.

In atherosclerosis where elastin destruction, perhaps as a result of leukocyte or macrophage elastases, is of biological significance, the inertness of elastin takes on considerable importance. The elastin lost from atherosclerotic arteries may not be replaced or if it is replaced, fiber formation may be unorganized and inappropriate for normal function. The degradation of elastin is therefore an extremely important factor in any potential repair of an injured artery. Another consequence of the damage to elastin mentioned previously relates to the chemotactic

properties of elastin derived peptides for macrophages.
This recruitment of macrophages may result in exacerbation
of atherosclerosis.

REFERENCES

1. Levene CI, Poole JCJ (1962) The collagen content of
    normal and atherosclerotic human aortic intima. Brit
    J Exp Path 43:469-471
2. Smith EB (1965) The influence of age and atheroscelero-
    sis on the chemistry of aortic intima. J Atheroscler
    Res 5:241-248
3. Bertelson S (1962) Hexosamine, hydroxyproline, and
    calcium levels in the intima of the human aorta as
    related to age and atherosclerotic changes. J
    Gerontol 17:24-26
4. Smith EB (1974) Acid glycosaminoglycan collagen and
    elastin content of normal artery, fatty streaks and
    plaques. Adv Exp Med Biol 43:125-139
5. Wagner WD, Clarkson TB (1975) Comparative primate
    atherosclerosis. II. A biochemical study of lipids,
    calcium, and collagen in atherosclerotic arteries.
    Exp Mol Pathol 23:96-121
6. Bornstein P, Sage H (1980) Structurally distinct
    collagen types. Ann Rev Biochem 49:957-1003
7. Miller EJ and Gay S (1982) Collagen: An overview.
    Methods Enzymol 82:3-32
8. Burgeson R (1982) Genetic heterogeneity of collagens.
    J Invest Dermatol 79(suppl 1):255-305
9. Cheah KSE (1985) Review Article. Collagen genes and
    inherited connective tissue disease. Biochem J
    229:287-303
10. van der Rest M, Mayne R, Ninomiya Y, Seidah NG,
    Chretien M, Olsen BR (1985) The structure of type
    IX collagen. J Biol Chem 260:220-225
11. Gay S, Balleisen L, Remberger K, Fietzek PP, Adelmann
    BC, Kuhn K (1975) Immunohistochemical evidence for the
    presence of collagen type III in human arterial walls,
    arterial thrombi, and in leukocytes, incubated with
    collagen in vitro. Klin Wschr 53:899-902
12. Gay S, Walter P, Kuhn K (1976) Characterization and
    distribution of collagen types in arterial hetero-
    grafts originating from the calf carotid. Klin Wschr
    54:889-894
13. McCullagh KG, Duance VC, Bishop KA (1980) The distri-
    bution of collagen types I, II and V (AB) in normal
    and atherosclerotic human aorta. J Pathol 130:45-55
14. Morton LF, Barnes MJ (1982) Collagen polymorphism
    in the normal and diseased blood vessel wall.
    Investigation of collagen Types I, III and V.
    Atherosclerosis 42:41-51
15. Sage H, Crouch E, Bornstein P (1979) Collagen synthe-
    sis by bovine aortic endothelial cells in culture.
    Biochemistry 18: 5433-5442
16. Sage H, Pritzl P, Bornstein P (1981) Secretory
    phenotypes of endothelial cells in culture: comparison
    of aortic, venous, capillary and corneal endothelium.
    Atherosclerosis 1:427-442

17. Sankey EA, Bown FE, Morton LF, Scott, Barnes MJ (1981)
    Analysis of the collagen types synthesized by bovine
    corneal endothelial cells in culture. Biochem J
    198:707-710
18. Tseng SC, Savion N, Gospodarowicz D, Stern R (1981)
    Characterization of collagen synthesized by cultured
    bovine corneal endothelial cells. J Biol Chem
    256:3361-3365
19. Sankey EA, Barnes MJ (1984) Comparison of the
    collagenous products synthesized in culture by pig
    aortic endothelial and smooth-muscle cells. Variability
    in endothelial-cell cultures. Biochem J 218:11-18
20. McCullagh KG, Balian G (1975) Collagen characteriza-
    tion and cell transformation in human atherosclerosis.
    Nature 258:73-75
21. Rauterberg J, Allam S, Brehmer V, Wirtz W, Hauss WH
    (1977) Characterization of the collagen synthesized
    by cultured human smooth muscle cells from fetal and
    adult aorta. Hoppe-Seyler's Z Physiol Chem 358:401-
    407
22. Ooshima A (1981) Collagen alpha B chain: increased
    proportion in human atherosclerosis. Science 213:
    666-668
23. Szymanowicz AG, Bellon G, Laurain-Guillaume G,
    Delvincourt T, Rawdoux A, Cavlet T, Borel JP (1982)
    An evaluation by sequential extraction of the pro-
    portions of collagen types from medium sized arteries.
    Artery 10:250-265
24. Hanson AN, Bentley JP (1983) Quantitation of type I
    to type III collagen ratios in small samples of human
    tendon, blood vessels and atherosclerotic plaque.
    Anal Biochem 130:32-40
25. Murata K, Motayama T, Kotake C (1986) Collagen types
    in various layers of human aorta and their changes
    with atherosclerotic process. Atherosclerosis 60:251-
    262
26. Chung E, Rhodes K, Miller EJ (1976) Isolation of
    three collagenous components of probable basement
    membrane origin from several tissues. Biochem
    Biophys Res Commun 71:1167-1174
27. Gay S, Martinez-Hernandez A, Rhodes RK, Miller EJ (1981)
    The collagenous exocytoskeleton of smooth muscle cells.
    Collagen Rel Res 1:377-384
28. Madri JA, Dreyer B, Pitlick FA, Furthmayr H (1980) The
    collagenous components of the subendothelium: Correla-
    tion of structure and function. Lab Invest 43:303-
    315
29. Martinez-Hernandez A, Gas S, Miller EJ (1982) Ultra-
    structural localization of type V collagen in rat
    kidney. J Cell Biol 92:343-349
30. Mayne R, Vail MS, Miller EJ (1978) Characterization
    of the collagen chains synthesized by cultured smooth
    muscle cells derived from rhesus monkey thoracic aorta.
    Biochemistry 17:446-452
31. Sankey EA, Bown FE, Morton LF, Scott DM, Barnes MJ
    (1981) Analysis of the collagen types synthesized by
    bovine corneal endothelial cells in culture. Biochem
    J 198:7-7-710

32. Trelstad RL, Lawley KR, Hayashi K, Ehrlich HP, Silver FH (1981) Type V collagen from the chick embryo: Biochemical, physiochemical and ultrastructural characteristics. Collagen Relat Res 1:39-52

33. Howard BV, Macarak EJ, Gunson D, Kefalides NA (1976) Characterization of the collagens synthesized by endothelial cells in culture. Proc Natl Acad Sci (US) 73:2361-2364

34. Jaffe EA, Minick CR, Adelmann BC, Becker CG, Nachman R (1976) Synthesis of basement membrane collagen by cultured human endothelial cells. J Exp Med 144:209-225

35. Gay S, Miller EJ (1983) What is collagen, what is not? Ultrastr Pathol 4:365-377

36. Holderbaum D, Ehrhart LA (1984) Modulation of Types I and III procollagen synthesis at various stages of arterial smooth muscle cell growth *in vitro*. Exp Cell Res 153:16-24

37. Barnes MJ (1985) Collagens in atherosclerosis. Collagen Rel Res 5:65-97

38. Krieg T, Muller PK (1977) The Marian's syndrome. *In vitro* study of collagen metabolism in tissue specimens of the aorta. Expt Cell Biol 45:207-221

39. Stenn KS, Madri JA, Roll FJ (1979) Migrating epidermis produces AB_2 collagen and requires continual collagen synthesis for movement. Nature 277:229-232

40. MuCullagh KG, Ehrhart LA (1974) Increased arterial collagen synthesis in experimental canine atherosclerosis. Atherosclerosis 19:13-28

41. Holderbaum D, Ehrhart LA, McCullagh KE (1976) Effects of hyperlipoproteinemic serum and exogenous proline concentration on collagen synthesis by isolated rabbit aortas. Proc Soc Exp Biol Med 150:365-367

42. St Clair RW, Jones DC, Hester SH (1983) Failure of hypercholesterolemic serum to stimulate collagen synthesis in aortic smooth muscle cells from two species of nonhuman primates having different rates of collagen synthesis (41716). Proc Soc Exp Med 174:137-142

43. Holderbaum D, Ehrhart LA (1984) Modulation of Types I and III procollagen synthesis at various stages of arterial smooth muscle cell growth *in vitro*. Exp Cell Res 153:16-24

44. Hosoda Y, Kawano K, Yamasawa F, Ishii T, Shibata T, Inayama S (1984) Age-dependent changes of collagen and elastin content in human aorta and pulmonary artery. Angiology 35:615-621

45. Fahrenbach WH, Sandberg LB, Cleary EG (1966) Ultrastructural studies on early elastogenesis. Anat Rec 155:563-576

46. Greenlee TK Jr, Ross R, Hartman JL (1966) The fine structure of elastin fibers. J Cell Biol 30:59-71

47. Karrer HE, Cox J (1961) Electron microscope study of developing chick embryo aorta. J Ultrastr Res 4:420-454

48. Rucker RB, Tinker D (1977) Structure and Metabolism of arterial elastin. Intern Rev Exptl Pathol 17:1-42

49. Foster JA (1982) Elastin structure and biosynthesis--an overview. Methods Enzymol 82:559-570

50. Rosenbloom J (1982) Elastin: Biosynthesis, structure, degradation and role in disease processes. Connect tissue Res 10:73-91
51. Ross (1973) The elastic fiber: A review. J Histochem Cytochem 21:199-208
52. Sandberg LB (1976) Elastin structure in health and disease. Int Rev Connect Tissue Res 7:159-199
53. Davidson JM, Crystal RG (1982) The molecular aspects of elastin gene expression. J Invest Dermatol 19: 133S-138S
54. Saunders NA, Grant ME (1985) The secretion of tro-poelastin by chick-embryo artery cells. Biochem J 230:217-225
55. Burnett W, Finnigan-Bunick A, Yoon K, Rosenbloom J (1982) Analysis of elastin gene expression in the developing chick aorta using cloned elastin cDNA. J Biol Chem 257:1569-1572
56. Burnett W, Yoon K, Finnigan-Bunick A, Rosembloom J (1982) Control of elastin synthesis. J Invest Dermatol 79:138S-145S
57. Foster JA, Rich CB, Fletcher S, Karr SR, Desa MD, Oliver T, Przybyla A (1981) Elastin biosynthesis in chick embryonic lung tissue. Comparison to chick aorta elastin. Biochemistry 20:3528-3535
58. Buckingham K, Khoo CS, Dubick M, Lefevre M, Cross C, Julian L and Rucker R (1981) Copper deficiency and elastin metabolism in avian lung. Proc Soc Exptl Biol Med 166:310-319
59. Burke JN, Ross R (1979) Synthesis of connective tissue macromolecules by smooth muscle. Intern Rev Connect Tissue Res 8:119-153
60. Snider R, Faris B, Vertitzki V, Moscaritolo R, Salcedol, Franzblau C (1981) Elastin biosynthesis and cross-link formation in rabbit aortic smooth muscle cell cultures. Biochemistry 20:2614-2618
61. Toselli P, Salcedo L, Oliver P, Franzflau C (1981) Formation of elastic fibers and elastin in rabbit aortic smooth muscle cell cultures. Connect Tissue Res 8:231-239
62. Kantor JO, Keller S, Parshley MS, Darnule TV, Karnule AT, Cerreta JM, Perrins GM, Mandel I (1980) Synthe-sis of crosslinked elastin by an endothelial cell culture. Biochem Giophys Res Commun 95:1381-1396
63. Carnes WH, Abraham PA, Buonassisi V (1979) Biosyn-thesis of elastin by an endothelial cell culture. Biochem Biophys Res Commun 90:1393-1399
64. Vaccaro C, Brody JS (1978) Ultrastructure of develop-ing alveoli. I. The role of the interstitial fibro-blast. Anat Rec 192:467-480
65. Partridge SM (1962) Elastin. Adv Protein Chem 17: 227-302
66. Partridge SM, Elsden DF, Thomas J (1963) Constitution of the crosslinkages in elastin. Nature 197:1297-1298
67. Partridge SM (1964) Biosynthesis of desmosine and isodesmosine cross-bridges in elastin. Biochem J 63:30-33
68. Partridge SM, Elsden DE, Thomas J, Dorfman A, Telser A, Ho P-L (1966) Incorporation of labelled lysine into the desmosine cross-bridges in elastin. Nature 209:399-400

69. Foster JA, Rubin L, Kagen HM, Franzblau C, Bruenger E, Sandberg LB (1974) Isolation and characterization of crosslinked peptides from elastin. J Biol Chem 249:6191-6196

70. Gerber GE, Amwar RA (1974) Structural studies cross-linked regions of elastin. J Biol Chem 249:5200-5207

71. Kagan HM, Hewitt NA, Salcedo LL, Franzblau C (1974) Catalytic activity of aortic lysyl oxidase in an insoluble enzyme-substrate complex. Biochim Biophys Acta 365:223-228

72. Harris ED (1976) Copper induced activation of aortic lysyl oxidase in vivo. Proc Natl Acad Sci (US) 73: 371-374

73. Smith DW, Sandberg LB, Leslie BH, Wolt TB, Minton ST, Myers B, Rucker RB (1981) Primary structure of a chick tropoelastin peptide: Evidence for a collagen-like amino acid sequence. Biochem Biophys Res Commun 103:880-885

74. Sandberg LB, Soskel NT, Wolt TB (1982) Structure of the elastic fiber: An overview. J Invest Dermatol 79:1285-1325

75. Harel S, Janoff A, Yu SU, Hurewitz A, Bergofsky EH (1980) Desmosine radioimmunoassay for measuring elastin degradation in vivo. Am Rev Respir Dis 112:769-773

76. Kramsch DM, Franzblau C, Hollander W (1971) The protein and lipid composition of arterial elastin and its relationship to lipid accumulation in the athero-sclerotic plaque. J Clin Invest 50:1666-1677

77. Kramsch DM, Hollander W (1973) The interaction of serum and arterial lipoporteins with elastin of the arterial intima and its role in the lipid accumulation in atherosclerotic plaques. J Clin Invest 52:236-247

78. Winlove CP, Parker KH, Ewins AR (1985) Reversible and irreversible interactions between elastin and plasma lipoproteins. Biochim Biophys Acta 838:374-380

79. Tokita K, Kanno K, Ikeda K (1977) Elastin sub-fraction as a binding site for lipids. Atherosclerosis 28:111-119

80. Guantieri V, Tamburro AM, Gordini DD (1983) Inter-actions of human and bovine elastins with lipids: their proteolysis by elastase. Connect Tissue Res 12:79-83

81. Chaudiere J, Derouette JC, Mendy F, Jacotot B, Robert L (1980) In vitro preparation of elastin triglyceride complexes: fatty acid uptake and modification of the susceptibility of elastase action. Atherosclerosis 36:183-247

82. Senior RM, Griffin GL, Mecham RP (1980) Chemotactic activity of elastin-derived peptides. J Clin Invest 66:859-862

83. Keeley FW, Partridge SM (1974) Amino acid composition and calcification of human aortic elastin. Athero-sclerosis 19:287-296

84. Robert L, Poullain N (1963) Etudes sur la structure de l'elastine et le mode d'action de l'elastase. I. Nouvelle, Methode de préparation de derives solubles de l'elastine. Bull Soc Chim Biol (Paris) 45:1317-1326

85. Jordan RE, Hewitt N, Lewis W, Kagan H, Franzblau C (1974) Regulation of elastase-catalyzed hydrolysis of insoluble elastin by synthetic and naturally occurring hydrophobic ligands. Biochemistry 13:3497-3502

86. Yu SY (1973) Calcification processes in atherosclerosis. In: Wagner WD, Clarkson TB (eds) Advances in Experimental Medicine and Biology. New York and London, Plenum Press, pp 403-425

87. Urry DW (1971) Neutral sites for calcium ion binding to elastin and collagen: A charge neutralization theory for calcification and its relationship to atherosclerosis. Proc Natl Acad Sci (US) 68:810-814

88. Kim KM (1976) Calcification of matrix vesicles in human aortic value and aortic media. Fed Proc 35:156-162

89. Rucker RB, Ford D, Diemann G, Tom K (1974) Additional evidence for the binding of calcium ions to elastin at neutral sites. Calc Tissue Res 14:317-325

90. Eisenstein R, Ayer JP, Papajiannis S, Hass GM, Ellis H (1964) Mineral binding by human arterial elastic tissue. Lab Invest 13(2):1198-1204

91. Janoff A, Scherer J (1968) Mediators of inflammation in leukocyte lysosomes. IX. Elastinolytic activity in granules of human polymorphonuclear leukocytes. J Exp Med 128:1137-1155

92. Banda MJ, Werb Z (1981) Mouse macrophage elastase. Purification and characterization as a metalloproteinase. Biochem J 193:589-605

93. Robert L, Jacob MP, Frances C, Godeau G, Horneback W (1984) Interaction between elastin and elastases and its role in the aging of the arterial wall, skin and other connective tissues. A review. Mech Ageing Dev 28(2-3):155-166

94. Bieth J (1981) Elastases: structure, function and pathological role. In: Bieth J, Collin-Lapinet, RL (eds) Frontiers of Matrix Biology, Vol 6, Basel: S Karger, pp 1-82

95. Hornebeck W, Legrand Y (1980) Possible implication of two elastinolytic proteases isolated from tissue aorta and blood platelets in atherosclerosis. In: Robert AM, Robert L (eds) Frontiers of Matrix Biology, Vol 8, Basel: S Karger, pp 199-215

13

Nature and Importance of Proteoglycans in the Atherosclerotic Plaque

G.S. Berenson, B. Radhakrishnamurthy, S.R. Srinivasan, P. Vijayagopal, and E.R. Dalferes, Jr.

INTRODUCTION

At the initial meeting on "Evolution of the Atherosclerotic Plaque" in 1963, the importance of specific glycosaminoglycans (GAG) (acid mucopolysaccharides) in atherosclerosis was shown (1). These complex sugars were noted to be an integral part of the arterial wall connective tissue matrix that changes with the type of atherosclerotic lesion. Although complex sugars were isolated from aorta about a century ago, it was not until the decade 1950-1960 (2) that characterization of the GAG fractions provided the opportunity to explore a pathobiologic role of these substances. Histochemical studies stimulated interest in complex sugars in atherosclerosis but did not allow their characterization. The considerable information that is now available from a variety of studies indicates that early in the formation of atherosclerotic lesions changes of GAG is part of the vascular connective tissue, followed by extensive lipid deposition and progression of lesions.

The arterial wall is composed of a highly organized connective tissue matrix formed by special vascular cells, smooth muscle and endothelial cells. Obviously, the metabolism of these cells dictates the composition of this matrix.

Supported by grants HL-02942 and the National Research and Demonstration Center-Arteriosclerosis (HL-15103) from the National Heart, Lung and Blood Institute of the United States Public Health Service.

The matrix itself contains interlacing fibrous structures, elastin and collagen, embedded within a gel of the complex carbohydrates. Further studies on these sugars show a major portion to be linked to protein as proteoglycans (PG). The carbohydrate-protein macromolecules (in the native state) are intricately related to the fibrous proteins. Much of the information on PG arises from earlier studies of cartilage chondromucoprotein (3), but with the introduction of dissociative extraction procedures by Sajdera and Hascall (4) characterization of arterial wall PG has now begun. Proteoglycans from blood vessel tissue are considerably different from material isolated from cartilage and probably because of their lower concentration in arterial tissue and because of their associations with fibrous proteins they are somewhat more difficult to isolate.

Current information on cardiovascular connective tissue carbohydrate-protein macromolecules and atherosclerosis has been recently reviewed (5). The intent of this discussion is to consider certain pertinent areas specifically relevant to the nature and biologic properties of PG of the arterial wall and related to the development of atherosclerotic lesions.

Proteoglycans

Proteoglycans (PG) are composed of protein and glycosaminoglycans (GAG) and are present in varying amounts in all connective tissues. They are primarily extracellular. But, both intracellular as well as cell membrane PG have been described. In the native state all GAG with the exception of hyaluronic acid are covalently linked to proteins (Figure 1). A striking feature of the PG is their heterogeneity in molecular size, protein and GAG composition. Even PG isolated from a single tissue have closely similar but distinct populations, and each population is polydisperse, containing molecules of varying size and charge.

There are at least two types of PG in the arterial wall: 1) isomeric chondroitin sulfate - or chondroitin sulfate-dermatan sulfate - PG (CS-DS-PG), and 2) heparan sulfate PG (HS-PG). The former is present in the aorta in greater amounts and is partly associated with collagen, while the latter is predominantly bound to elastin, and also

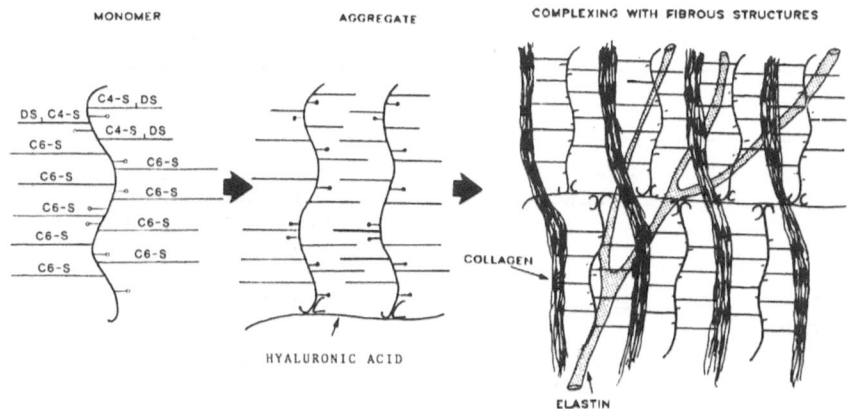

Figure 1. A schematic model of proteoglycan interaction with fibrous proteins in connective tissue of the arterial wall. Depicted are the microstructure, aggregation of proteoglycan, and complexing in the gel matrix of connective tissue with collagen and elastin in a more native state. (Reprinted by permission of Berenson, G.S. *et al*, and the American Journal of Medical Sciences 294;429-440, 1987).

occurs on the endothelial surface. The isolation of these substances by various extraction procedures including specific proteases to hydrolyze fibrous proteins suggest that the PG is strongly associated with the different fibrous proteins and may be "compartmentalized" in the tissue (Table 1).

　　1. Chondroitin Sulfate-Dermatan Sulfate Proteoglycan
　　Detailed chemical structure of a CS-DS-PG from bovine aorta has been reported (6). The PG contains two types of GAG chains: a) chondroitin 6-sulfate chains, and b) chondroitin 4-sulfate-dermatan sulfate hybrid chains. The core protein has a molecular weight of about 180,000. There are 12 GAG chains on the core protein. Nine chains are of chondroitin 6-sulfate, each with an average molecular weight of 49,000, and three chains with chondroitin 4-sulfate-dermatan sulfate with an average molecular weight of 37,000. The dermatan sulfate is linked to the protein core through chondroitin 4-sulfate (Figure 2).

　　Proteoglycan containing exclusively chondroitin 6-sulfate or dermatan sulfate chains as GAG were isolated from arterial cells grown in culture, and intact tissues from different species of animals (7,8). It is apparent that PG in the aorta are heterogeneous, and it is likely that microheterogeneity occurs in the GAG chains in a single PG species as suggested above.

Table 1. Characteristics of Proteoglycan Types in Aorta

	CS–DS–PG	HS–PG
Chemistry	GS-4, CS-6, DS (Galactosamine)	Polydisperse (Glucosamine) Microheterogeneity of Sulfonation, Acetyl, Uronate
Cellular Origin	SMC, Fibroblasts	Endothelial Cells
Occurrence	Extracellular Matrix	Membrane, Cellular
Matrix Fiber Association	Collagen	Elastin
Biology	LDL Binding Foam Cell Formation	Antithrombin Binding Lipoprotein Lipase Binding

Abbreviations: CS - chondroitin sulfate; DS - dermatan sulfate; HS - heparan sulfate; PG - proteoglycan; SMC - smooth muscle cells

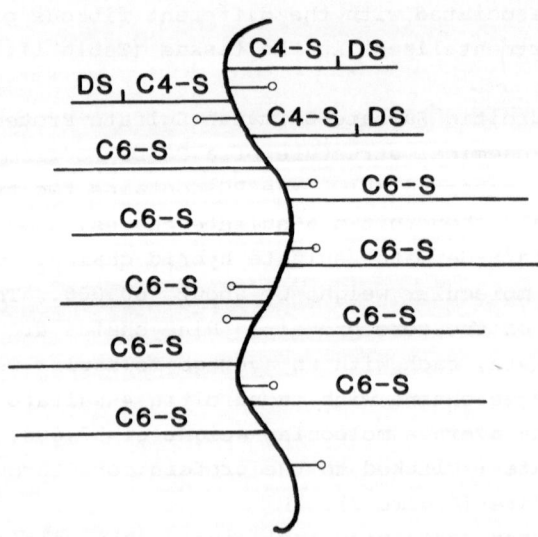

Figure 2. A tentative structure of chondroitin sulfate (CS)-dermatan sulfate (DS) proteoglycan from bovine aorta. Oligosaccharide side chains on the core protein are indicated. With permission, Radhakrishnamurthy B, Jeansonne N, Berenson GS (1986) Biochem Biophys Acta 882:85-96.

2. Heparan Sulfate Proteoglycan

Unlike CS-DS-PG, arterial HS-PG cannot be easily extracted by common dissociative solvents (9). Fibrous proteins of arterial tissue, specifically elastin, need to be
solubilized by elastase prior to extraction of the bulk of
this PG, as in Table 1. However, a small amount of HS-PG
can be extracted by dissociative solvents. The preparations
isolated by both methods have similar protein and GAG composition, except that the preparation from dissociative solvent
extraction has a somewhat higher molecular weight.

Link Protein and Proteoglycan Aggregation

Proteoglycans exist in the extracellular matrix as high
molecular weight aggregates. The aggregates are composed of
PG monomers, hyaluronic acid and link protein (s). Stabilization of the aggregate is a major function of the link
protein (10).

A link protein with a molecular weight of 49,000 was
isolated from bovine aorta CS-DS-PG aggregates and was shown
to be a glycoprotein (11). This link protein has a similar
aminoacid composition to that isolated from cartilage. As
in cartilage, the link protein enhances and stabilized aorta
PG aggregation in the presence of hyaluronic acid. Immunologic cross-reactivity of aorta link protein with cartilage
link protein 1 antibodies has also been observed (12).

Proteoglycan Changes in Atherosclerosis

Proteoglycan or GAG have been implicated in the pathogenesis of atherosclerosis for many years with changes noted
during development of lesions as well as with regression (5).
Although there are numerous studies of GAG, results obtained
by many investigators have been conflicting. Both increases
and decreases in total as well as in individual GAG concentrations have been observed due to variability involved in
experimental design as well as methodology. The discrepancy
in these observations are due to pooling of samples from
different age groups and with varying degrees of lesions, the
use of whole aorta vs intima-media preparations, and variations in chemical isolation and quantitation procedures.
Such observations are often only of a descriptive nature,

and have not provided specific leads as to their normal
function or their role in atherogenesis.

1. Human Studies

Fairly extensive studies on arterial GAG with atherosclerosis were performed in our laboratory (13). Considered
in relation to surface involvement with atherosclerosis the
concentration of total GAG increased as the involvement increased from 10 to 30% and as fatty streaks progress to
early fibrous plaques, but thereafter a decrease occurs with
further involvement and formation of unextractable tissue
and deposition of calcium salts. Of the individual GAG,
hyaluronic acid and heparan sulfate concentrations do not
change appreciably, while chondroitin 6-sulfate and dermatan
sulfate concentrations increase with increasing extensiveness
of fatty streaks. The chondroitin 6-sulfate increases
slightly in the fatty streaks but increases more in fibrous
plaques. Similar observations have been made on aortas from
experimental animals with diet-induced atherosclerosis (14).
The most consistent changes have been an increase in chondroitin and dermatan sulfates.

More recently, attention has been focused on the more
native state of GAG and the PG changes in atherosclerotic
aortas. We isolated PG from human fatty streaks and fibrous
plaques and compared their composition with PG from uninvolved
tissue (15). The wet tissues were sequentially extracted by
guanidine hydrochloride followed by hydrolysis of the tissue
with elastase. CS-DS-PG were predominant in guanidine hydrochloride extracts of the tissue. Most of the HS-PG were
released from the tissue by hydrolysis with elastase. The
PG concentration measured as uronate, was lower in fatty
streaks and fibrous plaques than in uninvolved tissue (0.58
and 0.48 vs 0.7 mg/g wet tissue), probably because of increased tissue concentration of lipids, collagen and calcium
salts in the lesions. The GAG composition of guanidine
hydrochloride extracted PG was similar in lesions and uninvolved tissue, but varied in the elastase hydrolyzed extracts. Gel filtration studies suggested the PG monomers from
lesions had greater molecular sizes than PG monomers from
uninvolved tissue. The studies indicate that alteration in

composition and an increase in molecular size of PG occur in atherosclerosis.

Wagner et al. (16) have observed that a chondroitin 6-sulfate PG from human atherosclerotic plaques had fewer but longer chondroitin sulfate chains per core protein and suggested a smaller overall monomer size in the atherosclerotic plaque.

2. Experimental Models

Because of limitations in obtaining human aorta tissue and possible degradation of core protein of PG before necropsy, we are currently studying PG changes in a rabbit model with diet-induced atherosclerosis. PG were radio-labelled with ^{35}S in organ culture and then extracted from tissue. A two-fold increase in ^{35}S incorporation into PG from atherosclerotic aorta occurred when compared to control animals. Proteoglycan monomers isolated from atherosclerotic aorta were larger in size than PG monomers from control rabbits (Figure 3). Greater amounts of chondroitin sulfates and dermatan sulfate and lesser amounts of heparan sulfate were noted in atherosclerotic aortas than in the controls. These findings are consistent with observations made in human and nonhuman primate tissues.

Glycosaminoglycans Changes During Regression of Lesions

The changes in GAG composition during regression depends to a large extent on the nature of the lesion and the amount of regression. At least a 50% increase of hyaluronic acid and a 40-70% decrease of chondroitin sulfates were observed in aortas with fatty streak lesions experimentally induced in rhesus monkeys. In lesions induced over a more prolonged period, regression resulted in an increase in both hyaluronic acid and heparan sulfate as well as a decrease of chondroitin sulfate.

The same trend of changes in the GAG composition occurred in an extensive study of cynomologous monkeys (17). In these animals diet-induced lesions were reduced by various anti-atherogenic regimens. Different treatments resulted in various degrees of regression. Although the mean total GAG concentration, per dry defatted tissue, did not differ

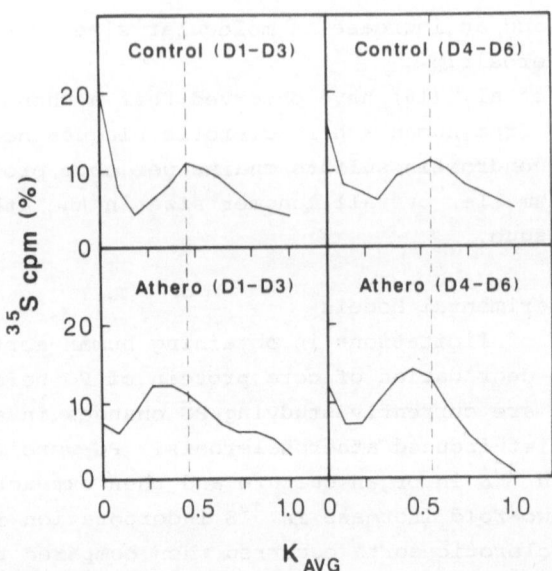

Figure 3. Gel filtration (sepharose CL-4B) of aorta proteo-glycan fractions from normal and atherosclerotic rabbits. Aortas were preincubated with (^{35}S) sulfate and extracted with 4.0 M guanidine HCl. Proteoglycans were fractionated by isopycnic density gradient centrifugation under disso-ciative conditions. Fractions representing bottom (D1-D3) and top (D4-6) gradients were pooled separately prior to gel filtration.

significantly among different treatment groups the changes significantly correlated with the severity of the lesions. As previously discussed, hyaluronic acid and heparan sulfate increased with the amount of regression and decreased in the vessels that persisted with greater severity of lesions.

These observations of GAG changes with disease provide the background for studies of PG, and are in concert with findings of materials isolated as proteoglycans.

Role of Proteoglycans in Atherosclerosis - Potential Mechanisms

The current concepts of the genesis of atherosclerosis focus on lipid infiltration and response to injury hypothe-sis (18). Both of these are not considered to be linked closely. Factors such as hemodynamic forces and hyperlipid-emia invoke damage to the endothelium, subsequently aggregation of platelets occur and smooth muscle cell proliferation ensues. In order to maintain integrity of the arterial wall synthesis of extracellular matrix components including PG occurs.

Although the lipids of atherosclerotic lesions are derived from plasma apo B-containing lipoproteins, the mechanisms of extracellular lipid accumulation is not clearly understood. Since an increase in lipid content of grossly normal intima with age is greater than the change of plasma lipid with age, mechanisms other than simple infiltration of plasma lipids into the vessel wall appear to be operative (Table 2). As indicated, proteoglycans likely play an important role in the accumulation of lipoprotein-derived lipids, both extracellularly and intracellularly.

Table 2. Proteoglycans and Atherosclerosis - Potential Mechanisms

---

1. Ion-exchange and molecular sieving - selective retention of lipoproteins (apo B).

2. Modification of low density lipoprotein size and charge - influence receptor-mediated uptake by smooth muscle cells and monocyte/macrophages.

3. Interaction with serine proteases - influence hemostatic properties.

4. Interaction with lipoprotein lipase - cholesteryl ester translocation from chylomicron remnants into arterial wall.

5. Aberrant fibrillogenesis of collagen and elastin - alterations in mechanical and physical properties.

Hemostatic Properties

It is well known that some GAG, e.g., heparin, heparan sulfate and dermatan sulfate, possess antithrombin and anti-coagulant activity. Arterial endothelial cell surface HS-PG might provide an antithrombogenic surface and inhibit platelet deposition as a protection to the endothelium.

Investigations of the hemostatic properties of a CS-DS-PG and a HS-PG from bovine aorta show that HS-PG have significantly more anticoagulant activity than CS-DS-PG in all clotting assays (19). HS-PG is also a more potent inhibitor of thrombin-induced platelet aggregation than CS-DS-PG. Both PG had no effect of ADP- and collagen-induced platelet aggregation. The protein core of the PG molecules is not essential for hemostatic properties. The anticoagulant activities of aorta PG appear to be due to the ability of GAG chains to

accelerate the inactivation of serine proteases by antithrombin III. PG might achieve this by increasing the binding affinity of these proteases for antithrombin III.

Recently, Kanaide et al. (20) observed that chondroitin
sulfate isolated from human atherosclerotic lesions had lower
anticoagulant activity than that obtained from normal aorta.
This suggests that the biologic properties of arterial PG
are altered in atherosclerosis.

Lipoprotein Lipase Binding

Lipoprotein lipase (LPL) is the key enzyme involved in
the hydrolysis of plasma chylomicrons and very low density
lipoprotein-triglycerides. LPL activity is localized at or
on the luminal endothelial surface of blood vessels. Even
though the nature of this localization is not clear, it
probably involves ionic interaction of LPL with some component of cell membranes, perhaps the HS-PG. Heparin or
heparin-like compounds are believed to affect the release
of LPL either by direct interaction with the enzyme or
competition for the LPL binding sites on the cell surface (21).
We observed that the CS-DS-PG from bovine aorta was about 60%
as active as heparin in releasing LPL in rabbits.

Lipoprotein-Proteoglycan Interaction

Subendothelial PG influences the transport of macromolecules across the arterial wall. The permeability and
retention of macromolecules such as lipoproteins, which enter
the matrix, may be modulated by molecular sieving, steric
exclusion, and electrostatic interaction. The permeating
components, especially LDL in excess amounts, contribute to
the microenvironment of cellular and connective tissue elements of the vessel wall.

A selective interaction of plasma apo B-containing lipoproteins occurs with certain arterial PG, especially the
chondroitin sulfate-dermatan sulfate type (22). The transfer
of lipids from LDL to fibrous proteins such as elastin (23)
could favor enrichment of the arterial wall with lipids. Yet,
the process of reverse cholesterol transport, as it occurs in
other tissues, likely counteracts with lipid build-up in the
vascular wall. While this may be the normal adaptive process,

focal tissue response to chronic injury may exaggerate the
lipid deposition by initiating alterations in cellular
metabolism, extracellular matrix characteristics, and rheo-
logical properties of the arterial wall. Recently, using a
rabbit model, we demonstrated that alterations in GAG metabolism in atherosclerosis are accompanied by an increase in
uptake of LDL by aorta (24). Our isolation of LDL-GAG (PG)
complexes intact from human atherosclerotic lesions as well
as from a rabbit model provides evidence for an *in vivo*
extracellular interaction (25,26).

In other studies (27), we demonstrated profound differences in LDL binding affinity among PG fractions that contain
isomeric chondroitin sulfates. Three preparations (D1, D2
and D3) obtained from bovine aorta that contained varying
amounts of chondroitin sulfates and dermatan sulfates were
isolated on the basis of buoyant density under dissociative
conditions. Quantitatively, fraction D3 with a sulfate to
hexosamine molar ratio of 1.05 had a greater affinity to LDL
than a fraction D1 with corresponding ratio of 0.73 (Figure 4).
Each of these PG fractions contained subpopulations or variants
with low and high affinity for LDL binding. Fraction D3 contained a high affinity PG that can be dissociated from LDL
only at an ionic strength of 1.0, which is even greater binding
affinity than occurs with heparin. Heparin is the most strongly binding GAG with LDL.

In fractions D1 and D2 the proportion of dermatan sulfate
increased in PG that were strongly bound to LDL, while fraction D3, the fraction with greatest affinity for LDL, contained
no dermatan sulfate; chondroitin 6-sulfate was the major iso-
mer in this higher affinity fraction. It appears that LDL
binding affinity of PG variants may depend not only on the
degree of sulfation (charge density) or constituent GAG but
on other chemical characteristics as well. These observations
indicate the heterogeneity of PG and it is likely that high
affinity PG variants are produced preferentially under conditions of injury and repair, which could lead to preferential
lipid accumulation.

The interaction of LDL particles with PG to form large
electronegative aggregates can also affect the arterial cellular metabolism in different ways. The reaction mechanism of

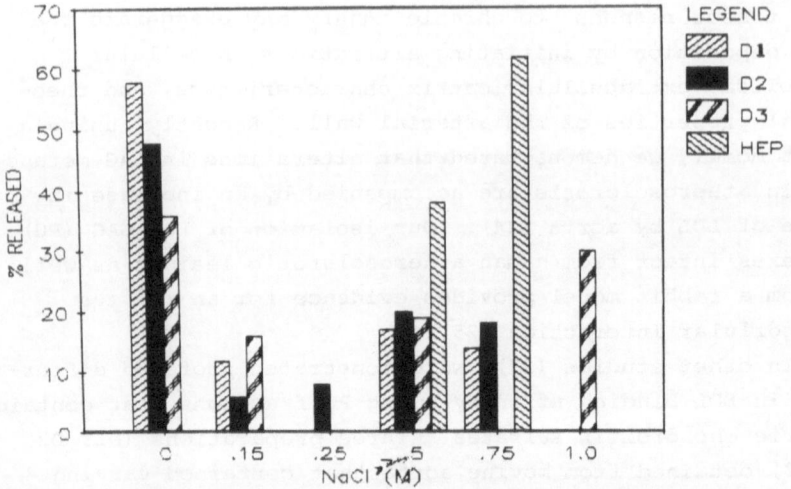

Figure 4. Binding affinity of bovine aorta proteoglycan
fractions (Dl-D3) to LDL. Proteoglycans were extracted with
4.0 M guanidine HCl, and fractionated by isopicnic density
gradient centrifugation under dissociative conditions.
Affinity chromatography of Dl, D2 and D3, representing bottom
gradient fractions, was performed by eluting the column with
increasing concentrations of NaCl. Heparin (Hep.) was included for comparison.

LDL-PG interactions involves an electrostatic binding of
basic amino groups of LDL protein (apo B) to polyanionic
groups of GAG (28). The same positively charged domains of
LDL are functionally essential for high affinity LDL receptor
binding by mesenchymal cells. Therefore, PG may significantly
inhibit the uptake of LDL by smooth muscle cells in the
contractile state. In these cells the LDL receptors are downregulated as the cholesterol content of the cell increases (29).
Resident macrophages of the arterial wall, from blood monocytes, avidly internalize the modified LDL by an alternate
receptor-mediated process devoid of down-regulation (30).
This results in cholesteryl ester accumulation within the
macrophage. The LDL-PG complexes can also be taken up by
macrophages (and possibly by transformed smooth muscle cells)
through a similar process, leading to a massive intracellular
cholesteryl ester accumulation as depicted schematically in
Figure 5.

ARTERIAL WALL PROTEOGLYCANS AND LIPID ACCUMMULATION

POTENTIAL MECHANISMS

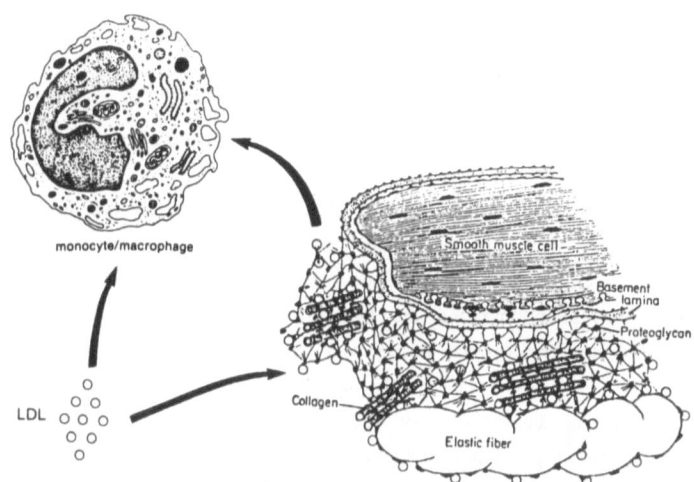

Figure 5. Potential role in extracellular and intracellular lipid accumulation in atherogenesis. With permission, Berenson GS, Radharkishnamurthy B, Srinivasan SR, Vijayagopal P, Dalferes Jr ER (1985) Ann NY Acad Sci 454:69-78.

Role of Proteoglycans in Foam Cell Formation

Atherosclerotic lesions contain a large number of foam cells, filled with cholesteryl ester. The foam cells partly originate from resident macrophages in the artery wall arising from blood monocytes. Monocytes enter the wall at sites of endothelial damage, or are deposited after transport through vasa vasorum (31). The *in vivo* mechanism for cholesteryl ester accumulation in macrophages and subsequent transformation into foam cells remains unclear. Since certain arterial wall PG readily form complexes with serum LDL, the question arises whether LDL-PG interactions promote internalization in macrophages. Recent studies strongly indicate such a possibility (32,33).

We (32) investigated the effect of complexes of LDL and CS-DS-PG preparations from bovine aorta on LDL degradation and cholesteryl ester accumulation in mouse peritoneal macrophages as a model. Both PG monomer and aggregate stimulated LDL degradation to different degrees. The PG aggregate-stimulated degradation of LDL was significantly higher than that mediated by PG monomer. Chloroquine, a known lysosomotropic agent, inhibits the PG-stimulated degradation of LDL.

The time-course of incorporation of $[^{14}C]$-oleate into cholesteryl $[^{14}C]$-oleate in the presence of native LDL and LDL-PG aggregate complex showed that the cells incubated with LDL-PG aggregate complex stimulate approximately an 80-fold increase in cholesteryl ester synthesis over cells incubated with LDL alone (Figure 6). This was confirmed morphologically by the presence of intracellular oil red O-positive droplets.

These studies show that the association of native PG aggregate but not the monomer with LDL is essential for the stimulation of LDL degradation and cholesterol ester accumulation. The mechanisms of recognition and uptake of LDL-PG complex by macrophages were not evident from these studies. Therefore, in order to test whether the degradation of LDL-PG complex is mediated by internalization through a specific binding site, degradation studies were conducted by incubating mouse peritoneal macrophages with increasing concentrations of the complex. Degradation data in the presence and absence of an excess of unlabeled LDL-PG complex showed that macrophages degraded LDL-PG complex with high affinity and saturability. A double reciprocal plot of data showed the apparent Km for degradation is 40 µg LDL cholesterol/mL. These results suggest that the complex is internalized through binding to a specific binding site. Furthermore, degradation of the complex does not occur at 4°C indicating that internalization of the complex is a prerequisite for degradation.

Pretreatment of macrophages with pronase and proteinase K markedly reduced LDL-PG complex degradation as compared to nontreated cells, showing that the binding site is protein in nature. Further, the observation that conconavalin A inhibited degradation of the complex, suggests that either the receptor is a glycoprotein or the complex is being blocked from binding to lysosomes.

A major question in studying the nature of the binding site for LDL-PG complex is whether the binding site is identical to or different from the receptor for native LDL, acetyl LDL and β-VLDL. Competitive LDL-PG degradation studies in macrophages in the presence or absence of an excess of unlabeled native LDL, acetyl LDL, β-VLDL and PG aggregate

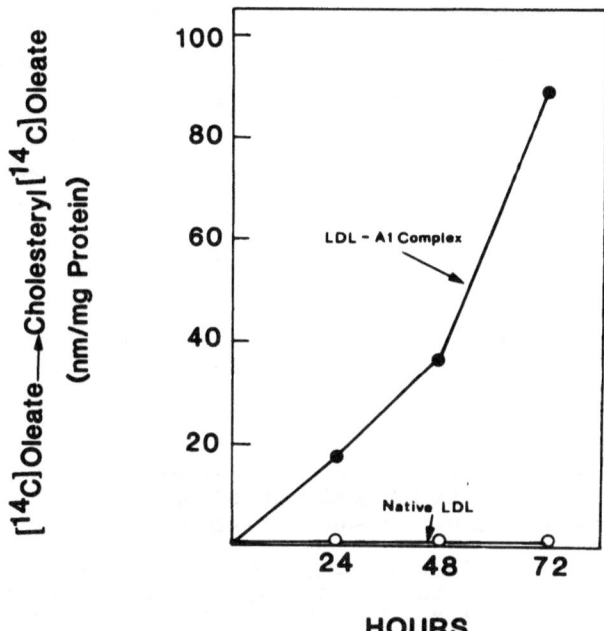

HOURS

Figure 6. Stimulation of cholesteryl ester formation in macrophages incubated with LDL-proteoglycan (Al) complexes. Monolayers of macrophages were incubated in 1 mL of medium A containing 0.2 mM [^{14}C] oleate-albumin (6520 cpm/nmol) and native LDL (95 μg/mL) or LDL proteoglycan complex (LDL, 95 μg and proteoglycan, 10.9 g uronic acid). The medium was replaced with fresh medium of identical composition every 24 hours. After incubation for 72 hours at 37°C, the cellular content of cholesteryl [^{14}C] oleate was determined. Each data point represents the average of triplicate assays, ●, LDL-Al complex; O, native LDL. With permission, Vijayagopal P, Srinivasan SR, Jones KM, Radhakrishnamurthy B, Berenson GS (1985) Biochim Biophys Acta 837:251-261.

showed that native LDL and PG do not compete with LDL-PG complex, but degradation of the complex is competitively inhibited by increasing concentrations of acetyl LDL and to some extent by β-VLDL (Figure 7). This suggests that LDL-PG complex is metabolized by the acetyl-LDL receptor. However, polyinosinic acid, a potent inhibitor of the binding and degradation of acetyl-LDL in macrophages, does not inhibit the degradation of LDL-PG complex. Therefore it is reasonable to conclude that while acetyl-LDL and LDL-PG complex may share

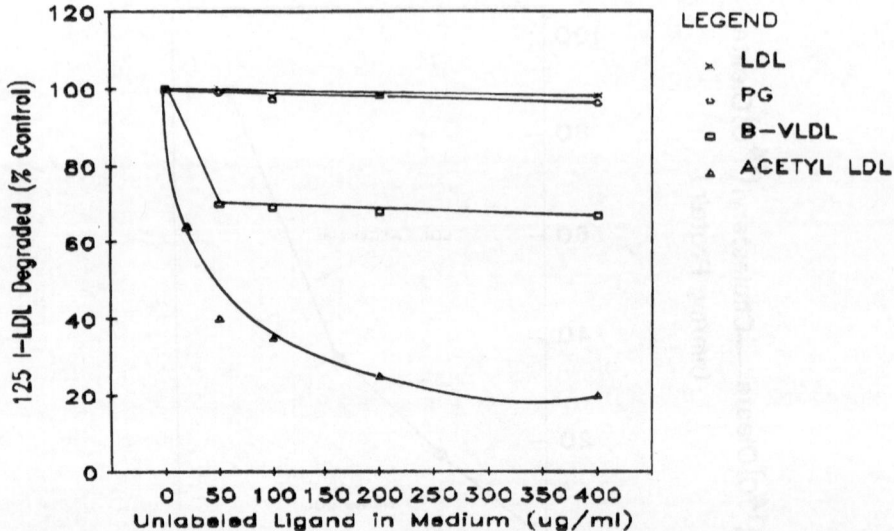

Figure 7. Ability of native LDL, acetyl-LDL, and β-VLDL and proteoglycan aggregate to inhibit the degradation of ^{125}-I-LDL-proteoglycan complex. Macrophage monolayers were incubated in 1 mL of Medium A containing ^{125}I-LDL-proteoglycan complex (50 μg/mL LDL cholesterol) and the indicated concentrations of nonradioactive native LDL, acetyl-LDL, β-VLDL and proteoglycan aggregate. After 5 hours at 37°C, the content of ^{125}I-labeled acid-soluble material in the culture medium was determined. The 100% value for degradation in the absence of any competing compound was 3.1 μg/mg protein; average of triplicate assays.

common binding determinants, the binding sites for these two ligands are not identical.

Degradation of LDL-PG complex was blocked by the monovalent carboxylic ionophore monensin, probably by disrupting either the delivery of the complex to lysosomes or the function of lysosomal enzymes. Monensin has been reported to inhibit the recycling of LDL receptor in fibroblasts (34) and recycling of acetyl-LDL receptor in rat liver endothelial cells (35). Further studies are needed to ascertain whether monensin also prevents the recycling of the receptor for LDL-PG complex.

Degradation of ^{125}I-LDL-proteoglycan complex was not suppressed by preincubation of cells with increasing amounts of unlabeled complex, suggesting that this process is not subject to down regulation. This observation also suggests that LDL-proteoglycan complex is not metabolized by the β-VLDL receptor since it is down regulated.

Thus, these studies provide some compelling evidence for a receptor-mediated pathway for the metabolism of LDL-proteoglycan complex in macrophages. Whether a similar process is operative *in vivo* in the case of human monocyte-derived macrophages of arterial wall remains to be seen. The evidence for a role for complexes of LDL and arterial wall proteoglycans in the pathophysiology of atherosclerosis is considerably strengthened by these observations.

Future Directions

Given current knowledge of structure-function relationships, several areas of investigation are germane to future work on cardiovascular proteoglycans. A common terminology needs to be established, based on better understanding of the heterogeneity of structure, for example CS-DS-PG (predominantly chondroitin sulfate containing proteoglycans), DS-CS-PG (predominantly dermatan sulfate containing proteoglycans), CS-PG (chondroitin sulfate proteoglycans) or DS-PG (dermatan sulfate proteoglycans). Proteoglycan homology of CS-4-DS linkage to protein core needs to be determined in vascular tissues from animal species (e.g., human, rabbit, monkey) as well as in different arteries (e.g., aorta, coronary arteries). Improved methods are needed for isolating HS-PG without use of enzymes like elastase. The influence of microheterogeneity of sulfation, acetylation and uronic acid composition on biologic functions also needs further study. Microheterogeneity can influence LDL interactions to induce macrophage uptake and alter hemostatic properties. Evaluating proteoglycan chemistry in susceptible and resistant animal species should help clarify the role of proteoglycan in atherosclerosis. Since synthesis and metabolism of proteoglycan will influence arterial lipoprotein metabolism, *in vitro* studies of proteoglycan metabolism in macrophages, smooth muscle and endothelial cells should complement the tissue studies. Overall, proteoglycans are important complex sugars found in the arterial wall, and they enter into a variety of biologic functions important to the integrity of the arterial wall.

REFERENCES

1. Berenson GS, Dalferes Jr ER, Robin R, Strong JP (1964) Mucopolysaccharides and atherosclerosis. In: Jones RJ (ed) Evolution of Atherosclerotic Plaque. Chicago: University of Chicago Press, pp. 139-150.

2. Morner CT (1895) Einige Beobachtungen uber die verbreitung der chondroitin schwefelsaure. Hoppe-Seyler's 2. Physiol Chem 20:357-364.

3. Malawistra I, Schubert M (1958) Chondromucoprotein: New extraction method and alkaline degradation. J Biol Chem 230:535-544.

4. Sajdera SW, Hascall VC (1969) Proteinpolysaccharide complex from bovine nasal cartilage. Comparison of low and high shear extraction procedures. J Biol Chem 244: 77-87.

5. Berenson GS, Radhakrishnamurthy B, Srinivasan SR, Vijayagopal P, Dalferes Jr ER, Sharma C (1984) Recent advances in molecular pathology: Carbohydrate-protein macromolecules and arterial wall integrity - A role in atherogenesis. Exp Molec Pathol 41:267-287.

6. Radhakrishnamurthy B, Jeansonne N, Berenson GS (1986) Organization of glycosaminoglycan chains in a chondroitin sulfate-dermatan sulfate proteoglycan from bovine aorta. Biochim Biophys Acta 882:85-96.

7. Wagner WD, Connor JR, Muldoon E (1982) High molecular weight proteoglycans biosynthesized in culture by pigeon aorta. Biochim Biophys Acta 717:132-142.

8. Rowe HA, Wagner WD (1985) Arterial dermatan sulfate-proteoglycan structure in atherosclerosis susceptible pigeons. Arteriosclerosis 5:101-109.

9. Radhakrishnamurthy B, Ruiz HA, Berenson GS (1977) Isolation and characterization of proteoglycans from bovine aorta. J Biol Chem 252:4831-4841.

10. Hardingham TE (1979) The role of link protein in the structure of cartilage proteoglycan aggregates. Biochem J 177:237.

11. Vijayagopal P, Radhakrishnamurthy B, Srinivasan SR, Berenson GS (1985) Isolation and characterization of a link protein from bovine aorta proteoglycan aggregate. Biochim Biophys Acta 839:110-118.

12. Gardell S, Baker J, Caterson B, Heinegard D, Roden L (1980) Link protein and a hyaluronic acid-binding region as components of aorta proteoglycan. Biochem Biophys Res Commun 95:1823.

13. Kumar V, Berenson GS, Ruiz H, Dalferes Jr ER, Strong JP (1967) Acid mucopolysaccharides of human aorta. Part 2. Variations with atherosclerotic involvement. J Atheroscler Res 7:583-590.

14. Radhakrishnamurthy B, Ruiz HA, Dalferes Jr ER, Srinivasan SR, Foster TA, Berenson GS (1982) Studies of arterial wall glycosaminoglycans and collagen during experimental regression of atherosclerotic lesions in cynomolgous monkeys. Lab Invest 47:153-159.

15. Dalferes Jr ER, Radhakrishnamurthy B, Ruiz H, Berenson GS (1987) Composition of proteoglycans from human atherosclerotic lesions. Exp & Molec Pathol 47:363-376.

16. Wagner WD, Salisbury BGJ, Rowe HA (1986) A proposed structure of chondroitin 6-sulfate proteoglycan of human normal and adjacent atherosclerotic plaque. Arteriosclerosis 6:407-417.

17. Radhakrishnamurthy B, Ruiz H, Dalferes Jr ER, Vesselinovitch D, Wissler RW, Berenson GS (1979) The effect of various dietary regimens and cholestyramine on aortic glycosaminoglycans during regression of atherosclerotic lesions in rhesus monkeys. Atherosclerosis 33:17-28.

18. Ross R (1981) Atherosclerosis: A problem of the biology of arterial wall cells and their interactions with blood components. Arteriosclerosis 1:293-311.

19. Vijayagopal P, Srinivasan SR, Radhakrishnamurthy B, Berenson GS (1983) Hemostatic properties and serum lipoprotein binding of a heparan sulfate proteoglycan from bovine aorta. Biochim Biophys Acta 758:70-83.

20. Kanaide H, Uranishi T, Nakashima Y, Nakamura M (1982) The anticoagulant effect of chondroitin sulfates isolated from normal and atherosclerotic regions of human aorta. Br J Exp Pathol 63:82-87.

21. Olivecroma T, Bengtsson G, Marklung SE, Lindahl M, Hook M (1977) Heparin-lipoprotein interactions. Fed Proc 36:60-65.

22. Vijayagopal P, Srinivasan SR, Radhakrishnamurthy B, Berenson GS (1981) Interaction of serum lipoprotein and a proteoglycan from bovine aorta. J Biol Chem 256:8234-8241.

23. Kramsch DM, Hollander W (1973) The interactions of serum and arterial lipoproteins with elastin of arterial intima and its role in the lipid accumulation in atherosclerotic plaques. J Clin Invest 52:232-247.

24. Srinivasan SR, Vijayagopal P, Dalferes Jr ER, Abbate B, Radhakrishnamurthy B, Berenson GS (1984) Dynamics of lipoprotein-glycosaminoglycan interactions in the atherosclerotic rabbit aorta in vivo. Biochim Biophys Acta 793:157-168.

25. Srinivasan SR, Dolan P, Radhakrishnamurthy B, Berenson GS (1972) Isolation of lipoprotein and mucopolysaccharide complexes from fatty streaks of human aortas. Atherosclerosis 16:95-104.

26. Srinivasan SR, Yost C, Berenson GS (1982) Lipoprotein-glycosaminoglycan interactions in aortas of rabbits fed atherogenic diets containing different fats. Atherosclerosis 43:289-301.

27. Srinivasan SR, Vijayagopal P, Eberle K, Radhakrishnamurthy B, Berenson GS (1986) Differences in low density lipoprotein binding among arterial chondroitin sulfate-dermatan sulfate proteoglycan variants. Arteriosclerosis 6:532a.

28. Iverius PH (1972) The interaction between human plasma lipoproteins and connective tissue glycosaminoglycans. J Biol Chem 247:2607-2613.

29. Brown MS, Kovanen PT, Goldstein JL (1981)   Regulation
    of plasma cholesterol by lipoprotein receptors.   Science
    212:628-635.
30. Brown MS, Goldstein JL (1983)   Lipoprotein metabolism
    in the macrophage: Implications for cholesterol depo-
    sition in atherosclerosis.   Ann Rev Biochem 52:223-261.
31. Fowler SE, Mayer EP, Greenspan P (1985)   Foam cells
    and atherogenesis.   Ann NY Acad Sci 454:79-90.
32. Vijayagopal P, Srinivasan SR, Jones KM, Radhakrishnamurthy
    B, Berenson GS (1985)   Complexes of low density lipopro-
    teins and arterial wall proteoglycan aggregates promote
    cholesteryl ester accumulation in mouse macrophages.
    Biochim Biophys Acta 837:251-261.
33. Salisbury BGJ, Falcone DJ, Minick CR (1985)   Insoluble
    low density lipoprotein-proteoglycan complexes enhance
    cholesteryl ester accumulation in macrophages.   Am J
    Pathol 120:6-11.
34. Basu SK, Goldstein J, Anderson RGW, Brown MS (1981)
    Monensin interrupts the recycling of low density lipo-
    protein receptors in human fibroblasts cell.   Cell
    24:493-502.
35. Blomhoff R, Devon CA, Eskild W, Helgerud P, Norum KR,
    Berg T (1984)   Clearance of acetyl low density lipo-
    protein by liver endothelial cells: Implications for
    hepatic cholesterol metabolism.   J Biol Chem 259:
    8898-8903.

14

Biochemical and Immunological Evidence for the Presence of Lipoprotein-Antilipoprotein Immune Complexes in Human Atherosclerotic Plaques

William Hollander, Antonio Lazzari, and Carl Franzblau

SUMMARY

Previous immunohistochemical studies of human atherosclerotic plaques have indicated a close association of the lipid protein complexes with the immunoglobulins (IgA, IgG, IgM) and complement (C3) contained in the lesion. The aim of the present studies was to determine whether the lipid-protein complexes or altered lipoproteins contained in the atherosclerotic plaque are present in the form of lipoprotein-antibody immune complexes.

The lipid-protein complexes were extracted from aortic atherosclerotic plaques into phosphate buffered saline and separated in the ultracentrifuge into a very low density fraction of d < 1.006 g/mL (VLDF) and a low density fraction of d 1.063–1.006 g/mL (LDF). LDF and VLDF were then purified by gel filtration on a Bio-Gel A-150 m column. The fractions were rich in cholesteryl ester and contained immunoreactive apo A-I, B, C-III and E as well as IgG, IgM, and C3. Small amounts of glycosaminoglycans (GAGs) consisting mainly of hyaluronic acid and chondroitin sulfate-C were detected in the fractions as was calcium. When examined by scanning electron microscope LDF and VLDF appeared heterogeneous in size and shape and showed surface irregularities and defects consistent with the appearance of aggregated and degraded lipoproteins. When mouse peritoneal macrophages were

Supported by NIH Grant HL 13262

incubated with LDF or VLDF, they accumulated cholesterol and cholesteryl ester and became foam cells. In contrast to the macrophages, smooth muscle cells did not accumulate lipid when incubated with LDF or VLDF. The uptake of the lipid-protein complexes by the macrophage appeared to be mediated by the protein component of the complexes since pretreatment of LDF or VLDF with pronase completely inhibited lipid deposition in the macrophage. Digestion of LDF or VLDF with chondroitinase ABC and hyaluronidase removed the GAG components of the complexes but it did not reduce lipid accumulation in the macrophage suggesting that the uptake of the complexes is not mediated by the dextran sulfate receptors of the macrophage. Competitive inhibition studies with opsonized sheep red blood cells suggest that the immune receptors (Fc and C3b receptors) of the macrophage may mediate the uptake of LDF and VLDF in a manner similar to that of an immune complex. The protein composition of foam cells isolated from atherosclerotic plaques, as revealed by immunohistochemical examination, appeared to be similar to that of the lipid-protein complexes and mouse peritoneal macrophages pre-incubated with these complexes suggesting that the complexes may play a role in the formation of macrophage derived foam cells in atherosclerotic lesions. The overall results of the study suggest that the lipid-protein complexes, which account for over 90% of the lipo-protein fractions isolated from atherosclerotic lesions, are altered plasma lipoproteins which have the biochemical and biological behavior of a lipoprotein-antibody immune complex.

INTRODUCTION

There is growing evidence that immunological factors may play a role in vascular disease (1). It has been shown that human atherosclerotic plaques contain a number of immune related proteins which include immunoglobulins A, G, and M and components of the complement system, such as C3, C3a, and C3c and the cytolytic complex of C5b-C9 (2-6). There also is some evidence that IgG antibodies may be synthesized by the diseased vessel (2,3). Inflammatory cells consisting mainly of lymphocytes and varying number of plasma cells also have been identified in atherosclerotic vessels (3,7-9). The relationship between these findings and the reports that autoantibodies and immune complexes may appear in the circulation of patients with hyperlipidemia and vascular disease has not been established (10-14).

In addition to humoral mediated immunity, there is evidence for the participation of cell mediated immune mechanisms in certain forms of vascular disease. Accelerated atherosclerosis has been described in human coronary vessels or coronary allograft recipients who have hypercholesterol-emia (15,16). Complicating atherosclerosis also has been observed in recipients of renal transplants (15,16). The accelerated atherosclerosis appears to be mediated at least in part by T-cell as well as autoantibodies directed against the endothelial cells. Recent studies suggest that T-cell mediated changes also may occur in naturally occurring atherosclerotic lesions (9).

The present studies were undertaken to determine whether the altered lipoproteins or lipid-protein complexes, previously described in the atherosclerotic plaques (17,18), may act as autoantigens and form immune complexes with IgG antibodies and complement contained in the lesion (1,2). The results of these studies confirm the presence of degraded and aggregated lipoproteins in the atherosclerotic plaque in close association with the immune-related proteins (17) and indicate that these lipoproteins behave biochemically and biologically like a lipoprotein-antibody immune complex.

METHODS

Isolation of Lipid-Protein Complexes

Samples of uncomplicated fatty-fibrous plaques were obtained from human aortas at autopsy within four hours after death and processed immediately as previously described (17, 18). Briefly, the intimal layer of the aortic specimens was homogenized, extracted into saline and separated into a low density fraction of d 1.063-1.006 g/mL (LDF) and a very low density fraction of d < 1.006 g/mL (VLDF). These fractions, which contain lipid-protein complexes, were purified by gel filtration on a Bio-Gel A-150 m column. Preservatives against bacterial contamination, oxidation and proteolysis were used during the preparation of the samples and included sodium azide (0.05%), EDTA (0.1%), reduced glutathione (0.05%), and E-amino caproic acid (0.13%).

Lipid and Protein Analyses

The biochemical analyses of the chromatographically purified lipid-protein complexes, LDF and VLDF, and the serum lipoproteins, LDL, and VLDL, were determined by methods previously described (17).

Briefly, the lipids were extracted from the Bio-Gel fractions with chloroform and methanol, 2:1 (v/v) and the cholesterol, cholesteryl ester (21), phospholipids (22), and triglycerides (23) were determined.

Protein was determined by the method of Lowry using bovine serum albumin as a standard (24). For fatty acid analysis, the lipids were extracted from the lipid-protein complexes with chloroform and methanol 2:1 (v/v) and isolated by chromatography on a 0.5 m silica gel plate in a 70:30:1 hexane-diethyl ether-acetic acid as previously described (17,25).

Glycosaminoglycans Analysis

The method for measuring glycosaminoglycans (GAG's) has been described previously in detail (26). Briefly, the lipid-protein complexes and serum lipoproteins were delipidated with chloroform/methanol (3:1) and digested with papain. A second proteolytic digestion was carried out with pronase. The digest was centrifuged and the supernatant was dissolved in water and analyzed for GAG's by two-dimensional electrophoresis (26,27).

Calcium Analysis

For calcium determination, an aliquot of delipidated minced tissue was ashed in Vycor vessles at 690°C for 24 hours. The ashed samples were dissolved in 1% lanthum chloride solution in 0.2 M HCL and analyzed for calcium by atomic spectrophotometry.

Immunochemical Analyses

The immunochemical analyses of the lipid-protein complexes and serum lipoproteins were carried out by the techniques of double immunodiffusion and immunoelectrophoresis (30,31) using goat antisera to apo-proteins A-I, B, C-III and E, immunoglobulins A, G, M and complement components Cla and C3. Immunochemical studies also were performed after delipidation and solubilization of the samples in sodium dodecyl sulfate (18).

Antisera to the delipidated and solubilized proteins of the lipid-protein complexes were raised in New Zealand white rabbits by the intramuscular injection of 1 to 1.5 mg of protein suspended in 0.5 mL of Freund's adjuvant. The injections were repeated at 1, 3, 5 and 6 weeks. One week after the last injection, the animals were bled and the raised antisera were tested by double immunodiffusion against the following specific antigens: apoproteins A, B, and E, immunoglobulins IgG and M and complement components C3 and Clq. Serum LDL and VLDL also were tested as antigens.

Electron Microscopy

The lipid-protein complexes and serum lipoproteins were fixed with 2% osmium tetroxide in 0.067 M phosphate buffer pH 7.4 (1:1 v/v). After gold coating in vacuum, samples were examined by scanning electron microscopy (Jelco U3). All procedures were done at less than $25^{O}C$ (32) and photographed at magnifications from 16,000 to 72,000.

Preparation of Mouse Peritoneal Macrophages

Female AKJ/R mice were obtained from the Jackson Laboratory (Bar Harbor, Maine). Peritoneal macrophages from the mice were isolated by the method of Edelson and Cohn (33). The cells were plated on tissue culture plastic slides containing eight chambers. After incubation in a humidified CO_2 (5%) incubator for one hour at $37^{O}C$, the non-adherent cells were removed by washing the chambers two times with pre-warmed RPMI-1640. The adherent cells were then used for the experiments.

Smooth Muscle Cell Isolation and Culture

Enzyme derived neonatal aortic rat and rabbit smooth muscle cells were isolated as described by Oakes and co-workers (34). Cells were seeded at 1.5 x 10^6/75 cm^2 flask in Dulbecco's Modified Eagle's Medium containing 317 g/L sodium bicarbonate, penicillin (100 units/mL) and streptomycin (100 µg/mL), and 0.1 µM non-essential amino acids with 10% fetal bovine serum. All experiments were performed on cells in second passage.

Isolation of Foam Cells from Atherosclerotic Lesions

Foam cells were isolated from the atherosclerotic aorta of humans (and monkey) by methods similar to those described by Schaffner and co-workers (35). The cells were suspended in RPMI-1640 and plated on tissue culture slides. The adherent cells were fixed with Bouin's fixative or pre-cooled methanol (-20°C). The slides fixed with Bouin's were stained with oil-red-O and the methanol fixed cells were used for immunofluorescence studies.

Uptake of Lipid-Protein Complexes by the Cultured Macrophage and Smooth Muscle Cell

Cultured peritoneal macrophages and smooth muscle cells were incubated with LDF or VLDF (0-360 µg/protein/mL) for 16 hours following which the cells were washed with pre-warmed RPMI-1640 and fixed with Bouin's solution. The cells were then stained with oil-red-O and the percent of cells with lipid droplets was determined. The incubations were carried out in RPMI-BSA at 37°C in a humidified chamber with 5% CO_2. Similar studies were carried out with chloroquine (0 to 15 µM) added to the incubation medium and with LDF or VLDF pretreated with pronase of chondroitinase ABC and bovine testicular hyaluronidase (26). The enzyme treated and untreated samples were then incubated with the isolated macrophages for 16 hours and the percent of cells with lipid droplets was determined.

The total and unesterified cholesterol content of the extracts was determined by the fluorometric enzymatic assay of Gamble and co-workers (36).

Effects of Lipid-Protein Complexes on Immunophagocytosis

Immunophagocytosis by macrophages was assessed with the use of opsonized sheep red blood cells as described by Schaffner and co-workers (35).

Erythrocytes coated with anti-sheep erythrocyte IgG are designated as EA-IgG and those coated with anti-sheep erythrocyte IgM plus complement as EA-IgM-C3. Opsonized blood cells (1×10^8 cells) were incubated with monolayers of macrophages contained in the tissue chambers in the presence or absence of increasing concentrations of LDF or VLDF (0-100 µg protein/mL). After one hour of incubation at $37^{\circ}C$ in a humidified chamber with 5% CO_2, the chambers were washed twice with PBS and fixed with Bouin's solution. The fixed slides were stained with hematoxylin and eosin and mounted under a coverslip. The findings were expressed as the percent of macrophages showing rosette formation.

Immunocytological Studies of Macrophages and Foam Cells

Immunofluorescent studies were performed on mouse macrophages pre-incubated with LDF or VLDF and on foam cells isolated from atherosclerotic plaques by the method of Coons and Kaplan (38). The primary antibodies used were monospecific and included goat anti-apoprotein A-I, B, C-III and E and mouse monoclonal antibodies to apo A, B, and E.

After fixation in methanol, the cells were incubated with the primary antibody and then with the secondary antibody which included fluorescein isothiocyanate (FITC) labeled F(ab')$_2$ anti-goat or anti-mouse IgG. Additional studies were performed with an affinity purified biotinylated secondary antibody followed by staining with FITC labeled avidin.

For detection of immunoglobulins, direct immunofluorescent examination of pre-fixed cells was performed using FITC labeled goat anti-human IgG or C3 and FITC labeled goat anti-human IgG, IgM, and IgA antisera (heavy and light chain specific) and protein A. The specificity of immunofluorescence staining was tested a) by using non-immune serum instead of the primary antibody, b) by absorption of FITC labeled antibody with specific antigen

and c) by blocking immunofluorescence of the cells by
pretreatment with unconjugated specific antisera.

Immunoperoxidase studies were also performed to confirm the findings with the immunofluorescent method. We
used the same primary antibody as described in the immunofluorescent studies. The secondary antibodies were peroxidase or biotin labeled. In the latter case peroxidase
labeled avidin was used before color development by the
addition of 3,3-diaminobenzidine.

RESULTS

Isolation of Lipid-Protein Complexes

The lipid-protein complexes extracted from fibrous
plaques were isolated by gel filtration on a Bio-Gel A-150 m
column following their separation in the ultracentrifuge
into a very low density fraction of d < 1.006 g/mL and a
low density fraction of d 1.063-1.006 g/mL.

When examined on the Bio-Gel column, the d < 1.006
fraction gave one peak which contained very low density
lipid-protein complexes designated as VLDF (Figure 1). The
elution volume of VLDF was smaller than that of tobacco
mosaic virus with a known molecular weight of 39×10^6kD.
When rechromatographed on a Bio-Gel A-50 M column, VLDF
eluted at the void volume.

The ultracentrifugically isolated d 1.063-1.006
fraction separated into two peaks on the Bio-Gel A-150 m
column (Figure 2). Peak 1 contained the low density lipid-
protein complexes designated as LDF, while peak 2 contained
an LDL like lipoprotein whose properties have been described
previously (17,18). Peak 1 had a smaller elution volume
than peak 2 whose elution pattern was approximately the
same as that of serum LDL. When examined on a Bio-Gel A-50 m
column LDL like VLDF eluted at the void volume. The lipid-
protein complexes, LDF and VLDF accounted for over 90% of
the ultracentrifugically isolated fractions from the plaque
while the LDL-like lipoprotein accounted for less than 10%
of the isolated fractions.

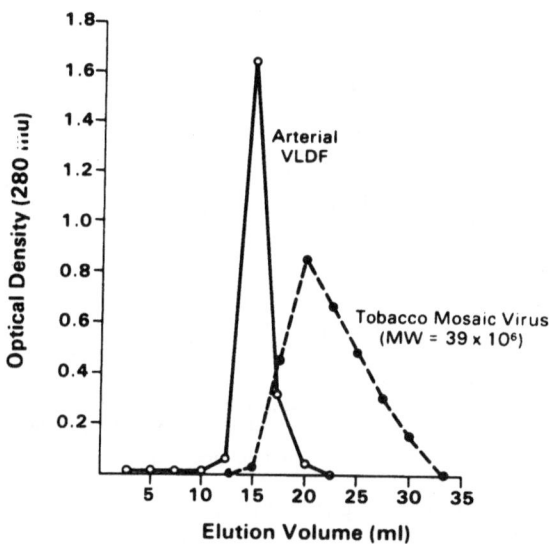

**Gel Filtration Pattern of Arterial Very
Low Density Fraction of d < 1.006 on
Bio-Gel A-150 m**

Figure 1. Gel filtration pattern of arterial very low
density fraction of d < 1.006 on Bio-Gel A-150 m column.
The fraction showed only one peak which contained the very
low density lipid-protein complexes (VLDF). VLDF, as
indicated by its elution volume, had a higher molecular
weight (MW) than tobacco mosaic virus with a known MW of
39×10^6 kD.

Biochemical Characteristics of Lipid-Protein Complexes

The composition of LDF and VLDF complexes are
summarized in Tables 1 and 2. The major lipid component
of the lipid-protein complexes was cholesterol which
constitutes 48.5% of LDF and 58.1% of VLDF. Most of the
cholesterol, 83%, was esterified in VLDF, while 53% was
esterified in LDF. Both fractions contained significant
amounts of phospholipids but only small amounts of triglycerides of less than 13%.

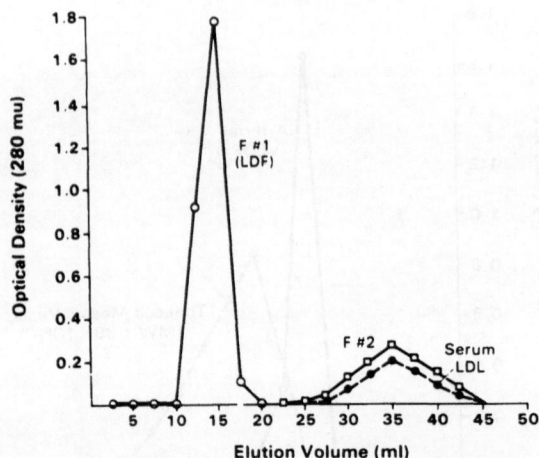

Figure 2. Gel filtration pattern of arterial low density
fraction of d 1.063-1.006 on Bio-Gel A-150 m column. The
fraction separated into a major peak which contained the
low density lipid protein complexes (LDF) and a minor peak
which contained an LDL-like lipoprotein with an elution
pattern similar to that of serum LDL.

The fatty acid composition of the cholesteryl ester
fraction of arterial LDF and VLDF appeared to be similar
with both fractions having a high ratio of linoleate to
oleate (Table 2).

LDF and VLDF contained 19.1% and 9.2% protein, respectively. The proteins in the intact fractions were not
immunochemically reactive and showed no reactions to the
antisera listed in Table 3. However, after delipidation
and solubilization of the complexes with SDS, a number of
different proteins were identified by double immunodiffusion.
These proteins included apolipoproteins A-I, B, C-III, and E,
immunoglobulins G, and M and complement component C3.

Table 1. Percent Composition of the Lipid-Protein Complexes
(LDF, VLDF) from Fibrous Plaques

	VLDF	LDF
Protein	9.2 ± 1.7	19.1 ± 1.4
Free Cholesterol	10.0 + 1.9	23.3 ± 3.0
Ester Cholesterol	48.1 + 4.5	25.2 ± 3.3
Phospholipids	18.3 ± 2.2	24.1 ± 2.9
Triglycerides	12.4 + 2.0	7.1 ± 0.3
GAGs*	1.4 ± 0.3	1.7 ± 0.3
Calcium	0.6 ± 0.1	0.5 ± 0.1

Mean ± SD, N = 5
* Chondroitin sulfate-C + hyaluronic acid

Table 2. Percent Fatty Acid Composition of Cholesteryl
Ester Fraction of Arterial LDF and VLDF

Fatty Acid	LDF	VLDF
14:0	3.1 ± 1.0	4.5 ± 0.8
16:0	18.2 ± 1.8	15.1 ± 1.7
16:1	5.5 ± 0.9	6.2 ± 1.1
18:0	3.8 ± 0.7	3.5 ± 0.7
18:1	23.1 ± 2.5	21.7 ± 3.1
18:2	42.5 ± 3.8	43.8 ± 4.5
18:3	1.4 ± 1.1	2.0 ± 1.2
20:4	2.4 ± 1.2	3.1 ± 1.3
18:2/18:1	1.8 ± 0.2*	2.0 ± 0.3*

Mean ± SD, N = 4
* Ratio of linoleate to oleate

Table 3. Analyses of Delipidated Arterial and Serum Lipoprotein Fractions by Double Immunodiffusion

| | | | Immunochemical Reaction | |
| Antisera | Arterial | | Serum | |
	LDF	VLDF	LDL	VLDL
Apo A-I	+	+	−	+
Apo B	+	+	+	+
Apo C-III	+	+	−	+
Apo E	+	+	−	+
IgG	+	+	−	−
IgM	+	+	−	−
C3	+	+	−	−
Albumin	+/−	+/−	−	−

These findings were supported by immunodiffusion and
immunoelectrophoretic studies in which rabbit antisera
raised against LDF and VLDF were reacted against known apoproteins, immunoglobulins, and complement.

Glycosaminoglycans (GAG) and calcium also were detected
in the lipid-protein complexes and constituted about 1.5% of
the complexes (Table 1). Chondroitin sulfate C and hyaluronic acid appeared to be the major GAG components as revealed
by two-dimensional electrophoresis and enzyme digestion with
chondroitinases ABC and hyaluronidase.

Electron Microscope Appearance of Lipid-Protein Complexes

When examined by scanning electron microscopy both LDF
and VLDF contained particles of different sizes and shapes.
The VLDF particles were generally larger than the LDF
particles, both of which showed surface irregularities and
surface defects consisting of pits and craters (Figure 3).
The latter findings are consistent with partial metabolic
degradation of the particles. The large size particles of
these fractions had a much larger diameter than the plasma

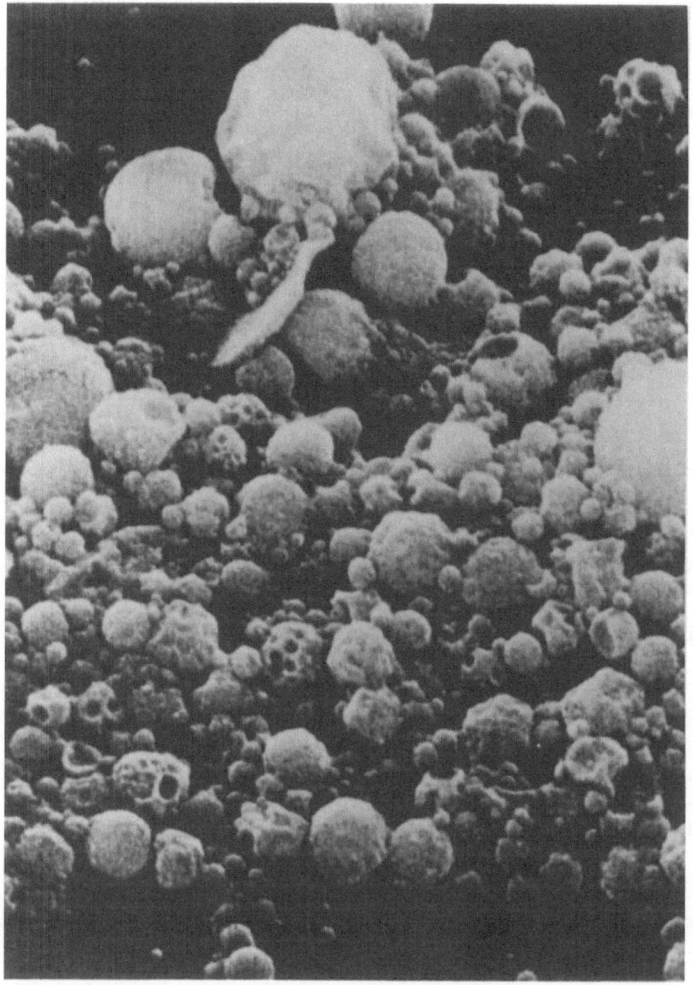

Figure 3. Scanning electron micrograph of VLDF isolated
from the atherosclerotic plaque. The fraction contained
large and small size particles with surface irregularities
and defects. The diameter of the larger particles was
greater than that of serum VLDL and averaged between
1.0 to 2.5 microns (x 22,000).

lipoproteins and averaged about 1.5 μm for VLDF and about
0.5 μm for LDF.

Uptake of Lipid-Protein Complexes by Peritoneal Macrophages
    When mouse peritoneal macrophages were incubated with
LDF or VLDF, they accumulated oil-red-O stainable lipid

droplets and became cholesteryl-ester rich cells (Table 4). The deposition of lipids in the cells increased with increasing concentrations of LDF and VLDF in the incubation medium (Figure 4). In contrast, peritoneal macrophages

Table 4. Free and Esterified Cholesterol Accumulation in Mouse Peritoneal Macrophages Incubated with LDF or VLDF Pretreated with Enzymes

| | Cholesterol (nmol/mg protein) | | | |
| | LDF | | VLDF | |
Incubation	Free	Ester	Free	Ester
Without LDF or VLDF	58	1	62	2
With LDF or VLDF	142	465	163	527
With LDF or VLDF Pre-treated with Pronase	66	2	74	3
With LDF or VLDF Pre-treated with Chondroiti-nases A, B, C and Hyaluronidase	137	454	156	502

Macrophages were incubated as indicated above in the presence and absence of LDF or VLDF at 180 µg protein/mL for 16 hours. Following incubation total cholesterol was measured in macrophage monolayers and esterified cholesterol was calculated as the difference between total and free cholesterol values. The above values are the average of duplicated determinations.

incubated with plasma LDL or VLDL in similar concentrations did not accumulate lipid droplets (data not shown). Chloroquine, a lysosomal inhibitor, enhanced the accumulation of stainable lipids in the macrophages incubated with LDF or VLDF (Figure 5). In contrast to the macrophage, smooth muscle cells isolated from the rabbit and rat aorta showed no lipid droplets when incubated with LDF or VLDF.

The removal of GAGs from LDF and VLDF by digestion with hyaluronidase and chondroitinase ABC prior to incubation did not alter the uptake of these complexes by the macrophage as indicated by the cholesterol content of the macrophages and the percentage of macrophages containing lipid droplets (Table 4, Figure 5). However, when LDF or VLDF was pretreated

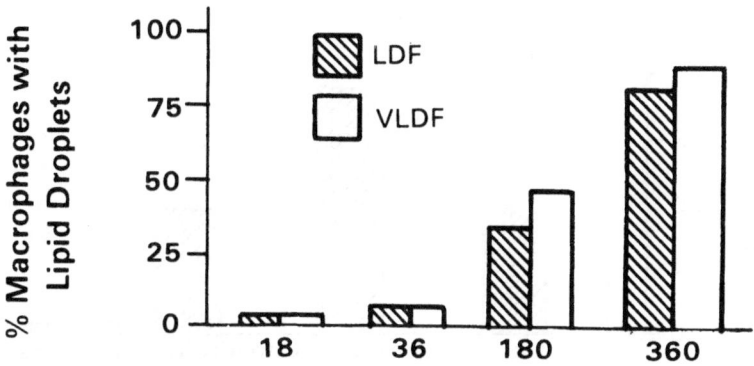

Protein Concentration (µg/ml)

Figure 4. Effect of increasing concentrations of LDF and VLDF on the lipid uptake by mouse peritoneal macrophages. The macrophages were incubated with the indicated concentrations of LDF and VLDF for 16 hours at 37°C. After incubation the cells were fixed, stained with oil-red-O and examined for lipid inclusions.

with pronase, lipid accumulation in the macrophage was completely suppressed (Table 4, Figure 5) suggesting that the uptake of these complexes by the macrophage is mediated through the protein moiety of the lipid protein complexes.

The uptake of the protein components of the lipid-protein complexes by the macrophage was demonstrable by immunofluorescence microscopy (Table 5). The immunoreactive proteins identified in the macrophage following incubation with LDF or VLDF included apo A-I, B, C-III and E as well as IgG and C3. The apoproteins and immune related proteins were detected in the cytoplasm of the macrophage as dense and discrete immunofluorescent deposits in close association

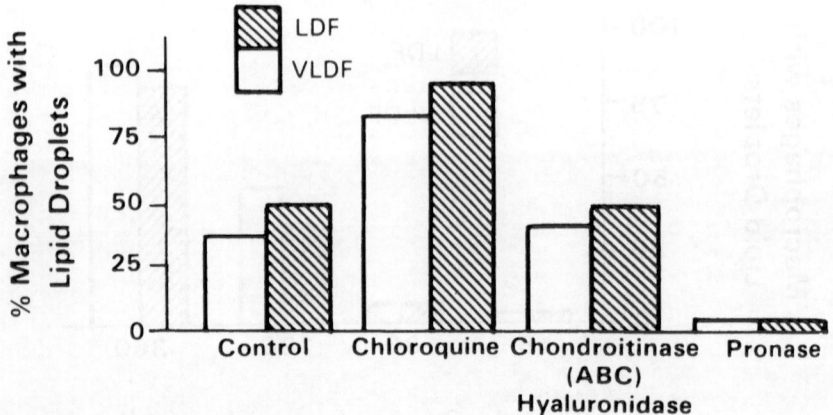

Figure 5. Effect of chloroquine and enzyme treatment of LDF
and VLDF on lipid accumulation in mouse macrophages. Monolayers of peritoneal macrophages were indubated with LDF or
VLDF (180 μg protein/mL) in the absence and presence of
chloroquine (10 μM) for 16 hours at 37°C. Macrophages also
were incubated with LDF or VLDF (180 μg protein/mL) pretreated with pronase (12 units/mg protein) or chondroitinase
ABC (4 units/mg protein) and testicular hyaluronidase (0.02
units/mg protein) for 16 hours at 37°C. The cells were
fixed in Bouin's solution, stained with oil-red-O and examined
for lipid inclusions. The above values are the average of
duplicate incubations.

with the lipids. Immunofluorescent staining for apo A-I,
B, C-III and IgG was not detectable in control macrophages
incubated without LDF or VLDF. Apo E and C3 were detected
inconsistently in a small number of the control cells which
showed faint staining. Similar findings were obtained using
the indirect immunoperoxidase method.

Since the lipid-protein complexes were shown to contain IgG and C3, the following studies were undertaken to
determine whether the complexes might bind to the immune
receptors (Fc and C3b receptors) of the macrophage.

The ability of the lipid-protein complexes (LDF, VLDF)
to inhibit immunophagocytosis of sheep red blood cells

Table 5.   Detection of Immune-Related Proteins and Apo-
           proteins in Mouse Peritoneal Macrophage Pre-
           incubated with LDF or VLDF and in Foam Cells
           Isolated from Atherosclerotic Plaques

Primary Antibody	Method	Mouse Peritoneal Macrophage	Plaque Foam Cell
Goat anti-human IgG, IgM and IgA	D	+	+
Goat anti-human IgG	D,P*	+	+
Goat anti-human C3	D,P	+	+
Protein A	D	+	
Goat anti-apo A	I	+	
Goat anti-apo B	I,P*	+	+
Goat anti-apo C-III	I	+	+
Goat anti-apo E	I,P*	+	
Mouse monoclonal anti-apo A	I*	+	+
Mouse monoclonal anti-apo B	I*,P	+	+
Mouse monoclonal anti-apo E	I*,P	+	+

D = Direct immunofluorescence method
I = Indirect immunofluorescence method
I* = Indirect immunofluorescence using a biotinylated
     secondary antibody and FITC labeled avidin
P = Indirect immunoperoxidase method
* = A biotinylated secondary antibody was used followed by
    staining with labeled avidin

(SRBC) coated with anti-SRBC IgG or IgM-C3 is summarized in
Figures 6 and 7. When the opsonized SRBC were incubated
with peritoneal macrophages in the absense of LDF or VLDF,
they adhered to the surface membrane of the macrophages
and formed rosettes. Large numbers of SRBC also were
ingested and phagocytized by the macrophage. However, when
LDF or VLDF was added to the incubation media, the binding
and phagocytosis of the coated SRBC was significantly
reduced. The inhibition of immunophagocytosis, as indicated

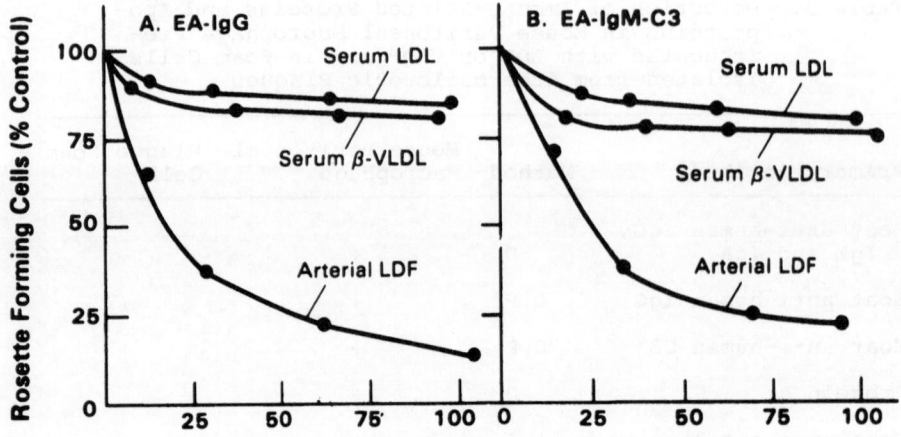

Figure 6. Ability of arterial LDF to inhibit immunophagocytosis of IgG and C3 coated sheep red blood cells by mouse
peritoneal macrophages. Each monolayer of macrophages was
incubated with the indicated concentrations of arterial LDF
and serum LDL and B-VLDL in 0.3 mL of RPMI-1640 containing
1% bovine sheep albumin for 30 minutes at 37ºC.   25 µL of
sheep red blood cells coated with anti-sheep erythrocyte
IgG or IgM-C3 (EA-IgG or EA-IgM-C3) was added in study A
and B respectively and the mixture was indubated for an
additional 60 minutes. The macrophage monolayers were
washed for an additional 60 minutes.   The macrophage monolayers were washed twice with RPMI-BSA, fixed with Bouin's
solution and stained with hematoxylin and eosin. 200 cells
were examined and the percent of macrophages forming
rosettes with sheep red blood cells was determined and
expressed as a percent of the values obtained in control
incubations without competing proteins. Each value represents the average of duplicate incubations.

by the number of rosette forming cells, increased as the
concentration of LDF or VLDF was increased in the incubation
media. In parallel studies serum LDL or B-VLDL had only
about a 15 to 20% inhibitory effect on immunophagocytosis

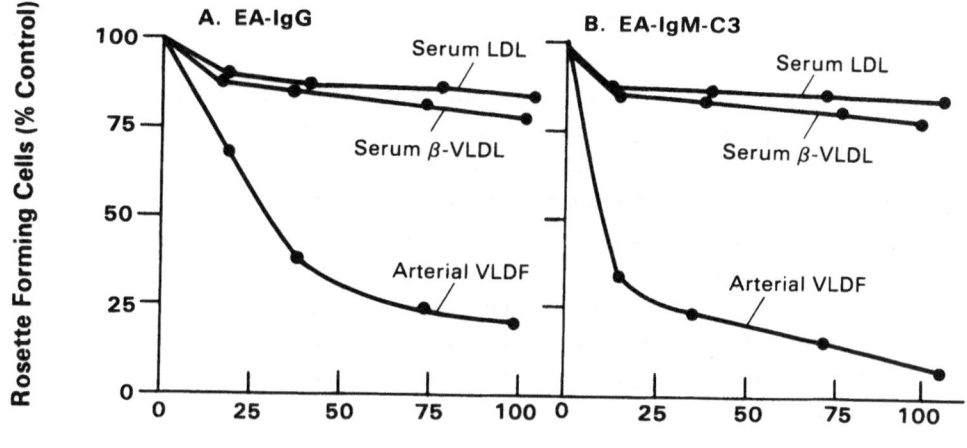

Figure 7. The ability of arterial VLDF to inhibit immunophagocytosis of IgG and C3 coated sheep red blood cells by
mouse peritoneal macrophages. Each monolayer of macrophages
was incubated with the indicated concentration of VLDF,
LDL, and B-VLDL in 0.3 mL of RPMI-1640 containing 1% bovine
serum albumin for 30 minutes at 37°C. 25 µL of sheep red
blood cells coated with anti-sheep erythrocyte IgG or IgM-
C3 (EA-IgG or EA-IgM-C3) was added in study A and B
respectively and the mixture was incubated for an additional
60 minutes. The macrophage monolayers were washed twice
with RPMI-BSA, fixed with Bouin's solution and stained with
hematoxylin and eosin. 200 cells were examined and the
percent of macrophages forming rosettes with the sheep red
blood cells as determined and expressed as a percent of the
values obtained in control incubations without competing
proteins. Each value represents the average of duplicate
incubations.

of the opsonized SRBC (Figures 6 and 7). These initial

studies suggest that the lipid-protein complexes are

capable of binding to the Fc and C3b receptors of the

macrophages.

Protein Composition of Plaque Foam Cells as Compared to the
Lipid-Protein Complexes

Foam cell isolated from atherosclerotic lesions of human
(as well as cynomolgus macaques) appeared to contain proteins
in common with LDF and VLDF and with peritoneal macrophages
pre-incubated with these proteins (Table 5). The proteins
identified in the plaque foam cell by immunofluorescent and
immunoperoxidase methods included IgG and C3 in as well as
apo A-I, B, C-III and E (Table 5).

These proteins were detected in the cytoplasm of the
cells as dense and granular immunofluorescent deposits
closely associated with the lipids.

DISCUSSION
The detection of apoproteins A-I, B, C-III and E in the
lipid-protein complexes (LDF, VLDF) isolated from atherosclerotic plaques suggests that the complexes are derived
from the plasma lipoproteins. The biochemical behavior
and ultrastructural appearance of the lipid-protein complexes
also support earlier studies suggesting that the complexes
represent insoluble and aggregated lipoproteins which have
become metabolically altered (17,18). In addition to
degradative changes in the plaque lipoproteins there is some
evidence for oxidative changes in these lipoproteins (19).

The origin of the lipid-protein complexes in the plaque
has not been established. However, they could be derived
from the lipoproteins taken up and metabolized by the foam
cells or from plasma lipoproteins trapped and metabolized in
the extracellular matrix. The presence of glycosaminoglycans
(GAG) and calcium in the lipid-protein complexes supports the
latter explanation and suggests that the 'trapping' or accumulation of LDF and VLDF in the plaque might be due to the
formation of insoluble lipoprotein-GAG complexes in the
extracellular matrix. The detection of chondroitin sulfate
and hyaluronic acid in the lipid-protein complexes are consistent with prior studies (17,39).

The finding of a high ratio of linoleate to oleate in
the cholesteryl ester fraction of LDF and VLDF also supports
the extracellular origin of the complexes since the ratio is

similar to that of plasma LDL and VLDF and much lower than
the ratio reported in foam cells (40). However, in support
of the foam cell origin of the lipid-protein complexes is the
ultrastructural appearance of the complexes which has some
similarities to that described for the lipid inclusions of
foam cells (32).

The demonstration that LDF and VLDF also contained IgG
and IgM antibodies and complement component C3, suggests
that these complexes may represent complement-fixing auto-
immune complexes in which IgG and IgM classes of antibodies
are directed against the degraded and altered lipoproteins
or apolipoproteins contained in LDF and VLDF. These
findings may be relative to the reports of other workers
(10-12) describing the presence of LDL-antibody immune
complexes in the circulation of humans with hyperlipidemia
and vascular disease. It is noteworthy that homologous
plasma LDL has been shown to be immunogenic after chemical
modification (41).

In addition to the biochemical composition, the
biological behavior of LDF and VLDF appeared to be consistent
with that of a lipoprotein-antibody immune complex. When
peritoneal macrophages were incubated with LDF or VLDF, they
accumulated cholesterol and cholesteryl esters and became
foam cells. Macrophages incubated with LDL-anti apo B immune
complexes also have been reported to respond similarly with
cholesteryl ester accumulation and transformation into foam
cells (12). In contrast to the macrophage, smooth muscle
cells which lack immune receptors did not accumulate lipid
or become foam cells when incubated with LDF or VLDF. These
findings suggest that the lipid-protein complexes, which
constitute more than 90% of the lipoproteins contained in
the plaque, may participate in the formation of macrophage
derived foam cells of the lesion.

The uptake of the LDF and VLDF by the macrophages
appears to be mediated by the protein component of the
complexes since pretreatment of LDF and VLDF with pronase
inhibited lipid deposition in the macrophage. Digestion
of LDF and VLDF with chondroitinases A, B, C and hyaluronidase removed the glycosaminoglycan components of the

complexes but it did not reduce the lipid accumulation in the macrophage. These findings suggest that the uptake of the complexes is not mediated by the dextran sulfate receptors of the macrophage described by Basu and co-workers (42).

The cell surface binding sites that initiate the uptake of the lipid-protein complexes has not been established. The competitive inhibition studies of Goldstein and co-workers indicate that the lipid-protein complexes compete only to a small degree with acetyl LDL for binding to the scavenger receptors of the macrophage (43). The present studies suggest that the complexes may be taken up via immune receptors of the macrophage in a manner similar to that of an immune complex. The findings that the lipid-protein complexes markedly inhibited immunophagocytosis of IgG and C3 coated sheep red blood cells (SRBC) support this interpretation and suggest that the complexes are able to compete with the opsonized SRBC for the Fc and C3b receptors of the macrophage. Conclusive evidence that LDF and VLDF are taken up via the immune receptors awaits the demonstration that the uptake of these complexes is inhibited by blockade of the immune receptors with specific antibodies.

The lipid-protein complexes, when taken up by the macrophages, appeared to be incompletely metabolized since the protein components of the complexes were detected in the cell after incubation with the macrophages. These proteins also were identified in the foam cells isolated from the atherosclerotic plaques and they included apoproteins A-I, B, C-III and E as well as IgG and C3. These and other findings discussed above are consistent with the concept that the lipid-protein complexes may be taken up and deposited in macrophage derived foam cells of the plaque as lipoprotein-antibody immune complexes. The presence of apo B and E in plaque foam cells also have been described by other workers (44,45). Apoprotein E as well as C3 could be natural protein components of foam cells derived from macrophages since these proteins have been shown to be synthesized and secreted by normal macrophages (46-48). Recently the synthesis of apoprotein E by smooth muscle cells also has been demonstrated (49), and thus, apo E also could be a natural component of smooth muscle derived foam cells. It is noteworthy that these same studies were unable to detect synthesis of apo A-I and apo B by aortic smooth muscle cells or macrophages.

REFERENCES

1. Hollander W, Colombo MA, Kramsch DM, and Kirkpatrick BJ (1974) Immunological aspects of atherosclerosis. Comparative pathology of the heart. Adv Cardiol 13: 192-207.
2. Hollander W, Colombo MA, Kirkpatrick BJ, Paddock J (1979) Soluble proteins in the human atherosclerotic plaque: With special reference to immunoglobulins, C3 complement component, α_1-antitrypsin and α_2-macroglobulin. Atherosclerosis 34:391-405.
3. Parums D, Mitchinson MJ (1981) Demonstration of immunoglobulin in the neighborhood of advanced atherosclerotic plaques. Atherosclerosis 38:211-216.
4. Hansson GK, Holm J, Kral JG (1984) Accumulation of IgG and complement factor C3 in human arterial endothelium and atherosclerotic lesions. Acta Pathol Microbiol Immunol Scand 92:429-435.
5. Vlaicu R, Rus HG, Niculescu F, Cristea A (1985) Immunoglobulins and complement components in human aortic atherosclerotic intima. Atherosclerosis 55:35-50.
6. Rus HG, Niculescu F, Constantinescu E, Cristea A, Vlaicu R (1986) Immunoelectron-microscopic localization of the terminal C5b-9 complement complex in human atherosclerotic fibrous plaque. Atherosclerosis 6: 35-42.
7. Schwartz CJ, Mitchell JRA (1962) Cellular infiltration of the human arterial adventitia associated with atheromatous plaques. Circulation 26:73-78.
8. Stratford N, Britten K, Gallagher P (1986) Inflammatory infiltrates in human coronary atherosclerosis. Atherosclerosis 59:271-276.
9. Jonasson L, Holm J, Skalli O, Bondjers G, Hansson GK (1986) Regional accumulations of T cells, macrophages and smooth muscle cells in the human atherosclerotic plaque. Arteriosclerosis 6:131-138.
10. Beaumont JL (1970) Autoimmune hyperlipidemia. In: Jones RJ (ed) Atherosclerosis. Berlin: Springer-Verlag, pp 166-176.
11. Szondy E, Horvath M, Mezey Z, Szekely J, Lengyel E, Fust G, Gero S (1983) Free and complexed anti-lipoprotein antibodies in vascular diseases. Atherosclerosis 49:67-77.
12. Klimov AN, Denisenko AD, Popov AV, Nagornev VA, Pleskov VM, Vinogradov AG, Densisenko TV, Magracheva EY, Kheifes GM, Kuznetzov AS (1985) Lipoprotein-antibody immune complexes: Their catabolism and role in foam cell formation. Atherosclerosis 58:1-15.

13. Romano EL, Camejo G, Soyano A (1984) Circulating immune complexes and antibodies to dietary antigens in patients with occlusive coronary lesions. Atherosclerosis 53:119.

14. Shingu M, Hurd ER (1981) Sera from patients with systemic lupus erythematosus reactive with human endothelial cells. J Rheumatol 8:581.

15. Caplan M, Hastillo A, Hess ML (1984) Immunologic mechanism in atherosclerotic process. Cardiovas Rev 5:713.

16. Preston RN (1979) Immunological aspects of atherosclerosis: A review. J Royal Soc Med 72:674.

17. Hollander W, Paddock J, Colombo MA (1979) Lipoproteins in human atherosclerotic vessels. I. Biochemical properties of arterial low density lipoproteins, very low density lipoproteins, and high density lipoproteins. Exp Mol Pathol 30:144-171.

18. Hollander W, Paddock J, Colombo MA (1979) Lipoproteins in human atherosclerotic vessels. II. Biochemical properties of the major apolipoproteins of arterial low density and very low density lipoproteins. Exp Mol Pathol 30:172-189.

19. Ball RY, Bindman JP, Carpenter KLH, Mitchinson MJ (1986) Oxidized low density lipoprotein induces caroid accumulation by murine peritoneal macrophages *in vitro*. Atherosclerosis 60:173-181.

20. Havel RJ, Eder HA, Bragdon JH (1955) The distribution and chemical composition of ultracentrifugally separated lipoproteins in human serum. J Clin Invest 34:1345-1353.

21. Schoenheimer R, Sperry WM (1934) A micromethod for the determination of free and combined cholesterol. J Biol Chem 106:745-760.

22. Youngberg GE, Youngberg MV (1930) Phosphorus metabolism. I. A system of blood phosphorus analysis. J Lab Clin Med 16:158-166.

23. Van Handel E, Zilversmit DB (1957) Micromethod for the direct determination of serum triglycerides. J Lab Clin Med 50:152.

24. Lowry OH, Rosebrough NJ, Farr AL, Randall RJ (1951) Protein measurement with the Folin reagent. J Biol Chem 193:265-275.

25. Metcalfe LD, Schmitz AA (1961) The rapid preparation of fatty acid esters for gas chromatographic analysis. Anal Chem 33:363-364.

26. Stevens RL, Colombo MA, Gonzales JJ, Hollander W, Schmid K (1976) The glycosaminoglycans of the human artery and their changes in atherosclerosis. J Clin Invest 58:470.

27. Hata R, Nagai Y (1973) A micro colorometric determination of acidic glycosaminoglycans by two-dimensional electrophoresis on a cellulose acetate strip. Anal Biochem 52:652.

28. Noble RP (1968) Electrophoretic separation of plasma lipoproteins in agarose gel. J Lipid Res 9:693.

29. Weber D, Osborn M (1969) The reliability of molecular weight determinations by duodecyl-sulphate polyacrylamide gel electrophoresis. J Biol Chem 244:4405-4412.

30. Ouchterlony O (1958) Diffusion-in-gel methods for immunological analysis. Progr Allergy 5:1-78.

31. Scheidegger JJ (1955) Une micro-method de l' immunoelectrophorese. Int Arch Allergy 7:103-110.

32. Insull W Jr, Hata Y (1971) Morphology of lipid rich organelles in tissues of man and rat. Proc IV Annual Scanning Electron Microscope Symposium, pp 337-341.

33. Edelson PJ, Cohn ZA (1976) Purification and cultivation of monocytes and macrophages. In: Bloom BR, David JR (eds) In vitro Methods in Cell-Mediated and Tumor Immunity. New York: Academic Press, Inc, pp 333-340.

34. Oakes BW, Batty AC, Handley CJ, Sandberg LB (1982) The synthesis of elastin, collagen, glycosaminoglycans by high density primary cultures of neonatal rat aortic smooth muscle: An ultrastructural and biochemical study. European J Cell 27:34-46.

35. Schaffner T, Taylor K. Burtucci EJ, Fisher-Dzoga K, Beeson JH, Glagov S, Wissler RW (1980) Arterial foam cells with distinctive immunomorphological and histochemical features of macrophages. Amer J Pathol 100:57.

36. Gamble W, Vaughn M, Avigan J (1978) Procedure for determination of free and total cholesterol in cultured cells. J Lipid Res 19:1068.

37. Griffin FM, Silverstein SC (1974) Segment response of the macrophage plasma membrane to a phagocytic stimulus. J Exp Med 139:323.

38. Coons AH, Kaplan MH (1950) Localization of antigen in tissue cells, Part 2. Improvements in a method for the detection of antigen by means of fluorescent antibody. J Exp Med 91:1

39. Srinivasan SR, Dolan P, Radhakrishnamurtry B, Berenson GS (1972) Isolation of lipoprotein-acid-mucopoly-saccharide complexes from fatty streaks of human aorta. Atherosclerosis 16:95-104.

40. Smith EB, Evans PH, Downham MD (1967) Lipid in the aortic intima: The correlation of morphological and chemical characteristics. J Atheroscler Res 7:171-186.

41. Steinbrecher UP, Fischer M, Witztum JL, Curtiss LK (1984) Immunogenicity of homologous low density lipoprotein after methylation, ethylation, acetylation and carbamylation. Generation of antibodies specific for derived lysine. J Lipid Res 24:1109.

42. Basu S, Brown MS, Ho YK, Goldstein JL (1979) Degradation of low density lipoprotein-dextran sulfate complexes associated with deposition of cholesteryl esters in mouse macrophages. J Biol Chem 254:7141.

43. Goldstein JL, Hoff HF, Yo YK, Basu S, Brown MS (1981) Stimulation of cholesteryl ester synthesis in macrophages by extracts of atherosclerotic human aortas and complexes of albumin/cholesteryl esters. Arteriosclerosis 1:210.

44. Yomantas S, Elner VM, Schaffner T, Wissler RW (1984) Immunohistochemical localization of apolipoprotein B in human atherosclerotic lesions. Arch Pathol Lab Med 108:374-378.

45. Murase T, Oka T, Yamada N, Mori N, Ishibashi S, Takaku F, Mori W (1986) Immunohistochemical localization of apolipoprotein E in atherosclerotic lesions of the aorta and coronary arteries. Atherosclerosis 60:1-6.
46. Nathan CF, Murray HW, Cohn ZA (1980) The macrophage as an effector cell. New Engl J Med 303:622-626.
47. Basu SK, Ho YK, Brown MS, Bilheimer DW, Anderson RW, Goldstein JL (1982) Biochemical and genetic studies of the apoprotein E secreted by mouse macrophages and human monocytes. J Biol Chem 257:9788-9795.
48. Werb Z, Chin JR (1983) Apoprotein E is synthesized by resident and thioglycollate-elicited macrophages but not by pyran copolymer of bacillus Calmette-Guerin activated macrophages. J Exp Med 158:1271-1293.
49. Driscoll DM, Getz GS (1984) Extrahepatic synthesis of apolipoprotein E. J Lipid Res 25:1368-1379.

15
Mechanisms of Calcification in Atherosclerosis

H.C. Anderson, D.H. McGregor and A. Tanimura

INTRODUCTION

Calcification of atherosclerotic plaque is widely
regarded by physicians and pathologists as a late manifestation of atherosclerosis. Such an attitude accords more
importance to the early events in atherogenesis, and fails
to properly take into account the morbidity-producing
potential of arterial calcification. Although there is some
evidence to suggest a degree of reversibility in mostly
lipid plaques, once infiltration of the plaque by insoluble
calcium phosphate salts has occurred, there may be little
likelihood of spontaneous reversal. Furthermore, the persistence of rigid mineral in the plaque causes a drastic
loss of local arterial elasticity, and may add permanence
and inflexibility to intimal surface irregularities which
in turn may promote local blood stasis, turbulence and
thrombus formation. Finally, breakdown of endothelial
integrity and arterial structure might be expected to occur
most frequently in association with rigid, calcified atherosclerotic plaques. The breakdown of endothelium exposes
blood to extrinsic factors of the coagulation cascade, and
is often associated with local thrombogenesis. Thrombogenesis may be tolerated in wide-bore arteries such as aorta,
but it severely compromises flow in smaller arteries, e.g.,
coronary and cerebral arteries, with devastating effects.
Therefore, there seems little justification to underestimate
the disease-producing potential of the calcification process
in atherosclerotic plaques.

Research supported by NIH Grant DE 05262

An interesting new development in mineralization research has been the discovery that there are similar features to the calcification process occurring in a variety of cardiovascular conditions including atherosclerotic plaque (1-5) arterial medial sclerosis (6), calcific cardiac valvular stenosis (7,8), and the calcification of bioprosthetic heart valves (9), and of pseudoneointima lining artificial heart and left ventricular assist devices (10). Indeed, a wide range of so-called pathological calcifications occurring at diverse sites share these features (11), including such calcific diseases as crystal deposition arthritis, calcifying tendonitis, calcinosis cutis, tympanosclerosis, and dental plaque and calculus. As a rule, all of these calcifications are brought about by the deposition of the same mineral salt, i.e., calcium phosphate, in the form of poorly crystaline hydroxyapatite, a molecule with 10 calcium atoms, 6 phosphates and 2 hydroxyls in the unit cell (12). Once formed, apatite crystals are highly insoluble in body fluids at physiological pH. They proliferate autocatalytically by homogeneous nucleation (a process in which initial crystals serve as nuclei or seeds for the formation of new crystals) in the presence or physiological concentrations of Ca^{2+} and PO_4^{3-} in the extracellular fluid (ECF).

A second common feature of virtually all forms of cardiovascular calcification is hydroxyapatite crystal initiation in association with cellular membranes, usually in the form of extracellular vesicles (11). Because of this common finding, an analogy has been drawn to the mechanism of skeletal calcification, described briefly in the next section, in which extracellular, cell-derived matrix vesicles serve as the initial submicroscopic site for hydroxyapatite mineral deposition (13,14). Studies of skeletal calcification have a long history, and are seemingly more advanced at present than studies of arterial calcification. Therefore, hypotheses and experimental techniques used to study skeletal calcification may be applicable to investigations of cardiovascular calcification.

Skeletal Calcification as a Model for Cardiovascular
Calcification

It is perhaps easiest to see and comprehend the basic
features of the mechanism of calcification of bones, cartilage and dentin by an examination of the process as it
occurs in the epiphyseal growth plate of growing long
bones (Figure 1). This is because there exists a unique
spacial orientation and geometric layering of cells and
matrix in the growth plate that reflects the timing of
cellular events in mineralization, i.e., the layering localizes progressive stages of the calcification process. In a
simplified view, extracellular vesicles are formed by
budding or perhaps selective cell disaggregation (13,14) in
upper levels of the growth plate, shortly after the cartilage
cells have undergone division. The exfoliated vesicles, (now
termed "matrix vesicles") are locked into the matrix by the
synthesis and deposition of new extracellular material consisting of a network of closely applied, small-diameter
collagen fibrils, and interspersed proteoglycan macromolecules. The first observable crystals of hydroxyapatite
appear by electron microscopy as electron-dense needles
within matrix vesicles (Figure 2). The crystals usually lie
against the inner surface of the vesicle membrane bilayer.

Phase I of calcification (Figure 2) is concerned with
the formation of the first crystals. The interior of the
matrix vesicle near its membrane is a favored site for first
crystal formation. Local factors that promote mineralization
at this site include: 1) the presence of a high concentration of calcium-binding acidic phospholipids (e.g., phosphatidyl serine) within the matrix vesicle membranes (15,16);
and 2) the increased activity of phosphatases, including
alkaline phosphatase (ALP) and related phosphatases, as the
vesicles approach the mineralization front (17). Matrix
vesicles are highly enriched in alkaline phosphatase, 5'-
AMPase, ATPase, inorganic pyrophosphatase and nucleoside
triphosphate pyrophosphohydrolase (17-22). These enzymes
are an integral part of the structure of the vesicle membrane (17,23-25). Although the exact molecular architecture
of the matrix vesicle membrane has not been elucidated, it
is likely that most of the required factors which are

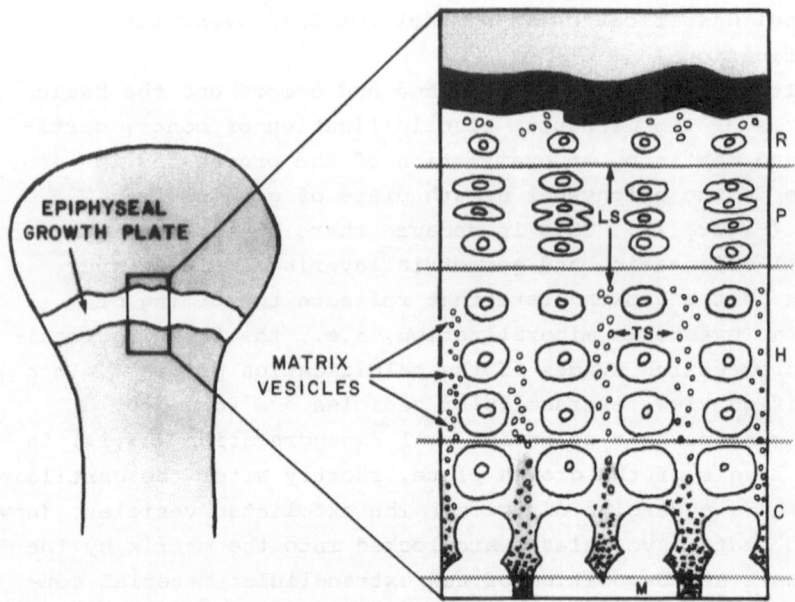

Figure 1. Diagram of the epiphyseal growth plate of a long
bone, the site at which growth in length occurs. The growth
plate is subdivided into the following anatomical regions:
The reserve zone (R), at the top of the growth plate, contains apparently inactive chondrocytes. The proliferative
zone (P) is a zone of active cell division where cell columns
first appear, thus allowing the matrix to be anatomically
subdivided into transverse matrix septa (TS), separating
cells within a column, and longitudinal septa (LS), separating
adjacent cell columns. The hypertropic zone (H) contains
enlarging chondrocytes and many matrix vesicles, found in
clusters in the longitudinal septa. The first mineral crystals arise within matrix vesicles of the hypertrophic zone
(see Figure 2). The calcifying zone (C) contains degenerating
chondrocytes. This is the level at which proliferating
mineral spreads from matrix vesicles radially outward to
infiltrate the interstices of the longitudinal septal matrix.
At the base of the growth plate lies the bony metaphysis (M)
with small vessels which remove the uncalcified transverse
matrix septa and degenerate cells, and leaving calcified
longitudinal septa upon which osteoblasts from the marrow
will deposit new bone (the primary spongiosa). (Reprinted
from "Calcium in Biological Systems", Plenum Publishing Corp.,
1985).

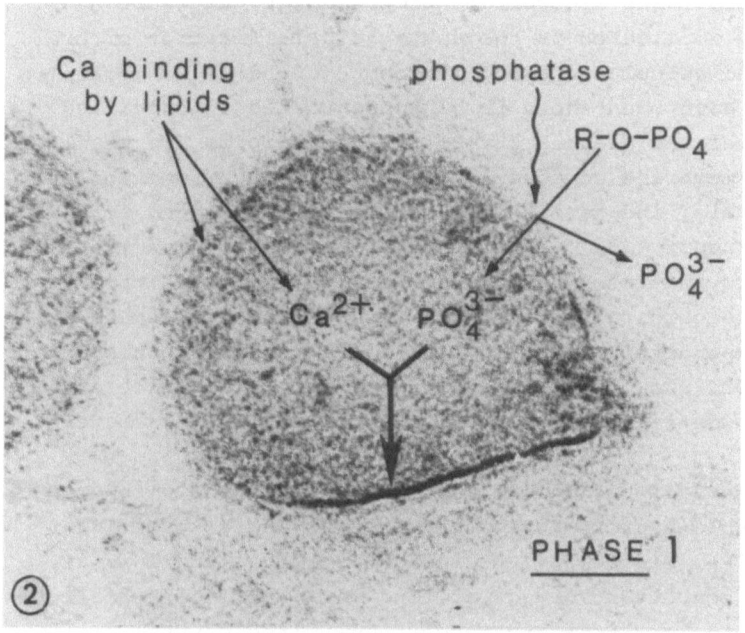

Figure 2. Scheme for mineralization in matrix vesicles. During phase 1, intravesicular calcium concentration is increased by its affinity for lipids of vesicle membrane and interior. Phosphatase (e.g., alkaline phosphatase, pyrophosphatase or adenosine triphosphatase) at the vesicle membrane acts on ester phosphate of matrix fluid or sap to produce a local increase in PO_4 concentration. These enzymes also might function as phosphotransferases, transferring PO_4 across the vesicle membrane. The intravesicular ionic product (Ca^{2+} x PO_4^{3-}) is thereby raised, resulting in initial deposition of $CaPO_4$ near membrane. (Uranyl acetate-lead citrate, reprinted with modification from Metab Bone Dis and Rel Res 1:83, 1978).

necessary to initiate mineralization are contained within this diaphanous bilayer.

It is important to note that calcification-promoting lipids, in addition to phosphatidyl serine, have been found in high concentration in matrix vesicles. Prominent among these are the calcium-phosphate-phospholipid complexes ($Ca-PO_4-PL$) seen in many types of skeletal and apatitic pathological calcifications (26-28). $Ca-PO_4-PL$ can initiate hydroxyapatite mineral deposition into metastable, serum-like calcium phosphate solutions, without enzymatic activity or an expenditure of energy (29). Also present in matrix

vesicle membranes are certain proteolipids that were
initially implicated in the apatitic calcification of oral,
plaque and calculus-causing microbes (30-33). Proteolipids
recently have been shown to be concentrated in calcified
atherosclerotic plaques (34,35). Proteolipids are usually
integral membrane components where they often function as
ion channels, and have been shown to be associated with
PO_4^{3-} transport (36). Bone proteolipids also have the
ability to initiate *in vitro* hydroxyapatite deposition from
serum-like calcifying solutions without phosphatase activity
or any expenditure of energy (31). As a part of this conference Dr. Daoud will discuss the presence and role of
proteolipids in atherosclerotic calcification in greater
detail.

Phase 2 of biological calcification begins with exposure
of insoluble hydroxyapatite crystals to the extracellular
fluid (ECF) (Figure 3). As indicated above, there is an
adequate concentration of Ca^{2+} and PO_4^{3-}, homeostatically
supplied in most ECFs, to support unlimited crystal proliferation. Under experimental *in vitro* conditions mineral
deposition continues until the supply of Ca^{2+} and PO_4^{3-} is
exhausted. Fortunately for the living animal there are many
extracellular factors which tend to limit and control the
rate and extent of Phase 2 calcification. Otherwise the
entire organism might become calcified by this relentless,
autocatalytic, physiochemical process. Among known factors
controlling progressive mineralization are: 1) Local ECF
pH which tends to be slightly elevated in growth plate
cartilage fluid (37). At non-skeletal sites a lower pH
would tend to retard mineral formation; 2) Proteoglycan
aggregates, which impede mineral deposition (38). Proteoglycan aggregates are decreased at mineralization sites in
the growth plate (38-40) and this tends to promote skeletal
mineralization; 3) Non-collagenous proteins with calcium-
binding affinity which also impede hydroxyapatite formation,
e.g., bone gla-protein (BGP), also known as "osteonectin"
(41,42), phosphoproteins (43), and the more recently
described "osteonectin" (42), which is believed to constitute
a bond between bone collagen and hydroxyapatite (44). None
of these skeletal calcium binding proteins has been shown

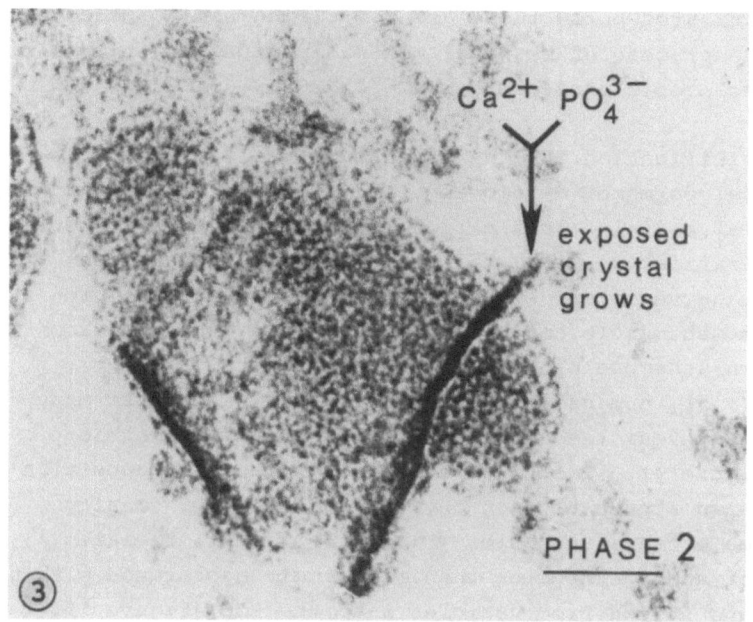

Figure 3. With accumulation and growth, intravesicular crystals are exposed to the extravesicular environment. Phase 2 begins with exposure of preformed apatite crystals to extravesicular fluid, which in normal animals is super-saturated with respect to apatite, enabling further crystal proliferation. Matrix vesicles pictured are in rat growth plate cartilage. (Uranyl acetate-lead citrate, reprinted with modification from Metab Bone Dis and Rel Res 1:83, 1978).

to initiate mineralization *in vivo* and all are known to impede hydroxyapatite mineral deposition *in vitro* (41-43); 4) Crystal-inhibiting polyphosphate molecules such as inorganic pyrophosphate (45), ATP (46) and the synthetic diphosphonates. The polyphosphates appear to "coat" crystal surfaces, thus preventing further crystal proliferation; and 5) Collagen, which in its native form is believed to promote apatite nucleation (47,48), and clearly plays a role in spacially orienting the newly formed crystals (48,49). It is likely that more than 99% of bone mineral is formed during Phase 2, i.e., during the phase of crystal proliferation. Thus all of the factors listed above can be expected to play important roles in the regulation of the calcification process.

As indicated below there are compelling similarities between the process of skeletal mineralization and that seen in atherosclerotic mineralization.

Initial Calcification in Atherosclerosis

Several forms of cardiovascular calcification, including arterial medial calcification (6,50) and atherosclerotic plaque calcification (1-4), are initiated in association with membrane vesicles derived from degenerate cells, presumably smooth muscle cells (Table 1). This has been shown to occur in atherosclerotic lesions of rabbits (3,5), chickens (3,5), humans (1-4), and swine (1). At first many extracellular vesicles cluster at the borders of elastic fibers (Figure 4). The first evidence of mineral deposition is seen as an apparently non-crystalline electron density within some of these vesicles (Figure 4). Small radial clusters of apatite needles then make their appearance within vesicles and spread from vesicles into the ECF (Figure 5). Clusters of apatite crystals grow radially by accumulation of new crystals at their surfaces to form larger mineral

Table 1. Extracellular Membrane-Vesicles in Cardiovascular Calcification

Site	Species	Authors
Aortic media	Human	Kim (6), Staubesand (50)
Aortic valve	Human	Kim and Huang (7), Kim et al. (8)
Pseudoneointima	Blood pump	Harasaki (10)
Bioprosthetic valve	Porcine	Schoen (9)
Atherosclerotic plaque	Human	Paegel (2), Tanimura (3-5)
	Rabbit	Tanimura (3-5)
	Chicken	Tanimura (3-5)
	Swine	Daoud (1)

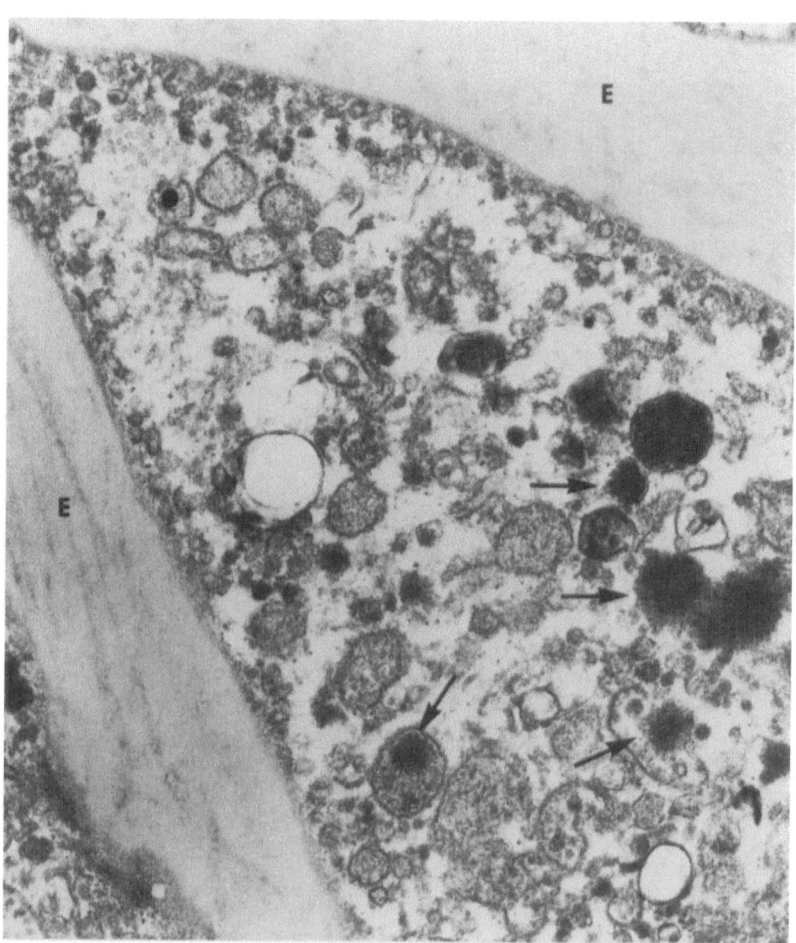

Figure 4. Human aortic intima. Adjacent to divergent
elastic fibers (E) are many small, intermediate and large
vesicles. The vesicles are limited by a single trilaminar
membrane and contain granular and globuler electron dense
material. There are associated clusters of electron dense
apparent mineral (arrows) within the vesicles and dispersed
among vesicles (x 78,000). (From Tanimura, et al., J Exp
Pathol 2:261, 1986).

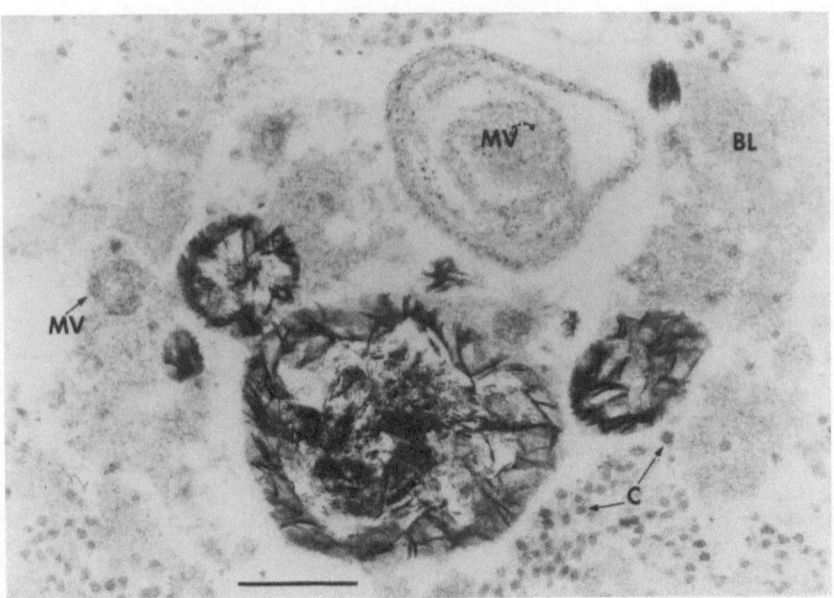

Figure 5. Chicken aortic intima, after three months of atherogenic diet. Several globular crystalline deposits, consistent with calcium hydroxyapatite, are seen in the extracellular matrix which also contains basal lamina-like material (BL), transected collagen fibrils (C) and a multi-lamellar vesicle-like structure (MV) studded with small electron dense particles. Bar = 0.5 μ. (x 79,000). (From Tanimura, et al., J Exp Pathol 2:275, 1986).

aggregates. The aggregates fuse to complete the mineralization of most intervening space. All of these features parallel what is seen in skeletal calcification.

There are notable differences, however, between calcifying arterial and skeletal matrix vesicles. Although skeletal matrix vesicles, particularly those of cartilage, are heterogeneous in size, shape and internal density (13), the arterial vesicles are even more variable in structure. This may be due to the fact that most arterial vesicles are presumed to be derived as cell debris from disrupted cells, while many skeletal matrix vesicles are thought to bud directly from the surface in intact cells. Skeletal matrix vesicles are enriched in alkakine phosphatase (ALP) and related phosphoesterases which have been shown to promote mineral initiation in a variety of *in vitro* systems (51-57). Although Tanimura and associates have demonstrated both ATPase and ALP in membranes of calcifying atherosclerotic vesicles by cytochemistry, these arterial vesicles have never been isolated, and thus the presence of phosphoesterase is not as yet biochemically confirmed. Finally, while the skeletal matrix vesicles are not particularly enriched in mitochondrial enzymes (51) and do not resemble mitochondria ultrastructurally, the calcifying cell debris of arterial intima, being derived from broken cells, may contain exocytosed mitochondria (7). Mitochondria have a well-known ability to concentrate calcium and phosphate to the point of mineral deposition (58,59).

Thus, there are a number of apparent structural and functional differences between skeletal and arterial matrix vesicles that may serve as the basis for real differences in their mechanisms of calcification. It will be possible to test these differences or similarities when methods are developed to study the biochemical and mineralizing properties of arterial vesicles in isolation, or under more defined conditions.

In the meantime, the phospholipids and proteolipids of atherosclerotic lesions have been extracted and studied in significant detail. Both $Ca-PO_4-PL$ (27) and proteolipid (34,35) have been shown to be present. Either or both could play an important role in mineral initiation. Although the subcellular location(s) of $Ca-PO_4-PL$ and proteolipid has not been determined, it is quite likely that proteolipid is associated with cellular membranes, as is the case with most biologically active proteolipids. Dr. Daoud has produced interesting new data (presented in this workshop) in which phospholipids and proteolipids of swine atheromas were extracted, separated biochemically and partially characterized. He has shown that these proteolipids can nucleate apatite *in vitro*. Thus, the stage seems to be set and methods at hand for a first look at the molecular structure and function of arterial "matrix vesicles" as related to calcification.

In the opinion of this author, experimentation directed toward an understanding of atherosclerotic calcification should be approached from the point of view of testing the

"vesicle hypothesis" of calcification which may be stated
as follows: In most instances of biological calcification,
i.e., in all normal skeletal tissues and in many calcific
diseases (such as atherosclerosis), mineral is initiated by
the action of membrane. Even if the vesicle hypothesis is
disproved for atherosclerotic calcification, it can nevertheless serve as a useful conceptual model designing experiments
for analysis of the mechanism of this form of pathological
calcification. New understanding of this phase of plaque
evolution will doubtless emerge.

REFERENCES

1. Daoud AS, Frank AS, Jarmolych J, Franco WT, Fritz KE
   (1985) Ultrastructural and elemental analyses of
   calcification of advanced aortic atherosclerosis.
   Exp Mol Pathol 43:687-697.
2. Paegel RD (1969) Ultrastructure of calcium deposits
   in atherosclerotic human aortas. J Ultrastr Res 26:
   412-423.
3. Tanimura A, McGregor DH, Anderson HC (1983) Matrix
   vesicles in atherosclerotic calcification. Proc Soc
   Exp Biol and Med 172:173-177.
4. Tanimura A, McGregor DH, Anderson HC (1986) Calcification in atherosclerosis. I. Human studies. J Exp
   Pathol 2:261-273.
5. Tanimura A, McGregor DH, Anderson HC (1986) Calcification in atherosclerosis. II. Animal studies. J
   Exp Pathol 2:275-297.
6. Kim KM (1976) Calcification of matrix vesicles in
   human aortic valve and aortic media. Fed Proc 35:
   156-162.
7. Kim KM, Huang SN (1972) Ultrastructural study of
   dystrophic calcification of human aortic valve. Lab
   Invest 26:481-482.
8. Kim KM, Yaligoresky JM, Mergner WJ, Jones RG, Pendergrass,
   RF, Trump BF (1976) Aging changes in the human aortic
   valve in relation to dystrophic calcification. Human
   Pathol 7:47-60.
9. Schoen FJ, Levy RJ, Nelson AC, Bernhard WF, Nashef A,
   Hawley M (1985) Mechanisms and progression of experimental bioprosthetic heart valve calcification. Lab
   Invest 52:523-532.
10. Harasaki H, Murray JD, McMahon J, Kiraly RJ, Fields A,
    Nose Y (1981) Calficication in left ventricular
    assist devices. Artificial Organs 5 (suppl):497-503.
11. Anderson HC (1983) Calcific diseases: A concept. Arch
    Pathol and Lab Med 107:341-348.
12. Posner AS (1969) Crystal chemistry of bone mineral.
    Physiol Rev 49:760-792.
13. Anderson HC (1969) Vesicles associated with calcifi-
    cation in the matrix of epiphyseal cartilage. J Cell
    Biol 41:59-72.
14. Bonucci E (1970) Fine structure and histochemistry of
    calcifying globules in epiphyseal cartilage. Z
    Zellforsch and Mikr Anat 103:192-217.

15. Peress NS, Anderson HC, Sajdera SW (1974) The lipids of matrix vesicles from bovine fetal epiphyseal cartilage. Calcif Tiss Res 14:275-281.
16. Wuthier RE (1975) Lipid composition of isolated carti-lage cells, membranes and matrix vesicles. Biochem Biophys Acta 409:128-143.
17. Matsuzawa T, Anderson HC (1971) Phosphatases of epiphy-seal cartilage studied by electron microscopic cyto-chemical methods. J Histochem and Cytochem 19:801-808.
18. Akisaka T, Gay CV (1985) Ultrastructural localization of calcium-activated adenosine triphosphatase (Ca+-ATPase) in growth plate cartilage. J Histochem and Cytochem 33:925-932.
19. Ali SY, Sajdera SW, Anderson HC (1970) Isolation and characterization of calcifying matrix vesicles from epiphyseal cartilage. Proc Natl Acad Sci USA 67:1513-1520.
20. Anderson HC, Matsuzawa T, Sajdera SW, Ali SY (1970) Membranous particles in calcifying cartilage matrix. Trans NY Acad Sci (Series II) 32:619-630.
21. Hsu HHT (1983) Purification and partial characterization of ATP pyrophosphohydrolase from fetal bovine epiphyseal cartilage. J Biol Chem 258:3463-3468.
22. Siegel SA, Hummel CF, Carty RP (1983) The role of nucleoside triphosphate pyrophosphohydrolase in *in vitro* nucleoside triphosphate-dependent matrix vesicle calci-fication. J Biol Chem 258:8601-8607.
23. Hsu HHT, Anderson HC (1978) Calcification of isolated matrix vesicles and reconstituted vesicles from fetal bovine cartilage. Proc Natl Acad Sci USA 75:3805-3808.
24. Kanabe S, Hsu HHT, Cecil RNA, Anderson HC (1983) Electron microscopic localization of adenosine triphos-phate (ATP)-hydrolysing activity in isolated matrix vesicles and reconstituted vesicles from calf cartilage. J Histochem and Cytochem 31:462-470.
25. Sajdera SW, Franklin S, Fortuna R (1976) Matrix vesicles of bovine fetal cartilage: Metabolic potential and solubilization with detergents. Fed Proc 35:154-155.
26. Boskey AL, Bullough PG (1984) Cartilage calcification: Normal and aberrant. Scan Elec Micros II:943-952.
27. Dimitrovsky E, Boskey AL, Minick CR, Posner AS (1981) Lipids associated with aortic calcification. Calcif Tiss Internat 33:314.
28. Wuthier RE, Gore ST (1977) Partition of inorganic ions and phospholipids in isolated cell, membrane and matrix vesicle fractions: Evidence for Ca-Pi-acidic phospho-lipid complexes. Calcif Tiss Res 24:163-171.
29. Boskey AL, Posner AS (1977) *In vitro* nucleation of hydroxyapatite by a bone calcium-phospholipid-phosphate complex. Calcif Tiss Res 22(5):197-201.
30. Boyan-Salyers BD, Boskey AL (1980) Relationship between proteolipids and calcium-phospholipid-phosphate complexes in *Bacterionema matruchotii* calcification. Calcif Tiss Intern 30:167-174.
31. Boyan BD, Landis WJ, Knight J, Dereszewski G, Zeagler J (1985) Microbial hydroxyapatite formation as a mode of proteolipid-dependent membrane-mediated calcification. Scan Elec Micros IV:1793-1800.

32. Ennever J, Vogel JJ, Rider LJ, Boyan-Salyers B (1976) Nucleation of microbiologic calcification by proteolipid. Proc Soc Exp Biol Med 152:147-150.
33. Ennever J, Boyan-Salyers B, Riggan LJ (1977) Proteolipid and bone matrix calcification. J Dent Res 56:967-970.
34. Romeo R, Augustyn JM, Fritz KE, Daoud AS (1984) Characterization of an apatite-inducing proteolipid from human aortic lesions. Arteriosclerosis 4:529a.
35. Ennever J, Vogel JJ, Riggan LJ (1980) Calcification by proteolipid from atherosclerotic aorta. Atherosclerosis 35:209-213.
36. Kessler RJ, Vaughn DA (1984) Divalent metal is required for both phosphate transport and phosphate binding to phosphorin, a proteolipid isolated from brush border membrane vesicle. J Biol Chem 259:9059-9063.
37. Howell DS, Pita JC, Marquez JF, Madruga JE (1968) Partition of calcium phosphate and protein in the fluid phase aspirated at calcifying sites in epiphyseal cartilage. J Clin Invest 47:1121-1132.
38. Cuervo LA, Pita JC, Howell DS (1973) Inhibition of calcium phosphate mineral growth by proteoglycan aggregate fractions in a synthetic lymph. Calcif Tiss Res 13:1-10.
39. Dziewaitkowski DD, Majznerski LL (1985) Role of proteo-glycans in endochondral ossification inhibition of calcification. Calcif Tiss Internat 37:460-464.
40. Hirschman A, Dziewaitkowski DD (1966) Protein-polysaccharide loss during endochondral ossification. Immunochemical evidence. Science 154:393-395.
41. Price PA, Otsuka AS, Poser JP, Kristaponis J, Raman N (1976) Characterization of α-carboxyglutamic acid-containing protein from bone. Proc Natl Acad Sci USA 73:1447-1451.
42. Romberg RW, Werness PG, Riggs, BL, Mann KG (1986) Inhibition of hydroxyapatite crystal growth by bone-specific and other calcium-binding proteins. Biochem 25:1176-1180.
43. Menanteau J, Neuman WF, Neuman MW (1982) A study of bone proteins which can prevent hydroxyapatite formation. Metal Bone Dis and Rel Res 4:157-162.
44. Termine JD, Kleinman HK, Whitson WS, Conn KM, McGarvey ML, Martin GR (1981) Osteonectin a bone specific protein linking mineral to collagen. Cell 26:99-105.
45. Fleish H, Russell RGG, Straumann F (1966) Effect of pyrophosphate on hydroxyapatite and its implications in calcium homeostasis. Nature 212:901-903.
46. Termine JD, Conn KM (1976) Inhibition of apatite formation by phosphorylated metabolites and macromole-cules. Calcif Tiss Res 22:149-157.
47. Glimcher MJ, Hodge AJ, Schmitt FD (1957) Macromolecular aggregation states in relation to mineralization. The collagen-hydroxyapatite system as studied *in vitro*. Proc Natl Acad Sci USA 43:860-866.
48. Glimcher MJ (1985) The role of collagen and phosphopro-teins in the calcification of bone and other collagenous tissues. In: Rubin RP, Weiss GB, Putney Jr JW (eds) Calcium in Biological Systems. New York: Plenum Press, pp. 607-616.

49. Dudley HR, Spiro D (1961) The fine structure of bone cells. J Biophys Biochem Cytol 11:627-649.

50. Staubesand J, Schmiebusch H, Seydewitz V, Steel F (1981) Matrix vesicles in the walls of arteries subjected to load-failure. In: Ascenzi A, Bonucci E, deBernard B (eds) Proc 3rd Intern Conf on Matrix Vesicles. Milano: Wichtig Editore srl, pp. 249-256.

51. Ali SY, Evans L (1973) The uptake of [^{45}Ca] calcium ions by matrix vesicles isolated from calcifying cartilage. Biochem J 134:647-650.

52. Anderson HC, Sajdera SW (1976) Calcification of rachitic cartilage to study matrix vesicle function. Fed Proc 35: 148-153.

53. Anderson HC, Hsu HHT (1978) A new method to measure ^{45}Ca accumulation by matrix vesicles in slices of rachitic growth plate cartilage. Metab Bone Dis and Rel Res 1:193-198.

54. Anderson HC, Kanabe S, Vaananen HK et al. (1984) Phosphatases and matrix vesicle calcification. In: Cohn DV, Potts Jr JT, Fujita T (eds) Endocrine Control of Bone and Calcium Metabolism. Amsterdam: Elsevier, pp. 410-413.

55. Fallon MD, Whyte MP, Tietlebaum SL (1980) Stereospecific inhibition of alkaline-phosphatese by L-tetramisole prevents *in vitro* cartilage calcification. Lav Invest 43:489-494.

56. Hsu HHT, Anderson HC (1977) A simple and defined method to study calcification by isolated matrix vesicles. Effect of ATP and vesicle phosphatase. Biochem Biophys Acta 500:162-172.

57. Murphree S, Hsu HHT, Anderson, HC (1982) The *in vitro* formation of crystalline apatite by matrix vesicles isolated from rachitic rat epiphyseal cartilage. Calcif Tiss Internat 34:562-568.

58. Greenawalt JW, Rossi C, Lehninger AL (1964) Effect of active accumulation of calcium and phosphations on the structure of rat liver mitochondria. J Cell Biol 2321-2338.

59. Jennings RB, Ganote CE, Reimer KA (1975) Ischemic tissue injury. Am J Pathol 81:179-198.

16

Characterization of Nucleating Proteolipids from Calcified and Non-Calcified Atherosclerotic Lesions

Rosemarie Romeo, Joan M. Augustyn, Gretchen Mandel, and Assaad S. Daoud

INTRODUCTION

Recent work (1-4) has shown that calcification of the atherosclerotic lesion occurs in extracellular membranous structures which are similar in ultrastructural appearance to the matrix vesicles identified by Anderson (5) and Bonocci (6) in the matrix of the epiphyseal growth plate in cartilage. It is now generally accepted that these matrix vesicles are the sites of initial extracellular calcification of all skeletal tissue and in many instances in pathologic calcification (7).

In a previous study (1) we have shown, by electron microscopy, that early calcification of the necrotic portion of the atheroma of swine abdominal aortas occurred primarily in degenerated cells or in matrix vesicle-like structures. Energy dispersive x-ray and line profile analyses showed that the major elements in the heavily calcified portions of the plaque were calcium and phosphorus. There was a direct relationship between the distribution and concentration of these elements, indicating that the mineral deposited was a calcium phosphate. Select area electron diffraction generated a pattern identical to that of calcium hydroxyapatite (HA) crystals. Calcification was not observed to occur on elastic tissue or collagen fibers.

Supported by the Veterans Administration and Grant No. 210038 NIHL.

The mechanism by which HA crystals are deposited in the matrix vesicles is still unknown. However, Ennever (8) has implicated a proteolipid, isolated from human aorta, in arterial calcification. This proteolipid, which is also present in bone (9), calcifying cartilage (10), calcifying bacteria (11) and dental calculi (12) has been shown to nucleate HA *in vitro*. Furthermore, *in vitro* calcification of matrix vesicles is proteolipid dependent (13).

In a preliminary study, carried out in collaboration with Ennever, we confirmed the presence of HA nucleating proteolipid in the calcified human and swine aortic athero-sclerotic lesions. The present study was carried out to determine if proteolipid is limited to calcified lesions or if it is present in normal tissue or non-calcified athero-sclerotic lesions.

MATERIALS AND METHODS
    1. Isolation of Proteolipid
    Human aortas were obtained at autopsy and stored at -20°C until sufficient quantity was obtained to begin isolation (usually 100 g wet weight). Aortas were then defrosted at 4°C overnight. The abdominal and thoracic aortas were stripped of adventitia and outer media. Calci-fied and non-calcified lesion areas were dissected from non-lesion areas. All three types of tissue were pooled and treated as separate samples. The tissue was cut into approx-imately 1 cm^2 sections and a total weight recorded. The extraction procedure was a modification of the method of Ennever (8), and can be summarized as follows: a) saline wash to remove soluble protein; b) decalcification with 2 N formic acid; c) removal of formic acid by exhaustive distilled water washes; d) lyophilization; e) extraction with chloroform:methanol:HCl (2:1:0.01;v:v:v) and f) pre-cipitation with acetone. Final purification of proteolipid was accomplished with a Bio-Sil TSK-250 gel filtration column (Bio-Rad) attached to a Perkin Elmer Series 10 liquid chromatograph. The sample was eluted with chloroform:metha-nol (2:1;v:v) in an isocratic manner at a flow rate of 1 mL per minute. Fractions were collected every 30 seconds and monitored for protein content by absorbance at 280 nm with a Perkin Elmer LC 85B spectrophotometric detector. As

applicable, fractions were pooled, dried under nitrogen and
stored at -20°C. The assessment of fraction purity was
determined by the reapplication of the individual fraction
to the TSK-250 column.

2. Determination of Apatite Inducing Proteolipid

Each TSK-250 fraction was analyzed for the ability to
form HA microcrystals in a solution of metastable calcium
phosphate (MCP) (14). At termination of incubation, samples
were washed with distilled deionized water and allowed to
air dry. Samples were then shipped to the Veterans Administration Crystal Identification Center in Milwaukee,
Wisconsin, where they were assessed for HA content with
x-ray diffraction.

3. Protein Quantitation

The protein content of the acetone precipitate or
purified proteolipid was measured with a modification of the
method of Lowry that is specific for proteolipids (16,17).

4. Lipid Quantitation

Total cholesterol content in the acetone precipitate
or purified proteolipid was determined according to the method
of Leffler (18). Triglyceride content was determined by
measurement of the glycerol moiety of the sample (19). Organic
phosphorus was determined by the method of Bartlett (20).

5. Morphologic Studies

Segments from calcified and non-calcified lesions and
from the non-lesion tissue were taken for light and electron
microscopic examination following formic acid decalcification
and delipidation with acidic chloroform-methanol. The sample
for light microscopy was fixed in buffered formaldehyde
solution, embedded in paraffin and sections were stained with
hematoxylin-eosin and Verhoeff-Van Gieson. The tissue for
electron microscopy was fixed in glutaraldehyde and post-fixed
in osmium tetroxide. The segments were embedded in epoxy
resin and sectioned on an ultramicrotome. Thick sections were
stained with toluidine blue and examined by light microscopy.

Finder grids were prepared from all three types of tissue and examined in a Phillips 300 transmission electron microscope.

Biochemical Results

1. Characterization of Acetone Precipitates

The protein content of calcified, non-calcified and non-lesion acetone precipitates, is shown in Table 1. The values are presented as micrograms of protein per milligram of dry weight of tissue (µg/mg dry weight). There was no apparent difference in protein values when the three lesion types were compared.

Table 1. Protein Content of Acetone Precipitates

Lesion Type	Protein µg/mg dry weight
Calcified	0.295
Non-Calcified	0.330
Non-Lesion	0.274

Differences were observed, however, when the lipid composition of the three precipitates were compared (Table 2). Cholesterol and triglyceride content are expressed as µg lipid/mg of dry weight of tissue, and phospholipid values are expressed as micromoles of total phosphorus per milligram of dry weight (µM/mg dry wgt).

As expected total cholesterol content was much greater in the calcified and non-calcified lesion precipitates than the total cholesterol values found in the non-lesion material. Phospholipid content was similar in all three types of tissue. The triglyceride content was highest in the calcified lesion precipitate and lowest in the non-lesion precipitate.

255

Table 2. Lipid Content of Acetone Precipitates

Lesion Type	Cholesterol µg/mg dry wgt	Triglyceride µg/mg dry wgt	Phospholipid µM/mg dry wgt
Calcified	4.88	1.040	0.005
Non-Calcified	4.25	0.102	0.005
Non-Lesion	0.34	0.067	0.003

2. Chromatographic Profiles

The three tissue types gave a similar profile following elution from the TSK-250 column. Calcified and non-calcified lesion and non-lesion precipitates were each characterized by three major peaks (Figure 1). The individual peaks from each precipitate were collected, dried under nitrogen and analyzed for their ability to nucleate, and their lipid amino acid content.

3. Nucleation

Each peak collected from the three lesion types was analyzed to determine its ability to nucleate HA *in vitro* (Table 3). Aliquots from peak 1 in all tissue types failed to induce HA; aliquots from peak 2, however, nucleated HA in all three tissue types. Aliquots from peak 3 from non-calcified lesion also induced the formation of HA but peak 3 in the other types of tissue did not induce formation of HA.

4. Lipid Characterization of Nucleating Peaks

A comparison of the lipid content of the nucleating peak common to all lesion types (i.e., peak 2) is presented in Table 4. Cholesterol and triglyceride are expressed as µg/µg protein, and phospholipid is expressed as µM/µg protein. There was an insufficient amount of peak 3 from non-calcified lesion to perform lipid characterization.

Cholesterol content in the non-calcified lesion peak was nearly twice that observed in the calcified lesion peak, while phospholipid content was highest in non-calcified and non-lesion tissue. There was insufficient material to determine triglyceride content in non-calcified lesion and non-lesion tissue.

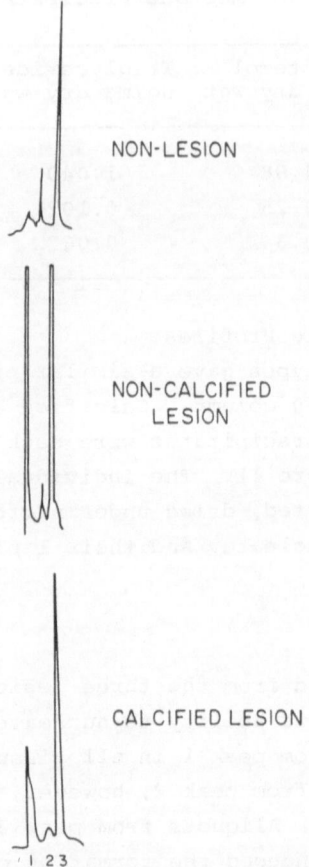

NON-LESION

NON-CALCIFIED
LESION

CALCIFIED LESION

1 2 3

Figure 1. TSK-250 Gel Filtration Chromatography of
Resolubilized Precipitates.

Morphologic Studies

Light microscopic examination of the paraffin-embedded
and of the toluidine blue stained epoxy-embedded thick sections
of tissue following formic acid treatment, showed no calcium
deposits in any of the sections examined including those from
the calcified lesions. However, a small focus of non-
mineralized osteoid tissue was noted in one of the toluidine
blue sections. The sections from both types of lesion showed
typical atheromata with necrotic core and fibrous cap. Cells
were demonstrable, although they stained poorly with both the
toluidine blue and hematoxylin-eosin stains. The sections
from the tissue subjected to acidic chloroform-methanol extraction, showed collapse of the tissue architecture with loss of

Table 3. *In vitro* Nucleation by Lesion Peaks

Lesion Type	Peak	Nucleates ?
Calcified	1	No
	2	Yes
	3	No
Non-Calcified	1	No
	2	Yes
	3	Yes
Non-Lesion	1	No
	2	Yes
	3	No

definition of the necrotic core. Only a few ill-defined cells could be observed.

Electron microscopic examination confirmed the results obtained with light microscopy. In the decalcified tissue, prior to the acidic chloroform-methanol extraction, there were no HA crystals observed in or outside the matrix vesicles. The vesicles were, in general, collapsed and their limiting membrane appeared thick and smudgy. The cell membranes were sometimes disrupted, but the cell shape appeared well preserved. Smooth muscle cells and foam cells were easily identifiable. The intracellular lipid inclusions were also well preserved; however, the myofilaments were not. The elastic tissue and collagen fibers showed the unusual ultra-structural appearance.

Table 4. Lipid Composition of Nucleating Peak 2

Lesion Type	Cholesterol µg/µg prot.	Triglyceride µg/µg prot.	Phospholipid µM/µg prot.
Calcified	19.34	0.76	0.002
Non-Calcified	33.12	QNS	0.025
Non-Lesion	1.15	QNS	0.044

The ultrastructural appearance of the tissue, following the acidic chloroform-methanol extraction, was extensively altered and none of the normal or pathological features were recognizable with certainty. Only amorphous material of various shapes, sizes and staining characteristics (Figure 2) was observed.

DISCUSSION

There is general agreement that *in vivo* calcification occurs in matrix vesicles. However, the mechanism of this calcification is still debatable. Several macromolecules, including proteoglycans (21), gamma-carboxy glutamic acid containing peptides and proteins (22), phosphoproteins (23), elastin that has been proteolytically modified (24) and proteolipids (8) have been reported to bind calcium. However, to date, only the proteolipid isolated by Ennever was found to nucleate HA *in vitro*. Proteolipid has been demonstrated in the matrix vesicles (13). Furthermore, *in vitro* calcification of matrix vesicles appears to be proteolipid dependent. Lyophilized matrix vesicles and matrix lipid extracts, containing calcifiable proteolipid, support HA formation in bicarbonate buffered metastable calcium phosphate solution, whereas the vesicle extracted residue and lipid extract, which do not contain calcifiable proteolipid, do not (13).

Our results showed that proteolipids, capable of nucleating HA *in vitro*, are present in the calcified atherosclerotic lesions. However, they are also present in non-calcified lesions and in the non-lesion tissue. These three types of tissue also contained fractions of proteolipid which do not nucleate HA *in vitro*. These findings, if extrapolated to the *in vivo* situation, suggest that either not all proteolipids promote calcification or that their HA nucleating activity is modulated by other factors present in the artery wall which may act as promoters or inhibitors of the nucleation process.

Boyan et al. (25,26) reported that bacterial calcification, which is also proteolipid dependent, involved the formation of calcium-phospholipid-phosphate complex ($CPLP_i$). Both proteolipid and $CPLP_i$ could be isolated from calcifying bacteria, whereas only proteolipids could be isolated from non-calcifying

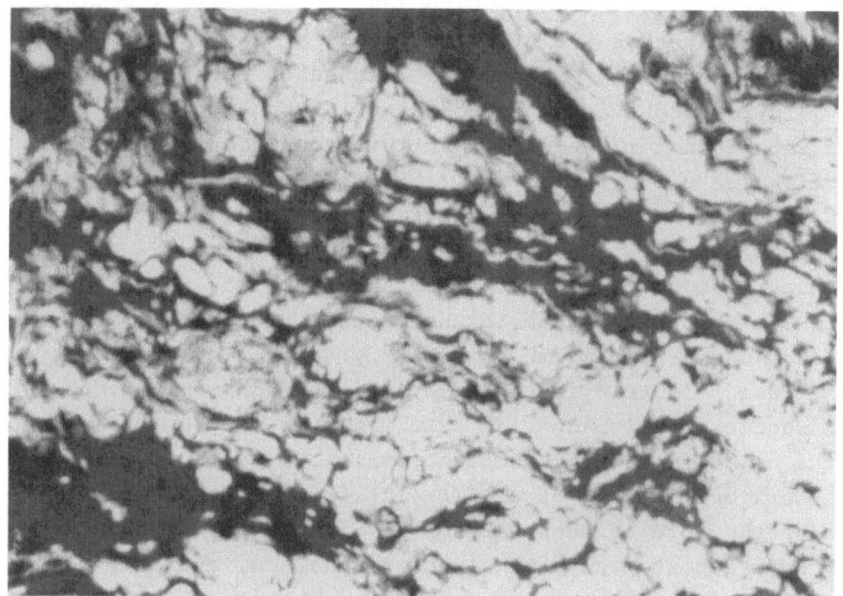

Figure 2.   Electron micrograph of a section from a calcified lesion after acidic chloroform-methanol extraction.   There are no hydroxyapatite crystals nor matrix vesicles present. The lesion features are extensively altered and none of the usual features are recognizable with certainty.   Only amorphous material of various shapes, sizes and staining characteristics are present. (x 20,000)

bacteria.   In the former, the proteolipid and $CPLP_i$ appeared to be two components of a single mineralizing entity in which the $CPLP_i$ is formed preferentially on phosphotidylserine and phosphoinositides of the proteolipids.   Phospholipid analysis of the two types of bacteria showed that the non-calcifying organisms are deficient in these acidic phospholipids, which explain their inability to form $CPLP_i$.   These investigators also suggested that the deficiency in acidic phospholipid in the proteolipid is probably due to differential segregation of the membrane lipid with respect to a different protein composition (25).

The ability of proteolipid to form HA *in vivo* may also be influenced by the presence of promoters or inhibitors of calcification in the microenvironment of the matrix vesicles. Among the promoters are elevated levels of Ca^{++} and PO_4^{3-}; while the inhibitors may include inadequate levels of Ca^{++}, PO_4^{3-}, pyrophosphate and adenosine triphosphate (ATP). Our data showed that the proteolipid fraction which nucleates HA *in vitro* was different in its lipid and amino acid composition (data not shown) among the two types of lesion and in the normal artery. We are now carrying out analysis of the phospholipids of proteolipids isolated from the three types of tissue in order to see if the proteolipid from the calcified lesions is richer in phosphotidylserine and phosphoinositides. If this is the case, a mechanism similar to that suggested for bacterial calcification, may be operative in the calcification of the atheroma.

Work by Anderson et al. (2-4,7) focuses special attention on the role of phosphatases in tissue calcification. They have reported that alkaline phosphatase, adenosine triphosphatase (ATPase), and other phosphatase enzymes are localized in the membrane of matrix vesicles. These enzymes are activated just before the onset of apatite deposition. Anderson suggested that Ca^{++} is attracted to the matrix vesicles by the acidic phospholipids which are known to be concentrated in these vesicles. The phosphatases may function as phosphotransferases leading to concentration of phosphate in the matrix vesicles. The high levels of Ca^{++} and phosphate in the confined microenvironment of the matrix vesicles would be sufficient to promote deposition of calcium apatite.

In conclusion, this study showed that *in vitro* HA nucleating proteolipids are present in normal and diseased arterial wall. These proteolipids differ from each other in their lipid and amino acid composition. The role of these proteolipids, and the significance of the differences in chemical composition, on the calcification process of the atheroma, remains to be elucidated. However, bacterial calcification studies suggest that the biochemical differences demonstrated in this study, may be important in atherosclerotic calcification.

REFERENCES

1. Daoud AS, Frank AS, Jarmolych J, Franco WT, Fritz KE (1985) Ultrastructural and elemental analysis of calcification of advanced swine aortic atherosclerosis. Exp Mol Path 43:337-347.

2. Tanimura A, McGregor DH, Anderson HC (1983) Matrix vesicles in atherosclerotic calcification. Proc Soc Exp Biol Med 172:173-177.

3. Tanimura A, McGregor DH, Anderson HC (1986) Calcification in atherosclerosis I. Human studies. J Exp Pathol 2(4):261-273.

4. Tanimura A, McGregor DH, Anderson HC (1986) Calcification in atherosclerosis II. Animan studies. J Exp Pathol 2(4):275-297.

5. Anderson HC (1969) Vesicles associated with calcification in the matrix of epiphyseal cartilage. J Cell Biol 41:59-72.

6. Bonucci E (1970) Fine structure and histochemistry of calcifying globules in epiphyseal cartilage. Z Zellforsch Mikrosk Anat 103:192-217.

7. Anderson HC (1983) Calcific diseases. A concept. Arch Pathol Lab Med 107:341-348.

8. Ennever J, Vogel JJ, Riggan LJ (1980) Calcification by proteolipid from atherosclerotic aorta. Atherosclerosis 35:209-213.

9. Ennever J, Vogel JJ, Levy BM (1974) Lipid and bone matrix calcification in vitro. Proc Soc Exp Bio Med 145:1386-1388.

10. Ennever J, Riggan LJ, Vogel JJ (1985) Proteolipid and collagen calcification, in vitro. Cytobios 39:151-157.

11. Ennever J, Vogel JJ, Ridge LJ, Boyan-Salyers BD (1976) Nucleation of microbiologic calcification by proteolipid. Proc Soc Exp Bio Med 152:147-150.

12. Ennever J, Vogel JJ, Riggan LJ, Paoloske SB (1977) Proteolipid and calculus matrix calcificafion in vitro. J Dent Res 56:140-142.

13. Boyan BD, Landis WJ, Knight J, Dereszewski G, Zeagler J (1984) Microbial hydroxyapatite formation as a model of proteolipid-dependent membrane-mediated calcification. Scan Elect Microsc IV:1793-1800.

14. Ennever J, Vogel JJ, Benson LA (1973) Lipid and calculus matrix calcification in vitro. J Dent Res 42:1056-1059.

15. Peters T, Reed RG (1980) The biosynthesis of rat serum alsumin. J Biol Chem 255:3156-3163.

16. Lowry OH, Rosebrough MJ, Farr AI, Randall RJ (1951) Protein measurement with the Folin Phenol Reagent. J Biol Chem 192:265-275.

17. Lees MB, Raxman S (1972) Modification of the Lowry Procedure for the analysis of proteolipid protein. Anal Biochem 47:184-192.

18. Leffler HH (1959) Estimation of cholesterol in serum. Am J Clin Pathol 31:310-313.

19. Van Hansel E, Zilversmit DB (1957) Micromethod for the direct determination of serum triglycerides. J Lab Clin Med 50:152-157.

20. Bartlett GR (1958) Colormetric assay methods for free and phosphorylated glyceric acids. J Biol Chem 234:469-471.

21. Wight TN (1980) Vessel proteoglycans and thrombo-genesis. In: Spart TH (ed) Progress in Hemostases and Thrombosis. Vol. 5, New York: Grune and Stratton, pp. 1-39.
22. Levy RJ, Lian JB, Gallop P (1979) Atherocalin, a μ-carboxyglutamic acid containing protein from athero-sclerotic plaque. Biochem Biophys Res Comm 91:41-79.
23. Keeley FW (1977) The extraction and partial characteri-zation of proteins released by decalcification from calcified human aortic plaques. Biochim Biophys Acta 494:384-394.
24. Hornebeck W, Patridge SM (1975) Conformational changes in fibrous elastin due to calcium ions. Eur J Biochem 51:73-78.
25. Boyan-Salyers BD, Boskey AL (1980) Relationship between proteolipids and calcium-phospholipid-phosphate com-plexes in bacterionema matruchotee calcification. Calcif Tissue Int 30:167-174.
26. Boyan BD, Boskey AL (1984) Co-isolation of proteolipids and calcium-phospholipid-phosphate complexes. Calcif Tissue Int 36:214-218.

Pathobiologic Processes

17
The Problems of Procedures for the Study of the Pathological Processes of Human Atherosclerosis

Robert W. Wissler

We are at an awkward stage in the study of the pathogenesis of atherosclerosis. We have learned a great deal
about the major processes which are probably involved in the
human atherosclerotic plaque (Figure 1). We know what to
study, and we can observe and quantitate most, if not all,
of the results of the processes in Figure 1. In other
words, procedures are available for quantitating components
of the human atherosclerotic plaque which reflect these
processes. But we really have difficulty in studying these
processes as they proceed in people.

The problems of studying processes in the human disease
are the result of a number of major features of the disease
entity itself. Some of the most prominent of these problems
are:

1. The inaccessibility during life of the major
    disease area - the inner portion of large and
    medium-sized arteries.
2. The slow rate of development of lesions of the
    disease - extending as it does over a period of
    months in the experimental animal, and over a
    period of years in the human.

Acknowledgements: The author is grateful for the editorial
assistance of Gertrud Friedman and the secretarial services
of LeAnn Morgan in preparing this manuscript. He also acknowledges the support of grants No. HL15062 and No. 33740, which
made possible the development of a number of the results and
the recent publications from this laboratory which are mentioned in this introduction.

PRINCIPAL PATHOLOGICAL PROCESSES

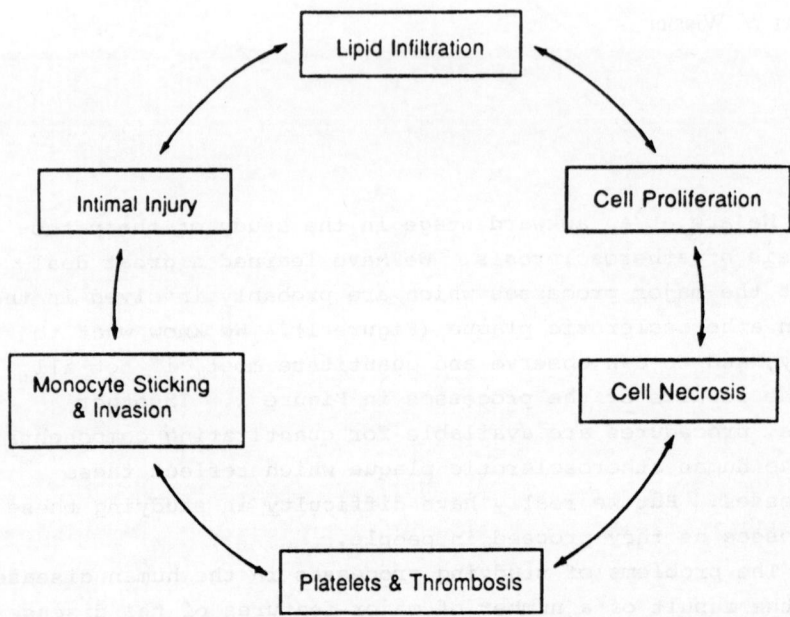

Figure 1. These processes all occur in human atherogenesis. They all probably play an important part in the progression of the plaque components which increase during the development of the human lesions. There is still much to learn about the sequence and the interaction of these processes, as well as the influence of the various risk factors on the relative prominence of each process in a given individual or lesion being studied.

3.   The relative infrequency with which suitable study material is obtained from standard areas of the human arterial tree. This problem is intensified by the focal nature of the disease and the relatively recent recognition of lesion "prone" and lesion "resistant" parts of the arterial tree (1).

There is old and recent evidence that infants and very small children develop fatty streaks in selected parts of the aorta. These appear to be associated with the nursing period and, according to the most recent meticulous study of atherogenesis in the early childhood period, they generally regress and disappear almost completely (2). There is little evidence of a progressive disease process in the intima until the late teens and early 20s, even in a relatively athero-sclerosis-vulnerable population like ours in the United States. Several studies in this county indicate that it is during this period, late in the second decade, that raised lesions begin to be evident. The nature of the changes in the endothelium, intima and sub-intima at this time are poorly understood. Evidence indicates that there are several microscopic types of fatty streaks evident at this time, and that this is after apo B and other lipoprotein fragments have accumulated in the intima, both extra- and intracellularly (3,4).

Fatty streaks appear to occur in all populations about this time, i.e., in those groups and nationalities which commonly develop progressive disease and those which do not. They also occur in many of the experimental animals which are used as models for atherosclerosis research, whether they have been subjected to manipulation, nutritional or otherwise, to produce hyperlipidemia.

Therefore, the most important processes and the most important questions which need to be answered about patho-genesis are related to progression, and not necessarily to the earliest lesions we can detect.

With these premises in mind, two major studies are now underway. One of these is centered in the United States. It involves 15 centers, and it is focusing on the specific quantitative changes which occur in the lesions of young people between 15 and 34 years, and the relationship of lesion features to risk factors (5). The other is a WHO study involving more than 20 countries, which is employing a protocol very similar to that of the United States study. It is sponsored and organized by the WHO with leadership provided by Nils Sternby in Sweden.

It is obvious that we can learn much by studying lesion components by quantitative methods. These observations will make it possible to define the major questions about pro-cesses which lead to progression and to stimulate the development of procedures, difficult as it may be, to study effectively the principal factors controlling the histo-genesis of the human disease.

Almost all of the overviews in this part of this volume are related to the processes which control the development of the major components of the plaque.

It is clear that we need additional procedures in order to study the processes of arterial lipid infiltration in people. Tracing influx and efflux of lipoproteins, cholesterol, and cholesteryl esters through the imperfect endothelial barrier is difficult *in vitro* and even in animal models, but it is doubly difficult *in vivo* in human subjects. Fortunately, some of the newer methods of tracing lipoproteins *in vivo* which are now being developed and applied to the study of human lesions may be helpful in this regard (6).

Arterial smooth muscle cell proliferation, which along with lipid infiltration constitutes a major process in atherogenesis in all species, is also very difficult to study in the free-living human subject; new procedures are called for. Fortunately, some of the innovative methods being employed by Gordon and Julie Campbell and coworkers (7,8), as well as some of the methods being reported by Giulio Gabbiani and coworkers (9,10) appear promising to detect cell changes associated with progressive atherogenesis. They are laying the groundwork for developing quantitative methods which may be valuable in measuring the cellular changes which mark the activation and progression of diffuse fibrous thickening of the intima, toward atherosclerosis.

These methods, and most of the methods now developed to measure cell deaths in both animal models (11) and in cell culture systems (12,13), will require further development before they can be used successfully in assessing cell proliferation and cell death (necrosis) in the arterial intima of free-living humans. As of now, they are of immense value in furthering the knowledge gained from the study of autopsies of young people.

The other important aspect of cell proliferation and cell death which will undoubtedly be investigated is the nature of the stimuli which emerge as most prominent for this part of the human disease process. It is now generally recognized that there are numerous sources of active stimulation of cell proliferation which may be active in atherogenesis (14,15,16) (Figure 2).

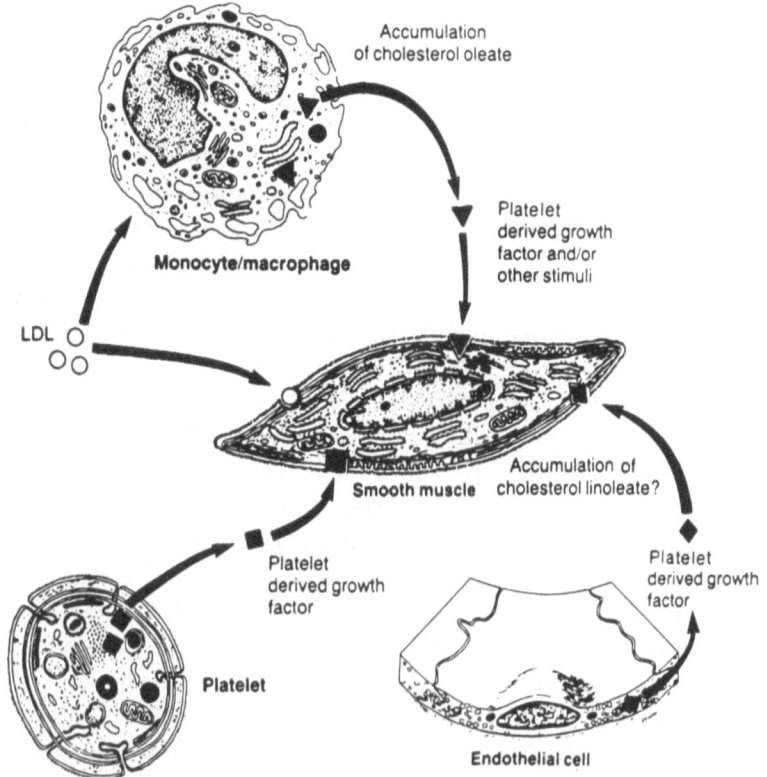

Figure 2. Sources of four growth stimulating factors which have been implicated in the arterial smooth muscle cell proliferation during atherosclerotic plaque formation (16) (With permission from Dr. Russell Ross and the American Heart Association, Inc.)

In fact, in addition to hyperlipidemic LDL and the three cellular sources from the artery, it now appears that smooth muscle cells themselves can be activated to produce a PDGF-like growth stimulating factor.

The most active field of investigation at present, relative to processes in the pathogenesis of atherosclerosis, is probably the one most in need of new procedures. It now appears likely that a major effect of hyperlipidemias of various types may be to alter the endothelium and some of the formed elements of the blood in such a way as to promote sticking of mononuclear cells and platelets (17-19). Here there are many paradoxes which require new procedures if we are to resolve them.

For example, even though several investigators have reported the use of antibodies to various parts of the monocyte-derived macrophage as a cell identification procedure, the results presented and published thus far indicate a very great variation in the proportions of the total cell population in the human plaque, which is made up of macrophages. Furthermore, when very carefully developed and tested enzyme methods for identification are utilized, the results are quite different. In general they indicate that, in fatty streaks from young people in the second and third decades, the percentage of total cells in the plaque which are derived from monocytes is almost always less than 10% and usually is about 1-3%. These fatty streaks from young people, age 15-34, are quite different in cellular composition compared to the transitory fatty streaks found in infancy. Furthermore, most of their cells stain with antibody to chicken gizzard alpha actin or to tropomyosin, which in our hands seem to be specific for phenotypically modulated smooth muscle cells.

Obviously, much more work is necessary before we will have methods with which we can study plaque cell populations in the living state, but the goal of learning more about the movement of monocytes and macrophages into and out of the plaque seems to be one which is worthy of further intensive investigation. The monocyte-derived macrophage, in spite of relatively small numbers, may be a very important cell in both the induction and regression of atherosclerosis, raising the possibility that numbers may not be nearly as important as cell kinetics and transport (20).

The circle of cell processes in atherogenesis (Figure 1) needs, for its completion, the role of intimal injury. Is it an early phenomenon or only a late one? The answer to this question will probably involve much of the latest work on lipid peroxidation, leukotrienes and free radical cell injury (21-23).

The following overviews in this part of this volume are designed to further clarify the knowledge which we have and to point out the areas which need further investigation. In many instances the challenge is to produce new procedures which will make it possible to study these processes more adequately in the live human subject.

REFERENCES

1. Cornhill JF (1984) Topographic probability mapping of aortic atherosclerosis. Report 763813/715703. Columbus: The Ohio State University Research Foundation.
2. Stary HC (1985) Macrophage foam cells in the coronary artery intima of human infants. Ann NY Acad Sci 454: 5-8.
3. Kao VCK, Wissler RW (1965) A study of the immunohisto-chemical localization of serum lipoproteins and other plasma proteins in human atherosclerotic lesions. Exp Mol Pathol 4:465-479.
4. Yomantas S, Elner VM, Schaffner T, Wi-sler RW (1984) Immunohistochemical localization of apolipoprotein B in human atherosclerotic lesions. Arch Pathol Lab Med 108:374-378.
5. Strong JP (1986) Coronary atherosclerosis in soldiers: A clue to the natural history of atherosclerosis in the young. JAMA 256:2863-2866.
6. Lees RS, Garabedian HD, Lees AM, et al. (1985) Technetium - 99m low density lipoproteins: Preparation and biodistribution. J Nucl Med 26:1056-1062.
7. Mosse PRL, Campbell GR, Wang ZL, Campbell JH (1985) Smooth muscle phenotypic expression in human carotid arteries. I. Comparison of cells from diffuse intimal thickenings adjacent to atheromatous plaques with those of the media. Lab Invest 53:556-562.
8. Campbell GR, Campbell JH (1985) Smooth muscle pheno-typic changes in arterial wall homeostasis: Implica-tions for the pathogenesis of atherosclerosis. Exp Mol Pathol 42:139-162.
9. Rungger-Brandle E, Gabbiani G (1983) The role of cyto-skeletal and cytocontractile elements in pathologic processes. Am J Pathol 110:361-392.
10. Kocher O, Gabbiani G (1986) Cytoskeletal features of normal and atheromatous human arterial smooth muscle cells. Hum Pathol 17:875-880.
11. Imai H, Werthessen NT, Taylor CB, Lee KT (1976) Angiotoxicity and arteriosclerosis due to contaminants of USP-grade cholesterol. Arch Pathol Lab Med 100:565-572.
12. Chen RM, Getz GS, Fischer-Dzoga K, Wissler RW (1977) The role of hyperlipidemic serum on the proliferation and necrosis of aortic medial cells *in vitro*. Exp Mol Pathol 26:359-374.
13. Morel DW, Di Corleto PE, Chisolm GM (1984) Endothe-lial and smooth muscle cells alter low density lipo-protein *in vitro* by free radical oxidation. Arterio-sclerosis 4:357-364.

14. Wissler RW (1979)   Interactions of low-density lipo-
    proteins from hypercholesterolemic serum with arterial
    wall cells and their extracellular products in athero-
    genesis and regression. In: Scanu AM, Wissler RW,
    Getz GS (eds) The Biochemistry of Atherosclerosis.
    New York: Marcel Dekker, Inc., pp. 345-368.
15. Wissler RW, Fischer Dzoga K, Bates SR, Chen RM (1981)
    Arterial smooth muscle cells in tissue culture. In:
    Schwartz CJ, Werthessen NT, Wolf S (eds) Structure
    and Function of the Circulation, Volume III. New York:
    Plenum Press, pp. 427-474.
16. Ross R (1981) Atherosclerosis: A problem of the
    biology of arterial wall cells and their interactions
    with blood components. Arteriosclerosis 1:293-311.
17. Carvalho AC, Colman RW, Lees RS (1974) Platelet
    function in hyperlipoproteinemia. N Engl J Med 290:434-
    438.
18. Henriksen T, Evensen SA, Carlander B (1979) Injury to
    human endothelial cells in culture induced by low
    density lipoproteins. Scand J Clin Lab Lnvest 39:361-368.
19. Bevilacqua MP, Pober JS, Wheeler ME, Cotran RS,
    Gimbrone Jr MA (1985) Interleukin 1 acts on cultured
    human vascular endothelium to increase the adhesion of
    polymorphonuclear leukocytes, monocytes, and related
    leukocyte cell lines. J Clin Invest 76:2003-2011.
20. Wissler RW, Vesselinovitch D, Davis HR (1987) Cellular
    components of the progressive atherosclerotic process.
    In: Olsson A, Gresham GA (eds) The Biology and Clinical
    Science of Atherosclerosis. Edinburgh: Livingston,
    pp. 51-73.
21. Steinbrecher UP, Parathasarathy S, Leake DS, Witztum JL,
    Steinberg D (1984) Modification of low density lipo-
    protein by endothelial cells involves lipid peroxidation
    and degradation of low density lipoprotein phospholipids.
    Proc Natl Acad Sci USA 81:3883-3887.
22. Parathasarathy S, Steinbrecher UP, Barnett J, Witztum JL,
    Steinberg D (1985) Essential role of phospholipase A_2
    activity in endothelial cell-induced modification of low
    density lipoprotein. Proc Natl Acad Sci USA 82:3000-3004.
23. Steinberg D (1986) Lipoproteins and atherogenesis:
    Current concepts. In: Hallgren B, Levin O, Rossner S,
    Vessby B (eds) Diet and Prevention of Coronary Heart
    Disease and Cancer. New York: Raven Press, pp. 95-112.

18
Problems and Progress in Understanding "Endothelial Permeability" and Mass Transport in Human Arteries

Donald L. Fry

Study of vascular transmural mass transport and its relationship to atherogenesis poses a variety of difficult practical and conceptual problems. The practical problems of research in this area are particularly difficult. If interpretable observations of arterial transmural transport are to be made, it is necessary to measure or control a very large number of variables, e.g., transmural pressure, blood concentration of the transported species, transmural concentration distribution, blood flow, etc. This extent of experimental control is virtually impossible to achieve in the living animal, particularly in man. One practical solution appears to be the development of an *in vitro*, metabolically-supported vessel system in which some acceptable control of variables is possible. Although there has been some progress in this direction (1), there are many unresolved problems. Most notably, it is not clear which physical and biochemical parameters (in addition to the obvious variables mentioned above) must be controlled to simulate adequately the *in vivo* situation. What subtle factors must be controlled to support normal arterial cellular function? How do we control sepsis over long periods of time in such a system?

Acknowledgement. The author gratefully acknowledges Cheuch Hou and Edward Herderick for their valuable programming assistance and data processing; and Carolyn Groff for the fine artwork and untiring assistance in the preparation of this manuscript. This research was supported by the National Heart, Lung, and Blood Institute Research Grants HL-29095 and HL-33760.

In human studies, how do we resolve the ethical and legal issues associated with the nontherapeutic use of donor tissue for this purpose?

Apart from these practical questions, this area of research also poses a number of challenging conceptual problems. One of the most challenging of these is the possible role of "endothelial permeability" or, more generally, the roles of mass transport in atherogenesis. Some of the evidence supporting the importance of mass transport in atherogenesis may be summarized as follows: First, epidemiological studies have shown that increased serum low density lipoprotein (LDL) concentration and increased blood pressure each correlate with the apparent rate of lesion development (2). Second, the concentration of LDL in lesions has been shown to be higher than at other sites in the vessel (3,4). Third, parenterally administered ^{125}I-LDL has been shown to accumulate preferentially in the lesions of patients (5). Fourth, it has been shown in various animal species that the normal topographic pattern of intimal Evans blue dye (EBD) uptake following parenteral administration of the dye is very similar to the pattern of intimal lipid staining following cholesterol feeding in these same species (6,7). Fifth, the topographic pattern of EBD staining also correlates with the uptakes of various plasma proteins (8,9). Thus, the evidence supports the assumption that atherogenesis develops in subendothelial tissues that are poorly protected from various assumed atherogenic plasma substances (atherogens) such as low density lipoprotein (LDL) as well as other contributing atherogens such as mitogenic factors, viruses, chemotactic agents, immune complexes, etc. (10-17). Accordingly, one might expect that regions of greatest endothelial permeability would be the regions of most severe disease. One might also expect the intimal tissue concentration of the atherogen in such regions to approach, but not exceed, the blood concentration. As summarized below, it has been shown that neither expectation appears to be correct.

Minick et al. (18) studied atherogenesis and endothelial regeneration in the ballooned deendothelialized cholesterol-fed rabbit. They found that atheromata developed preferentially under the newly regenerating endothelial surface and, paradoxically, tended to spare the remaining highly permeable deendothelialized areas even though these regions continued to be exposed to the hypercholesterolemic blood. The latter is of considerable interest since it suggests that chronic exposure of the intimal tissue to the normal or even elevated level of serum cholesterol is insufficient to cause severe atherosclerosis. On the other hand, preferential involvement of the reendothelialized regions suggests that atherogenesis may be fostered by conditions associated with the newly regenerating endothelial surface. The newly regenerating endothelial surface has been studied in ballooned deendothelialized rats by Schwartz et al. (19). They found that the intercellular junctions of the regenerating surface layer remained open for about eight weeks, suggesting that the same may have been true for the study of Minick et al. of the region of endothelium at the advancing edge of the regenerating surface. In a study that may be related to the foregoing, Smith and Staples (4) measured the serum protein composition of arterial interstitial fluids from necropsy specimens. They reported that the average interstitial fluid concentration of unbound LDL in lesion areas tended to be greater than the corresponding blood plasma concentrations. Three possible explanations for this observation would be: 1) synthesis *in situ* (for which there is no evidence), 2) decreased apparent activity coefficient for LDL in the interstitial milieu, and 3) interstitial macromolecular sieving.

Sieving of albumin and LDL has been studied in the deendothelialized *in vitro* porcine artery preparation (1). These studies examined the uptake and intimal interfacial concentrations of ^{125}I-LDL and ^{125}I-albumin as a function of pressure and stirring (simulated flow). It was found that in the pressurized, nonstirred situation the intimal interfacial concentration of each protein was greater than its concentration in the bulk phase of the serum and that the corresponding arterial uptakes were also greater from the unstirred than the stirred serum. These data show that both LDL and albumin (or molecular forms derived from these) are sieved in the superficial intimal layers of the *in vitro* porcine arterial preparation under pressurized conditions.

Thus, the literature to date appears to be consistent with the hypothesis that atherogenesis is fostered by some poorly defined, aberrant set of mass transport processes characterized by increased intimal concentration of LDL, perhaps due to intimal interstitial sieving and some form of endothelial dysfunction associated, among other things, with injury and regrowth. In an effort to gain better insight into possible transport processes that might explain some of the foregoing observations, it will be helpful to examine certain mass transport concepts and simple models.

Some Concepts Regarding Atherogenesis and Mass Transport

Atherogenesis

Atherogenesis may be viewed as a system of vascular interstitial chemical reactions in which a particular reactant, an "atherogenic" substance (or atherogen), enters the input end of the reaction system and causes a cascade of chemical events that result in an end product that we recognize as a component of an atherosclerotic lesion (20). This system may be represented by a reaction scheme such as follows:

$$A \text{ (atherogen)} + B \text{ (e.g., binding site)} \underset{k_b}{\overset{k_f}{\rightleftarrows}} C \text{ (intermediate product)}$$

$$C + D \rightarrow \ldots \rightarrow \text{Lesion Component} \qquad (1)$$

in which substance A, an atherogen, reacts with B to produce an intermediate product, C. This allows C to react with D and so on ultimately leading to the formation of the lesion component. All else being equal, the rate at which the final product, the lesion component, is formed will vary monotonically with the chemically-active interstitial concentration of A.

Chemical Activity, Concentration, and the Distribution
Coefficient

The chemically-active concentration of A in the interstitial fluid at a point (x) in the tissue is called the
chemical activity [a(x), mol cm^{-3}] of A at x (20-22). The
relationship between the chemical activity [a(x)] and the
corresponding volume-averaged tissue concentration [c(x),
mol cm^{-3}] at x can be seen from the following considerations (21). Tissue concentration can be measured directly
as the quantity of atherogen per unit volume of tissue at x.
The corresponding chemical activity, however, must be inferred from the measured concentration and the "solute equilibrium distribution coefficient". The tissue solute distribution coefficient [ε(x)] is defined as the ratio of the
tissue equilibrium concentration [c(x)$_{equil}$] of the molecular
species of interest (atherogen) to the corresponding chemical
activity (a$_0$) of the species in the equilibrating solution.
Thus,

$$\varepsilon(x) = c(x)_{equil}/a_0 \tag{2}$$

Although ε is determined in the equilibrium state, it may be
used also, subject to certain defined conditions (21,22), in
nonequilibrium states to relate the chemical activity (a) at
a point to the corresponding local concentration. Thus, in
general,

$$a(x) = c(x)/\varepsilon(x) \tag{3}$$

It can be seen from Equation 3 that $1/\varepsilon(x)$ acts like an
activity coefficient to relate c(x) to a(x) in a tissue
system. As discussed elsewhere (21), the quantity $1/\varepsilon(x)$
takes into account the solvent fractional volume (ε_w) in
the tissue that is available to the solute as well as the
apparent activity coefficient (γ) for the solute in that
fractional volume, i.e.,

$$1/\varepsilon = \gamma/\varepsilon_w \tag{4}$$

It helps to see the relationships among $a(x)$, $c(x)$, and
$\varepsilon(x)$ more clearly by digressing for a moment to visualize
the following simple experiment to measure $\varepsilon(x)$. Referring
to the upper portion of Figure 1, a "homogeneous" slab of
arterial tissue is submersed in a chamber of serum containing a concentration, c_0, of atherogen so that we may observe
the transmural concentration distributions [$c(x)$] of the
atherogen as these evolve with time (T). Concentration
[$c(x)$] is shown on the ordinate and the location (x) across
the wall is shown on the abscissa with $x = 0$ at the intimal
surface and $x = H$ at the adventitial surface. The family
of curves that is shown represents the transmural concentration distributions, $c(x)$, at increasing times (T_1, T_2, ...)
after submersion of the tissue into the serum. Note that
after sufficient time ($\sim T_\infty$) the concentration distribution
no longer changes with time and becomes uniform across the
tissue at the equilibrium concentration [$c(x)_{equil}$]. At
this point the chemically-active concentration of atherogen
in the interstitial fluids everywhere in the tissue has
become equal to that (a_0) in the serum reagent, i.e., there
no longer are any activity gradients to cause change.

The chemical activity (a_0) of the atherogen in the serum
phase is defined by $a_0 = \gamma_0 c_0$ in which γ_0 is the activity
coefficient. Therefore, in accordance with Equation 2,
$\varepsilon(x) = c(x)_{equil}/\gamma_0 c_0$. Moreover, at times less than T_∞,
$a(x) = c(x)/\varepsilon(x)$ in accordance with Equation 3. The family
of $a(x)/a_0$ curves in the lower portion of Figure 1 was
calculated in this manner from the corresponding $c(x)/c_0$
curves shown in the upper portion of the Figure. Note that,
unlike concentration, chemical activity is continuous across
the intimal and adventitial interfaces, i.e., the $a(x)/a_0$
contours do not have discontinuous values at interfaces.

Mass Transport

As noted with regard to Equation 1, the chemical activity
[$a(x)$] of a particular atherogen (a) may be assumed to be one
of the main driving forces for development of the corresponding
lesion component. Thus, the transmural $a(x)$ contour may be
considered to represent a potential for lesion development
or potential "risk" at each point (x) across the wall. Since
these contours are determined by the interaction of the pro-

CONCENTRATION, ACTIVITY, AND THE
DISTRIBUTION COEFFICIENT (ε)

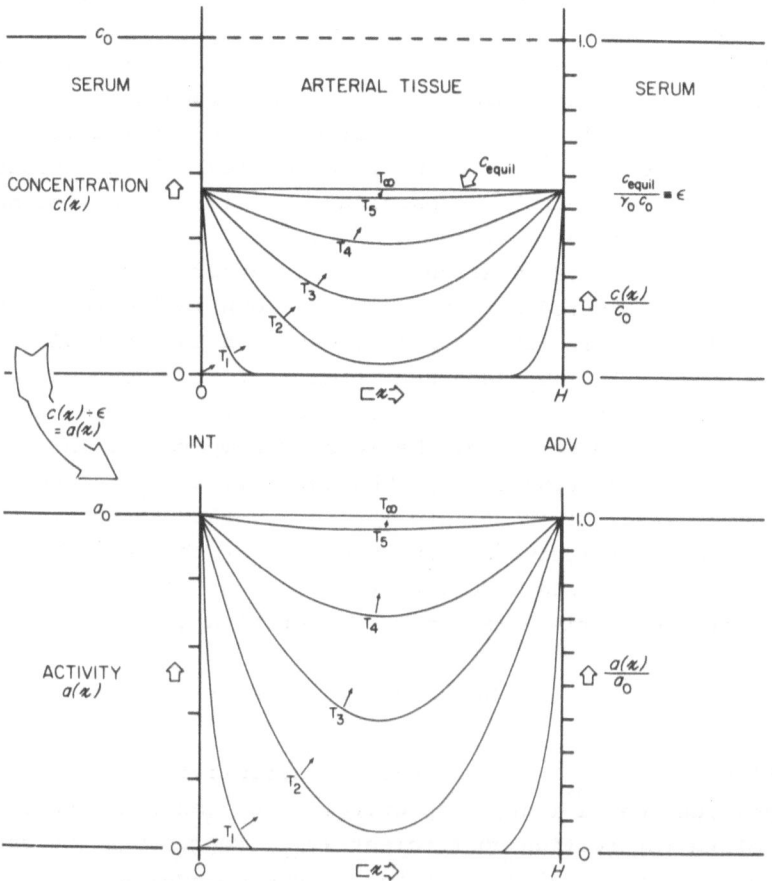

Figure 1.   Diagram depicting experiment showing relationships
among concentration [c(x)], chemical activity [a(x)], and
the distribution coefficient (ε) in a homogeneous slab of
arterial tissue at various times (T_1, T_2, ...) following
submersion in serum reagent containing a concentration (c_0)
of atherogen; γ_0 is the activity coefficient, and a_0 is the
corresponding chemical activity of atherogen in reagent,
x is transmural distance from intimal surface (x = 0);
adventitial interface is located at x = H.

cesses of mass transport with structural barriers to this
transport, it is of interest to explore simple examples of
this type of interactions. Such considerations may provide
further insight into some of the extrinsic conditions and
physical features of an artery that may increase the risk

of atherogenesis. In this regard, interest will be focused
on how an atherogen is transported and accumulates across a
multilayered vascular wall such as shown in Figure 2. For
reference purposes the x axis of a Cartesian coordinate
system is shown extending from the blood-endothelial interface at x = 0 to the media-adventitia interface at x = H.
Subscripts, ℓ, will be used to designate the particular
layer being considered. We shall be particularly interested
in factors that control the magnitude of a(x) in the intimal
layer (ℓ = 2) of this structure.

A formula for calculation of a(x) contours across a
stylized multilayered artery (such as shown in Figure 2) is
described elsewhere (20,23) and is based on the following
assumptions: 1) The transmural flux (J_ℓ) of atherogen has
reached steady state. 2) Of the factors that determine
a(x), chemical reactions may be ignored compared to the
effect of mass transport. 3) The total flux (J_ℓ) across a
particular (ℓth) layer of interest, e.g., the intimal layer,
consists of a diffusive component driven by the activity
gradient ($-\partial a/\partial x$) and a convective component that is carried
by the pressure-driven transmural water flux (J_v), i.e.,

$$J_\ell = -D_\ell \partial a/\partial x + f_{A\ell} J_v a_\ell \tag{5}$$

in which D_ℓ and $f_{A\ell}$ are the apparent diffusivity and apparent
retardation coefficient, respectively, for the ℓth layer.
The solute retardation coefficient ($f_{A\ell}$) represents the ratio
of the convective velocity of the solute molecules to the
velocity of the associated solvent (water) molecules. If
$f_{A\ell}$ is equal to 1, it means that the solute molecules are
moving through the ℓth tissue layer with the same velocity
as the water. Values less than 1 indicate that the convective motion of the solute molecules is less than that of
the water, i.e., solute velocity is being hindered by the
sieving effect of tissue. A corollary is that the magnitude
of f_A will tend to vary inversely with the size of the
atherogen. A second corollary is that if f_A for the ℓth
layer is larger than the f_A for the next [(ℓ + 1)th] layer,
the solute concentration and chemical activity will tend to

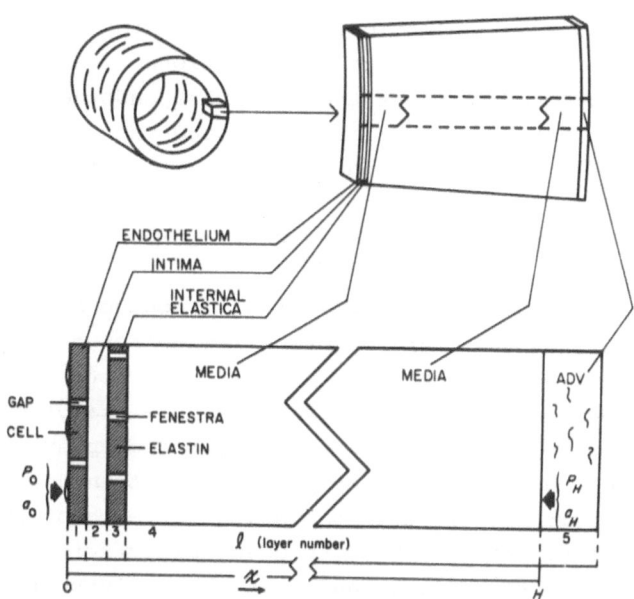

Figure 2. Schematic diagram of multilayered arterial wall
showing x axis of coordinate system extending from x = 0 at
luminal surface to x = H at adventitial interface and
traversing layer numbers ℓ = 1 through 4. Layers ℓ = 1 and
3 shown as two-phase systems and ℓ = 2 and 4 as single phase
systems. P_0 and P_H are pressures and a_0 and a_H are chemical
activities at luminal (x = 0) and adventitial (x = H) interfaces, respectively.

build up in the ℓth layer due to the added retardation of
the convected solute at the interface with the (ℓ + 1) layer.
This accumulation creates an increased "chemical pressure"
for diffusion from the interface in both directions. Thus
the magnitude of the increased chemical activity and diffusive
fluxes from such an interface will depend not only on the
differences between the two f_A's for the two layers but also
on the two diffusivities (D_ℓ's). 4) Referring to Figure 2,
the endothelial surface (ℓ = 1) is a two-phase layer consisting of equispaced endothelial cells separated by intercellular gaps containing matrix material. The fractional
area of the surface covered by cells is α_{el} and that covered
by the intervening intercellular gaps is α_{ml}. Thus, if the
intercellular gaps are closed, α_{ml} = 0; if they occupy 50%
of the intimal surface, α_{ml} = 0.5; and if the cells have
shrunk to mere points (endothelial denudation), α_{ml} = 1.

The assumptions and mathematical details of how the fractional areas, α_m and α_ℓ, enter into the computations of D_ℓ, $f_{A\ell}$, and J_v in Equation 5 to represent the two-phase endothelial (and internal elastica) layer in Figure 2 exceed the scope of the present report and may be found elsewhere (21-23).

Conditions of Aberrant Mass Transport that Might Lead to Atherogenesis

Schematic examples of transmural a(x) contours based on the above stylized model are described below for certain simple, single and progressively multilayered arterial structural configurations of interest. These examples were chosen in a step-wise sequence of increasing complexity to illustrate the physics of the component mass transport processes that could lead to atherogenesis. In each of these cases, it will be assumed that the chemical activity in the bulk phase of the blood is a_0 and that the activity in the interstitial fluids at the abluminal (adventitial) interface is a_H as indicated in Figure 2. In these diagrams, the a(x) contours will be on the ordinate and transmural distance (x) will appear on the abscissa with x = 0 at the blood-luminal interface and x = H at the abluminal interface with the adventitial interstitial fluids as also shown in Figure 2. As will be indicated in the following illustrative examples, the blood phase will be assumed either to be stirred (flowing) or non-stirred; the transmural pressure, P, $(P_0 - P_H$ in Figure 2) will be assumed to be either zero or 100 mmHg.

Case No. 1

Effect of pressure on transmural chemical activity distributions [a(x)] across a single layer, homogeneous arterial media (without endothelial cells, intimal layer, or internal elastica) in contact with stirred blood. The steady-state a(x) curve for the unpressurized (P = 0) case, i.e., the case in which flux is driven only by diffusion (first term on right of Equation 5), appears as the lower sloping straight line in Figure 3. In this situation, a(x) varies linearly across the wall from a_0 at the blood interface to a_H at the adventitial interface. The upper a(x) curve is

EFFECT OF PRESSURE

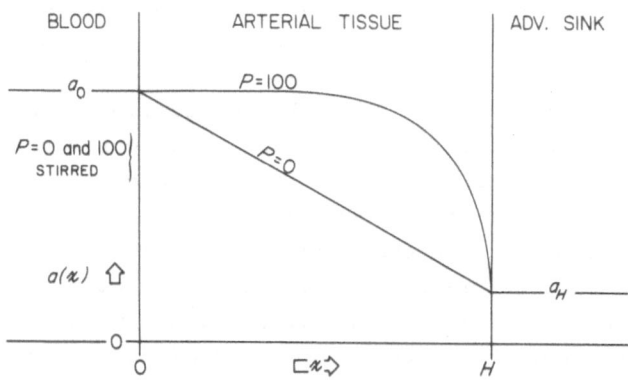

Figure 3. Effect of pressure. Diagrammatic representation of the steady-state arterial transmural (x, abscissa) chemical activity distributions [a(x), ordinate] across simple homogeneous single-layered artery from stirred blood for no transmural pressure (P = 0, simple diffusion) and for transmural pressure of 100 mmHg (P = 100, diffusion and convection). a_0 and a_H are chemical activities of liquids at luminal and abluminal interfaces, respectively, as noted in Figure 2.

for the pressurized (P = 100) situation. In this case, the transmural flux is the sum of the diffusive and the pressure-driven convective components represented by the respective two terms on the right of Equation 5. Unlike the P =0 curve, this curve is concave toward the abscissa but, like the P = 0 curve, extends from a_0 on the left to a_H on the right. Note that a(x) is continuous across each interface, and in the present example a(x) never exceeds the chemical activity (a_0) in the bulk phase of the blood. We shall return to this important point in the next example in which we compare the effect on a(x) of stirring and not stirring the blood in the pressurized situation.

Case No. 2
Effect of stirring on the chemical activity distribution [a(x)] across the single layered, pressurized wall (media)

that was considered in Case No. 1. Referring to Figure 4, the lower a(x) curve is the a(x) for the pressurized stirred and the upper curve for the pressurized non-stirred case. Note that the curve for the non-stirred case begins to rise above a_0 before entering the tissue phase due to molecular sieving at the interface. As explained earlier, sieving occurs at such an interface if the convective retardation coefficient of the wall (f_{A2}) is smaller than that (f_{A1}) of the blood. Thus all of the convective flux that is presented to the wall cannot be accommodated across the interface. As a result, the concentration of the sieved species in the non-stirred situation builds up at the interface until chemical activity gradients build up to create compensating diffusive fluxes away from the sieving site to balance the rate of sieving. Thus the excess flux diffuses back toward the blood phase down the gradient shown to the left of the interface for the non-stirred case.

In the stirred case, the solute is still sieved at the interface, but the sieved molecules are immediately washed away by the flow (stirring). As a result, the chemical activity at the interface does not rise but remains at the value (a_0) of the bulk reagent as if the retardation coefficients were identical on both sides of the interface and sieving were not occurring.

As mentioned earlier, recent work (1) has confirmed the existence of this sieving phenomenon in the *in vitro*, deendothelialized porcine artery preparation. It was shown that the intimal surface concentrations of both ^{125}I-LDL and ^{125}I-albumin in the pressurized, non-stirred situation were greater than the corresponding a_0 and that stirring abolished the difference. Moreover, it was shown that the uptake of each of these proteins, which is proportional to the area between the a(x) contour and the abscissa, was greater for the pressurized non-stirred case than for the stirred case as indicated by the greater elevation of the non-stirred a(x) curve in Figure 4. The significance of the foregoing will be seen better in the following example.

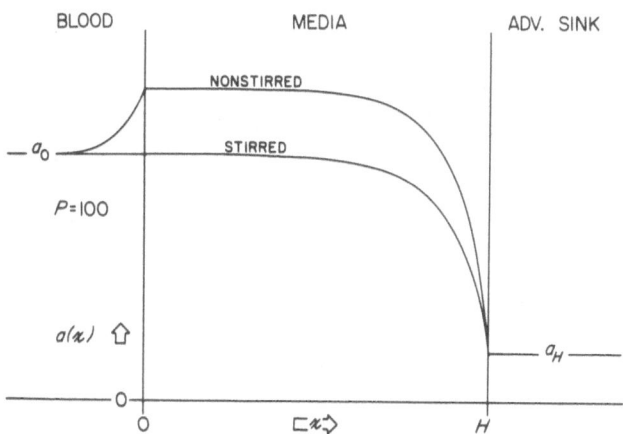

Figure 4. Effect of stirring: Steady-state a(x) contours for pressurized, stirred [same as p = 100 a(x) in Figure 3] and unstirred blood reagent. Otherwise identical to model in Figure 3.

Case No. 3

Effect of adding a porous intimal layer (without endothelial cells), e.g., thrombus, to the single layered wall (media) that was considered in Case No. 2. In the previous case, it was shown that if the adjacent blood flow washed away the sieved species, the tissue chemical activity did not rise above that (a_0) of the bulk phase of the blood. If, on the other hand, a porous layer such as thrombus (24) is placed on the intimal surface, a different situation arises as indicated by the a(x) contour shown in Figure 5. The porous layer allows the convective flux of atherogen to proceed to the original interface virtually unsieved. Like the previous case, it becomes sieved at this interface. However, unlike the previous case, the associated buildup of sieved atherogen at the interface will occur whether the adjacent blood phase is stirred or not since the site of sieving is sequestered by the intervening porous layer from the mixing effects of the adjacent flow. As also discussed in the previous case, the magnitude of a(x) at the interface

EFFECT OF POROUS INTIMAL LAYER

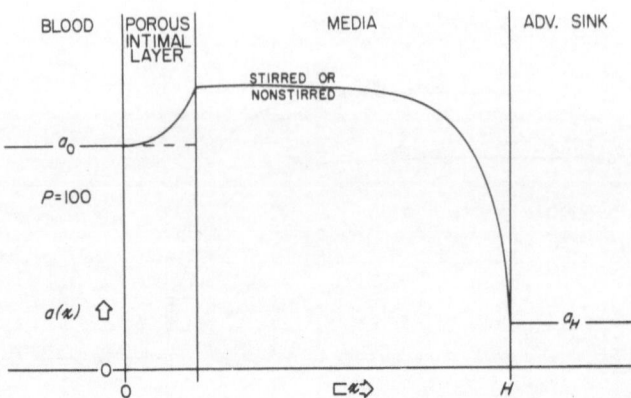

Figure 5. Effect of adding a porous intimal layer and otherwise identical to model in Figure 4. Note that a(x) contour is unaffected by stirring and is identical to un-stirred a(x) in Figure 4.

will depend not only on the rate of sieving but also on the diffusive resistance of the retrograde flux path (porous layer) back to the blood. It will be recalled that a tentative conclusion drawn from the review of evidence presented earlier was that an increased rate of atherogenesis may require an interstitial concentration of atherogen that is significantly elevated above that of the blood. The situation illustrated above appears to provide a simple transport mechanism for achieving such an elevation.

Case No. 4
Effect of adding an internal elastica (IE) layer to the double layered wall (medial layer plus intimal layer without endothelial cells) that was considered in Case No. 3. Atherogenesis is common in the intimal layer but is uncommon in the medial layer unless a_0 is extremely high (e.g., hypercholesterolemia) or unless the IE has become fragmented. Thus, it appears that there is something special about the barrier function of the first elastic lamina in elastic

arteries or IE in muscular arteries. In view of this, it is
of interest to examine the effect of adding an IE layer
between the porous intimal layer and the media of the
example illustrated in Figure 5 for Case No. 3. The IE
layer will be assumed to have a low diffusivity and to be
a more efficient molecular sieve than considered above to
stimulate the observations that the IE appears to be a major
barrier to transport.

Referring to Figure 6, the resulting $a(x)$ contour is
seen to rise progressively in the porous intimal layer to
a higher peak value at the IE interface than seen in
Case No. 3, and then drop precipitously across the IE to
a low value at the interface with the media (due to dilution
with ultrafiltrate from the more efficient IE "sieve"). The
contour then remains at a relatively low value across the
media rising finally to the value, a_H, at the abluminal
boundary as the dilute flux of ultrafiltrate meets the
retrograde diffusive flux from the more concentrated adventitial interstitial fluids. The addition of the IE has
radically changed the shape of the $a(x)$ contour and increased
the peak intimal $a(x)$. (The peak would have been even higher
in the non-stirred case which has been omitted for simpli-
city.) This new $a(x)$ configuration is consistent with the
common observation that the atherosclerotic process is most
severe in the intimal layer and tends to spare the media.
It is of interest next to complete the picture by adding the
final layer, the endothelial surface, to illustrate its
important and paradoxical role.

Case No. 5

The effect of adding an endothelial cell layer to the
three-layered wall shown in Case No. 4. As mentioned earlier
the mathematical model, upon which these illustrative examples
are based, includes provision for study of the effect of
varying the fractional area (α_{ml}) of the endothelial intercellular gaps. A family of $a(x)$ contours for selected values
of endothelial gap fractional area (α_{ml}) appears in Figure 7
with the corresponding values of α_{ml} shown at the left of
each curve. Note that Case No. 4 corresponds to the $\alpha_{ml} = 1$

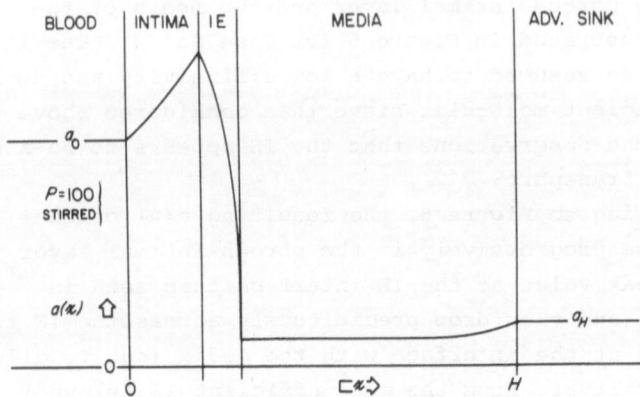

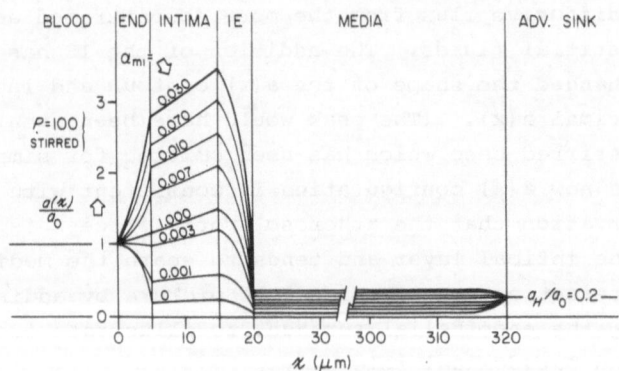

Figure 6. Effect of interposing internal elastica (IE) layer between intimal and medial layers of model shown in Figure 5: Note that addition of IE radically changes shape and magnitude of $a(x)$.

Figure 7. Effect of adding an endothelial layer (END) with varying endothelial intercellular gaps to model shown in Figure 6: α_{ml} is fractional area of the endothelial intercellular gaps. Family of $a(x)$ contours is shown for different values of α_{ml} as noted on left. See also text and Figure 2.

isopleth in this family, i.e., to the situation in which
the endothelial cells have disappeared. Referring to the
$\alpha_{m1} = 0.03$ isopleth, it can be seen that the greatest
intimal chemical activity does not occur with total endothelial loss ($\alpha_{m1} = 1$), which corresponds to the greatest
"endothelial permeability," but, paradoxically occurs at a
fractional gap area (α_{m1}) of only 0.03. To the extent that
the interstitial chemical activity represents the potential
for intimal atherogenesis, the greater risk in this particular case occurs when 97% of the surface is covered with
endothelial cells separated by small gaps and not when
the endothelial cells have disappeared completely. In
addition, it can be seen that the a(x) across the media
remain low for all values of α_{m1} which is consistent with
the observed sparing of this part of the wall. Finally,
it is of interest to note that no part of the wall appears
to be at increased risk when the intercellular gaps are
completely closed, i.e., when $\alpha_{m1} = 0$. The foregoing
illustrative exercise, as well as more comprehensive studies
with the model (20) seem to point to the following conclusions (taken from reference 20):

It appears that sites along the arterial tree that are
characterized 1) by subtle changes in endothelial permeability (simulated in the model with slightly opened endothelial junctions) and 2) by subadjacent interstitial
sieving would be predicted to be at increased risk of atherogenesis even in the presence of well-stirred or flowing blood
and in the absence of other risk factors. Referring to the
a(x)/a_0 contour in Figure 7 for $\alpha_{m1} = 0.03$ as an example of
the foregoing situation, chemical activity distributions can
be formed that may fuel at least three types of atherogenic
processes: 1) Cellular migration: chemical activity
gradients of chemotactic atherogens are formed that could
favor migration of cellular elements such as monocytes (16) from
plasma and of smooth muscle cells (25) from the media to the
intima-internal elastica interface. 2) Cellular proliferation: the larger mitogenic and mutagenic atherogens (11,15)
achieve a maximum intimal chemical activity near the internal
elastica interface. 3) Cholesteryl ester accumulation: the

chemical activity of a cholesterol-bearing atherogen (e.g., βVLDL, "modified LDL", etc.) will have a similar distribution to the above, thereby feeding the chain of processes leading to increased cholesteryl ester formation at the same site (26-28). Thus, the endothelial surface with slightly open junctions acting in concert with a subjacent macromolecular sieve, such as the internal elastica, may shape the chemical activity distributions of an ensemble of atherogens that would favor an accelerated genesis of the intimal components of an arteriosclerotic lesion and, depending on the selectivity (f_A) of the sieve and types of atherogens present, could specify the histological architecture of the lesion (fibrous, foam cell, etc.).

REFERENCES

1. Fry DL, Cornhill JF, Sharma H, Pap JM, Mitschelen J (1986) Uptake of low density lipoprotein, albumin, and water by deendothelialized *in vitro* minipig aorta. Arteriosclerosis 6:475-490.

2. Gorton T, Sorlie P, Kannel WB (1971) The Framingham Study: An epidemiological investigation of cardiovascular disease. Section 27. Washington, DC: US Government Printing Office.

3. Hoff HF, Heideman CL, Jackson RL, Bayardo RJ, Kim HS, Gotto AM Jr (1975) Localization patterns of plasma apolipoproteins in human atherosclerotic lesions. Circ Res 37:72-79.

4. Smith EB, Staples EM (1982) Plasma protein concentrations in interstitial fluid from human aortas. Proc Roy Soc Lond Ser B 217:59-75.

5. Lees RS, Isaacsohn J, Lees AM, Fischman AJ, Strauss HW, Barlai-Kovach M (1985) Imaging of atherosclerosis with technitium-99m labelled low density lipoproteins in human subjects. Circulation 72(Suppl III):III-198.

6. Fry DL (1976) Hemodynamic forces in atherogenesis. In: Scheinberg R (ed) Cerebrovascular Diseases. New York: Raven Press, pp. 77-97.

7. Gerrity RG, Naito HK, Richardson M, Schwartz CJ (1979) Dietary induced atherogenesis in swine. Morphology of the intima in prelesion stages. Am J Pathol 95:775-792.

8. Bell FP, Adamson IL, Schwartz CJ (1974) Aortic endothelial permeability to albumin: Focal and regional patterns of uptake and transmural distribution of 131-I-albumin in the young pig. Exptl Molec Pathol 20:57-68.

9. Bell FP, Gallus AS, Schwartz CJ (1974) Focal and regional patterns of uptake and the transmural distribution of 131-I-fibrinogen in the pig aorta *in vivo*. Exptl Molec Pathol 20:281-292.

10. Ross R, Glomset J, Kariya B, Harker L (1974) A platelet-dependent serum factor that simulates proliferation of arterial smooth muscle cells *in vitro*. Proc Natl Acad Sci 71:1207-1210.
11. Fless GM, Kirchhausen T, Fisher-Dzoga K. Wissler RW, Scanu AM (1982) Serum low density lipoproteins with mitogenic effect on cultured aortic smooth muscle cells. Atherosclerosis 41:171-183.
12. Gotto AM Jr (1979) Status report: Plasma lipids, lipoproteins, and coronary artery disease. Atherosclerosis Rev 4:17-28.
13. Smith EB, Staples EM, Dietz HS, Smith RH (1979) Role of endothelium in sequestration of lipoprotein and fibrinogen in aortic lesions, thrombi, and graft pseudo-intimas. Lancet 2:812-816.
14. Walton KW, Williamson N (1968) Histological and immunofluorescent studies on the evolution of the human atheromatous plaque. J Athero Res 8:599-624.
15. Benditt EP (1977) Implications of the monoclonal character of human atherosclerosic plaques. Am J Pathol 86:693-702.
16. Gerrity RG, Goss JA, Soby L (1985) Control of monocyte recruitment by chemotactic factor(s) in lesion prone areas of swine aorta. Arteriosclerosis 5:55-66.
17. Becker CG (1978) The thrombotic process and atherogenesis in specific arterial injury:immunologic injury. In: Chandler AB, et al. (eds) Advances in Experimental Medicine and Biology, Volume 104. New York: Plenum Press, pp. 371-378.
18. Minick CR, Stemerman MB, Insull W Jr (1977) Effect of regenerated endothelium on lipid accumulation in the arterial wall. Proc Natl Acad Sci 74:1724-1728.
19. Schwartz SM, Stemerman MB, Benditt EP (1975) The aortic intima: II. Repair of the aortic lining after mechanical denudation. Am J Pathol 81:15-42.
20. Fry DL (1987) Mass transport, atherogenesis, and risk. Arteriosclerosis 17:88-100.
21. Fry DL (1983) Effect of pressure and stirring on *in vitro* aortic transmural 125-I-albumin transport. Am J Physiol 245:H977-H991.
22. Fry DL (1985) Mathematical models of arterial transmural transport. Am J Physiol 284:H240-H263.
23. Fry DL (1985) Steady-state macromolecular transport across a multilayered arterial wall. Math Modelling (Int'l J) 6:353-368.
24. Duguid JB (1948) Thrombosis as a factor in the pathogenesis of aortic atherogenesis. J Pathol Bact 60:57-61.
25. Grotendorst GR, Seppa HEJ, Kleinman HK, Martin GR (1981) Attachment of smooth muscle cells to collagen and their migration toward platelet-derived growth factor. Proc Natl Acad Sci 78:3669-3672.
26. Innerarity TL, Arnold KS, Weisgraber KH, Mahley RW (1986) Apolipoprotein E is the determinant that mediates the receptor uptake of β-very low density lipoproteins by mouse macrophages. Arteriosclerosis 6:114-122.
27. Brown MS, Ho, YK, Goldstein JL (1980) The cholesteryl ester cycle in macrophage foam cells. Continual hydrolysis and reesterification on cytoplasmic cholesteryl esters. J Biol Chem 255:9344-9352.
28. Mazzone T, Chait A (1982) Autogegulation of the modified low density lipoprotein receptor in human monocyte-derived macrophages. Arteriosclerosis 2:487-492.

19

Accumulating Evidence from Human Artery Studies of What Gets Transported and What Accumulates Relative to Atherogenesis

Elspeth B. Smith

The simple concept that endothelium acts as a barrier
to plasma macromolecules is no longer tenable. Instead,
endothelium appears to provide a sophisticated transport
system, and the main barrier is situated at the internal
elastic lamina (IEL). In experimental animals the endothelium virtually lies on the IEL, making accurate study of
their separate functions extremely difficult. Endothelium
and IEL are separated by the diffusely thickened intima of
the adult human aorta and coronary arteries. Unfortunately,
in human subjects it is usually only possible to measure
the steady state concentration of plasma macromolecules,
which represents the resultant of influx, efflux, reversible
and irreversible binding and destruction.

Virtually all plasma proteins are present in intima,
and their concentrations are directly related to plasma
concentration and molecular mass (M_r). Expression of concentration as microliters of the patients own plasma demonstrates the relative retention of the proteins, and it can
be seen in Table 1 that this decreased with decreasing M_r.
There are just two major exceptions - fibronectin and
plasminogen. Retention of fibronectin was 6-8 times the
expected level, probably reflecting both reversible binding

Acknowledgements: The author's work was supported by grants
from the British Heart Foundation and the Medical Research
Council. The names of the author's co-workers are cited in
the references.

Table 1. Relative Retention of Plasma Macromolecules in
Normal Intima

	M_r (x 10^{-3})	% of LDL Retention
LDL-ApoB	2700	100
α_2-macroglobulin	720	43
Fibronectin	440	200-300
Fibrinogen	340	[33][a]
HDL$_2$ ApoA	360	12[b] (+12)[c]
HDL$_3$	170	
Transferrin	76	35
Prothrombin	72	38
Albumin	67	21
Antithrombin III	65	28
α_2-antiplasmin	65	25
α_1-antitrypsin	54	18
Plasminogen	91	Not found in 70% of samples

[a] About 50% fibrinogen; remainder fibrin/fibrinogen
degradation products (FDP).

[b] HDL$_{2+3}$

[c] Component of slow mobility, containing apoAl only

to some component of the connective tissue matrix and local
synthesis. We failed to recover plasminogen from 75% of
samples despite normal plasma levels (1,2), a finding that
we still do not understand.

Macromolecules in Interstitial Fluid

In a tissue sample macromolecules may be free in the
interstitial fluid or reversibly or irreversibly associated
with cell surfaces and the connective tissue matrix.   In
terms of atherogenesis we are concerned primarily with
factors that influence smooth muscle cell metabolism,
particularly stimulation of cell proliferation and collagen
synthesis. These factors must, therefore, be in the
interstitial fluid (IF), which provides the immediate
nutritive environment of the cells.

The concentration of LDL and two other marker proteins, α_2-macroglobulin (α_2-M) and albumin, in IF from normal areas of human aortic intima is shown in Table 2, expressed as percent of concentration in the patient's own plasma. In IF the concentration of LDL, measured as apo-B, is twice the plasma concentration, whereas albumin is half the plasma concentration; virtually no apo-B is found in medial IF (3). Absolute concentrations of apo-B in plasma and IF are highly correlated, but the relative concentration in IF remains constant over a plasma LDL range of 180-630mg/100 ml. However, relative concentration showed a significant correlation with age, increasing by about 1% per annum over the age range 31-96 years (p = 0.005).

In early proliferative lesions there is a doubling of interstitial fluid space, but little change in the concentration of macromolecules in the IF (Table 3). As lesions apparently mature the interstitial fluid volume decreases again and there is a reciprocal increase in macromolecule concentration (p = 0.01) (4,5). The results suggest that changes in intimal matrix may be of greater importance than change in trans-endothelial transport in determining steady state concentrations in early human lesions.

Trans-endothelial Transport and Endothelial Injury

At the ultrastructural level, transport of LDL has been visualized across rat and rabbit aortic endothelium (6,7). In rat aorta some LDL is taken up by receptor mediated endocytosis. The amount appeared to be independent of LDL concentration in the perfusion medium. Some LDL is taken up into plasmalemmal vesicles and crosses the endothelial cell by transcytosis; the amount transported depended on LDL concentration and appeared to be a nonsaturable process. This exactly parallels our findings on the relation between plasma and intimal concentrations of macromolecules in human aorta (3). In chemical studies plasma clearances were the same for native LDL and reductively methylated LDL, which is not recognized by the LDL receptor (8).

Table 2. Concentration of Plasma Proteins in Interstitial
Fluid from Normal Aortic Intima and Media

	Percent of Plasma Concentration		
Sample	LDL	α_2-M	Albumin
Intima			
Men (n = 22)	212 $\pm$ 54[a]	115 $\pm$ 32	55 $\pm$ 16
Women (n = 22)	219 $\pm$ 67	114 $\pm$ 48	53 $\pm$ 15
Media (n = 11)	0 (n = 7)	11 $\pm$ 2	18 $\pm$ 6
	trace (n = 4)		

[a] Standard deviation

A major source of confusion has been failure to
differentiate between flux and steady state concentration.
Experimental endothelial denudation, which probably also
results in damage to the IEL, produces rapid flux but
equally rapid re-equilibration, whereas in re-endothelialized
areas there is progressive accumulation of LDL (9).

In the early stages of cholesterol feeding in rabbits
Simionescu et al. (7) found enhanced uptake and deposition
of lipoprotein and lipid while endothelium remained morphologically intact and no platelet involvement was detected.
Stemmerman et al. (10) found no loss of endothelium or
separation between endothelial cells in foci of increased
uptake of horse radish peroxidase and LDL in normal rabbit
aorta.

Changes of Macromolecules in Intima: Degradation or Complex
Formation

Fibrinogen undergoes extensive changes within the
intima (Figure 1). Some is probably converted to insoluble
fibrin, which is present in virtually all samples of
intima (11), and both fibrinogen and fibrin appear to be
degraded because the soluble fraction contains unchanged
fibrinogen, high M_r components which may be fragments X and
Y derived from fibrinogen, and fragment D-dimer, which must
be derived from cross-linked fibrin (12).

Table 3. Relationship Between the Amount of LDL in Tissue, and Interstitial Fluid Concentration and Volume

	Concentration		Distribution Volume[c]
	μLPS[a] Tissue/100 mg d.t.[b]	IF % of plasma conc.	mg Water/100 mg d.t.
Normal			
Intima	860 ± 99	226 ± 15	397 ± 33
Media	<3	0 - trace	-
Proliferative Lesions			
Gelatinous	2024 ± 352	330 ± 35	644 ± 81
Transitional	1085 ± 195	432 ± 98	255 ± 47
White fibrous (caps only)	128 ± 28	118 ± 26	129 ± 34

a PS = patient's own serum

b 100 mg lipid-extracted dry tissue

c Distribution volume approximates to the IF space

**Woman aged 62 — extract of pooled
small gelatinous lesions**

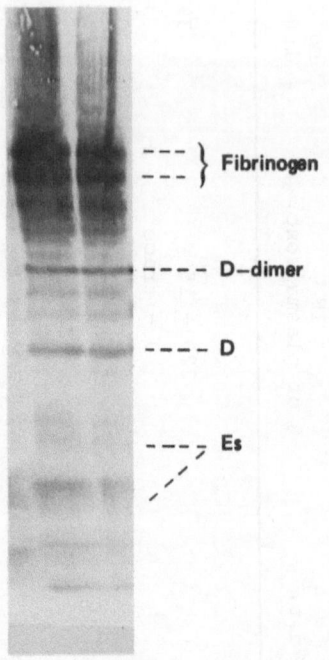

**Separated by SDS—PAGE and immuno-blotted
for fibrinogen-related antigens**

Figure 1. Fibrin/fibrinogen-related antigens in intimal
extract showing the characteristic range of large and small
FDPs.

HDL also appears to undergo major change, with loss of
components with the electrophoretic characteristics of HDL_2
and HDL_3 and appearance of a component with slower electrophoretic mobility and higher density, which contains apo-Al
but not apo-A-II (13,14).

Obviously, a question of major interest is the fate of
LDL, and here the situation is very unclear. In homogenates,
which presumably contain other extracellular particles such

as perifibrous lipid (PFL) as well as intact LDL, Hoff and
Gaubatz (15) found increased net negative charge and changed
composition in the LDL fraction. On isoelectric focusing
from whole tissue we found a component that focused with
plasma LDL (peak A) and an apo-B-containing component that
was too large to enter a 3.4% polyacrylamide gel (peak B).
In normal intima, A was the major peak but in lesions the
proportion of peak A decreased and peak B increased, suggesting some form of aggregation (16). However, on agarose
electrophoresis of intimal interstitial fluid we found no
consistent change in net negative charge of LDL in normal
intima or fatty streaks. In some samples mobility was
increased, and in others it was the same as the subject's
plasma LDL. In early gelatinous thickenings there was,
however, a consistent slight decrease in net negative
charge (17).

It is frequently asserted that LDL forms reversible
complexes with glycosaminoglycans (GAG) in intima, and this
accounts for its high concentration, but our studies on human
intima have not provided support for this idea. The virtually linear relation between relative retention and molecular
mass (M_r) suggests molecular sieving, not specific binding
(18). Comparison of the ratios of LDL to other macromolecules in interstitial fluid and whole tissue should reveal
reversible binding. The tissue will contain both LDL that
is free in the interstitial fluid and reversibly bound LDL,
whereas the interstitial fluid will contain the free fraction only. There is no increase in the ratios LDL/α_2-
macroglobulin or LDL/albumin in tissue compared with free
IF (Table 4). This is in marked contrast to fibronectin;
the ratio LDL/fibronectin was consistently and significantly
lower in tissue than in interstitial fluid, and indicated
that about half the fibronectin was reversibly associated
with some component of the tissue (1,3,4). Absence of
specific reversible complex formation does not mean that
GAG have no role - they probably have a major influence on
the volume of the interstitial space and the distribution
volume of the macromolecules within it (18).

Table 4. Ratios of LDL to other Macromolecules in Interstitial Fluid and Whole Intimal Tissue

	Interstitial Fluid	Tissue
LDL/α_2-M		
Normal intima (n = 11)	1.94	1.80
Gel lesions (n = 11)	1.77	1.15
LDL/albumin		
Normal intima (n = 11)	4.10	3.25
Gel lesions (n = 11)	5.13	3.80
LDL/fibronectin		
Normal intima (n = 6)	9.40	5.2
Gel lesions (n = 15)	9.80	5.2

Flux Into Human Intima

Recently, Stender and Hjelms (19) examined uptake of
labelled free and ester cholesterol into macroscopically
normal human ascending aorta over time periods ranging from
0.2 to 114 hours before surgical excision. The results are
difficult to interpret because all lipoprotein fractions
were labelled, there appeared to be both exchange and
esterification of free cholesterol and hydrolysis of
cholesterol ester. At time periods of less than one hour
the counts in the inner intima/media layer were too low to
measure influx, and in the 24-114 hour periods the counts
presumably no longer represent influx but approach steady-
state conditions. However, in all cases the amount of
cholesterol that entered the inner intima/media layer per
unit time was far greater than the amount that had accumulated over the patient's lifetime, thus there must be
extensive efflux although these experiments do not tell us
if the efflux is in the form of intact lipoprotein or free
or esterified cholesterol. However, in their experimental
studies with apo-B-labelled LDL, Carew et al. (20) concluded that only 10-20% of apo-B was degraded, and 80% must
re-equilibrate by bi-directional transfer.

Model of Intimal Steady State

Any model must take into account endothelial trans-cytosis and molecular sieving. It is assumed that plasma-lemmal vesicles equilibrate with plasma or interstitial fluid at the luminal or abluminal surfaces, move randomly across the cell by Brownian motion, and that a proportion will then re-equilibrate at the other side, resulting in net transfer of solutes from high concentration to lower concentration fluids. Obviously, this mechanism could not produce a two-fold concentration of LDL in the immediate sub-endothelial space, and I postulate (Figure 2) that the macromolecules are carried through the endothelial basement membrane by convective transport in the trans-arterial water flow. They encounter a major barrier at the IEL, and escape into the media at rates that are inversely proportional to molecular mass.

Very little LDL enters the normal media, therefore there must be efflux back across the endothelium. There is evidence that the basement membrane provides a significant molecular sieve (21). The convective outward transport (influx) of macromolecules will be mainly independent of M_r, but efflux back into the lumen will require diffusion across the basement membrane into the sub-endothelial space and be highly dependent on M_r. Thus for LDL a two-fold concentration gradient develops before influx and efflux come into equilibrium.

Perhaps future studies should be less concerned with the morphology and lipid metabolism of the endothelial cells themselves, and concentrate more on the basement membrane. Haust (22) observed increases in basement membrane-like material in lesions; increase in thickness and density of basement membrane might be a factor in trapping even higher concentrations of LDL in lesions.

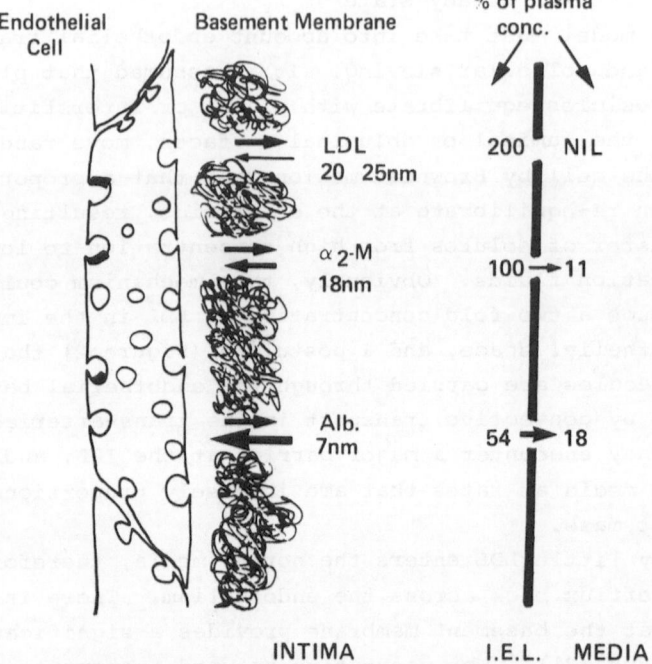

Figure 2. Hypothetical scheme depicting the steady state in intima. Following transcytosis macromolecules are carried outwards across the endothelial basement membrane by convective transport at approximately equal rates. The rate of efflux by reverse transcytosis is dependent on diffusion back across the basement membrane, and this is inversely related to molecular diameter.

REFERENCES

1. Smith EB, Ashall C (1986) Fibronectin distribution in human aortic intima and atherosclerotic lesions: Concentration of soluble and collagenase-releasable fractions. Biochim Biophys Acta 880:10-15.
2. Smith EB, Ashall C (1985) Fibrinolysis and plasminogen concentration in aortic intima in relation to death following myocardial infarction. Atherosclerosis 55: 171-186.
3. Smith EB, Staples EM (1982) Plasma protein concentration in interstitial fluid from human aortas. Proc R Soc Lond B 217:59-75.

4. Smith EB, Ashall C (1983) Low density lipoprotein concentration in interstitial fluid from human athero-sclerotic lesions: Relation to theories of endothelial damage and lipoprotein binding. Biochim Biophys Acta 754:249-257.
5. Smith EB, Ashall C (1984) Compartmentalization of water in human atherosclerotic lesions. Arterio-sclerosis 4:21-27.
6. Vasile E, Simionescu M, Simionescu N (1983) Visuali-zation of the binding, endocytosis and transcytosis of low-density lipoprotein in the arterial endothelium in situ. J Cell Biol 96:1677-1689.
7. Simionescu N, Vasile E, Lupu F, Popescu G, Simionescu M (1986) Accumulation of extracellular cholesterol-rich liposomes in the arterial intima and cardiac valves of the hyperlipidemic rabbit. Am J Pathol 123:109-125.
8. Wiklund O, Carew TE, Steinberg D (1985) Role of the low density lipoprotein receptor in penetration of low density lipoprotein into rabbit aortic wall. Arterio-sclerosis 5:135-141.
9. Falcone DJ, Hajjar DP, Minick CR (1984) Lipoprotein and albumin accumulation in re-endothelialized and de-endothelialized aorta. Am J Pathol 114:112-120.
10. Stemmerman MB, Morrel EM, Burke KR, Colton CK, Smith KA, Lees RS (1986) Local variation in arterial wall permeability to low density lipoprotein in normal rabbit aorta. Arteriosclerosis 6:64-69.
11. Smith EB, Alexander KM, Massie IB (1976) Insoluble "fibrin" in human aortic intima. Quantitative studies on the relationship between insoluble "fibrin", soluble fibrinogen and LD-lipoprotein. Atherosclerosis 23:19-39.
12. Smith EB (1986) Fibrinogen, fibrin and fibrin degrada-tion products in relation to atherosclerosis. In: Fidge NH, Nesterl PJ (eds), Atherosclerosis VII. Amsterdam: Excerpta Medica, pp. 459-462.
13. Heideman CL, Hoff HF (1982) Lipoproteins containing apolipoprotein Al extracted from human aortas. Biochim Biophys Acta 711:431-444.
14. Smith EB, Ashall C, Walker JE (1984) High density lipo-protein (HDL) subfractions in interstitial fluid from human aortic intima and atherosclerotic lesions. Biochem Soc Trans 12:843-844.
15. Hoff HF, Gaubatz JW (1982) Isolation, purification and characterization of a lipoprotein containing apo B from the human aorta. Atherosclerosis 42:273-297.
16. Smith EB, Dietz HS, Craig IB (1979) Characterization of free and tightly bound lipoprotein in intima by thin layer isoelectric focusing. Atherosclerosis 33:329-342.
17. Smith EB, Ashall C (1983) Variability of the electro-phoretic mobility of low density lipoprotein - Compari-son of interstitial fluid from human aortic intima and serum. Atherosclerosis 49:89-98.
18. Smith EB, Staples EM (1982) Intimal and medial plasma protein concentrations and endothelial function. Atherosclerosis 41:295-308.
19. Stender S, Hjelms E (1984) In vivo influx of free and esterified plasma cholesterol into human aortic tissue without atherosclerotic lesions. J Clin Invest 74:1871-1881.

20. Carew TE, Pittman RC, Marchand ER, Steinberg D (1984) Measurement *in vivo* of irreversible degradation of low density lipoprotein in the rabbit aorta. Arteriosclerosis 4:214-224.

21. Johansson BR (1979) Capillary permeability to interstitial microinjections of macromolecules, and influence of hydrostatic pressure on endothelial ultrastructure. Acta Physiol Scand, Suppl 463:45-50.

22. Haust MD (1977) Connective tissue in atherosclerosis. In: Schettler G, Goto Y, Hata Y, Klose G (eds), Atherosclerosis IV. Berlin: Springer-Verlag, pp. 30-35.

20

How Hemodynamic Forces in the Human Affect the Topography and Development of Atherosclerosis

Morton H. Friedman

The purpose of this presentation is to address two questions regarding the role of hemodynamic forces in the atherosclerotic process. The first, relates to the influence of hemodynamics on atherosclerotic <u>development</u>, i.e., what is the response, particularly the pathologic response, of the vessel wall to its hemodynamic environment? The second, is related to hemodynamic influences on the <u>topography</u> of atherosclerosis, i.e., what is the distribution of hemo-dynamic variables, particularly those that might have an adverse effect on the vessel wall? Consistent with the purpose of this meeting, both of these questions will be addressed with as much emphasis as possible on the <u>human</u> lesion. As charged, I will discuss what we know about the answers to these two questions, why we do not know more, and what it is that we need to be able to do to fill the gaps in our knowledge.

The Response of the Human Vessel Wall to Hemodynamic Forces

Most of the recent and best controlled studies of the response of vascular cells to hemodynamic forces have been carried out in cell culture using primarily non-human cells. From these experiments, we know some of the hemodynamic factors to which these cells respond. They respond to shear stress; that is, the drag on the cells by fluid moving past

Prepared with support from the National Institutes of Health, Grant HL-34626.

them. In an artery, the shear at the blood vessel wall is caused by the flow flowing through the lumen. Vascular endothelium in culture responds specifically to oscillatory components in the shear environment, as will be illustrated shortly. Recently, Davies and coworkers (1) showed that turbulence increases the turnover rate of bovine aortic endothelial cells in culture.

The responses of vascular cells to these hemodynamic stresses are diverse. Perhaps the most widely studied response is change in shape (2,3). Endothelial cells in culture exposed to constant unidirectional shear stresses become elongated and line up with the direction of flow. Morphologic changes within the cell are also seen. Exposure to steady laminar shear can cause stress fibers in the cytoskeleton of cultured bovine aortic endothelial cells to hypertrophy and align with the outside flow (MA Gimbrone, personal communication). Metabolic changes can also be induced by shear stress. Frangos, et al. (4) examined the effect of shear stress on prostacyclin production by human umbilical vein endothelial cells. The production rate was increased markedly when a steady shear stress of 10 dynes per square centimeter - which is in the physiological range of time-average stresses in man (5) - was applied to these cells. When a sinusoidally varying shear stress, 2 dynes per square centimeter in amplitude, was superimposed on the steady shear, so that the stress to which the cells were exposed oscillated with a frequency of 1 Hz between 8 and 12 dynes per square centimeter, prostacyclin production rate was doubled. Some of these responses have also been noted in animal experiments.

Although we have learned a great deal about the response of vascular cells, primarily endothelial cells, in culture to hemodynamic stresses, we have not been very successful in making the connection between these observations and the role of hemodynamics in the development of the human lesion. A major reason for this failure relates to the second question that was posed above.

The *In vivo* Distribution of Hemodynamic Variables

Sites in the arterial tree that appear predisposed to atherosclerosis are sites at which the hemodynamics is often unusual. It should be recognized, however, that, apart from the effect of spatial variations in the hemodynamic environment, hemodynamics can influence the topography of the disease if the arterial vulnerability to hemodynamic stress varies from site to site. Very little is known about these latter variations.

Using techniques such as ultrasound, we can assess the more global hemodynamic parameters in human arteries that are not too deep within the body. We know also in a general way how hemodynamic variables are distributed among vascular beds and organ systems, and we have a general notion of the distribution of hemodynamic variables within specific vascular geometric configurations. For instance, we know that at a branch shear stresses are likely to be higher along the flow divider than along the outer walls.

We know also that there are considerable differences in the hemodynamic environment at sites separated by only millimeters, that is, over distances commensurate with the focal lesion. There is also considerable variation among individuals in hemodynamic forces at corresponding sites.

This variability is illustrated in Figure 1, which shows the profiles of maximum instantaneous shear rate along the outer walls of four human aortic bifurcations. These shear rates were obtained by laser Doppler anemometry in flow-through vascular casts whose silhouettes are also shown in the figure. The flows through the casts were pulsatile and physiologically realistic. In simple tubular branches of uniform diameter, the shear rate profile at the lateral walls passes through a minimum near the level of the flow divider tip (Z = 0 in Figure 1). It can be seen from the figure that such is not always the case for real arterial branches. In some vessels (e.g., AB-9) the shear rate changes hardly at all or increases monotonically with Z. In other vessels, such as AB-4, minima are seen but can occur either proximal or distal to the flow divider tip.

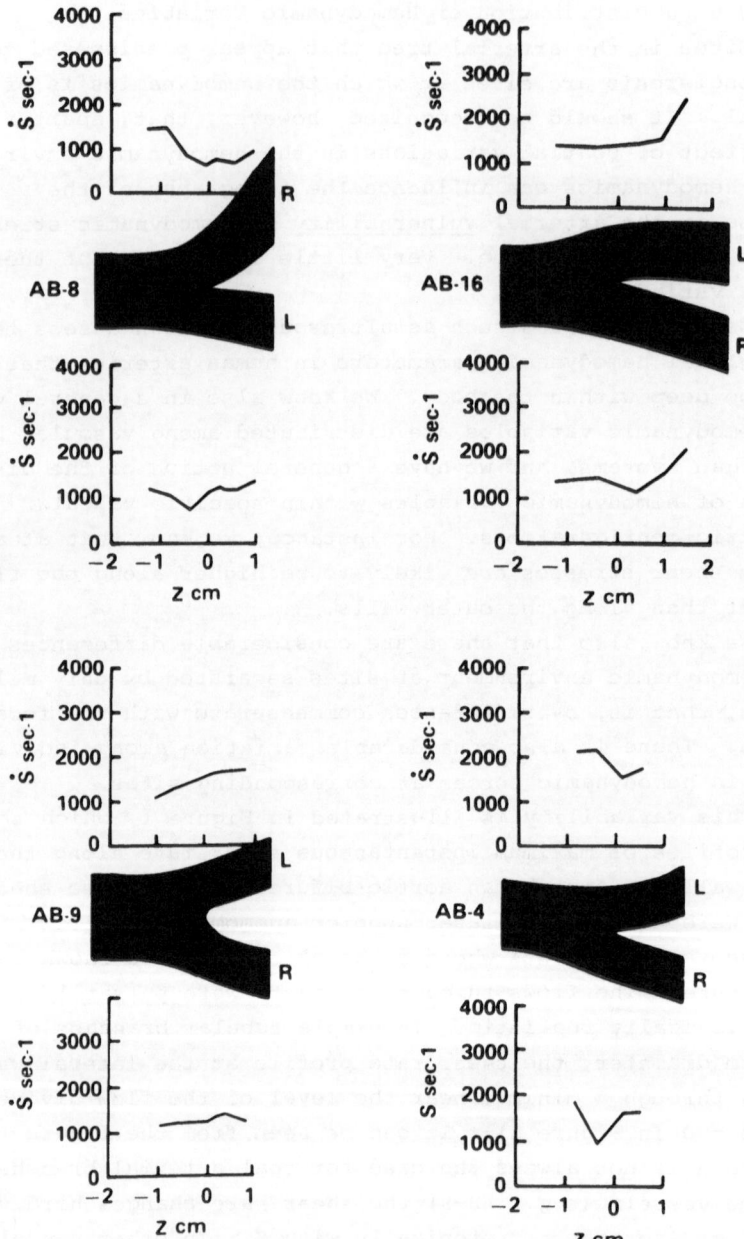

Figure 1. Variation of maximum instantaneous shear rate with distance along the lateral walls of four human aortic bifurcations. The silhouettes of the bifurcations are traced from flow-through casts of the vessel segments.

As a result of this variability, we cannot <u>predict</u> the distribution of hemodynamic variables in any individual with the resolution that we would like. The limitations this imposes on the search for the role of hemodynamics in human atherosclerosis will be discussed next, along with some other problems.

Problems in Assessing the Role of Hemodynamics in Atherosclerosis, and Some Attempted Solutions

To relate the results of cell culture experimentation to the development of human vascular disease, it is necessary to demonstrate in man an association between hemodynamic factors, including those known to affect cells in culture, and the evolving atherosclerotic lesion. Because of the spatial variability of both the *in vivo* flow variables and the disease, the hemodynamic and corresponding pathologic measurements must be well resolved spatially. In trying to meet this requirement, we encounter a number of significant problems:

1. As noted earlier, there is a considerable individual variability in the distribution of hemodynamic quantities in real arteries. This means that the hemodynamic data that we need to establish the relation between hemodynamics and atherosclerosis must be <u>measured</u>, because we cannot know, without measuring, the hemodynamic environment at any parti-cular site in a given vessel.

2. The distribution of lesions varies among individuals and, in any particular individual, probably varies with time as well. Thus, our need to measure *in vivo* hemodynamics is paralleled by a similar need with respect to plaques.

3. Human hemodynamic data must be measured with a resolution comparable to the scale of the focal disease to which it presumably contributes. We cannot meet this require-ment with available noninvasive technology.

4. Finally, we cannot visualize early atherosclerotic disease *in vivo* using current imaging technology, so we can-not follow the course of the disease at any given site.

Because of these problems, there have been very few studies in which <u>hemodynamics</u> and <u>atherosclerosis</u> in <u>the</u> <u>human</u> <u>species</u> have been addressed simultaneously. We are confronted with variability in both hemodynamics and vessel pathology, and our ability to measure either of these quantities in living man is inadequate.

The approaches to dealing with the variability problem are of two kinds. The first of these is the method traditionally used to deal with biological variability. Hemodynamics and pathology are quantitated in a sufficiently large population, the results are averaged and relationships are sought among the averages. The second approach is to compare hemodynamics and pathology in a series of individuals. Since we cannot measure hemodynamics with sufficient resolution *in vivo*, the common recourse has been to *ex vivo* measurements or to measurements in casts or models of arterial segments. Since casts replicate the arteries of a particular individual, experiments in casts are best suited to the "individual vessel" approach to dealing with the variability problem. This is clearly also the case for experiments with *ex vivo* specimens. In this latter category, mention should be made of measurements by Karino (6) of particle paths in human carotid, cerebral and basilar artery fiburcations made transparent with methyl salicylate.

Models, on the other hand, are made to be representative of the average geometry of a segment of interest, and therefore are more suitable to the "average vessel" approach to the variability problem. Vascular models have ranged from simple tubular constructions to more complex shapes whose dimensions are derived from collected autopsy material.

Because of our inability to measure early lesions *in vivo*, we usually get only one look at any specimen, at autopsy. This can seriously limit our understanding if, as some evidence suggests (7), the time dependence of the atherosclerotic process is complex.

The best example of the use of averaging to examining the relationship between hemodynamic shear and human vascular morphology is the work reported by Ku et al. (8). These investigators measured the intimal thickness at twenty standard sites in twelve human carotid bifurcations. Intimal thickness has been the most commonly used morphological measure in studies such as this, because of the association between intimal thickening and early atherosclerotic development. The average thickness at each of the twenty sites was computed and correlated against hemodynamic measurements in a Plexiglas model whose geometry was representative of the bifurcation. Thus the average intimal thicknesses in the twelve vessels were correlated against what could be regarded as the hemodynamics in an _average_ of the vessel geometries.

The limitations of this technique are two-fold. First, one loses the information that may be available from individual variability in the location and progression of intimal thickening. A second limitation of the averaging approach is that it implicitly assumes that all specimens are from the same population; this may not be the case, as we shall discuss shortly.

The alternative route, which we have chosen, is to investigate the relation between hemodynamics and wall morphology in a series of vessels. The results are then synthesized into a self-consistent picture of the vessel response. Naturally, we cannot use models to quantitate the hemodynamics in these specimens, because we must retain the particular contours of each vessel. Therefore, we carry out our experiments in flow-through casts of human arterial segments. Figure 2 illustrates this approach. In this figure, the upper left-hand panel is a Silastic mold of the lumen of a human aortic bifurcation. This is the segment of the vasculature with which we have worked most extensively; we are also using coronary artery bifurcations from human hearts. Two sites are indicated on the mold. The upper right-hand panel shows the velocity profiles at those sites, measured using laser Doppler anemometry near the wall of the cast made from the mold. We have worked with both rigid and elastic casts. The lower panels show the histology of the corresponding sites in the vessel from which the mold was made. We then seek correlations between a variety of hemodynamic measurements made in the cast and morphologic measurements made on the original vessel.

A principal limitation of this technique is that it is time consuming. Presumably, the offsetting benefit is the realism of the data that are obtained.

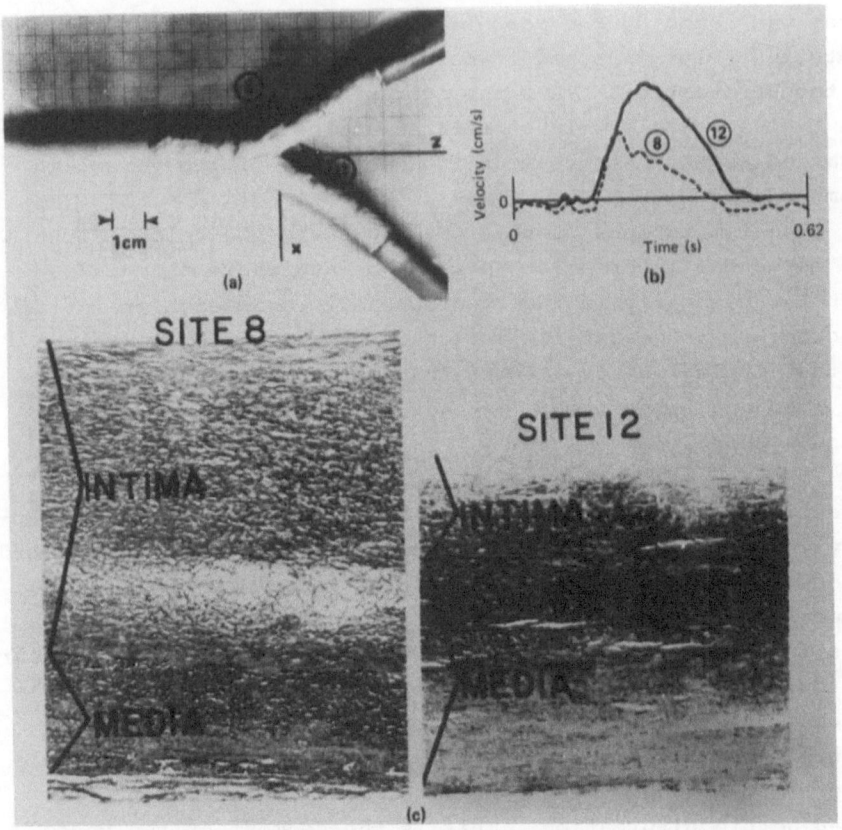

Figure 2. (a). Mold of an aortic bifurcation. Two sites
are marked. (b). Velocity histories at the two sites marked
in (a); the velocities were measured 0.058 cm from the wall
of a cast made from the mold in (a). The maximum velocity
at Site 12 was 137 cm/s. (c). Histology at the two sites in
the original vessel. Verhoeff-van Gieson stain.

The Association Between Hemodynamics and Atherosclerosis in
Man

What have we learned from studies such as those that have
just been described, with respect to the associations between
hemodynamics and atherosclerosis in man? First, we know which
hemodynamic features are not essential for atherogenesis. The
most authentic hemodynamic experiments use realistic flow
waves and fluid dynamic scaling to insure that the fluid
dynamic phenomena seen in the experiments are representative
of those that are present in vivo. These experiments show

that there is essentially no turbulence in most of the normal cardiovascular system and certainly no turbulence at many of the sites at which lesions occur relatively early in life. Turbulence cannot be a necessary initiator of the lesion. Turbulence in more severely occluded vessels may play a role in the _evolution_ of the plaque. A second phenomenon that does not occur in the vasculature at many sites where lesions are found is separation. Separated flows _per se_ are not necessary to atherogenesis; however, certain features associated with flow separation, such as relatively protracted periods of low wall shear, or variability in the direction and magnitude of the shear stress at the wall, may indeed be important in the disease process.

Because turbulence and separation are not essential to the atherosclerotic process, much effort has been directed toward understanding the role of wall shear stress. Our experiments indicate that the relationship between shear and the intimal thickening process is complex and time-dependent. A sketch showing our current thinking on this subject is shown in Figure 3. At any site in the vessel, the relationship between intimal thickness and time depends on the shear at that point, but thickening does not progress at a constant rate. Indeed, our data suggest that sites exposed to higher shear stresses initially thicken more quickly, but sites exposed to lower shears eventually reach greater thicknesses and therefore may be more prone to disease.

The behavior shown in Figure 3 offers an explanation of what has sometimes been called "high shear-low shear controversy". Some investigators have found that sites associated with high shear have thicker intimas, whereas other experimenters have reported the opposite. Figure 3 shows that either of these results can be obtained, depending on the extent to which the thickening process has progressed at the time of the experiment. This time-dependent character of the relation between thickness and shear rate, suggested by our "individual vessel" experiments (7), would not be revealed by "average vessel" experiments, since an implicit assumption in the averaging process is that the dependence of intimal thickness on shear rate is the same for all specimens.

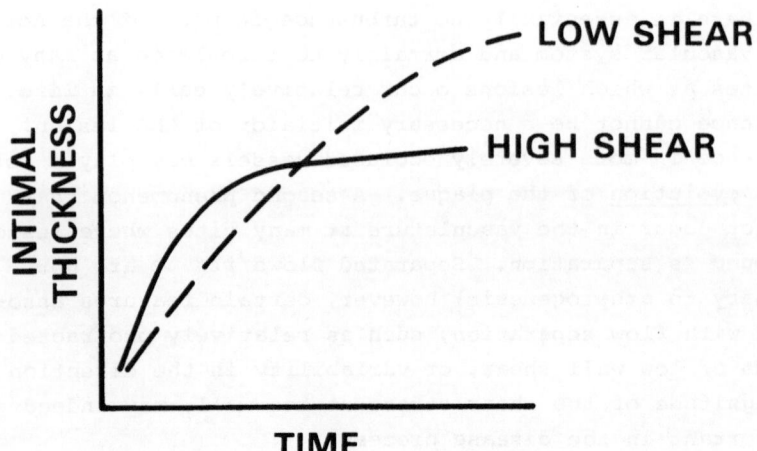

Figure 3. Sketch of the variation with shear rate of
intimal thickening over time, as inferred from data like
those in Figure 2.

A Model of Intimal Thickening Under Shear

We have developed a very simple model of intimal thickening which includes a selection of the biological processes
that take place in the arterial wall and which explains how
curves of thickness versus time for different shear rates
can cross. The model is illustrated in Figure 4. In this
model, the number density of smooth muscle cells per unit
surface area initially increases with time, as a result of
migration and proliferation. The model is blind to the
site of origin (intima or media) of the earliest cells. The
accumulation rate remains constant until a limiting number
density of cells (n_{si} in the figure) is reached. After this
point, the number density of smooth muscle cells remains
constant. The cells produce matrix in proportion to their
number.

Lipoprotein enters the intima from the blood. Free
lipoprotein can be consumed by smooth muscle cells and is
bound by the matrix elaborated by those cells. Monocytes
enter the wall, transform to macrophages and consume

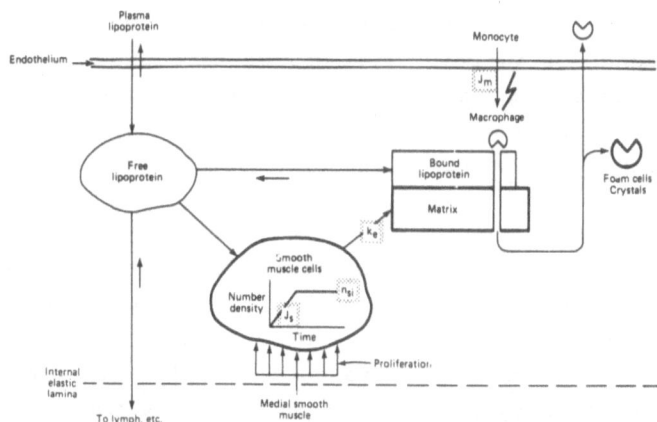

Figure 4. Model of shear-dependent intimal thickening. The
parameters on stippled backgrounds are allowed to vary with
wall shear. The heavily outlined compartments contribute
to intimal thickness.

extracellular lipid. The macrophages either exit into the
blood or remain in the intima and form foam cells. The
thickness of the intima is made up of contributions from
the smooth muscle cells, extracellular matrix and foam
cells.

This model has been translated mathematically into a
set of equations, which we have used to correlate our
experimental data. The four parameters indicated in Figure 4
are allowed to vary with shear rate. These include the rate
of accumulation of smooth muscle cells, the smooth muscle
cell number density at inhibition, the rate constant for the
expression of matrix by smooth muscle, and the monocyte entry
rate. We are incorporating a chemotactic term into the model,
so that the monocyte recruitment rate can depend in part on
the number density of smooth muscle cells. When this model

is applied to our experimental results, it demonstrates that
the dependence of intimal thickness on time shown schematically in Figure 3 can arise if thickening is governed by
by multiple competing shear-dependent processes, some of which
tend to promote thickening, and others of which inhibit it.

Closing Thoughts

Let me conclude with some closing thoughts about the
importance of hemodynamic mechanisms in atherosclerosis.
One fact that becomes very clear on examining hemodynamic
data from a large variety of vascular models and segments
is that, by and large, the hemodynamic environment is
qualitatively similar throughout the systemic arterial
system. Thus, it is not likely that hemodynamic forces
cause particular biological processes to take place at some
sites and not at others. Rather, hemodynamics affects the
biology of the arterial wall in degree such that the rates
of certain flow-dependent processes are caused to proceed
more rapidly at some sites than at others. Put another way,
hemodynamics is a mediator of the evolution of the arterial
intima. It is this mediation that we are trying to understand by modeling the processes that take place in the wall.
We "close the loop" with the cell culture experiments by
incorporating in the model the processes and mechanisms
they suggest. Our understanding of the role of hemodynamics
in atherogenesis and atherosclerotic development cannot increase any faster than our knowledge of the biology of the
vessel wall.

Even without knowing which hemodynamic phenomena are
significant in atherogenesis, we can be certain that these
phenomena depend on the geometry of the channel through which
the blood is flowing. This is fundamental fluid mechanics.
Thus, if particular hemodynamic environments are indeed
atherogenic, then geometric features that promote these
environments in susceptible vessels can increase the risk
of early or more rapidly progressing disease in their
neighborhood. We have used the term "geometric risk factor"
to denote such features of the arterial tree (9,10). The
identification of geometric risk factors might help us to
understand the considerable variability among individuals

in the progression of atherosclerosis that remains even
after the more widely accepted risk factors have been taken
into account.

REFERENCES

1. Davies PF, Remuzzi A, Gordon EJ, Dewey CF, Gimbrone MA
    (1986) Turbulent fluid shear stress induces vascular
    endothelial cell turnover *in vitro*. Proc Natl Acad
    Sci USA 83:2114-2117.
2. Dewey CF (1984) Effect of fluid flow on living vascular
    cells. J Biomech Eng 106:31-35.
3. Levesque MJ, Nerem RM (1985) The elongation and orien-
    tation of cultured endothelial cells in response to
    shear stress. J Biomech Eng 107:341-347.
4. Frangos JA, Eskin SG, McIntire LV, Ives CL (1985)
    Flow effects on prostacyclin production by cultured
    human endothelial cells. Science 227:1477-1479.
5. Friedman MH, Hutchins GM, Bargeron CB, Deters OJ,
    Mark FF (1981) Correlation between intimal thickness
    and fluid shear in human arteries. Atherosclerosis
    39:425-436.
6. Karino T (1986) Microscopic structure of disturbed
    flows in the arterial and venous systems, and its
    implication in the localization of vascular diseases.
    Intl Angiology 5:297-313.
7. Friedman MH, Deters OJ, Bargeron CB, Hutchins GM,
    Mark FF (1986) Shear-dependent thickening of the
    human arterial intima. Atherosclerosis 60:161-171.
8. Ku DN, Giddens DP, Zarins CK, Glagov S (1985)
    Pulsatile flow and atherosclerosis in the human
    carotid bifurcation. Arteriosclerosis 5:293-302.
9. Friedman MH, O'Brien V, Ehrlich LW (1975) Calcula-
    tions of pulsatile flow through a branch; implications
    for the hemodynamics of atherogenesis. Circ Res 36:
    277-285.
10. Friedman MH, Deters OJ, Mark FF, Bargeron CB, Hutchins
    GM (1983) Arterial geometry affects hemodynamics; a
    potential risk factor for atherosclerosis. Athero-
    sclerosis 46:225-231.

21

What do we find in Human Atherosclerosis that Provides Insight into the Hemodynamic Factors in Atherogenesis?

Christopher K. Zarins, Seymour Glagov, and Don P. Giddens

INTRODUCTION

A prominent feature of human atherosclerosis is that despite a number of systemic influences, plaque deposition tends to be a focal process with predominant localization at arterial branch points and bifurcations. Furthermore, certain arteries such as the carotid and coronary arteries and those of the lower extremity are particularly prone to plaque formation while others such as those of the upper extremity are rarely affected. Both the focal and selective distribution of plaques have been attributed to local differences in hemodynamic conditions. For many years it was thought that high shear stress damaged the endothelium and was an initiating factor in plaque formation (1,2). The proposed relationship among high shear stress, endothelial injury and plaque deposition was based on *in vitro* experimental observations and *in vivo* observations in experimental animals. Not until the distribution of human atherosclerotic plaques was studied by making precise quantitative correlations of plaque localization with hemodynamic conditions did it become apparent that quite the opposite was true (3). Plaques tend to form in areas of low and oscillating shear stress and not in areas of high shear stress. Thus, attempts to gain insight into the role of hemodynamic factors in atherogenesis need to begin with the study of the human

Supported by NHLBI Grant HL-15062 and NSF Grant CME 7921551

atherosclerotic plaque. *In vitro* observations and animal experiments permit control of variables and precision in measurements but findings must be correlated with direct observations of human atherosclerotic lesions in order to avoid erroneous conclusions. In particular, the study of those human arteries which are highly susceptible to plaque formation, such as the carotid bifurcation, coronary arteries and lower extremity arteries, should provide important clues to hemodynamic influences which can then be tested in animal and *in vitro* models.

Human Carotid Artery Bifurcation

The human carotid artery is well suited for the study of the relationships between hemodynamic factors and athero-sclerotic plaque formation. It is particularly susceptible to plaque formation in the region of the bifurcation where the common carotid artery divides to form the internal and external carotid arteries. Localized intimal thickening in this area is found early in life (4) and localized athero-sclerotic plaque is found commonly in adults (5). It is remarkable that large, complex and complicated plaques may form at the carotid bifurcation, while the proximal common carotid artery and the distal internal carotid artery are largely free of lesions (6). Plaques occur primarily along the outer wall of the internal carotid artery in the region of the carotid sinus opposite the bifurcation flow divider. This is the site of early asymptomatic plaque formation, as well as the site of complex clinically significant stenoses and ulcerations.

The geometry of the carotid artery may contribute to the susceptibility of this region to atherosclerosis. In addition to hemodynamic disturbances produced by the branching angles of the bifurcation, hemodynamic alterations are also created by the internal carotid sinus. The sinus is a localized dilation of the origin of the internal carotid artery at the bifurcation. This segment has twice the cross-sectional area of the distal internal carotid artery and as a result, hemodynamic disturbances such as flow separation and velocity and shear stress disorders develop and may play important roles in the local control of plaque development.

Flow visualization studies using both steady and pulsatile flow models have shown that as flow from the common carotid artery enters the carotid bifurcation, stream lines are compressed towards the bifurcation flow divider and towards the inner wall of the internal carotid artery where flow is rapid and laminar and shear stress is high (Figure 1) (7). Human carotid plaques do not form initially along the inner wall of the carotid sinus. Along the outer wall of the sinus a large region of flow separation develops in which flow velocity and shear stress are low (Figure 1). The earliest carotid intimal thickenings and plaques develop in this region, as do late complicated and clinically significant carotid lesions (Figure 2). In the region of flow separation along the outer wall there is a reversal of axial flow and slow movement upstream. However, the region of separation is not simply a zone of stasis and recirculation but a zone of complex secondary flow patterns including counter rotating helical trajectories (Figure 3). Flow reattaches distally in the sinus and in the distal internal carotid artery. This area is almost always free of plaque.

Studies of dye washout and particle trajectories in precise scale models reveal that dye is carried rapidly along the inner wall but is cleared very slowly from the outer region of the carotid sinus (7). Particles transported to this region of slow flow and flow separation would thus have more time to interact with the vessel wall. Time-dependent lipid particle-vessel wall interactions would thus be facilitated in the slow flow region favoring transport of particles into the vessel wall and plaque formation. We have suggested the term increased residence time to denote the likely effect of low and complex shear rates on particles in susceptible regions. The implication of increased residence time is that this condition could be the mechanistic potentiating hemodynamic factor for the initiation of atherosclerotic plaques. Blood borne cellular elements which may play a role in atherogenesis are also likely to have an increased probability of adhesion to the vessel wall in

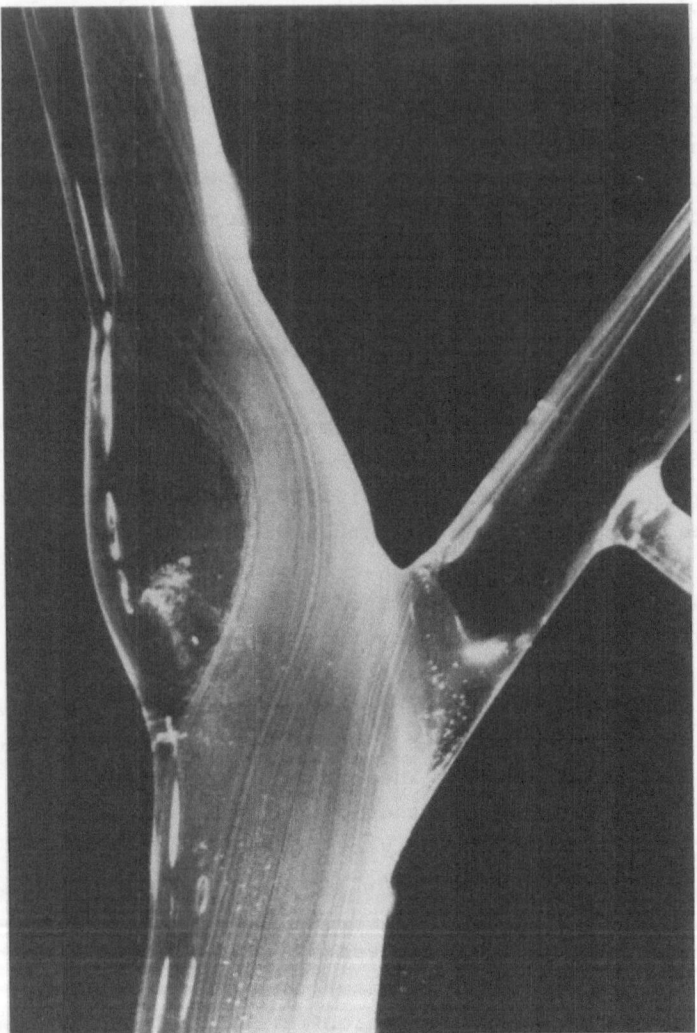

Figure 1. Hydrogen bubble flow visualization in a model
carotid bifurcation demonstrating a large area of flow
separation on the outer wall of the internal carotid sinus.
Flow is skewed towards the bifurcation flow divider. Wall
shear stress is high and unidirectional along the inner
wall and low and oscillating along the outer wall. Plaques
form in the area of low and oscillating shear stress and
not in the high shear stress areas. (Reproduced with permission of the American Heart Association, Inc. and
Circulation Research, Volume 53, pages 502-514, 1983).

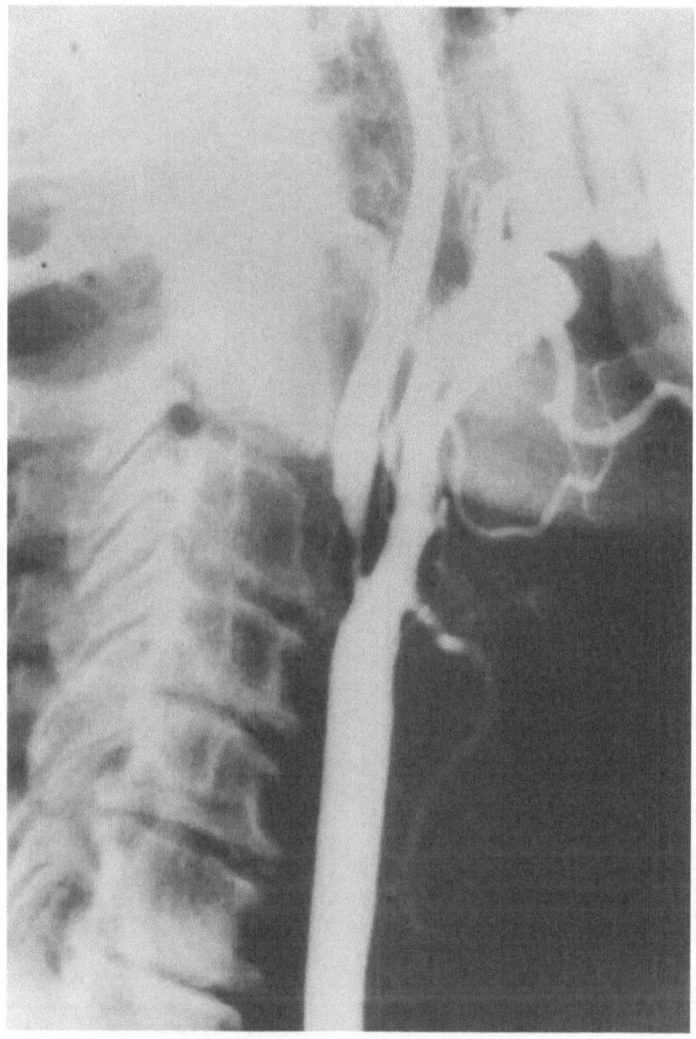

Figure 2. Angiogram of carotid bifurcation demonstrating plaque formation along the outer wall of the carotid sinus where wall shear stress is low.

regions of increased residence time. Flow separation has been shown to favor the deposition of platelets in *in vitro* studies (8). Angiographic and ultrasound studies in patients have confirmed the presence of flow separation and stasis in the outer wall region of the carotid bifurcation which is prone to plaque formation (9,10).

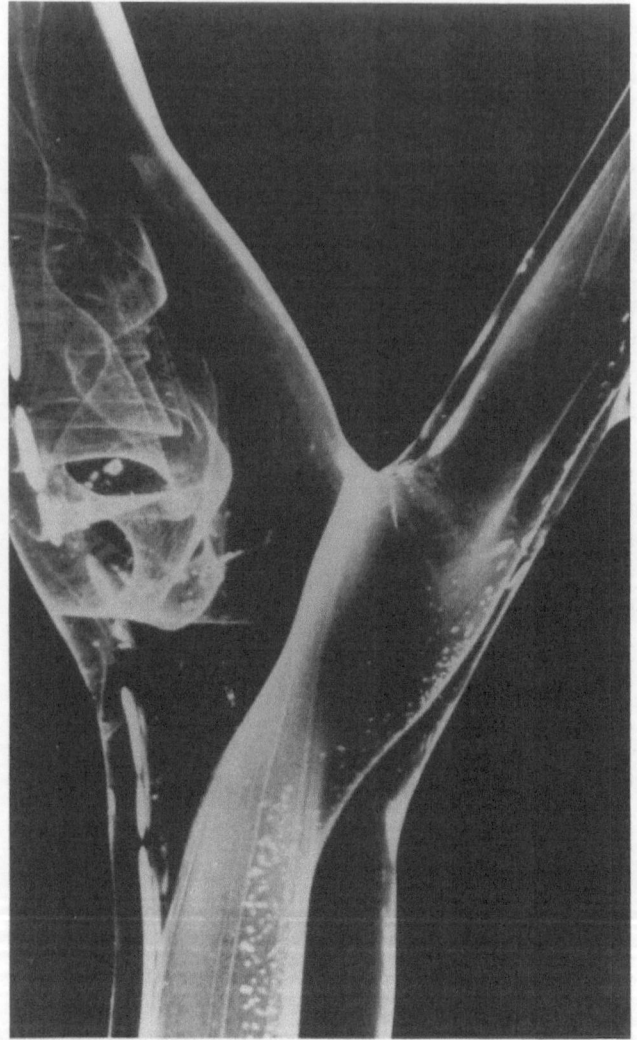

Figure 3. Hydrogen bubble flow visualization demonstrating
flow disturbance along the outer wall of the carotid bifurcation.   This is an area of oscillation in shear stress
direction and prolonged particle residence time.   Both
factors may be important in plaque formation.

<u>Quantitative</u> <u>studies</u> of wall shear stress in accurate
scale models of the carotid bifurcation using laser Doppler
anemometry reveal that flow velocity, and therefore shear
stress, is high along the inner wall of the carotid bifurcation and very low along the outer wall (3).   Correlative

studies reveal an inverse relationship between the absolute
level of wall shear stress and plaque formation in the human
carotid artery bifurcation (3). Such an inverse relationship
has also been demonstrated in experimental studies using
aortic coarctation in primates (11). Quantitative flow
studies in model systems under conditions of pulsatile flow
have suggested that oscillation in the direction of wall
shear stress may also be important in plaque formation (12).
Along the inner wall of a model carotid bifurcation where
shear stress is high, flow and shear stress are undirectional.
However, along the outer wall of the carotid sinus, there is
flow reversal during late systole and oscillation in the
shear stress directional vector (13). Fluid velocity oscil-
lates about a mean shear stress value close to zero along the
outer wall of the carotid sinus and further induced increased
residence time. Despite the absence of a clear region of
stasis or an area of permanent boundary layer separation,
fluid convection is delayed and fluid elements near the outer
wall are trapped for several pulse cycles (12).

Variations in shear stress direction associated with
pulsatile flow may also lead to increased endothelial permeability (14). The oscillating shear stress pattern may cause
an increased ingress of plasma constituents through the endothelial monolayer by affecting the stability of intercellular
junctions. Unidirectional shear, on the other hand, may be
well tolerated regardless of the magnitude of shear stress
and could conceivably induce firmer intercellular attachment
sites than would be present in regions of low and oscillating
shear.

Quantitative model flow studies correlated to early
plaque localization in the human carotid artery bifurcation
have revealed that early plaque deposition occurs in regions
characterized by flow separation, stasis, increased particle
residence time, low mean shear stress and oscillation in
shear stress direction. As plaques enlarge, however, the
geometric configuration of the bifurcation and carotid sinus
is modified and new flow patterns are likely to develop.
These conditions may favor plaque formation on the side and
inner walls of the carotid sinus rather than the outer wall.
In its most advanced and stenotic form, carotid atherosclerosis

may involve the entire circumference of the carotid sinus
including the region of the flow divider. Nevertheless,
plaques are usually largest and most complicated at the
outer and side walls of the carotid bifurcation. The hemodynamic conditions which exist at the carotid bifurcation
may also influence the surface characteristics of existing
carotid plaques and contribute to their tendency to ulcerate
and embolize. Thus, as a stenosis develops in the carotid
bifurcation, the low shear stress condition which promotes
plaque formation may change to a high shear stress or
turbulent condition which would contribute to erosion of
the endothelial surface and/or disruption of the fibrous
cap with subsequent plaque ulceration, embolization and
thrombosis.

We need, therefore, to study not only the hemodynamic
factors which potentiate or induce plaque formation, but
also those which contribute to plaque progression, stenosis,
and complication.

Human Coronary Arteries

Human coronary arteries are particularly prone to
atherosclerosis. As in the carotid artery, coronary plaques
tend to be focal and are more severe at branch points. The
bifurcation of the left main coronary artery into the left
anterior descending and circumflex branches is very commonly
involved. Plaque distribution at this bifurcation occurs on
the outer wall of the bifurcation opposite the flow divider
(15) in a pattern very similar to that described for the
carotid bifurcation. Similar hemodynamic factors may be
involved.

Hemodynamic conditions in the coronary circulation are
more complex than at the carotid bifurcation. During systole,
coronary arterial flow decreases initially during the iso-
volumetric contraction and rapid ejection phases. Flow
increases briefly when peak systolic aortic pressure exceeds
intra-coronary pressure and then decreases again during the
remainder of systole as intramyocardial pressure increases
the resistance to flow (16). With tachycardia, there is
reversal of flow during systole. During diastolic iso-
volumetric relaxation, coronary flow accelerates rapidly

as intramyocardial and intraventricular pressures decline.
Coronary flow then decreases slowly as aortic pressure
falls and intraventricular pressure builds again late in
diastole (17). Thus, during each cardiac cycle, the
coronary arteries are subjected to two systolic and one
diastolic episode of flow acceleration and deceleration.
If oscillating flow conditions and oscillation of shear
stress direction is an important factor in plaque localization, the coronary arteries may be at greater risk than
the carotid bifurcation or other systemic arteries since
they are exposed to more than twice the number of fluctuations in flow direction. Additional predisposing hemodynamic
features include the marked excursions in blood flow during
the cardiac cycle, the geometric configuration of the
vessels and their branches, the mechanical torsion and
flexion of the vessels associated with cardiac motion,
and the special reactivity of coronary artery smooth muscle
to vasoactive substances and nervous impulses. Individual
variation in these factors may account for individual
differences in lesion distribution.

The phasic fluctuations in coronary blood flow occur
predominantly in systole (18). As heart rate increases, the
number of systoles increases and the time spent in diastole,
when coronary flow is greatest, decreases (19). Thus, the
frequency and magnitude of oscillations in shear stress
direction is directly dependent on heart rate. Reduction
in heart rate would reduce the number of oscillating events
experienced by the coronary arteries. Thus, even modest
changes in heart rate could have significant cumulative
effects on conditions in the coronary arteries. The magnitude of this is demonstrated when one considers the effect
of lowering average heart rate from 80 beats/minute to
60 beats/minute. During a one-year period, the number of
systoles and hence oscillating events, would be reduced by
10.5 million.

In order to test the hypothesis that heart rate is an
important risk factor in the development of coronary atherosclerosis, we produced sinoatrial node ablation in cynomolgus
monkeys. This resulted in 20 percent reduction in mean heart
rate and a reduction in the magnitude of heart rate

fluctuation. After six months on an atherogenic diet, animals with a low heart rate had a 50 percent reduction in intimal plaque area, 50 percent reduction in maximum lesion area, and 50 percent reduction in percent stenosis (20). Thus, heart rate reduction had significant protective effect on coronary atherosclerosis in atherosclerotic monkeys.

Clinical studies have also directly implicated heart rate as an independent risk factor in human coronary atherosclerosis. A number of major prospective clinical studies have found high heart rates in men at rest to be predictive of future manifestation of coronary heart disease (21,22). Conversely low heart rates have been reported to protect against the development of coronary atherosclerosis (23). Although increased resting heart rate in sedentary men also seems to correlate significantly with an atherogenic lipid profile (24), both theoretical and experimental evidence suggests that hemodynamic factors associated with cyclic myocardial contraction selectively predispose coronary arteries to atherosclerosis. Hemodynamic factors such as hypertension, altered shear stress and flow disturbances have also been implicated in plaque localization and progression in several locations including the coronary arteries (25), but a selective effect on the coronary tree has not been emphasized.

Lower Extremity Arteries

The arteries of the lower extremities frequently develop atherosclerotic plaques while vessels of similar size in the upper extremities are usually spared. In addition to differences in hydrostatic pressure, the arteries of the lower extremities are subjected to more marked variations in flow rate depending on the level of physical activity. This may be most marked in the abdominal aorta which is particularly vulnerable to early and rapid development of atherosclerosis compared to the thoracic and suprarenal aorta. One-quarter of the cardiac output is delivered to the renal arteires at rest (26). Renal artery flow, together with celiac and superior mesenteric artery flow, thus results in a constant high volume flow

through the suprarenal aorta. In contrast, the volume of
blood flow in the aorta below the renal arteries is greatly
dependent on the muscular activity of the lower extremities.
The infrarenal abdominal aorta may be the appropriate size
for a physically active bipedal existence, but with an
increasingly sedentary life-style in our society, the infrarenal aorta may be subjected to a relatively slower flow
velocity than the suprarenal aorta during a major portion
of the day. This effect may be further accentuated by the
tendency of the aorta to dilate with age. Thus a slower
flow pattern in the abdominal aorta may tend to favor intimal
proliferation and the ingress of lipids with the formation
of atherosclerotic plaques in a manner similar to that which
exists at the outer wall of the carotid sinus.

Cigarette smoking and diabetes mellitus are the risk
factors most closely associated with atherosclerotic disease
of the lower extremities. The manner in which these factors
and the special hemodynamic conditions of lower extremity
arteries are mutually enhancing remains to be elucidated
and would be a fruitful area for futher investigation. Of
the arteries of the lower extremity, the superficial femoral
artery is most commonly the site of multiple stenotic lesions,
while the profunda femoris tends to be spared. The superficial femoral artery is a major conduit with relatively few
proximal branches, and flow velocity is likely to be relatively slow on the average, varying in relation to activity
of the calf muscles during walking or running. The profunda
femoris is a smaller muscular vessel with many branches to
the thigh muscles. Flow velocity is likely to be relatively
high under normal conditions. Plaques in the superficial
femoral artery have not been shown to occur preferentially
at branching sites, but stenotic lesions tend to appear
earliest at the adductor hiatus where the vessel is straight
and branches are few. Repeated mechanical trauma, limitations
on vessel compliance or enlargement associated with the
closely applied adductor magnus tendon may contribute to
the selective localization of occlusive disease in this
position.

There are no suitable animal models to study the complexities of lower extremity atherosclerosis and hemo-dynamic conditions. However, new techniques or noninvasive plaque detection in humans using Duplex ultrasound imaging devices permit accurate local hemodynamic assessment, as well as lesion assessment and may lead to new insights on the role of hemodynamic factors in peripheral athero-sclerosis.

Artery Wall Adaptation

Another important feature of human atherosclerosis is the adaptive response of the artery wall to enlarging intimal plaques. Intimal plaque deposition does not always lead to lumen stenosis if arteries can enlarge and thus compensate for the effect of plaque encroachment on lumen diameter. Hemodynamic forces appear to be important in the determina-tion of artery size. In embryonic development, vascular channels with high flow enlarge while those with low flow become smaller and atrophy (27). Many vessels in high flow positions, such as arteries feeding an arteriovenous fistula (28), autogenous aortorenal bypass grafts (29), and collateral arteries carrying flow about an obstruction tend to enlarge in response to increases in flow. Conversely, lumen diameter is reduced in vessels with low flow, such as in arteries distal to arteriovenous fistulae, in arteries supplying atrophic or amputated extremities or in vascular bypass grafts that are too large in relation to the run-off bed.

Immediately after establishing an experimental arterio-venous fistula in monkeys, blood flow and flow velocity were greatly increased in the proximal arteries and wall shear stress was markedly elevated. However, after six months, the proximal arteries had dilated and wall shear stress had returned to normal levels of 15 dynes/cm^2 despite the per-sistence of a ten-fold increase in volume of flow and a 2.5-fold increase in flow velocity (27).

Since wall shear stress is inversely related to the cube of the lumen radius, alterations in lumen radius can effectively regulate wall shear stress under widely varying conditions of flow. Wall shear stress appears to range between 10 and 20 dynes/cm^2 throughout the vascular tree from the aorta to the capillary level and may serve as a regulator of lumen diameter (30). These flow dependent alterations in vessel diameter appear to be endothelium dependent and may result in both increases (31) and decreases (32) in vessel size.

In experimental diet-induced atherosclerosis in monkeys, as intimal plaques enlarge, coronary arteries enlarge and maintain a near normal lumen diameter (25,33). Similar observations have been made on human coronary arteries indicating that these arteries tend to enlarge as lesions develop (34). However, there appears to be a limit to artery enlargement after which further plaque deposition results in lumen stenosis. This limit appears to occur when intimal plaque area is approximately 40% of the area encompassed by the internal elastic lamina (35). Thus the development of a stenosis may depend upon the rate of plaque deposition on the one hand, which would tend to narrow the lumen, and the rate of artery dilation, which would tend to maintain a normal lumen. The mechanism by which the adaptive process is achieved is not clear. Possible explanations include effects of the plaque directly upon the subjacent wall, as well as effects of altered flow on the opposite intact portion of the wall. Early uncomplicated plaques tend to be eccentric with lumen surfaces conforming to the general curvature of the vessel, while the artery lumen maintains a circular or slightly oval cross-section (36). Plaques are therefore crescentic on cross-section. As the lesion is sequestered from the lumen, the underlying wall is usually thinned and both plaque and wall tend to bulge outward (36,37). This outward extension could be the result of compressive forces exerted by the developing plaque or result from atrophy of the underlying wall due to inter-ference with diffusion from the lumen into the media. Alternately, the intact artery wall opposite the developing plaque may respond by circumferential extension, thereby enlarging the artery. Such a reaction could be induced by the increased flow velocity resulting from narrowing of the lumen by the enlarging plaque.

CONCLUSION

The study of the human atherosclerotic plaques is essential to the understanding of local conditions and hemo-dynamic forces which account for the unique localization patterns of atherosclerosis. Human lesions should provide the data in which we may define the natural history of human atherosclerosis in order to reach an understanding of the processes of plaque progression and plaque regression. The clinically important features of human atherosclerotic plaques such as the formation of stenoses, plaque hemorrhages, ulcerations and thromboses can best be studied by examining human lesions. The validity of carefully controlled experi-mental studies must be ascertained by appropriate correlation with data from human atherosclerotic lesions. Such corre-lation will provide new insights into plaque pathogenesis and artery wall adaptation.

REFERENCES

1. Fry DL (1973) Responses of arterial wall to certain physical factors. In: Atherogenesis, Initiating Factors. Ciba Foundation Symposium. Amsterdam Scientific, pp. 93-125.
2. Ross R, Glomset J (1986) The pathogenesis of athero-sclerosis. New Engl J Med 295:369.
3. Zairns CK, Giddens DP, Bharadvaj BK, et al. (1983) Carotid bifurcation atherosclerosis: Quantitation of plaque localization with flow velocity profiles and wall shear stress. Circ Res 53:502-514.
4. Peterson RE, Livingston KE, Escobar A (1960) Develop-ment and distribution of gross atherosclerotic lesions at cervical carotid bifurcation. Neurology 10:955.
5. McGill HC, et al. (1968) General findings of the International Atherosclerosis Project. Lab Invest 18:498.
6. Heath D, Smith P, Harris P, et al. (1973) The athero-sclerotic human carotid sinus. J Pathol 110:49.
7. Bharadvaj BK, Mabon RF, Giddens DP (1982a) Steady flow in a model of the human carotid bifurcation, Part I. Flow visualization. J Biochem 15:349-362.
8. Partnentier EM, Morton WA, Petschek HE (1981) Platelet aggregate formation in a region of separated blood flow. Phys Fluids 20:2012-2021.
9. Benditt EP (1974) Evidence for a monoclonal origin of human atherosclerotic plaques and some implications. Circulation 50:650-652.
10. Ku DN, Giddens DP, Phillips DJ, et al. (1985) Hemo-dynamics of the normal human carotid bifurcation: In vitro and in vivo studies. Ultrasound in Med and Biol (11)1:13-26.

11. Zarins CK, Bomberger RA, Glagov S (1981) Localization of stenosis: Increased flow velocity inhibits atherogenesis. Circulation 64(Suppl II):221-227.
12. Ku DN, Zarins CK, Giddens DP, et al. (1985) Pulsatile flow and atherosclerosis in the human carotid bifurcation: Positive correlation between plaque localization and low and oscillating shear stress. Arteriosclerosis 5:292-302.
13. Ku DN, Giddens DP (1983) Pulsatile flow in a model carotid bifurcation. Arteriosclerosis 3:31-39.
14. Fry DL (1976) Hemodynamic forces in atherogenesis. In: Steinberg P Cerebrovascular Diseases. Raven Press, pp. 77-95.
15. Svidland A (1983) The localization of sudanophilic and fibrous plaques in the main left coronary bifurcation. Atherosclerosis 48:139-145.
16. Granata L, Olsson RA, Huvos A, Gregg DE (1965) Coronary inflow and oxygen usage following cardiac sympathetic nerve stimulator and unanesthetized dogs. Circ Res 16:114.
17. Gregg DE, Khouri EM, Rayford CR (1965) Systemic and coronary energetics in the resting unanesthetized dog. Circ Res 16:102.
18. Laurent D, Bolenc-Williams C, Williams FL, Katz LN (1956) Effects of heart rate on coronary flow and cardiac oxygen consumption. Am J Physiol 185:355-364.
19. Boudoulas H, Rittgers SE, Lewis RP, Leier CV, Weissler Am (1979) Changes in diastolic time with various pharmacologic agents. Circulation 60:164-169.
20. Beere PA, Glagov S, Zarins CK (1984) Retarding effect of lowered heart rate on coronary atherosclerosis. Science 226:180-182.
21. Schroll M, Hagerup LM (1977) Risk factors of myocardial infarction and death in men aged 50 at entry. Dan Med Bull 24:252.
22. Dyer AR, Persky V, Stamler J, et al. (1980) Heart rate as a prognostic factor for coronary heart disease and mortality: Findings in three Chicago epidemiologic studies. Am J Epidemiol 112:736.
23. Williams PT, Wood PD, Haskell WL, Vranizan KM (1982. The effects of running mileage and duration on plasma lipoprotein levels. JAMA 247:2674.
24. Williams PT, Haskell WL, Vranizan KM, et al. (1985) Associations of resting heart rate with concentrations of lipoprotein subfractions in sedentary men. Circulation 71:441.
25. Glagov S (1972) Hemodynamic risk factors: Mechanical stress, mural architecture, medial nutrition and the vulnerability of arteries to atherosclerosis. In: Wissler RW, Geer JC (eds) The Pathogenesis of Atherosclerosis. Baltimore: Williams and Wilkens, pp. 164-199.
26. Guyton AC (1961) Textbook of Medical Physiology (2nd edition). Philadelphia and London: Saunders, p. 356.
27. Zarins CK, Zatina MA, Giddens DP, Ku DN, Glagov S (1987) Shear stress regulation of artery lumen diameter in experimental atherogenesis. J Vasc Surg 5(3):413-420.
28. Schumacker HB Jr (1970) Aneurysm development and degenerative changes in dilated artery proximal to arteriovenous fistual. Surg Gynecol Obstet 130:636.

29. Szilagyi DE, Elliott JP, Hageman JH, Smith RF, Dall'Oloma CA (1973) Biologic fate of autogenous vein implants as arterial substitutes. Surgery 178:232.
30. Kamiya A, Togawa T (1980) Adaptive regulation of wall shear stress to flow change in the canine carotid artery. Am J Physiol 239(Heart Circ Physiol 8):H14-H21.
31. Smeisko V, Kozik J, Dolezel S (1985) Role of endothelium in the control of arterial diameter by blood flow. Blood Vessles 22:247-251.
32. Langille BL, O'Donnell F (1986) Reductions in arterial diameter produced by chronic diseases in blood flow are endothelial-dependent. Science 231:405-407.
33. Bond MD, Adams MR, Bullock BC (1981) Complicating factors in evaluating coronary artery atherosclerosis. Artery 9:21.
34. Glagov S, Weisenberg E, Kolletis C, Stankunavicius R, Zarins CK (1986) Compensatory enlargement of human atherosclerotic coronary arteries prevents narrowing of the lumen. FASEB 45(3):583.
35. Glagov S, Weisenberg E, Zarins CK, Kolletis G, Stankunavicius R (1987) Compensatory enlargement of human atherosclerotic coronary arteries. New Engl J Med 316:1371-1375.
36. Glagov S, Zarins CK (1983) Quantitating atherosclerosis: Problems of definition. In: Bond MG, Insull W, Glagov S, Chandler AB, Cornhill F (eds) Clinical Diagnosis of Atherosclerosis: Quantitative Methods of Evaluation. New York: Springer-Verlag, pp. 11-35.
37. Crawford T, Levene CL (1953) Medial thinning in atheroma. J Pathol Bact 66:19.

22

Cell Births and Cell Deaths in the Human Atherosclerotic Plaque as Evaluated from Human Studies

W.A. Thomas and D.N. Kim

At the outset it must be said that there are very little quantitative data on cell births and deaths in human atherogenesis. Therefore my presentation must be of necessity largely speculative.

We know that cell births occur in human atherogenesis because we find occasional cells in mitosis and because it is the only reasonable way to account for most of the great increase in smooth muscle cells (SMC) that is observed. We know that cell deaths occur because we can find cell debris in increasing quantities as the lesions progress. In addition we have direct evidence from hyperlipidemic (HL) diet induced atherogenesis in swine that cell births and deaths are a very important part of the process and these data are very likely relevant for man.

When investigators study early atherogenesis they begin with the flat yellow fatty streak which is perhaps the first grossly visible manifestation. This virtually guarantees that the most prominent early microscopic feature will be fat filled cells both of SMC and monocyte origin. We prefer to begin our study prior to the appearance of grossly visible lesions and in fact before lesions can even be identified with certainty microscopically. This means that our studies must begin at sites of predilection for atherosclerosis. Fortunately there are sites of predilection that are clearly recognizable and that appears to be the source for most of the lesions that become clinically significant. These are sites of normal intimal thickening which we have chosen to call intimal cellular masses (ICM) to emphasize their cellular component (1-25).

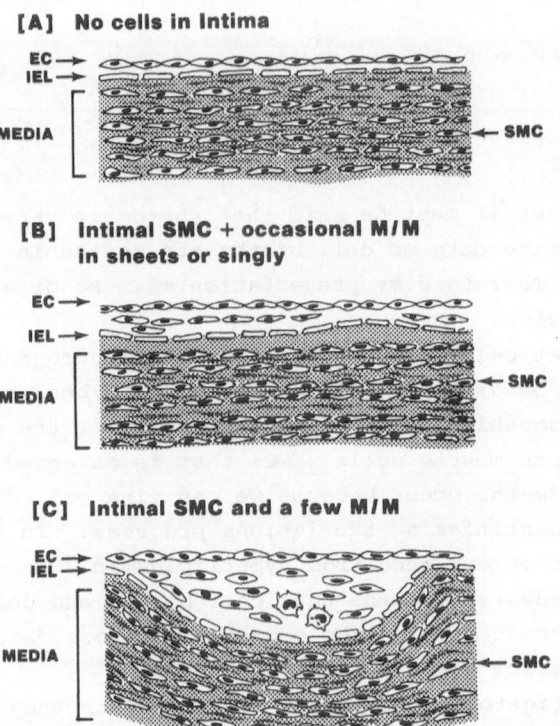

Figure 1. Normal arterial intima in a young person. In most arteries, there are only a few cells in the intima between the endothelial cells (EC) and the internal elastic lamina (IEL). In some sites, there are masses of cells, smooth muscle cells (SMC) and monocyte-macrophages (M/M), in the intima referred to by us as intimal cellular masses (ICM). The matrix and other non-cellular elements in the intima are not illustrated.

In Figure 1 are shown the different forms the arterial intima may take in the normal state. In most anatomic sites there are masses of cells in the intima referred to by us as ICM. Two sites of predilection for ICM are the first portion of the coronary arteries and the distal portion of the abdominal aorta and our attention has been directed mostly to these sites. However these are by no means the only sites in which the ICM are found. In the normal state the ICM cells

are mostly SMC but they also contain scattered monocyte/
macrophages (M/M). We are presenting the ICM in the drawing
as flat on the surface and seemingly pushed into the underlying media because this is the way they appear in arteries
fixed under pressure (and presumably also in the living state)

They are present from birth; grow rapidly in the first
few months of life, then very slowly; cell types are mostly
SMC with a few macrophages (9,10,18,24).

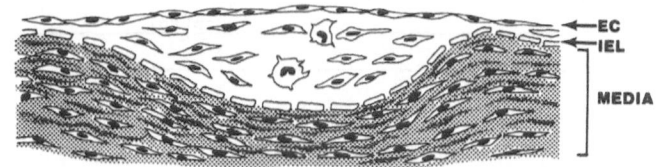

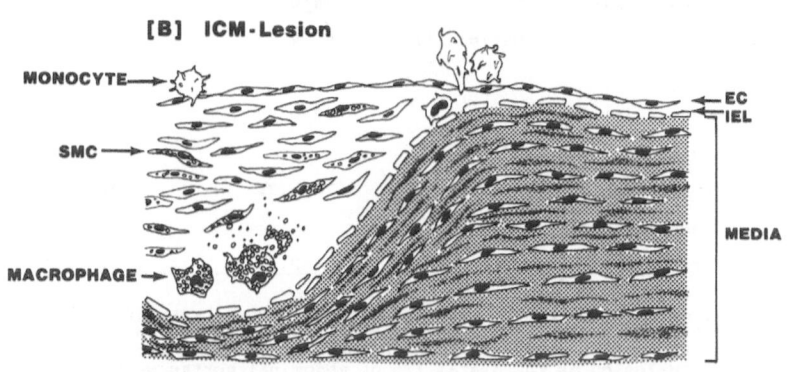

Figure 2. Early atherogenesis. Transformation of a normal
ICM (A) into an ICM-lesion (B). The number of smooth muscle cells and macrophages is increased. Both smooth muscle
cells and macrophages contain lipid vacuoles.

In Figure 2 we show here a normal ICM being transformed
into an ICM-lesion.

What are the distinctions between the normal ICM and
an ICM-lesion? These are subtle and in the early stages
of lesion development a sharp dividing line cannot be drawn.
Fat accumulation begins early but this may also occur to
some extent in otherwise normal ICM. In the experiemtnal
animal increased replicative activity as indicated by

tritiated thymidine labeling indices occurs very early after starting an atherogenic diet and this is quickly followed by an increase in ICM cell numbers. The early increase in cell numbers can be ascertained in experimental animals on a statistical basis by comparison of values at a given anatomical site between atherogenic diet-fed and control animals (12,14,15,17,20-23). In man this is more difficult with currently available data.

Table 1. Data on [3]HTdR Labeling Indices of Abdominal Aortas of Young Swine[a]

	Control	HL
n	34	21
ICM or ICM lesion		
LI observed (%)	0.64+0.09[b]	2.13+0.29
LI required for observed		
with no loss(%)	0.58+0.15	1.79+0.17
Cell loss index per S period (%)	0.06+0.17	0.34+0.33
Media		
LI observed (%)	0.42+0.09	0.70+0.09
LI required for observed		
increase with no loss (%)	0.28+0.20	0.38+0.21
Cell loss index per		
S period (%)	0.14+0.22	0.32+0.23

[a] Two-month-old male Yorkshire swine were fed a hyperlipidemic diet for 3 months. Terminally tritiated thymidine was given 2 hours before sacrifice. The numbers of cells in the intima or ICM-lesion of the distal 1/5 of abdominal aortas were counted. The labeling indices (LI) were determined after autoradiography.

[b] Mean ± standard error of mean

In Table 1 we show some data related to replicative activity in normal ICM and early ICM-lesions in young swine at 3 months on an atherogenic diet which is probably also applicable to man (23). We are using tritiated thymidine labeling indices ([3]HTdR LI) as an index of replicative activity. Even in the normal state the ICM have higher [3]HTdR LI than do the cells in the normal media. Shortly after beginning the HL diet the [3]HTdR LI increase and by 4 months on the diet they are about as high as they are ever going to be. Also in the swine the number of ICM-lesion cells increases to an average 8-fold greater numbers than in

the normal ICM. By making certain reasonable assumptions
we can calculate the LIs required to give the observed
increase in cell numbers (23). By comparing the values with
the observed average LI we can obtain some idea regarding
cell loss presumably by cell deaths. This calculation does
not take into account entry of cells by infiltration from
the blood stream (monocyte) or from the media (SMC) which
would make the cell loss values greater to the extent that
entry from outside the intimal compartment is numerically
important. We have also carried out transmission electron
microscopy counts of dead cells in the intimas of similar
HL swine and have found increased numbers of dead cell forms
as early as 3 days on HL diets (26-28). In experimental
animals we assume the ICM are normal when they are in animals
on diets that do not lead to the development of atherosc_lero-
tic lesions. In man we have a more difficult and perhaps
an impossible problem when we try to arrive at a definition
of the normal state in regard to the arterial intima. In
the early 1960's we looked for a human population in which
clinically significant atherosclerosis was virtually absent
and we found one in the black population of Uganda, East
Africa (29-30). In Figure 3 we contrast values for maximum
intimal thicknesses of the first portion of coronary arteries between black Ugandans and white New Yorkers aged 16-
40. You can see that the intimas are far thicker in the
New Yorkers which would correspond to a far greater number
of intimal cells than in the East Africans. We assume that
the values for the New Yorkers reflect the extent of athero-
slcerosis at this age and that the values for the Africans
represent something approaching the normal state.

In Figure 4 we present corresponding data for younger
members of the same two populations beginning with newborns.
Again we assume that the African values represent something
approaching the normal ICM state. The values for the New
Yorkers in the younger age groups are not significantly
different from those of the Africans suggesting that the
early increases in cell numbers represent mostly normal growth.
The main point of this figure is to show that the intima of
the proximal portion of the coronary arteries is a substantial

entity even in the presumed near normal state in man as it
is in some experimental animals. These data would be more
useful if we had counted intimal nuclei per cross section
instead of only measuring maximal thickness but we can
reasonably assume that there is at least a rough correspondence between maximum thickness and cell numbers.

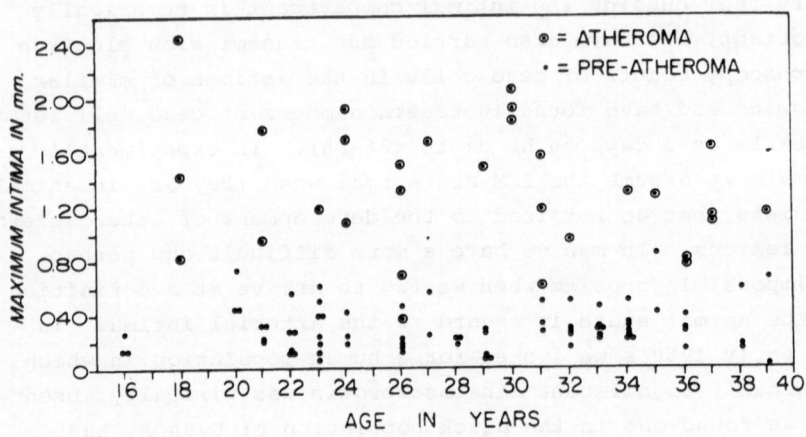

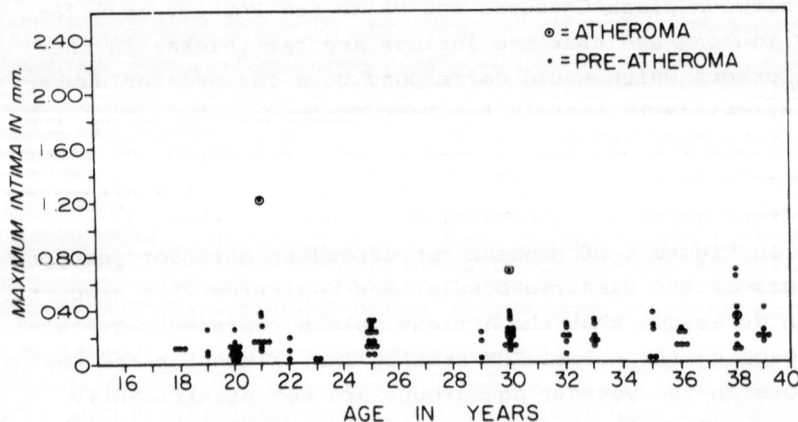

Figure 3. Scattergrams of the numbers of pre-atheroma and
atheroma lesions and maximum intimal thickness of the proximal segments of coronary arteries of black Ugandans (Africans)
and white New Yorkers (Americans) aged 16-40 years (30).

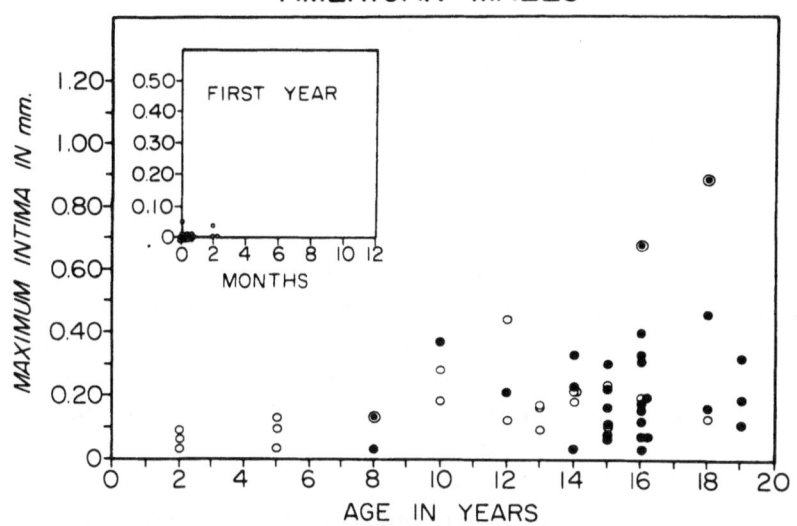

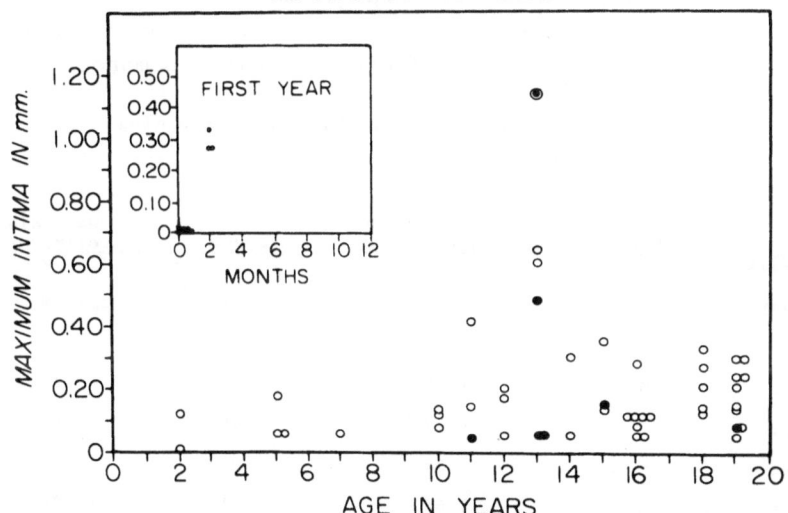

Figure 4. Scattergrams of the numbers of atheroma, pre-
atheroma with fat and pre-atheroma lesions and maximum intimal
thicknesses of the proximal segments of coronary arteries in
young black male East Africans (African Males) and white
New Yorkers (American Males) aged 0-20 years. Insets are
values for the ages of 0 to 12 months (29).

In Table 2 are shown some values for ICM and ICM-
lesions of the proximal portion of the left anterior descending coronary artery obtained from recent routine autopsies
on individuals from newborns to 39 years of age in Albany,
New York. The cross sectional area and the nuclear profile
per cross section (Np/Cx used as an index of ICM or ICM-
lesion cell numbers) roughly correspond. The percentage of
lesion occupied by lipid rich necrotic debris was obtained
by point counting and reflects cell necrosis and extracellular lipid accumulation. Even at 5 years of age the ICM
is a substantial entity and may show necrotic debris (11,13,
16). This may indicate that we are already dealing with a
pathologic process but much more data are needed for this
aspect to be properly evaluated. The increase in intimal
cell numbers with age presumably represents in part an excess
of cell births over cell deaths and in part infiltration of
monocytes from the blood stream into the intima. It should
be noted that the monocyte/macrophages also replicate in the
intima in both man and experimental animals (10,18). This
is shown by Stary in man using mitotic figures and by us in
unpublished observations in swine using combined monoclonal

Table 2. Data on First Segment of Left Anterior Descending
(LAD) Coronary

Age	Sex	ICM or lesion Cx Area (mm^2)	Np/Cx[a]	Necrosis Area(%ICM)
0(NB)b	M	0.001	3	0
1 day	F	0	0	0
1 yr	M	0.01	10	0
5 yr	M	1.09	1621	20
26yr	F	0.97	2096	14
26yr	M	2.53	4603	10
31yr	M	1.68	2916	0.2
36yr	M	2.22	2236	10
39yr	F	1.20	1663	0

a: Nuclear profiles per cross section

b: Newborn

antibody techniques for identifying monocyte/macrophages
and tritiated thymidine for labeling cells synthesizing
DNA. How much of the increase represents normal development
and how much atherogenesis remains to be seen.

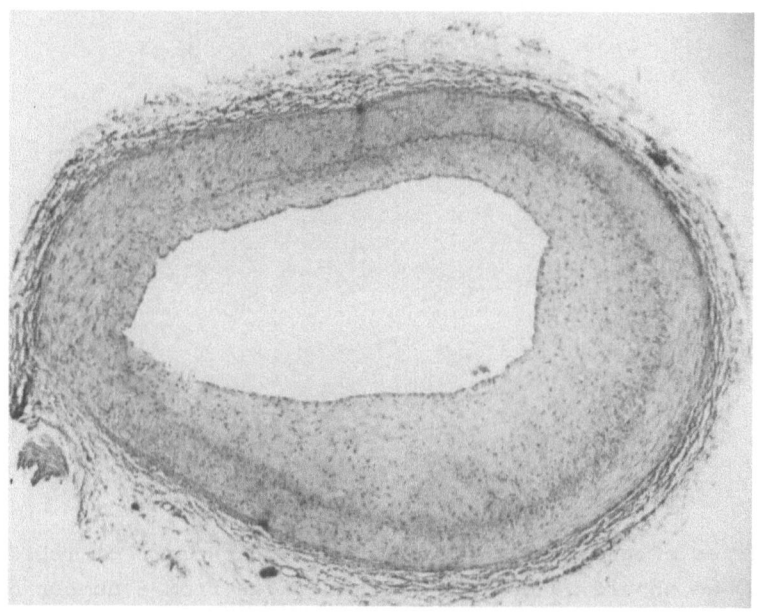

Figure 5. A proximal segment of left anterior descending
branch of the coronary artery of a 5-year-old male. The
intima is thicker than the media. Immersion fixed, paraffin
section, H & E stain, X 40.

In Figure 6 we show a higher magnification of the same
presumed normal artery. We are suggesting that with aging
in human populations living on high fat high cholesterol
diets these ICM become transformed into atherosclerotic
lesions and that increased cell births and deaths are a very
important part of the transformation. The exact point at
which such an ICM becomes an ICM lesion is difficult to
define.

In Table 3 we are illustrating a type of calculation
that can be made to give ball-park figures regarding quantity
of cell replicative activity needed to provide an observed
increase in intimal cell numbers (23). We are using for
illustration the nuclear profiles per cross section for LAD

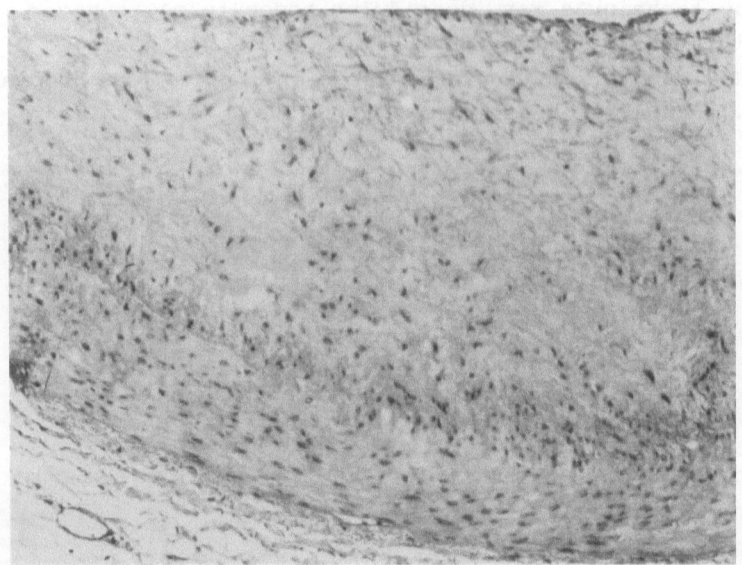

Figure 6. A higher magnification of the same coronary
artery as in Figure 5. Intima contains sparsely distributed
cells and abundant matrix elements. H & E stain, X 128.

coronaries of the 1-year-old and the 5-year-old from Table 2.
Ideally we should be dealing with averages from a number of
individuals and should take into account growth in length of
the artery as well as the cross sectional dimension. However
this simplified example will suffice to illustrate the
approach. Although the results are expressed in terms of
the commonly understood tritiated thymidine labeling indices
it will be apparent that it is not necessary to use tritiated
thymidine but only to count cells. The increase over the
4 years is by a factor of 1621 Np/Cx divided by 10 Np/Cx. A
pulse of tritiated thymidine labels all cells that are in S
period, the DNA synthesis portion of the cell cycle; hence
one "S period's worth". If the S period of the intimal cells
is approximately 12 hours as it is in swine we would label a
half days worth. If we assume that each labeled cell divides
and produces an additional cell the increase per half day
would be a multiple of 1 + the fraction labeled. The
increase for n S periods with the same average LI would be
by a factor of this multiple to the nth power. The n for
4 years in this illustration is 2920.

Table 3. Ball Park Estimate of Average Net Labeling
Index (LI) Required in Human to Increase LAD
Np/Cx from 10 to 1621 Over a 4-Year-Period

1. Increase is 1621/10 = 162-fold.
2. Increase per S period is (1 + LI as a fraction) -fold.
3. Increase for n S periods is $(1 + LI \text{ as a decimal})^n$.
4. Assuming S period as 12 hrs there are 2 x 365 x 4 = 2920
    S periods in 4 years.
5. Then $(1 + LI \text{ as a fraction})^{2920}$ = 162.
6. 1 + LI as a fraction = 2920 $\sqrt{162}$.
7. Average LI = 0.17% which is well within the range of
    the plausible.

The equation then reads as shown in the Table. We can
solve for LI by taking the 2920th root of 162. It turns out
to be 0.17% which is well within the range of the plausible.
Judging from observations in swine the actual labeling indices
in human ICM and ICM-lesions are probably substantially
higher than this allowing for a considerable number of cell
deaths. The main point of this exercise is to show that
quite plausible cell replication rates can in theory account
for all of the enormous increase in cells observed in developing atherosclerotic lesions. This is not meant to imply
that no contribution is made from other sources. Infiltration of monocyte from the blood stream is also undoubtedly
a factor.

Now we shall discuss briefly the possibility of the
excessive cell replications representing neoplastic activity.
This idea dates back to the Benditts' observation that
monotypic foci could be found in the atherosclerotic plaques
of black women who were heterozygous for G-6-PD which was
confirmed by us and others (31-39).

Some have concluded from this that atherosclerotic
lesions are neoplastic in origin. However, we favor the
alternative that the monotypism is reflecting the superior
survival characteristics of one phenotype over the other in
a given environment. We think it is much more likely that
atherosclerosis is mainly a hyperplastic process (35-39).

Table 4.   Hypotheses Regarding Causes for Hyperplasia of
            Cells in ICM

---

1. Ultimate cause probably excessive lipoproteins (LP)
    of particular types.
2. These result in excessive production of growth factors
    (GF) by ICM cells or increased entry from the blood
    stream.
3. Stimulation of GF production by particular LPs, maybe
    secondary to killing of cells or by direct interaction
    with ICM SMC and/or Monocyte/Macrophages or by other
    means.

In Table 4 we present some hypotheses regarding the
presumed hyperplasia of cells in the ICM. The ultimate
cause is probably excessive lipoproteins of particular
types. This results in excessive production of growth
factors. Stimulation of excessive production of growth factors by particular lipoproteins could be secondary to cell
injury or by direct interaction with the target cells themselves or by other means.

REFERENCES
1. Dock W (1946) The predilection of atherosclerosis for the
    coronary arteries. JAMA 131:875-878
2. Schornagel HE (1956) Intimal thickening in the coronary
    arteries in infants. Arch Pathol 62:427-432
3. Moon HD (1957) Coronary arteries in fetuses, infants, and
    juveniles. Circulation 16:263-267
4. Stehbens WE (1960) Focal intimal proliferation in the
    cerebral arteries. Am J Path 36:289-301
5. Neufeld HN, Wagenvoort CA, and Edwards JE (1962) Coronary
    arteries in fetuses, infants, juveniles, and young adults.
    Lab Invest 11:837-844
6. Geer JC, McGill HC, Robertson WB, and Strong JP (1968)
    Histologic characteristics of coronary artery fatty streaks.
    Lab Invest 18:565-570
7. Getz GS, Vesselinovitch D, and Wissler RW (1969) A
    dynamic pathology of atherosclerosis. Am J Med 46:657-673
8. Haust MD (1971) The morphogenesis and fate of potential
    and early atherosclerotic lesions in man. Hum Path
    2:1-29
9. Stary HC and Strong JP (1976) Coronary artery fine
    structure in Rhesus monkeys: Nonatherosclerotic intimal·
    thickening. Prim Med 9:321-358

10. Stary HC (1976) Coronary artery fine structure in Rhesus monkeys: The early atherosclerotic lesion and its progression. Prim Med 9:359-395

11. Velican C and Velican D (1976) Intimal thickening in developing coronary arteries and its relevance to atherosclerotic involvement. Atherosclerosis 23:345-355

12. Thomas WA, Reiner JM, Florentin RA, and Scott RF (1979) Population dynamics of arterial cells during atherogenesis. VIII. Separation of the roles of injury and growth stimulation in early aortic atherogenesis in swine originating in preexisting intimal smooth cell masses. Exptl Mol Pathol 31:124-144

13. Velican D and Velican C (1979) Study of fibrous plaques occurring in the coronary arteries of children. Atherosclerosis 33:201-215

14. Scott RF, Thomas WA, Lee WM, Reiner JM, and Florentin RA (1979) Distribution of intimal smooth muscle cell masses and their relationship to early atherosclerosis in abdominal aortas of young swine. Atherosclerosis 34:291-301

15. Thomas WA, Kim DN, Lee KT, Reiner JM, and Schmee J (1983) Population dynamics of arterial cells during atherogenesis. Part 13 Mitogenic and cytotoxic effects of a hyperlipidemic (HL) diet on cells in advanced lesions in the abdominal aortas of swine fed an HL diet for 270-345 days. Exptl Mol Pathol 39:257-270

16. Velican C and Velican D (1983) Progression of coronary atherosclerosis from adolescence to mature adults. Atherosclerosis 47:131-144

17. Kim DN, Lee KT, Schmee J and Thomas WA (1983) Anti-proliferative effect of pyridinolcarbomate and of aspirin in the early stages of atherogenesis in swine. Atherosclerosis 48:1-13

18. Stary HC (1983) Structure and ultrastructure of the coronary artery intima in children and young adults up to age 29. In: Atherosclerosis VI. Proceedings of the Sixth International Symposium. Schettler FG et al (eds) Springer-Verlag, Berlin/Heidelberg/New York, pp 82-86

19. Grottum P, Svindland A and Walloe L (1983) Localization of atherosclerotic lesions in the bifurcation of the main left coronary artery. Atherosclerosis 47:55-62

20. Kim DN, Schmee J, Lee KT, and Thomas WA (1984) Hypo-atherogenic effect of dietary corn oil exceeds hypo-cholesterolemic effect in swine. Atherosclerosis 52:101-113

21. Kim DN, Lee KT, Schmee J, Thomas WA (1984) Quantification of intimal cell masses and atherosclerotic lesions in coronary arteries of control and hyperlipidemic swine. Atherosclerosis 52:115-122

22. Kim DN, Schmee J, Lee KT, and Thomas WA (1985) Intimal cell masses in the abdominal aortas of swine fed a low-fat, low-cholesterol diet for up to twelve years of age. Atherosclerosis 55:151-159

23. Kim DN, Schmee J, Lee KT, and Thomas WA (1985) Intimal cell mass (ICM)-derived atherosclerotic lesions in the abdominal aorta of hyperlipidemic (HL) swine. I. Cell of origin, cell divisions and cell losses in first 90 days on HL diet. Atherosclerosis 56:169-188

24. Imai H, Connell CE, Lee KT, Kim DN, and Thomas WA (1985) Differential counts by electron microscopy of cell types

in normal intimal cell masses in swine abdominal aortas.
Exptl Mol Pathol 42:377-388

25. Cornhill JF, Barrett WA, Herderick EE, Mahley RW, and
Fry DL (1985) Topographic study of sudanophilic lesions
in cholesterol-fed minipigs by image analysis. Arteriosclerosis 5:415-426

26. Imai H and Thomas WA (1968) Cerebral atherosclerosis
in swine: Role of necrosis in progression of diet-
induced lesions from proliferative to atheromatous
stage. Exptl Mol Pathol 8:330-357

27. Imai H, Lee SK, Pastori SJ, and Thomas WA (1970)
Degeneration of arterial smooth muscle cells: Ultrastructural study of smooth muscle cell death in control
and cholesterol-fed animals. Virchows Arch Abt A Path
Anat 350:183-204

28. Imai H, Werthessen NT, Taylor CB, and Lee KT (1976)
Angiotoxicity and arteriosclerosis due to contaminants
of USP-grade cholesterol. Arch Pathol Lab Med 100:
565-572

29. Scott RF, Florentin RA, Daoud AS, Morrison ES, Jones
RM, and Hutt MSR (1966) Coronary arteries of children
and young adults. A comparison of lipids and anatomic
features in New Yorkers and East Africans. Exptl
Mol Pathol 5:12-42

30. Daoud A, Jarmolych J, Zumbo O, Fani K and Florentin R
(1964) "Preatheroma" phase of coronary atherosclerosis
in man. Exptl Mol Pathol 3:475-484

31. Benditt EP and Benditt JM (1973) Evidence for a monoclonal origin of human atherosclerotic plaques. Proc
Natl Acad Sci USA 70:1753-1756

32. Pearson TA, Wang A, Solez K, and Hiptinstall RH (1975)
Clonal characteristics of fibrous plaques and fatty
streaks from human aortas. Am J Pathol 81:379-388

33. Pearson TA, Dillman JM, Solez K, and Hiptinstall RH
(1978) Clonal markers in the study of origin and
growth of human atherosclerotic lesions. Circ Res
43:10-18

34. Pearson TA, Dillman JM, Solez K, Hiptinstall RH (1978)
Clonal characteristics in layers of human atherosclerotic plaques. Am J Pathol 93:93-102

35. Thomas WA, Reiner JM, Janakidevi K, Florentin RA, and
Lee KT (1979) Population dynamics of arterial cells
during atherogenesis. X. Study of monotypism in
atherosclerotic lesions of black women heterozygous
for glucose-6-phosphate dehydrogenase (G-6-PD). Exptl
Mol Pathol 31:367-386

36. Lee KT, Thomas WA, Janakidevi K, Droms M, Reiner JM
and Borg KY (1981) Mosaicism in female hybrid hares
heterozygous for glucose-6-phosphate dehydrogenase
(G-6-PD). I. General properties of a hybrid hare model
with special reference to atherogenesis. Exptl Mol Pathol
34:191-201

37. Janakidevi K, Lee KT, Thomas WA, Reiner JM, and Murray
CD (1981) Mosaicism in female hybrid hares hetero-
zygous for glucose-6-phosphate dehydrogenase (G-6-PD).
II. Changes in the ratios of G-6-PD types in skin
fibroblast carried through multiple passages. Exptl
Mol Pathol 34:202-208

38. Murray CD, Lee Kt, Thomas WA, Reiner JM, and
     Janakidevi K (1981) Mosaicism in female hybrid hares
     heterozygous for glucose-6-phosphate dehydrogenase
     (G-6-PD). III. Changes in the ratios of G-6-PD types
     in skin fibroblast exposed to 25-hydroxy cholesterol.
     Exptl Mol Pathol 34:209-215
39. Thomas WA, and Kim DN (1983) Biology of disease:
     Atherosclerosis as a hyperplastic and/or neoplastic
     process. Lab Invest 48:245-255

23

Immunocytochemical Analysis of the Cellular Composition of Atherosclerotic Lesions in the Human Aorta

Toyohiro Tsukada, Michael E. Rosenfeld, Allen M. Gown, and Russell Ross

ABSTRACT

This report presents the results of immunocytochemical analyses of the cellular composition of atherosclerotic lesions in the human aorta. Aortae obtained at autopsy were immunostained with monoclonal antibodies against human alveolar macrophages (HAM-56), muscle actin (HHF35), the T-200 antigen of lymphocytes and monocytes, and the factor VIII related antigen of endothelial cells. Based on the immunostaining characteristics, three broad categories of lesions were observed. These include: the fibro-fatty lesion, the fibrous lesion, and the advanced lesion. The advantages of using monoclonal antibody techniques over traditional morphologic and histochemical approaches are also discussed.

INTRODUCTION

Microscopic observations of atherosclerotic lesions have been recorded for many decades. However, our capacity to demonstrate the cellular composition of the lesions is relatively recent (1-6). Traditionally, analyses of the cellular composition of lesions have relied on electron microscopic and histologic approaches and cell types were determined based on characteristic morphologic and histo-chemical features (5-11). Smooth muscle cells were recog-nized by their elongate or thin "pancake-like" shapes, cytoplasmic myofilaments and dense bodies, and surrounding basal laminae (5,7). Macrophages were distinguished from smooth muscle cells by their numerous lamellipodia, absence of basal laminae, and large number of cytoplasmic dense bodies representing primary and secondary lysosomes (7). In addition, histochemical markers such as non-specific esterase (8), peroxidase (9), and acid lipase (9,10) as well as F_c and C_3 receptors (11) have been used to identify macrophages at the light microscopic level. Each of these traditional approaches for identification of cell types within atherosclerotic lesions are problematic. At the ultrastructural level, the large amount of preparation time and high resolution have severely limited the size of the sample that can feasibly be studied. Further, in many cases (such as with foam cells or transverse sections) cytoplasmic constituents are obscured making cellular identification ambiguous at best. The use of histochemical approaches is also accompanied by certain limitations. For example, the reliance on frozen sections reduces the tissue preservation and quality of the resulting morphology. Many of the histo-chemical markers are non-specific causing additional ambi-guity in the interpretation of the data.

Recent immunocytochemical techniques utilizing cell type specific monoclonal antibodies have alleviated many of the problems cited above. In this report, we present the results of our immunocytochemical investigations of the distribution of various cell types within human atheroscler-otic plaques, using monoclonal antibodies specific for smooth muscle cells (12), macrophages (13), lymphocytes (14), and endothelial cells (15).

MATERIALS AND METHODS

Sources of Antibodies

Antibody HHF35 is a monocloanl anti-actin antibody generated in our laboratories that recognizes α- and λ-actin isotypes common to all muscle cells (12). It does not react with fibroblasts, endothelial cells, lymphocytes, monocytes or macrophages (13). Antibody HAM-56 is an anti-monocyte/-macrophage monoclonal antibody generated against normal human alveolar macrophages obtained via lung lavage (13).

It recognizes peripheral blood monocytes, cultured and
tissue alveolar macrophages, other tissue macrophages such
as Kupffer cells and macrophages of the lymph nodes. It
does not recognize T or B lymphocytes, granulocytes or
platelets (13). Both antibodies HHF35 and HAM-56 were
generated using a modification of the Köhler-Milstein
hybridoma techniques (14). Monoclonal antibody to the T-200
antigen present on T and B lymphocytes and monocytes (15)
were obtained commercially (Dako, Santa Barbara, CA). Monoclonal antibodies to factor VIII related antigen, an
endothelial-cell specific marker (16), were purchased from
Cappel Laboratories (Malvern, PA).

Tissue Procurement

Segments of aorta were obtained from the surgical and
autopsy pathology services of University Hospital, Seattle.
Autopsy material was obtained within 12 hours of death
(range: 4-12 hours). Patients ranged in age from 34 to
58 years with a total of 96 specimens obtained from 68
individuals. Aortic segments containing small atherosclerotic lesions of 0.2-2.0 cm diameter that were raised, gray
and with or without evidence of an atheromatous base, were
dissected out and immersed in Methanol-Carnoy's fixative
(60% methanol, 30% chloroform, 10% glacial acetic acid)
over night. Fatty streaks or dots were not included in
the study. All tissue segments were sequentially transferred to absolute methanol, 70% methanol, and PBS prior
to embedding in paraffin.

Immunocytochemistry

An avidin-biotin-immunoperoxidase system was used
[with or without a nickel chloride color intensification
(17)] on deparaffinized tissue sections as previously
described (12,13).

RESULTS

Based on the staining patterns observed in serial
sections using monoclonal antibodies specific for smooth
monocyte/macrophages, lymphocyte/monocytes and endothelial
cells, we have deduced that there are three broad categories

of atherosclerotic lesions in the human aorta. In addition,
we have analyzed areas of normal human aorta as a basis of
comparison. Table 1 shows that the normal aorta is primarily composed of HHF35 positive smooth muscle cells and contains an intact endothelium. The first category of atherosclerotic lesion is the fibro-fatty lesion and is composed
predominantly of monocyte/macrophages, many of which are
extensively vacuolated (foam cells) (Figure 1A-1D). There
are also small numbers of lymphocytes present (T-200 positive
by HAM-56 negative) and occasionally an intact endothelium.
The intactness of the endothelium was quite variable with
all of the lesion categories observed and may reflect both
denudation of the endothelium and artifact induced during
procurement and processing of the tissue.

The second category of lesion observed was the fibrous
lesion. This type of lesion contained a much higher percentage of smooth muscle cells than a fibro-fatty lesion and,
in most cases many of the smooth muscle cells were organized
into a well defined fibrous cap. The fibrous lesions also
contained significant numbers of HAM-56 positive cells
situated both immediately beneath the endothelium and within
the core of the lesions. Fibrous lesions also frequently
contained measurable numbers of anti T-200 positive lymphocytes.

The final category of lesions was the advanced lesion.
Hematoxylin and eosin staining most often revealed a very
complex, heterogenous morphology indicating that modifications
due to thrombosis and subsequent organization, and massive
intimal thickening had occurred. Foam cells of both smooth
muscle and macrophage origin were generally present. Frequently the advanced lesions contained areas of fibrous cap,
shoulder regions and atheromatous core zones with each region
displaying extreme variability in cellular composition. The
fibrous cap zones frequently resembled the complete fibrous
lesion, containing large numbers of smooth muscle cells with
variable numbers of macrophages and lymphocytes. The shoulder
regions were frequently richer in macrophages and lymphocytes
suggesting that they are similar to fibro-fatty lesions. These
shoulder regions occasionally exhibited areas of neovascularization as defined by the presence of Factor VIII related
antigen positive cells outlining a vessel (Figure 2). The

Table 1. Cellular Composition of Human Aortic Atherosclerotic Lesions

	Smooth Muscle Cells[a]	Monocyte/ Macrophages[b]	Lymphocytes/ Monocytes[c]	Endothelium[d]
Normal aorta	Predominant	Minimal	Minimal	Intact
Fibro-fatty lesion	Minimal	Predominant	Small numbers present	Variable
Fibrous lesion	Variable numbers present	Variable numbers present	Small numbers present	Variable
Advanced lesion	Variable numbers present	Variable numbers present	Small numbers present	Surface - variable Presence of intimal and medial neo-vascularization

[a] As defined by HHF35 positivity

[b] As defined by HAM-56 positivity

[c] As defined by T-200 positivity

[d] As defined by Factor VIII related antigen positivity

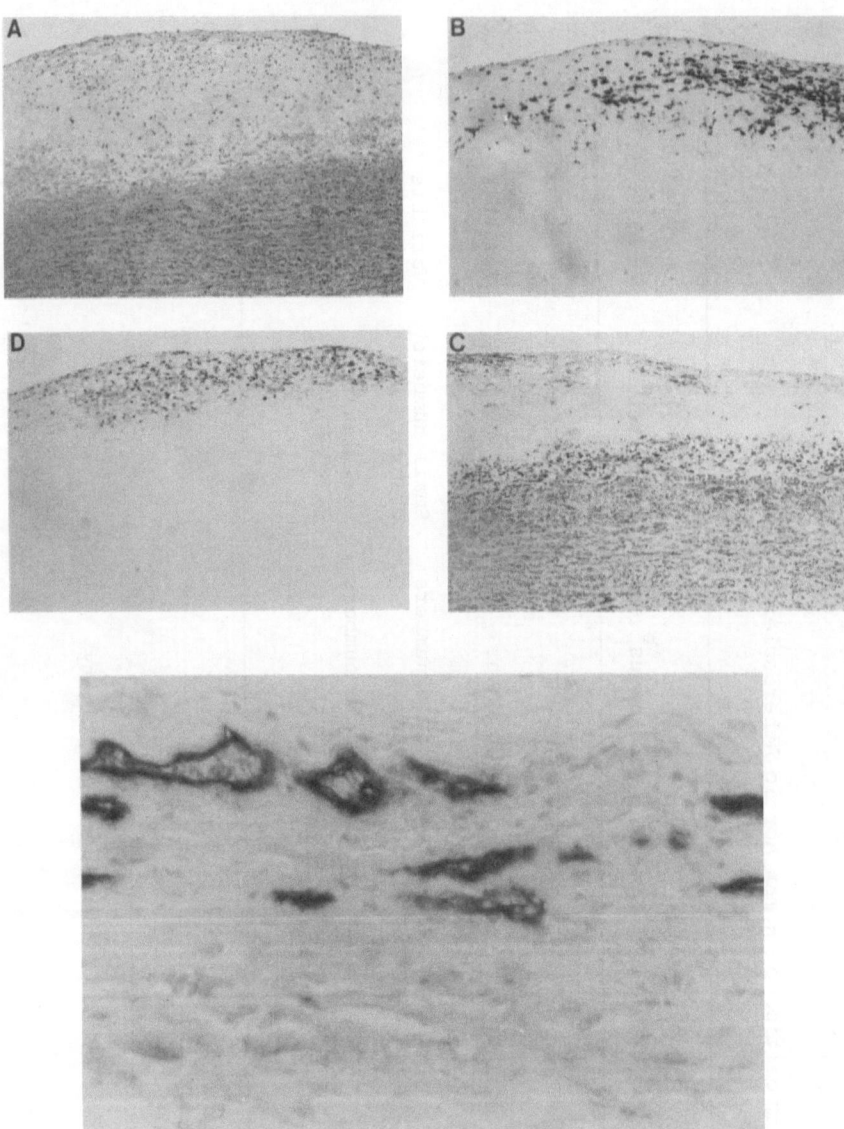

Figure 1. Immunocytochemical analysis of the cellular composition of a fibro-fatty lesion. Figures 1A-1D are serial sections reacted with (a) H & E, (b) HAM-56), (c) HHF35, (d) Anti-T-200 antigen. (x 138).
Figure 2. Neovascularization in the intima of an advanced lesion. This section was immunostained with an anti-factor VIII related antigen monoclonal antibody (x 947).

atheromatous core region was generally the least cellular, but contained hypertrophied HAM-56 and HHF35 positive foam cells. The advanced lesions also contained areas of deep neovascularization within foci of smooth muscle cells in the media.

DISCUSSION

The results of this study have demonstrated the applicability of monoclonal antibody techniques to the analysis of the cellular composition of human atherosclerotic lesions. Although we have focused only on the lesions of the aorta, we have observed several characteristic types of lesions that may also be descriptive of the cellular compositions of atherosclerotic lesions at other locations. We have observed lesions that are primarily composed of monocyte/macrophages (fibro-fatty lesions). This lesion may represent a transitional type of lesion, one between the early fatty streak and more advanced fibro-proliferative lesions. We have observed lesions that contain mixed populations of blood-borne cells together with smooth muscle cells frequently organized into a fibrous cap. Finally, we have observed lesions of very heterogeneous and complex cellular composition and organization that frequently contained areas of intimal and medial neovascularization. This study has demonstrated the difficulty in generalizing about the cellular composition of the human atherosclerotic lesion as witnessed by the extreme variability that exists from individual to individual, lesion to lesion, and within individual lesions.

Although previous studies with cell specific markers, including monoclonal antibodies have been published (8-10, 18-21), we feel that we have expanded on previous results in several ways:

1. The development of higher specific monoclonal antibodies for both smooth muscle cells and macrophages has enabled us to distinguish foam cells derived from the two different cell types without relying on morphologic or histochemical criteria. In addition, as opposed to previously published studies with cell specific monoclonal antibodies (18-21) our antibodies recognize hypertrophied and necrotic foam cells within the atheromatous core region of advanced lesions.

2. We are able to use these antibodies in well preserved tissue sections thus maintaining the overall morphology and cellular organization of the lesions. Antibodies
HHF35 and HAM-56 can also be used with plastic embedded and
aldehyde fixed tissue and cross react with nonhuman primate
and rabbit cells facilitating inter-species comparisons.

3. The simultaneous use of antibodies specific for the
four major cell types within the atherosclerotic lesion has
enabled us to account for and document the distribution of
a very large percentage of the total number of cells present
within the artery wall and has allowed us to demonstrate the
presence of neovascularization in areas of both the intima
and media.

REFERENCES

1. Parker F (1958) An electron microscope study of
    coronary arteries. Am J Anat 103:247-273.
2. Geer JC, McGill HC, Strong JP (1961) The fine
    structure of human atherosclerotic lesions. Am J
    Pathol 38:263-287.
3. Geer JC (1965) Fine structure of human aortic intimal
    thickening and fatty streaks. Lab Invest 14:1764-1793.
4. Ghidoni JJ, O'Neal RM (1967) Recent advances in
    molecular pathology: A review: Ultrastructure of
    human atheroma. Exp Mol Pathol 7:378-406.
5. Geer JC, Haust MD (1972) Smooth Muscle Cells in
    Atherosclerosis. Monographs on Atherosclerosis,
    Volume 2. Pollak OJ, Simms HS, Kirk SE (eds) Basel-
    New York: S Karger.
6. Huff HF, Heideman CL, Ganbotz JW, Schff DW, Titus JL,
    Gotto Jr AM (1978) Correlation of apolipoprotein B
    retention with the structure of atherosclerotic plaques
    from human aortas. Lab Invest 38:560-567.
7. Ross R, Wight TN, Strandness E, Thiele B (1984) Human
    atherosclerosis I. Cell constitution and characteristics
    of advanced lesions of the superficial femoral artery.
    Am J Pathol 114:79-83.
8. Fritz KE, Daoud AS, Jormolych J (1980) Non-specific
    esterase activity during regression of swine aortic
    atherosclerosis. Artery 7:352-366.
9. Schaffner T, Taylor K, Bartucci EJ, Fischer-Dzoga K,
    Beeson JH, Glagov S, Wissler RW (1980) Arterial foam
    cells exhibit distinctive immunomorphologic and histo-
    chemical features of macrophages. Am J Pathol 100:57-80.
10. Davis HR, Vesselinovitch D, Wissler RW (1984) Histo-
    chemical detection and quantification of macrophages in
    rhesus and cynomologus monkey atherosclerotic lesions.
    J Histochem Cytochem 32:1319-1377.
11. Fowler S, Shio H, Haley NJ (1979) Characterization
    of lipid-laden aortic cells from cholesterol-fed
    rabbits: IV. Investigation of macrophage-like pro-
    perties of aortic cell populations. Lab Invest 41:
    372-378.

12. Tsukada T, Tippins D, Gordon D, Ross R, Gown AM (1987) HHF35: A muscle-actin specific monoclonal antibody. Am J Pathol 126:51-60.

13. Gown AM, Tsukada T, Ross R (1986) Human atherosclerosis. Immunocytochemical analysis of the cellular composition of human atherosclerotic lesions. Am J Pathol 125:191-207.

14. Gown AM, Vogel AM (1982) Monoclonal antibodies to intermediate filament proteins of human cells: Unique and cross-reacting antibodies. J Cell Biol 95:414-424.

15. Dalchau R, Kirkely J, Fabre JW (1980) Monoclonal antibody to a human leukocyte-specific membrane glycoprotein probably homologous to the leukocyte-common (L-C) antigen of the rat. Eur J Immunol 10:737-744.

16. Hoyer LW, de Los Santos RP, Hoyer JR (1973) Antihemophiliac factor antigen localization in endothelial cells by immunofluorescent microscopy. J Clin Invest 52:2737-2744.

17. Hsu SM, Soban E (1982) Color modification of diaminobenzidine (DAB) precipitation by metallic ions and its application for double immunohistochemistry. J Histochem Cytochem 30:1079-1082.

18. Watanabe T, Yoshikawa Y, Nagafuchi Y, Toyoshima H, Watanabe T (1985) Role of macrophages in atherosclerosis: Sequential observations of cholesterol-induced rabbit aortic lesions by the immunoperoxidase technique using monoclonal antimacrophage antibody. Lab Invest 53:80-90.

19. Klurfeld DM (1985) Identification of foam cells in human atherosclerotic lesions as macrophages using monoclonal antibodies. Arch Pathol Lab Med 109:445-449.

20. Agel NM, Ball RY, Waldman H, Mitchinson MJ (1985) Identification of macrophages and smooth muscle cells in human atherosclerosis using monoclonal antibodies. J Pathol 146:197-204.

21. Jonasson L, Holm J, Skalli O, Bondjers G, Hansson GK (1986) Regional accumulation of T cells, macrophages and smooth muscle cells in human atherosclerotic plaque. Arteriosclerosis 6:131-138.

24

An Overview of Thrombosis and Platelet Involvement in the Development of the Human Atherosclerotic Plaque

A. Bleakley Chandler

INTRODUCTION

Thrombi that form on the walls of arteries may persist to become incorporated into the intima and thereby participate in atherogenesis. As a mural thrombus is incorporated by overgrowth of new endothelium, it may be converted to plaque tissue by arterial wall cells, which organize the thrombus. The main cells that organize a thrombus are intimal smooth muscle or myointimal cells. Unresolved and unorganized remnants of a thrombus may undergo fatty change and calcification. Thus, as a thrombus is converted to an atherosclerotic plaque it loses its identity and the lesion becomes decreasingly recognizable as thrombotic in origin. During the thrombotic process, platelets react with the arterial wall and participate in the formation of thrombi. Platelets, as well as monocytes, which also occur in thrombi (1), might contribute further to atherogenesis by the release of growth factors that stimulate the proliferation of intimal smooth muscle cells (2,3), which are a prominent feature of atherosclerotic plaques (4-6). These cells take part in early plaque development and are present in fatty streaks. They may continue to proliferate, produce collagen and progressively enlarge the plaque. In addition, like macrophages, they accumulate lipid as part of plaque development (5,7,8). Proliferation of myointimal cells may involve the thrombotic process or other atherogenic stimuli. The role of thrombi and their plasma and cellular

constituents in human atherogenesis will be considered here
in detail.

Thrombosis and Atherogenesis

The pathologist Carl von Rokitansky first postulated
over 100 years ago what has become widely known as the
thrombogenic hypothesis of atherosclerosis (9). Rokitansky
proposed that the disease is the result of an excessive
intimal deposition of blood components, including fibrin.
He maintained that localized thickening, atheromatous change
and calcification of the arterial wall are due to the
repeated deposition of blood elements and their subsequent
metamorphosis and degeneration on the lining membrane of the
vascular wall. This hypothesis was not generally accepted
at the time. The main objection was that the lesion of
atherosclerosis is in the intima not on the surface and,
therefore, could not be due to a surface deposit (10). This
seemingly important objection turned out to be unfounded
when it was shown that endothelium can grow over a thrombus
and incorporate it into the intima.

In his Harvey Lecture of 1912, Mallory (11) pointed out
that endothelial cells quickly cover over any fibrin within
the lumen. He considered fibrous plaques of the aorta
usually, perhaps always, to be formed by the organization of
thrombi. Fibrin in thrombi was thought to be a strong
stimulus to the production of connective tissue and he
likened the process to the formation of thick plates of
fibrous tissue on the surface of the spleen following acute
infections. As Rokitansky has previously observed, Mallory
noted that plaques are often stratified; the connective
tissue, replacing two or more layers of fibrin formed at
different times could be recognized like the layers marking
the annual growth of a tree. Clark and his colleagues (12)
studied atherosclerotic lesions in the aorta and coronary
arteries and concluded that the hyalinized bands of fibrinoid
in plaques are thrombotic in nature. They observed a gradual
transition from masses that were clearly mural surface
deposits to those covered by endothelium and collagenous
tissue. These observations were confirmed and extended by
Duguid (13,14), who considered transitional lesions of this

sort the essential link in the chain of evidence that
connects thrombosis with atherogenesis (Figure 1).

Duguid (13,15) further demonstrated that occlusive as
well as mural thrombi can be converted to atherosclerotic
plaques. An occlusive thrombus can first retract to a
mural or parietal position to create a single channel
between the thrombus and opposing vessel wall. Like other
mural thrombi, the retracted thrombus then becomes incorporated into the arterial wall as an eccentric plaque. This
process has been repeatedly demonstrated in the experimental
animal (16) and more recently by clinical angiographic
studies (17-19). It is clear from these observations that
although an occlusive thrombus may be a terminal event, it
need not be.

Organization and Atherosclerotic Metamorphosis of Thrombi

The arterial wall reacts to a thrombus by organizing
or converting it to living tissue. Organization takes place
by an ingrowth of connective tissue while adjacent endothelium grows over the thrombus to reestablish continuity of
the vascular lining (13). Small mural thrombi are organized
by an avascular process (14,20,21) whereas larger thrombi
tend to become vascularized by an ingrowth of capillary
sprouts from the newly formed overlying endothelium (4,20,22).
The connective tissue, which is fibromuscular in character,
is largely derived from smooth muscle cells (4,23-25).
Thrombi that have formed over atherosclerotic plaques may
be invaded by underlying smooth muscle cells of the plaque,
which have been shown to be capable of multiplication by
in vitro studies (26,27). In vitro, arterial smooth muscle
cells synthesize collagen types I, III, IV, V and VI (28-30),
elastic fiber microfibrils (31), glycosaminoglycans and
proteoglycans (32). Endothelial cells also may contribute
to the connective tissue matrix by undergoing phenotypic
modulation or metaplasia (25,33) (Figure 2). Endothelial
cells synthesize in vitro both basement membrane type IV
and pericellular type V collagen (29,34-36) as well as
elastin, elastic microfibrils (34), glycosaminoglycans (37)
and glycoproteins (35,36,38). The production of type V
collagen by endothelial cells may have added significance in

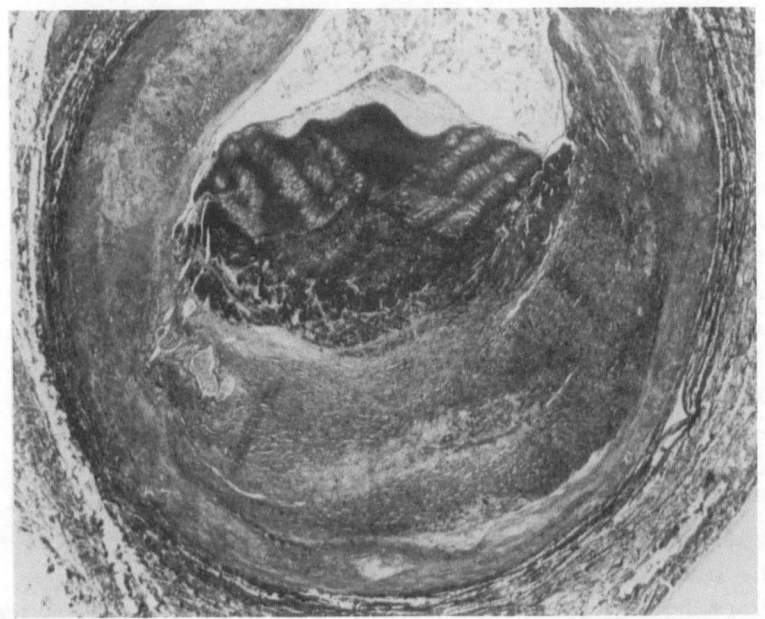

Figure 1. Layered thrombus of a coronary artery. Three
distinct layers of differing age are discernible in the
thrombus. The upper most recent layer has radiating platelet
columns connected by fibrin, while the middle layer consists
mainly of compact fibrin. The deepest oldest hyaline layer
is being organized by connective tissue and capillaries
extending from the fibrous plaque below, which merges with
the organizing thrombus. PTAH (x 16).

thromboatherogenesis in that it is now known to be a fibrillar
interstitial collagen (39,40), which along with the major
interstitial collagens I and III is concentrated in atherosclerotic plaques (41,42).

Monoclonal growth

In relation to the Benditt's monoclonal genetic mutation
theory of plaque origin (43), it is of interest to note that
the cells organizing a thrombus tend to become monoclonal as
measured by sex-linked enzyme markers (44). The monoclonal
theory suggests that atherosclerotic plaques arise by the
proliferation of a single clone of cells. The Monoclonality
of the majority of fibrous plaques has been cited as evidence
that thrombi cannot play a role in atherogenesis (45) on the
basis that the cells organizing a thrombus would be polyclonal.

363

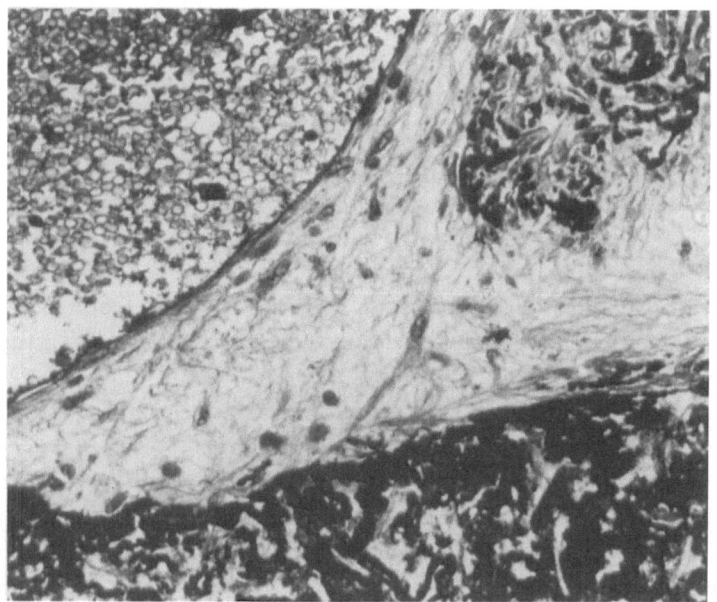

Figure 2. Organizing endothelialized thrombus. A large
stellate cell with cytoplasmic myofibrils in the center of
the field and similar cells to the left, just beneath the
lumen and regenerated endothelium, are associated with a
delicate fibrillar connective tissue replacing the black-
stained thrombus. The subendothelial location of these
cells suggests they are modified endothelial cells, which as
discussed in the text, may participate in the production of
the extracellular connective tissue matrix. Several monocyte/
macrophages in the matrix can be seen just to the left of
the large stellate cell. PSR-TP Levanol (x 256).

Pearson and his associates (44) provided objective evidence
in their study that monoclonal characteristics similar to
those in fibrous plaques develop in arterial thrombi as they
become organized.

Rate of Metamorphosis
The rate of each reaction engaged in metamorphis of a
thrombus could significantly influence the type of lesion
that develops. The amount of thrombus incorporated into the
arterial wall is determined by the rate of endothelialization
relative to that of thrombolysis (46). Endothelial regeneration in man is fairly slow, taking up to eight days to cover
such small areas as an arterial needle puncture wound (47).
Since the rate of endothelialization seems relatively constant,

the size of the initial thrombus could materially affect the outcome. Mural microthrombi that are not lysed probably are rapidly incorporated and quickly lose their identity. Conversely, a large thrombus would be more slowly organized and more likely to retain unresolved thrombic remnants in its center for a long time (20). How rapidly an occlusive thrombus in man can retract to an eccentric parietal position is not presently known. Experimental occlusive coronary thrombi in the dog, however, can retract by one week after formation, and become converted to eccentric fibrous plaques by six weeks (48).

Variable Composition of Thrombi and Plaques

Atherosclerotic plaques vary in composition from those that are sclerotic and largely fibromuscular to those that contain much lipid and are atheromatous. Many transitional forms exist between these extremes. Thrombi also vary considerably in composition, but all thrombic elements - fibrin, cellular elements and plasma - influence plaque development. Fresh arterial thrombi characteristically contain numerous platelets. The recently described growth factor derived from platelets (49) may stimulate smooth muscle cells to proliferate and make collagen. Monocytes in thrombi (1), may release a similar growth factor (50). Fibrin in thrombi seems to actively stimulate the production of collagen (4,11, 51) perhaps by serving as a scaffold on which smooth muscle cells grow (52). During lysis, fibrin may also release bound thrombin (53), which has been shown to enhance endothelial cell growth *in vitro* (54).

Lipid in Thrombi and Platelets

Crawford and Levene (20) observed that the sequestered remnants of an incompletely organized thrombus may undergo regressive changes to grummous fatty material (Figure 3). Both cellular elements and plasma lipids contribute to the fat content of thrombi. Plasma lipids may be entrapped in a forming thrombus and continue to be absorbed as it is organized (55,56). Among the cellular elements in thrombi, platelets are a major source of lipid (57,58). They are especially rich in cholesterol (59), which seems to be present in

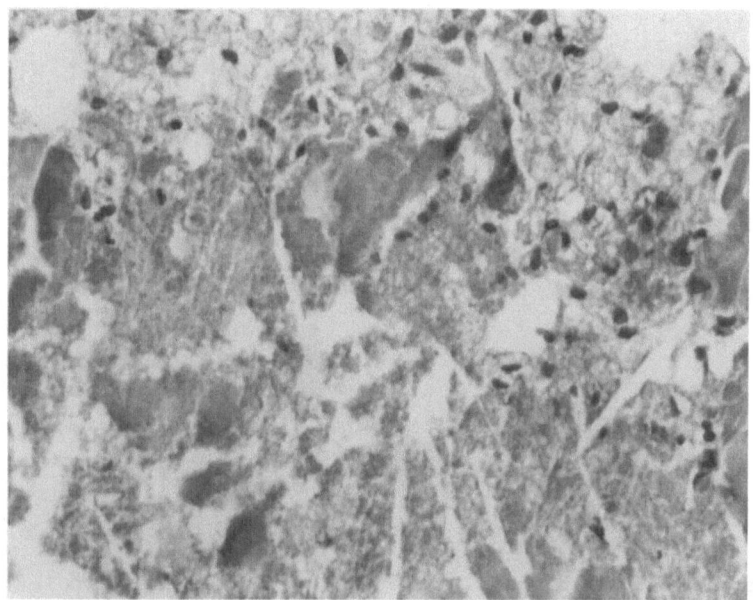

Figure 3. Fatty change of a thrombus. In the central region of an organizing occlusive renal artery thrombus, estimated by history to be 6 months old, cholesterol clefts have developed in unresolved degenerating thrombis remnants. Foam cells are at the top of the field. PTAH (x 256).

platelets in proportion to plasma levels (60). Foam cells characteristic of those in atherosclerotic plaques can be derived from macrophages that have phagocytized lipid-rich platelets (57) (Figure 4). Platelet derivatives have been frequently detected in these cells by immunohistology in atherosclerotic lesions (61). Although cholesterol in plate-lets is not esterified as much as it is in plasma and in plaques (62), it has been shown by *in vitro* experiments that macrophages can interact with platelets to accumulate and esterify cholesterol (63), including that of plasma lipo-proteins (64). Ross and his associates (27) have described the presence of lipid inclusions in smooth muscle cells as well as in macrophages of organizing thrombi. Kruth (personal communication) has shown recently that activated platelets also may release cholesterol, which could be taken up by both cell types.

The variable features of atherosclerosis thus find their counterparts in the cellular and plasma constituents of

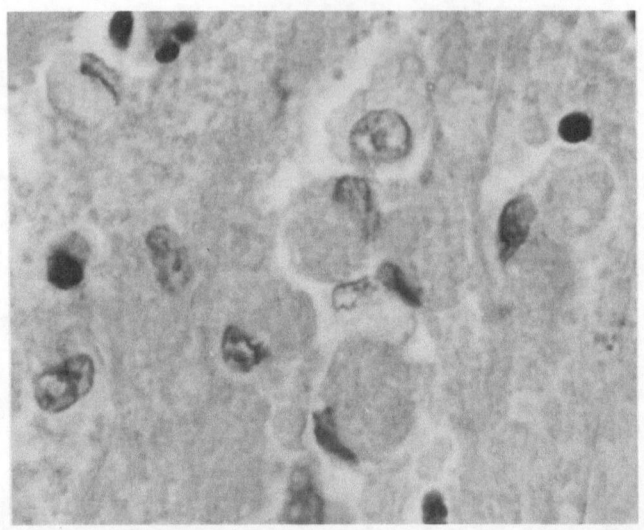

Figure 4. Phagocytized platelets. Monocytes in platelet columns of a thrombus have become distended with platelets that have been phagocytized. Some of the monocytic macrophages have become vacuolated foam cells as the lipid-rich platelets within their cytoplasm have disintegrated. Hematoxylin and eosin (x 240).

thrombi and in the arterial wall cells that organize and convert them to plaques. At the same time, it must be emphasized that metamorphosis of thrombi to plaques is recognized as only one of several mechanisms of atherogenesis, none of which need be mutually exclusive of the other (65).

Progressive and Recurrent Thrombus in Atherosclerosis

Thrombus is not simply an isolated event in the course of atherosclerosis, it is intimately involved in continued development of the lesion. The stratified appearance of many plaques suggests that they were formed by repeated deposits of thrombi (11-13). Clark and his colleagues (12) and others (4,13,66) have emphasized that recurrent thrombosis is an important factor in the pathogenesis of progressive atherosclerotic stenosis of coronary arteries. Deeper layers of thrombus are organized and converted into plaque as fresh uppermost layers are deposited. This form of episodic, and often silent, plaque growth may extend over months or years (66) (Figure 5).

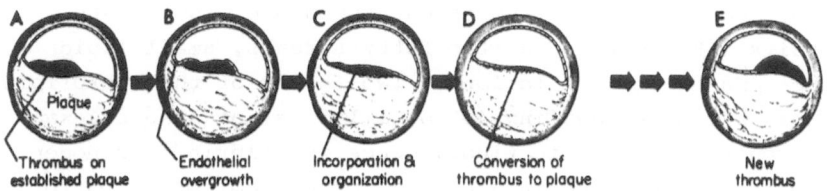

Figure 5. Thrombotic build-up of plaque. Diagram illustrating the incorporation of a mural thrombus over a plaque by endothelial overgrowth and conversion to plaque by organization. This process may be subclinical and repeatedly occur.

Significance of Thrombosis in Plaque Development

Since the evidence of the thrombotic origin of an atherosclerotic plaque is obscured as a result of metamorphosis of the thrombus, it is difficult to ascertain the true contribution of thrombosis to plaque development. For this reason, any estimate of the incidence of incorporated thrombi in plaques is likely to be an underestimate. A survey in 1975 of roughly 400 cases reported over the previous 40 years gave quantitative data about participation of thrombi in atherogenesis (67). Most quantitative studies have assessed the frequency with which thrombi can be identified in established plaques, particularly in aortic lesions. Thrombotic components are most often identified within fibrous and fibrofatty plaques. The relative frequency of reported cases exhibiting thrombotic components in the aorta varies widely from one series to another, from 30 to 89 percent, whereas the reported frequency of thrombotic elements in aortic lesions of those cases with thrombi varies over a narrow range, from 40 to 45 percent (67).

By means of immunofluorescent techniques, Woolf and Carstairs (68) compared aortic fatty streaks, small lipid plaques and fibrolipid lesions. Two-thirds of the fibrolipid plaques, a figure equaling 45% of all types of plaques examined, contained specific fluorescence for fibrin/fibrinogen antigen. Fluorescence in a banded, often laminated, pattern suggested it was thrombotic fibrin rather than fibrin/fibrinogen derived from infiltration or hemmorhage. Platelet antigen also was detected in the same areas in about one-half of these plaques. In the fatty streaks and small lipid plaques, a diffuse pattern of fluorescence specific for fibrin/fibrinogen antigen, but not platelet antigen, was thought to represent fibrinogen that had infiltrated along with plasma from the lumen. Although thrombosis does not appear to be a factor in the pathogenesis of superficial fatty streaks, the possibility that fatty streaks provide a base for thrombus formation and subsequent growth of the lesions should not be excluded (69,70).

Initiation of Plaques by Thrombi

There is limited evidence that thrombosis is a factor in the inception of atherosclerotic lesions. Occasional small mural thrombi, either uncovered or in varying stages of incorporation, have been observed on apparently healthy vessel walls (14,16,70-72), but undetected and preexistent submicroscopic changes could be present in a seemingly normal artery (71). Interpretation of possible early thrombotic lesions may be further complicated by reaction of the intima to the overlying thrombus. Jørgensen and his coworkers (73) correlated the presence of aortic microthrombi with focal intimal edema and suggested that the edematous lesions resulted from injury to the vascular lining by the thrombi. Regardless of their mode of origin, small thrombotic-vascular lesions could represent an incipient stage of atherosclerosis. Unequivocal and strong support for the concept that thrombi can initiate plaque formation on a normal vessel wall is recognized in thromboembolism. In man (74) and in the experimental animal (16,58), plaques can be derived from thromboemboli that have lodged in previously normal arteries.

Age of Onset

Little information is available on the age when thrombi begin to contribute to plaque growth. In an autopsy study conducted in this laboratory on the main division of the left coronary artery in 9 cases ranging in age from 12 to 30 years, superficial microthrombi were found to be incorporated by endothelium in plaques of coronary arteries only after the age of 25 years (75). Uncovered thrombi were found as early as 12 years of age, both on fibrous plaques and minimally altered arterial walls (75) (Figure 6). In a series of 400 evenly distributed cases from 1-40 years of age reported by Velican and Velican (76), both surface and incorporated microthrombi were observed on and in thickened intimas and developing atherosclerotic plaques of coronary arteries with increasing frequency from a rate of 2% at 11-15 years to 22% at 36-40 years of age.

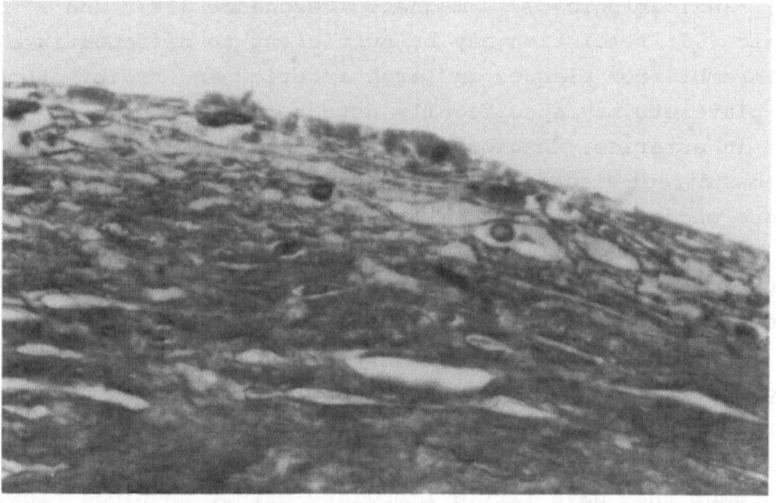

Figure 6. Microthrombus of a coronary artery. The micro-thrombus is largely comprised of aggregated platelets formed over a superficial foam cell collection of a fibrous plaque from a subject 30 years of age. Endothelium is not evident beneath the thrombus in this plane of section. PASH-Allochrome (x 400).

These observations on the frequency of intimal thrombotic lesions, while still incomplete and limited by the exclusion of thrombi that have lost their identity in the conversion process, nevertheless, provide substantial evidence that thrombosis is an important factor in the long-term development of arterial plaques. Moreover, factors might exist in some subsets of the population that increase the rate of production of thrombi or impede and prevent their resolution so that, in effect, the thrombi accumulate and produce advanced atherosclerosis (58).

Correlative Clinical-Pathologic Assessment

The possobility of extending classical morphologic studies of arterial thrombi by *in vivo* imaging techniques is a recent development. X-ray angiographic procedures, angioscopy, magnetic resonance, radioisotopic and ultrasonic imaging all may be applied to the study of thrombi and thrombotic-vascular lesions. Angiographic (77), magnetic resonance (78), and ultrasonic (79) resolution may be sufficient to differentiate recent thrombi from plaques in large arteries and radioisotope-labeled platelets may specifically detect these thrombotic elements in arteries. Angioscopy is a new clinical technique that allows direct visualization of intraluminal thrombi and the plaque surface (80).

In vivo imaging will allow longitudinal studies in individual patients as well as correlative morphologic assessment when lesions are excised or are studied at autopsy. Clinically silent lesions may be detected and followed before becoming overtly manifest, making possible a much more accurate assessment of the contribution of thrombi to the growth and development of plaques, especially by small recurring mural thrombi that have little immediate effect on blood flow. Davis and his associates (81) have shown that some but not all plaques accumulate [111]Indium-labeled platelets, suggesting that some lesions either have a different natural history from others or represent lesions at different stages of development. With multiple imaging methods for *in vivo* detection of thrombi now at hand or on the horizon, it should soon be feasible to monitor antithrombotic measures directed toward reduction of the long-term effects of thrombosis on plaque growth.

The Platelet-Derived Growth Factor and Atherogenesis

A series of studies by Ross and his associates and subsequently by other investigators has led to a concept of
atherogenesis whereby a growth factor released from platelets
interacting with an injured arterial wall stimulates intimal
smooth muscle cells to proliferate and synthesize collagen
(49,82-85). The evidence in support of this concept is
derived from *in vitro* studies and from studies in the
experimental animal under conditions of thrombocytopenia or
platelet inhibition (2,3,86).

The platelet-derived growth factor was discovered
following the observation that monkey arterial smooth muscle
cells remain quiescent when cultured in a medium containing
serum derived from platelet-free plasma, whereas cells cultured in a medium containing serum derived either from
clotted whole blood or from platelet-free plasma with an
added extract of platelets are stimulated to proliferate (49).
Subsequently, it was demonstrated that this mitogenic factor
is a basic polypeptide hormone (3,87) located in the alpha
granules of the platelet (88,89). The platelet appears
simply to be a carrier of the hormone, which is produced elsewhere possibly in the megakaryocyte (3,50).

Kaplan and his coworkers (89) commented on the remarkably
specific delivery system for this hormone, which is released
only where needed at sites of injury. Upon release of platelet
constituents, the hormone may initiate replication of connective tissue cells and the reparative process. Unfortunately,
the healing response often overreacts, or leaves in its wake
the nidus on which pathologic processes begin. The potential
effects of this growth factor fit nicely into Virchow's concept of injury and repair as it applies to atherosclerosis
(2,86); indeed, thrombosis itself is a reparative process,
often being an exaggerated response to vascular injury.

A related aspect of platelet interaction with the vessel
wall to take into account is the release of lytic enzymes and
vasoactive amines by platelets, which may injure the endothelium, make it more permeable, and thus allow such agents
as the platelet-derived growth factor to have access to the
subendothelial intima (73,90). This aspect of platelet behavior, when placed against the background of evidence that

platelets also protect and nourish endothelium is paradoxical, and serves to illustrate the paucity of knowledge
in this area (90).

At present, it is difficult to assess fully the significance of the platelet-derived and other related growth factors
in human atherogenesis (2,3). The platelet-derived growth
factor may be one of several mitogens, including additional
ones from plasma, the monocyte/macrophage and endothelial
cell that stimulate smooth muscle cells to proliferate and
participate in plaque development. Recent *in vitro* studies
have shown that activated monocytes and macrophages may
synthesize and secrete a platelet-like growth factor (50,91)
and that endothelial cells produce a similar substance (92,
93) which may be released by action of thrombin on the
cell (94).

Regardless of the ultimate significance of growth factors
in atherosclerosis, it remains clear that thrombi, which contain platelets, monocytes and plasma (1,95), are organized by
smooth muscle and endothelial cells and may so contribute to
atherogenesis. Hence, there is reason to anticipate that as
intensive investigation of these factors continues, therapeutic intervention and prophylaxis of thromboarterial disease
by antithrombotic and platelet inhibitory measures will be
increasingly evaluated.

REFERENCES

1. Chandler AB (1969) The anatomy of a thrombus. In:
   Sherry S, Brinkhous KM, Genton E, Stengle, JM (eds)
   Thrombosis. Washington: National Academy of Sciences,
   pp. 279-299.
2. Ross R (1986) The pathogenesis of atherosclerosis -
   An update. N Engl J Med 314:488-500.
3. Ross R, Rained EW, Bowen-Pope DF (1986) The biology of
   platelet-derived growth factor. Cell 46:155-169.
4. Morgan AD (1956) The Pathogenesis of Coronary Occlusion.
   Oxford: Blackwell Scientific Pub., pp. 1-171.
5. Geer JC, Haust MD (1972) Smooth Muscle Cells in Atherogenesis. Basel: Karger, pp. 1-140.
6. Campbell GR, Campbell JH (1985) Smooth muscle phenotypic changes in arterial wall homeostasis: Implications
   for the pathogenesis of atherosclerosis. Exp Mol Path
   42:139-162.
7. Geer JC, McGill Jr HC, Strong JP (1961) The fine
   structure of human atherosclerotic lesions. Am J Pathol
   38:263-287.

8. Bierman EL, Albers JJ (1975) Lipoprotein uptake by cultured human arterial smooth muscle cells. Biochim Biophys Acta 388:198-202.
9. Rokitansky C (1855) A Manual of Pathological Anatomy, Volume 4. Swaine WE, Sieveking E, Moore CH, Day GE (translators). Philadelphia: Blanchard & Lee, pp. 198-207.
10. Long ER (1933) The development of our knowledge of arteriosclerosis. In: Cowdry EV (ed) Arteriosclerosis. New York: MacMillan, pp. 19-52.
11. Mallory FB (1912-1913) The infectous lesions of blood vessels. In: The Harvey Lecutres. Philadelphia: JB Lippincott, pp. 150-166.
12. Clark E, Graef I, Chasis H (1936) Thrombosis of the aorta and coronary arteries with special reference to "fibrinoid" lesions. Arch Pathol 22:183-212.
13. Duguid JB (1946) Thrombosis as a factor in the pathogenesis of coronary atherosclerosis. J Pathol Bac 58: 207-212.
14. Duguid JB (1949) Thrombosis as a factor in the pathogenesis of aortic atherosclerosis. J Pathol Bac 60: 57-61.
15. Duguid JB (1949) Pathogenesis of atherosclerosis. Lancet 2:925-927.
16. Chandler AB (1970) Thrombosis and the development of atherosclerotic lesions. In: Jones RJ (ed) Atherosclerosis: Procedings of the Second International Symposium. New York: Springer-Verlag, pp. 88-93.
17. Henderson RR, Hansing CE, Razavi M, Rowe GG (1973) Resolution of an obstructive coronary lesion as demonstrated by selective angiography in a patient with transmural myocardial infarction. Am J Card 31:785-788.
18. Kavanagh-Gray D (1974) Angiographic evidence of coronary occlusion and resolution. CMA J 110:945-946.
19. DeWood MA, Notske RN, Simpson CS, Stifter WF, Shields JP (1985) Prevalence and significance of spontaneous thrombolysis in transmural myocardial infarction. Eur Heart J 6(Suppl E):33-42.
20. Crawford T, Levene CI (1952) Incorporation of fibrin in the aortic intima. J Pathol Bact 64:523-528.
21. Heard BE (1949) Mural thrombosis in the renal artery and its relation to atherosclerosis. J Pathol Bact 61: 635-637.
22. Geiringer E (1951) Intimal vascularization and atherosclerosis. J Pathol Bact 63:201-211.
23. More RH, Movat HZ, Haust MC (1957) Role of mural fibrin thrombi of the aorta in the genesis of arteriosclerotic plaques. Report of two cases. Arch Pathol 63:612-620.
24. Haust MD, More RH, Movat HZ (1959) The mechanism of fibrosis in arteriosclerosis. Am J Pathol 35:265-273.
25. Haust MD, More RH, Movat HZ (1960) The role of smooth muscle cells in the fibrogenesis of arteriosclerosis. Am J Pathol 37:377-389.
26. Eskin SG, Sybers HD, Lester JW, Navarro LT, Gotto Jr AM, DeBakey ME (1981) Human smooth muscle cells cultured from atherosclerotic plaques and uninvolved vessel wall. In vitro 17:713-718.

27. Ross R, Wight TN, Strandness E, Thiele B (1984) Human atherosclerosis. I. Cell constitution and characteristics of advanced lesions of the superficial femoral artery. Am J Pathol 114:79-93.

28. Layman DL, Epstein Jr EH, Dodson RF, Titus JL (1977) Biosynthesis of type I and III collagens by cultured smooth muscle cells from human aorta. Proc Natl Acad Sci USA 74:671-675.

29. Madri JA, Dreyer B, Pitlick FA, Furthmayr H (1980) The collagenous components of the subendothelium. Lab Invest 43:303-315.

30. Von Der Mark H, Aumailley M, Wick G, Fleishmajer T, Timpl R (1984) Immunochemistry, genuine size and tissue localization of collagen IV. Eur J Biochem 142:493-502.

31. Gimbrone Jr MA, Cotran RS (1975) Human vascular smooth muscle in culture. Lab Invest 33:16-27.

32. Tammi M, Ronnemaa T, Vihersaari T, Lehtonen A, Vikari J (1979) High density lipoproteinemia due to vigorous physical work inhibits the incorporation of (3H) thymidine and the synthesis of glycosaminoglycans by human aortic smooth muscle cells in culture. Atherosclerosis 32:23-32.

33. Altschul R (1954) Endothelium, Its Development, Morphology, Function, and Pathology. New York: MacMillan, pp. 1-157.

34. Jaffee EA, Minick CR, Adelman B, Becker CG, Nachman R (1976) Synthesis of basement membrane collagen by cultured human endothelial cells. J Exp Med 144:209-225.

35. Sage H, Bornstein P (1982) Endothelial cells from umbilical vein and a hemangioendothelioma secrete base-membrane largely to the exclusion of interstitial pro-collagens. Arteriosclerosis 2:27-36.

36. Fry G, Parsons T, Hoak J, Sage H, Gingrich RD, Ercolani L, Nghiem D, Czervionke R (1984) Properties of cultured endothelium from adult human vessels. Arteriosclerosis 4:4-13.

37. Gordon PB, Conn G, Hatcher VB (1985) Glycosaminoglycan production in cultures of early and late passage human endothelial cells: The influence of an anionic endothelial cell growth factor and the extracellular matrix. J Cell Phys 125:596-607.

38. Jaffee EA, Weksler BB (1979) Recovery of endothelial cell prostacyclin production after inhibition by low dose of aspirin. J Clin Invest 63:532-535.

39. Modesti A, Kalebic T, Scarpa S, Togo S, Grotendorst G, Liotta LL, Triche TJ (1984) Type V collagen in human amnion is a 12 nm fibrillar component of the pericellular interstitium. Eur J Cell Biol 35:246-255.

40. Schuppan D, Becker J, Boehm H, Hahn EG (1986) Immuno-fluorescent localization of type-V collagen as a fibrillar component of the interstitial connective tissue of human mucosa, artery and liver. Cell Tissue Res 243:535-543.

41. McCullagh KG, Duance VC, Bishop KA (1980) The distribution of collagen types I, III, and V (AB) in normal and atherosclerotic human aorta. J Pathol 130:45-55.

42. Morton LF, Barnes MJ (1982) Collagen polymorphism in the normal and diseased blood vessel wall. Atherosclerosis 42:41-51.

43. Benditt EP, Benditt JM (1973) Evidence for a mono-
    clonal origin of human atherosclerotic plaques. Proc
    Natl Acad Sci USA 70:1753-1756.
44. Pearson TA, Solez K, Dillman J, Heptinstall RH (1979)
    Monoclonal characteristics of organizing arterial thrombi:
    Significance in the origin and growth of human athero-
    sclerotic plaques. Lancet 1:7-11.
45. Benditt EP (1974) Evidence for a monoclonal origin of
    human atherosclerotic plaques and some implications.
    Circulation 50:650-652.
46. Davies MJ, Woolf N, Bradley JPW (1960) Endotheliali-
    sation of experimentally produced mural thrombi in
    the pig aorta. J Pathol 97:589-594.
47. Crawford T (1956) The healing of puncture wounds in
    arteries. J Pathol Bact 72:547-552.
48. Pope JT, Chandler AB, Asokan SK, Pollard D (1974)
    Metamorphosis of experimental coronary thrombi into
    arteriosclerotic plaques. Circulation 50(Suppl III):
    295 (abstract).
49. Ross R, Glomset JA, Kariya B, Harker LA (1974) A
    platelet-dependent serum factor that stimulates the pro-
    liferation of arterial smooth muscle cells *in vitro*.
    Proc Natl Acad Sci USA 71:1207-1210.
50. Shomokado K, Raines EW, Madtes DK, Barrett TB, Benditt
    EP, Ross R (1985) A significant part of macrophage-
    derived growth factor consists of at least two forms
    of PDGF. Cell 43:277-286.
51. Haust MD, Movat HZ, More RH (1956) The role of fibrin
    thrombi in the genesis of the common white plaque in
    arteriosclerosis. Circulation 14:483 (abstract).
52. Smith EB (1986) Fibrinogen, fibrin and fibrin degrada-
    tion products in relation to atherosclerosis. Clinics
    in Haematology 15:355-370.
53. Francis CW, Markham Jr RE, Barlow GH, Florack TM,
    Dobrznski DM, Marder VJ (1983) Thrombin activity of
    fibrin thrombi and soluble plasmic derivatives. J Lab
    Clin Med 102:220-230.
54. Gospodarowicz D, Brown KD, Birdwell CR, Zetter BR (1978)
    Control of proliferation of human vascular cells. J
    Cell Biol 77:774-788.
55. Woolf N, Pilkington JRE, Carstairs KC (1966) The
    occurrence of lipoproteins in thrombi. J Pathol Bact
    91:383-387.
56. Scott PJ, Hurley PJ (1969) Incorporation of radioiodina-
    ted serum albumin and low-density lipoprotein into human
    thrombi *in vivo*. J Pathol 97:603-609.
57. Chandler AB, Hand RA (1961) Phagocytized platelets; a
    source of lipids in human thrombi and atherosclerotic
    plaques. Science 134:946-947.
58. Hand RA, Chandler AB (1962) Atherosclerotic metamorpho-
    sis of autologous pulmonary thromboemboli in the rabbit.
    Am J Pathol 40:469-486.
59. Andreoli VM, Maffei F, Tonon GC (1973/1974) Platelet
    lipid modification induced by fatty acids: Experimental
    studies and correlations with human neuropathology.
    Haemostasis 2:118-140.
60. Shastri KM, Carvalho ACA, Lees RS (1980) Platelet
    function and platelet lipid composition in the dyslipo-
    proteinemias. J Lipid Res 21:467-472.

61. Sevitt S (1986) Platelets and foam cells in the evolution of atherosclerosis - Histological and immunohistological studies of human lesions. Atherosclerosis 61: 107-115.

62. Smith EB (1967) Quantitative and qualitative comparison of the lipids in platelets, aortic intima, and mural thrombi. Cardiovasc Res 1:111-115.

63. Curtiss LK, Black AS, Takagi Y, Plow EF (1987) A new mechanism for foam cell generation in atherosclerotic lesions. J Clin Invest 80:367-373.

64. Fogelman AM, Schechter I, Seager J, Hokom M, Child JS, Edwards PA (1980) Malondialdehyde alteration of low density lipoproteins leads to cholesteryl ester accumulation in human monocyte-macrophages. Proc Natl Acad Sci USA 77:2214-2218.

65. McMillan GC (1978) The process from normal to lesion. In: Chandler AB, Eurenius K, McMillan GC, Nelson GB, Schwartz CJ, Wessler S (eds) The Thrombotic Process in Atherogenesis. New York: Plenum, pp. 3-10.

66. Crawford T (1986) Thrombotic occlusion and the plaque. In: Jones RJ (ed) Evolution of the Atherosclerotic Plaque. Chicago: Univ. Chicago Press, pp. 279-290.

67. Chandler AB, Pope JT (1975) Arterial thrombosis in atherogenesis: A survey of the frequency of incorporation of thrombi into atherosclerotic plaques. In: Hautvast JGAJ, Hermus RJJ, van der Haar F (eds) Blood and Arterial Wall in Atherogenesis and Arterial Thrombosis. Leiden: E.J. Brill, pp. 110-118.

68. Woolf N, Carstairs KC (1967) Infiltration and thrombosis in Atherogenesis. A study using immunofluorescent techniques. Am J Pathol 51:373-386.

69. Woolf N (1961) The distribution of fibrin within the aortic intima. A immunohistochemical study. Am J Pathol 39:521-532.

70. Haust MD (1971) The morphogenesis and fate of potential and early atherosclerotic lesions in man. Human Pathol 2:1-29.

71. Movat HZ, Haust MD, More RH (1959) The morphologic elements in the early lesions of arteriosclerosis. Am J Pathol 35:93-101.

72. McMillan GC (1965) The onset of plaque formation in arteriosclerosis. Acta Cardiol (Suppl II):43-62.

73. Jørgensen L, Pakcham MA, Rowsell HC, Mustard JF (1972) Deposition of formed elements of blood on the intima and signs of intimal injury in the aorta of rabbit, pig and man. Lab Invest 27:341-350.

74. Barnard PJ (1954) Pulmonary arteriosclerosis and cor pulmonale due to recurrent thromboembolism. Circulation 10:343-361.

75. Chandler AB (1972) Thrombosis in the development of coronary atherosclerosis. In: Likoff W, Segal BL, Insull Jr W, Moyer JH (eds) Atherosclerosis and Coronary Heart Disease. New York: Grune and Stratton, pp. 28-34.

76. Velican C, Velican D (1980) The precursors of coronary atherosclerotic plaques in subjects up to 40 years old. Atherosclerosis 37:33-46.

77. DeWood MA, Spores J, Notske R, et al. (1980) Prevalence of total coronary occlusion during the early hours of transmural myocardial infarction. N Engl J Med 303:897-902.

78. Valk PE, Hale JD, Kaufman L, Crooks LE, Higgins CB (1985)   MR imaging of the aorta with three-dimensional vessel reconstruction: Validation by angiography. Radiology 157:721-725.
79. McKinney WM, Harpold GJ (1982)   B-Mode ultrasound inter-rogation of arteries. In: Bond MG, Insull W, Glagov S, Chandler AB, Cornhill JF (eds)   Clinical Diagnosis of Atherosclerosis. New York: Springer-Verlag, pp. 173-182.
80. Sherman CT, Litvack F, Grundfest W, et al. (1986)   Coro-nary angioscopy in patients with unstable angina pectoris. N Engl J Med 315:913-919.
81. Davis II HH, Siegel BA, Sherman LA, et al. (1980) Scintigraphic detection of carotid atherosclerosis with indium-111-labeled autologous platelets. Circulation 61:982-988.
82. Ross R, Glomset JA (1976)   The pathogenesis of athero-sclerosis. N Engl J Med 295:369-377 and 420-425.
83. Rutherford RB, Ross R (1976)   Platelet factors stimulate fibroblasts and smooth muscle cells quiescent in plasma serum to proliferate. J Cell Biol 69:196-203.
84. Burke JM, Ross R (1977)   Collagen synthesis by monkey arterial smooth muscle cells during proliferation and quiescence in culture. Exp Cell Res 107:387-395.
85. Witte LD, Kaplan KL, Nossel HL, Lages BA, Weiss HJ, Goodman DS (1978)   Studies of the release from human platelets of the growth factor for cultured human arterial smooth muscle cells. Circ Res 42:402-409.
86. Friedman RJ, Burns ER (1978)   Role of platelets in the proliferative response of the injured artery. Progress in Hemostasis and Thrombosis 4:249-278.
87. Antoniades HN, Scher CD, Stiles CD (1979)   Purification of human platelet-derived growth factor. Proc Natl Acad Sci USA 76:1809-1813.
88. Kaplan KL, Broekman MJ, Chernoff A, Lesznik GR, Drillings M (1979)   Platelet α-granule proteins: Studies on release and subcellular localization. Blood 53:604-618.
89. Kaplan DR, Chao FC, Stiles CD, Antoniades HN, Scher CD (1979)   Platelet α-granules contain a growth factor for fibroblasts. Blood 53:1043-1052.
90. Majno G, Joris I (1978)   Endothelium 1977: A review. In: Chandler AB, Eurenius K, McMillan GC, Nelson DB, Schwartz CJ, Wessler S (eds)   The Thrombotic Process in Atherogenesis. New York: Plenum, pp. 169-225, 481-526.
91. Glenn KC, Ross R (1981)   Human monocyte-derived growth factor(s) for mesenchymal cells: Activation of secretion by endotoxin and concanavalin A.   Cell 25:603-615.
92. DiCorleto PE, Bowen-Pope DF (1983)   Cultured endothelial cells produce a platelet-derived growth factor-like pro-tein.   Proc Natl Acad Sci USA 80:1919-1923.
93. Collins T, Ginsbrug D, Boss JM, Orkin SH, Pober JS (1985) Cultured human endothelial cells express platelet-derived growth factor B chain: cDNA cloning and structural analysis. Nature 316:748-750.
94. Harlan JM, Thompson PJ, Ross R, Bowen-Pope DF (1986) β-thrombin induces release of PDGF-like molecule(s) by cultured human endothelial cells. J Cell Biol 103:1129-1133.
95. Iga Y, Stella SR, Chandler AB (1984)   Molecular exchange between blood and *in vitro* thrombi. Haemostasis 14:361-366.

25
Observations Regarding the Thrombotic Process in Human Subjects

Marcus A. DeWood, Pierre P. Leimgruber, and William F. Stifter

INTRODUCTION

Whereas atherosclerosis of the coronary arteries frequently is manifested as chronic stable angina, many patients
rapidly evolve to acute ischemic syndromes. The mechanisms
by which this conversion from a stable state to clinically
unstable coronary artery disease usually occurs because of
severe coronary stenosis by occlusive plaque (1). For the
past several years the contribution of coronary thrombosis
to acute ischemic syndromes and the interaction of coronary
thrombus with underlying plaque has been debated (2). Importantly, the fate of the occlusive thrombus in patients
has remained unclear. Many authors have concluded that
whether or not thrombosis spontaneously resolves, there is
some incorporation into the arterial wall which contributes
to the underlying plaque itself (3-7). This phenomenon may
correlate with waxing and waning of ischemic symptoms.

The underlying factors contributing to the generation
of coronary thrombosis are unknown. Nevertheless, recent
clinical data (8-10) based on arteriographic findings with
and without thrombolytic agents have emphasized the important
contribution of coronary thrombosis.

The preceding speaker has presented data suggesting
coronary thrombosis can undergo organization and incorporation

Supported in part by the Deaconess and Sacred Heart Medical
Center Foundations and the Inland Empire Heart Research
Foundation.

into the arterial wall and, in part, contribute to the atherosclerotic plaque. Furthermore, occlusive thrombi may become nonocclusive and then undergo subsequent transformation into atherosclerotic plaque.

The purpose of this short paper is to review clinical data regarding the behavior of coronary occlusion and thrombosis in acute ischemic syndromes. Furthermore we have attempted to explore the relationship between spontaneous thrombolysis and clot retraction in evolution of the human atherosclerotic plaque.

METHODS

Clinical Acute Ischemic Syndromes

In order to correlate histologic and clinical data we will present information on three major acute syndromes: Q-wave (transmural) infarction, non-Q-wave (non-transmural or subendocardial) infarction and early unstable angina pectoris.

Q-Wave Myocardial Infarction

As early as 1970 we began to perform coronary arteriography on patients in the early hours of Q-wave infarction. Infarction was defined clinically by (1) very discrete onset of chest pain in conjunction with electrocardiographic ST segment elevation that evolved to Q-waves. As is shown in Figure 1a, total coronary occlusion was frequently discovered. Figure 1b demonstrates that staining was observed at the point of occlusion and later (Figure 1c) resolution of this total coronary occlusion was observed at the point of an atherosclerotic plaque.

We investigated 517 patients with coronary arteriography within 24 hours of symptom onset of Q-wave infarction (11). The results are presented in Figure 2. As is shown, coronary thrombus was observed by arteriography (either by staining or by an intraluminal filling defect consistent with thrombus) in 80% of the 368 patients studied within the first six hours of symptom onset. As is shown in Figure 2, the prevalence of coronary thrombus fell significantly over the next several hours in patient groups that showed similar characteristics

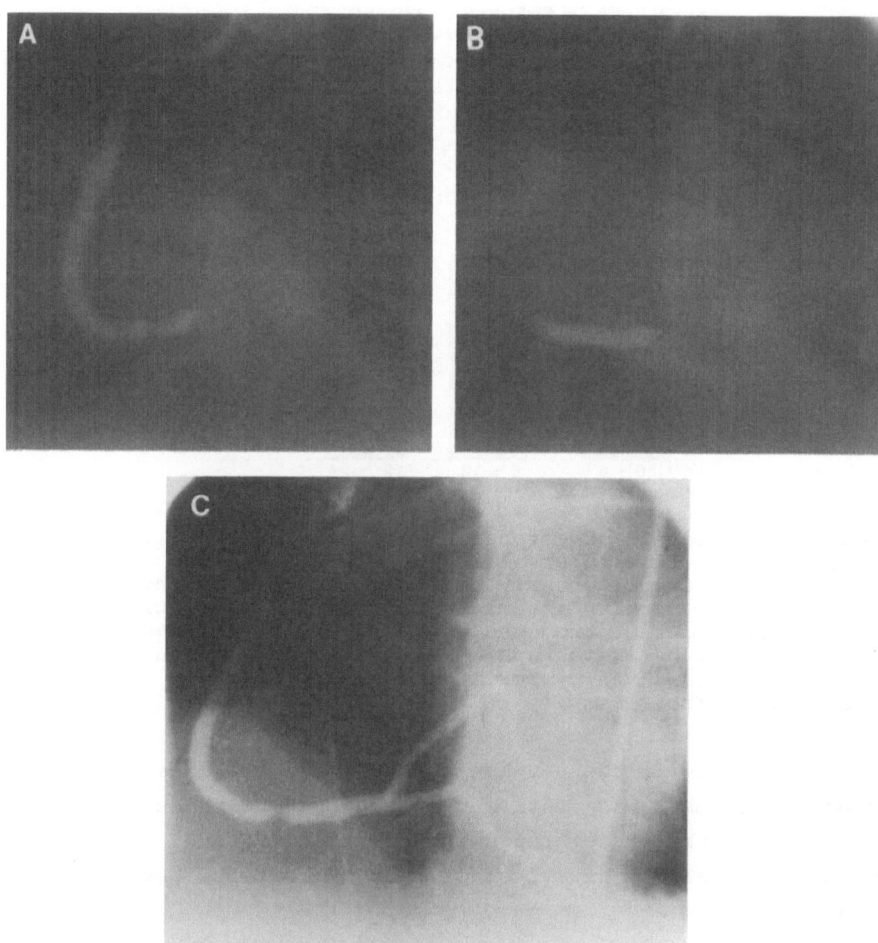

Figure 1a.   Coronary occlusion of a right coronary artery in
the first two hours after symptom onset in Q-wave infarction.
Figure 1b.   Cineangiographic evidence of a thrombus causative
of the acute myocardial infarction.
Figure 1c.   Resolution of thrombotic occlusion with remaining
plaque upon restudy.
Reprinted from Circulation, 68(II)I39-I49, 1983 by permission
of the American Heart Association, Inc.

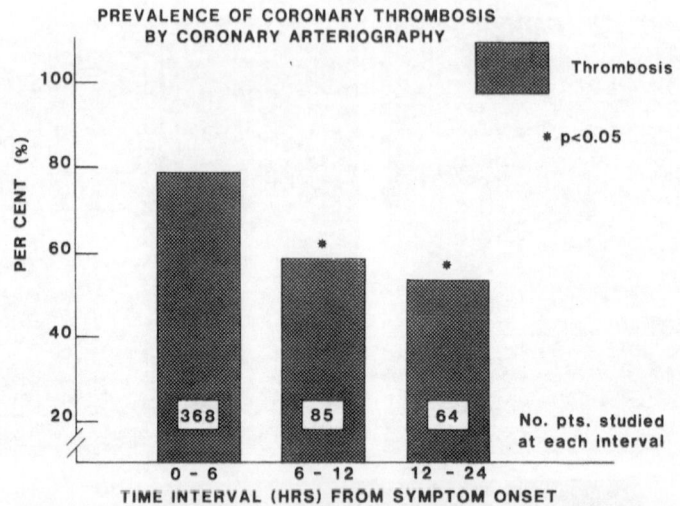

PREVALENCE OF CORONARY THROMBOSIS
BY CORONARY ARTERIOGRAPHY

Figure 2. Evidence of coronary occlusion in groups studied
during various time intervals. There was a decline in the
prevalence of total coronary occlusion as well as the
prevalence of coronary thrombosis suggesting that coronary
thrombus may retract from the vessel wall in the less
visible figure by angiography. Reprinted from Circulation,
68 (II) I39-I49, 1983 by permission of the American Heart
Association, Inc.

as the patients in the 0-6 hour group. The presence of
coronary thrombus was confirmed during open heart surgery by
retrieval of thrombus through the arteriotomy site. These
thrombi were almost always at or near the site of severe
stenosis.

Non-Q-Wave Myocardial Infarction
During the period from 1974 to 1984, we also investigated the coronary arteriographic findings in 341 patients
who had sustained a non-Q-wave myocardial infarction. Usually we observed subtotal occlusion as is depicted in Figure 3.
There was lesser prevalence of coronary thrombus and coronary
occlusion in the non-Q-wave infarct group, but in approximately
one-third of the patients coronary thrombus was observed.
Depicted in Figure 4 is the finding of an increased prevalence
of coronary occlusion and a decreased frequency of subtotal
coronary occlusion in comparable groups in whom coronary
arteriography was performed during the acute ischemic syndrome.
Because there was increase in coronary closure over time, it

383

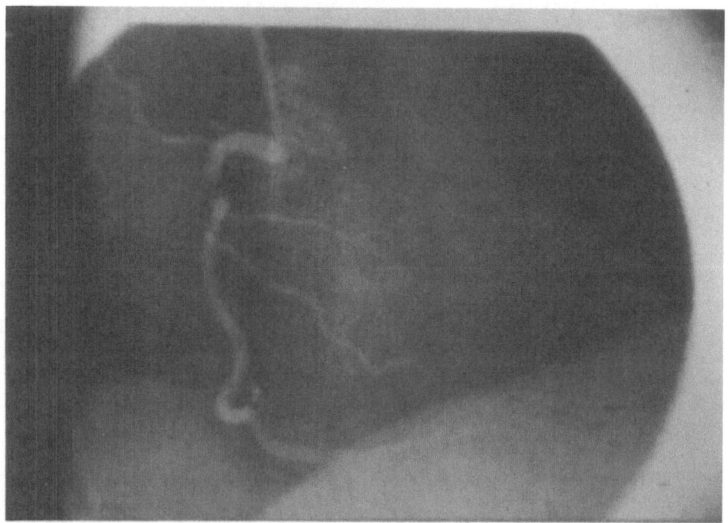

Figure 3. This figure demonstrates subtotal coronary
occlusion with a thrombus of the right coronary artery in a
patient with non-Q-wave myocardial infarction.

appeared to us that there was a dynamic behavior at the site
of coronary stenosis suggestive of rapidly progressive disease
in an unstable area of the coronary anatomy.

Importantly, of the 341 patients, more than 70% had
waxing and waning of chest pain and symptomatology that was
much less precise than the patients with Q-wave infarcts who
generally presented with a well defined sentinal event requiring hospitalization. As with the Q-wave infarct group,
thrombus was extracted (although much less frequently) in some
of these patients.

Unstable Angina Pectoris
From 1972 to 1983 (13) we studied more than one thousand
patients by coronary arteriography and left ventriculography
in the various states of unstable angina. Unstable angina
was defined as intermittent chest pain syndromes without
laboratory evidence of myocardial necrosis and no evolution
of Q-waves on the electrocardiogram. The coronary arteriographic findings were similar to those associated with the
non-Q-wave group and the two groups were very similar in their
clinical presentation. The only major finding that distinguished

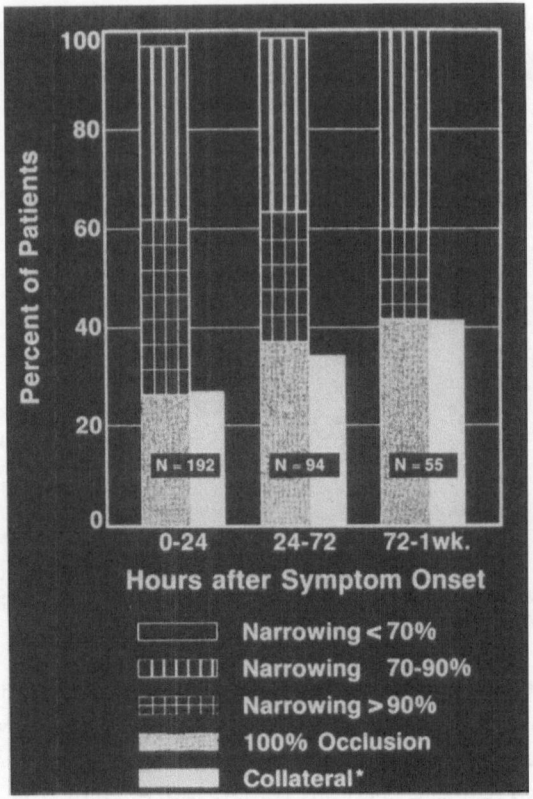

Figure 4. This figure demonstrates an increase in coronary
occlusion over time in patients with non-Q-wave infarction.
It also demonstrates a decrease in subtotal coronary occlusion.
This syndrome correlated with prolonged symptomatology with
waxing and waning of chest pain. Reprinted by permission
of the New England Journal of Medicine, 325; 417-423, 1986.

between the two syndromes was laboratory evidence of myocardial damage defined as abnormal elevation of MB creatine
kinase in peripheral blood samples. In these patients, we
observed a much more prolonged clinical course with multiple
bouts of chest discomfort. We now know that these bouts of
chest discomfort may correlate with thrombus that is too small
to be detected by coronary arteriograms but can be seen by
intraoperative angioscopy (14). We also found thrombi in
patients with unstable angina. These occurred much less than
in Q-wave and non-Q-wave infarctions but the clinical course
of these patients seemed to correlate with the non-Q-wave
infarct group.

Histologic Findings of Thrombi During Acute Ischemic Syndrome

To determine whether or not we could correlate histologic findings with the clinical states, thrombi were submitted in patients undergoing coronary bypass surgery as a therapy for Q-wave infarction, non-Q-wave infarction, and unstable angina pectoris. The thrombi were analyzed blindly and the analysis was done without knowledge of the clinical state.

Thrombosis in Q-wave Myocardial Infarction

To retrieve coronary thrombi in Q-wave myocardial infarction, a Fogarty Catheter was passed into the infarct related vessel to extract the clot. This syndrome usually had an abrupt onset with a well defined clinical event. It appeared that only a minority of patients had experienced antecedent waxing and waning of symptoms. When the thrombus was retrieved, it was submitted for histologic examination. Slices were taken from the leading edge backwards into the thrombus. As is shown in Figure 5, the distal tip of the thrombus demonstrated acute inflammatory cells but the majority of the portion of the thrombus was made up of fresh platelet fibrin mass. As is shown in Figure 5, the red blood cells usually retained their morphology in the acute Q-wave infarcts. The central portion of the thrombus was occupied by smaller degrees of acute inflammatory cells and there was more fibrin-platelet lines interspersed with areas of red blood cells typical of acute arterial thrombi.

Thrombosis in Non-Q-Wave Infarction

The clinical picture in non-Q-wave infarct patients was quite different from Q-wave infarct patients. These patients were less likely to have a discrete event but had waxing and waning of chest pain. As is shown in Figure 6, these non-Q-wave infarcts had far more organization of thrombus and fewer white cells. This was mixed with fresh areas of thrombus, however, and the histologic findings demonstrated organized thrombus with variable amounts of red blood cells, fibrin, and acute inflammatory cells. This is further demonstrated in Figure 7.

Insofar as patients with non-Q-wave infarcts were con-cerned, interaction of the thrombus at the vessel wall was

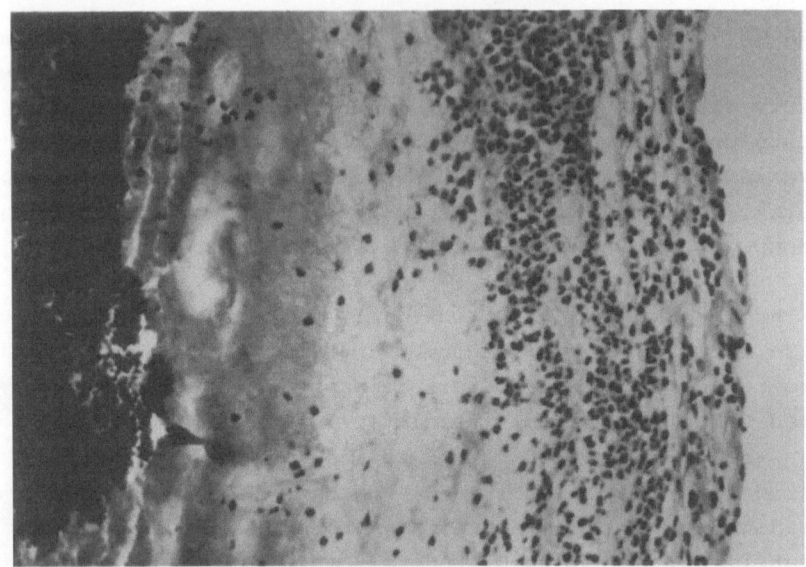

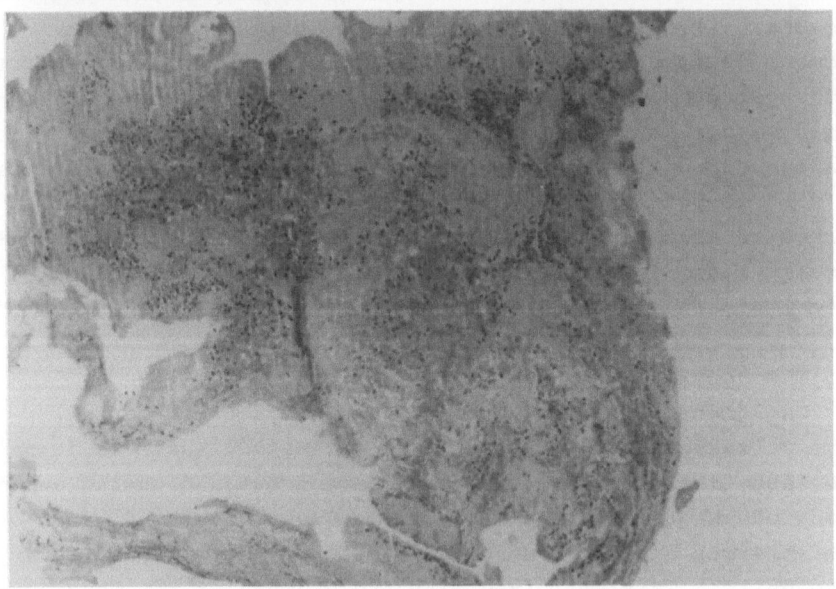

Figure 5. This figure demonstrates the distal tip of a fresh thrombus in Q-wave infarction. Note the acute inflammatory cells followed by red blood cells and fibrin.
Figure 6. This figure demonstrates a thrombus taken from a patient with a recent onset of symptoms. Fresh as well as organized areas in the thrombus are present.

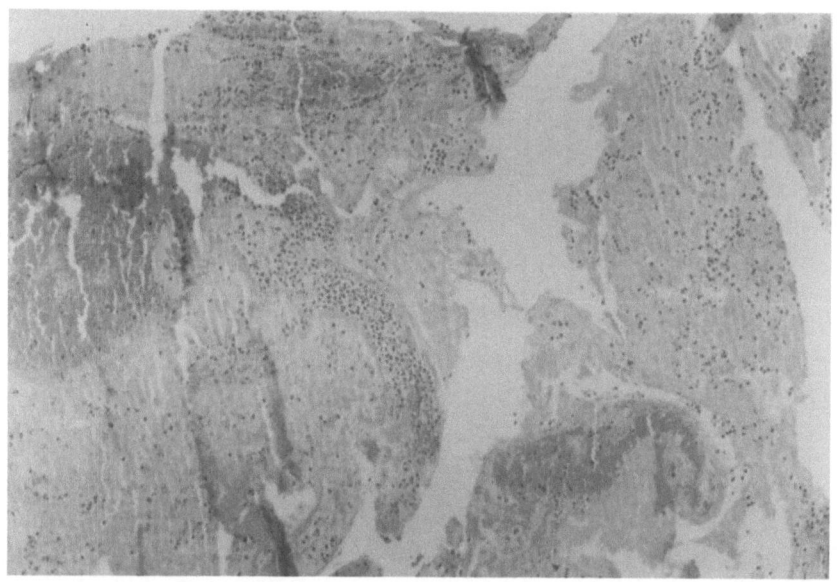

Figure 7. Demonstrates a different area from the same patient. As can be shown there is acute inflammation present as well as more organized area of thrombus.

different as well. In patients who had a prolonged clinical course, the fibrin red blood cell mesh clearly was interactive with ruptured plaque and frequently appeared to be undergoing reabsorption into the area of plaque on the vessel wall. This is demonstrated in Figure 8.

Thrombosis in Unstable Angina

Patients with unstable angina clinically resembled the group with non-Q-wave myocardial infarction. Recent observations have demonstrated that there is less angiographic evidence of coronary thrombus than in non-Q-wave or Q-wave infarctions (15). Nevertheless, angioscopic findings support the concept that thrombus may be present in the absence of angiography (14). The thrombi we retrieved from patients who had undergone operation for very early unstable angina pectoris indicated very acute inflammation with significant amounts of fibrin and platelets. This is demonstrated in Figure 9.

By contrast, patients who had a prolonged course of unstable angina and were treated approximately a week after

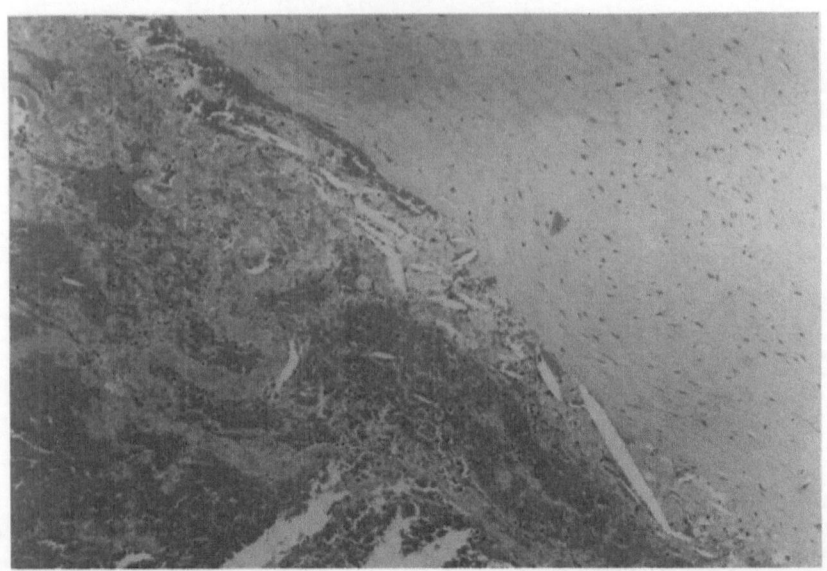

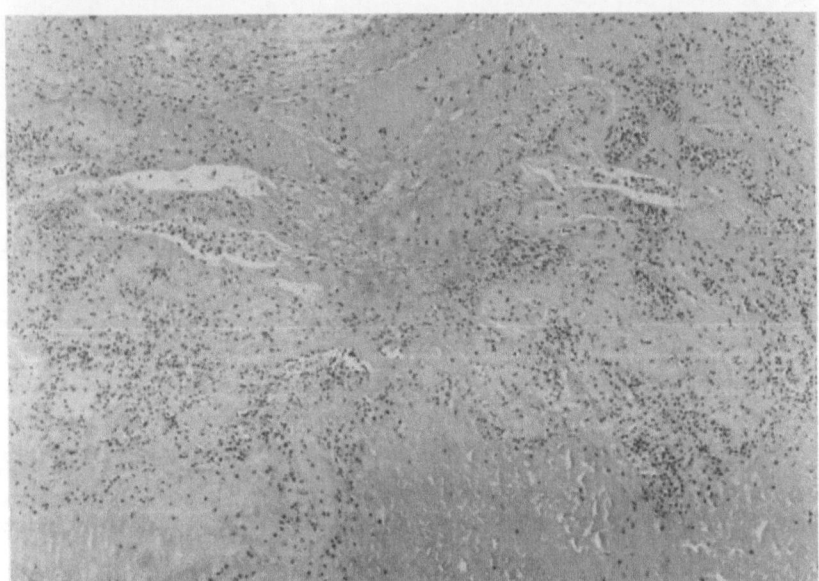

Figure 8.   Demonstrates vessel wall (right) and cholesterol
clefts at the atherosclerotic plaque interacting platelet
and fibrin.   Note that the red blood cells have lost their
distinct morphology and there are few acute inflammatory
cells present.
Figure 9.   Demonstrates a patient with early unstable angina
pectoris that had occurred after waxing and waning of chest
pain.   As is shown, there are significant portions of acute
inflammatory cells as well as areas of older thrombus present.

symptoms began, frequently had old organized thrombus in conjunction with fresh clot once again made up of some inflammatory cells but mostly fibrin, platelets, and red blood
cells. This is demonstrated in Figure 10.

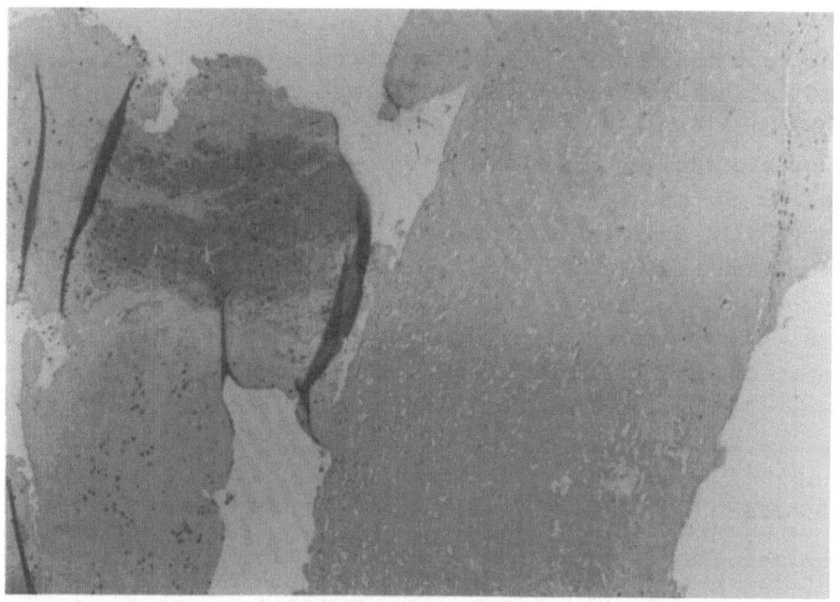

Figure 10. Shows newer thrombus on the left and older throm-
but on the right. This was taken from a patient with unstable angina pectoris that had occurred for approximately
one week. The pain had augmented which required open heart
surgery (with thrombectomy) despite maximum medical therapy.

DISCUSSION

The goals of this paper were to review the correlation of the clinical states and histologic findings associated in three acute ischemic syndromes. In the acute
Q-wave myocardial infarction, we found mostly polymorphonuclear inflammatory cells with fibrin and platelets almost
entirely composed of fresh thrombus. By contrast, in the
non-Q-wave infarcts, there was a variable degree of new
and old thrombus in uneven stages of organization. There
appeared to be a waxing and waning of intermittent symptoms
associated with the non-Q-wave infarcts, especially if allowed to progress with ischemia. Early treatment of non-Q-wave
infarcts did demonstrate thrombi that were significantly

different from thrombi extracted early in Q-wave infarctions.
Thrombi harvested later in the course of Q-wave infarcts
demonstrated usually less total occlusion and there was evidence of retraction from the vessel wall with significant
interaction with the underlying atherosclerotic plaque.

Likewise, if thrombi were harvested early from patients
with recent onset of symptoms, the thrombi generally yielded
fibrin, platelets, and red blood cells. These also occurred
as nonocclusive thrombi. In patients with prolonged symptoms
of unstable angina, there was evidence of ongoing mixture of
organized thrombus as well as new formation of thrombus.

Overall, there appears to be a rough correlation between
symptoms and histologic findings, especially if the duration
of symptoms is carefully evaluated. In fresh thrombus, interaction with the underlying atherosclerotic plaque and episodes
of chest discomfort appear to be associated with variable
degrees of "layering" of fibrin platelets, red blood cells,
and acute inflammatory cells.

REFERENCES

1. Alison HW, Russell Jr RO, Mantle JA, Kouchoukos NT,
    Moraski RE, Rackley CE (1978) Coronary anatomy and
    arteriography in patients with unstable angina pectoris.
    Am J Cardiol 41:209.
2. Chandler AB, Chapman I, Erhardt LR, et al. (1974)
    Coronary thrombosis in myocardial infarction. Report
    of a workshop on the role of coronary thrombosis in
    the pathogenesis of myocardial infarction. Am J
    Cardiol 34:823-833.
3. Duguid JB (1949) Pathogenesis of atherosclerosis.
    Lancet 2:925-935.
4. Crawford T (1967) The pathogenesis of atherosclerosis:
    A reassessment of the thrombogenic hypothesis. In:
    Crawford T (ed) Modern Trends in Pathology, Volume 2.
    London: Appleton-Century-Crofts, pp. 238-251.
5. Chandler AB (1970) Thrombosis and the development of
    atherosclerotic lesions. In: Jones RJ (ed) Second
    International Symposium on Atherosclerosis. New York:
    Springer-Verlag, pp. 88-93.
6. French JE (1971) Atherogenesis and thrombosis. Semin
    Hematol 8:84-90.
7. Friedman M (1971) The coronary thrombosis: Its origin
    and fate. Human Pathol 2:81-128.
8. DeWood MA, Spores J, Notske R, et al. (1980) Prevalence
    of total coronary occlusion during the early hours of
    transmural myocardial infarction. N Engl J Med 303:
    897-902.
9. Ganz W, Buchbinder N, Marcus H, et al. (1981) Intra-
    coronary thrombolysis in evolving myocardial infarction.
    Am Heart J 101:4-13.

10. Mathey DG, Kuck K-H, Tilsner V, et al. (1981) Non-surgical coronary artery recanalization in acute trans-mural myocardial infarction. Circulation 63:489-497.

11. DeWood MA, Spores J, Hensley GR, et al. (1983) Coronary arteriographic findings in acute transmural myocardial infarction. Circulation 68:I39-I49.

12. DeWood MA, Stifter WF, Simpson CS, et al. (1986) Coronary arteriographic findings soon after non-Q-wave myocardial infarction. N Engl J Med 315:417-423.

13. DeWood MA, Grunwald RP, O'Grady WP, Shield JP (1983) The role in surgery in unstable angina and acute myo-cardial infarction. In: Wagner GS (ed) Acute Myo-cardial Ischemia and Infarction. Berlin and New York: Martinus Nishoff Co.

14. Sherman CT, Litvack F, Grundfest W, et al. (1986) Coronary angioscopy in patients with unstable angina pectoris. N Engl J Med 315:913-919.

15. Bresnahan DR, Davis JL, Holmes Jr DR, Smith HC (1985) Angiographic occurrence and clinical correlates of intraluminal coronary thrombus: Role of unstable angina. J Am Coll Cardiol 6:285-289.

26

Plaque Hemorrhages, Their Genesis and Their Role in Supra-Plaque Thrombosis and Atherogenesis

Paris Constantinides

The last and most lethal step in the evolution of
advanced atherosclerosis in coronary arteries is thrombosis
in diseased vessels - something that practically never occurs
in normal arteries.

In a small number of cases thrombosis is easy to explain
because it develops over an obviously ulcerated plaque, but
in the great majority of cases it has no obvious microscopic
basis since the thrombus seems to develop over plaques with
perfectly <u>intact</u> caps. In most of these arteries there is a
hemorrhagic gruel underneath the cap (Figure 1), as already
pointed out by Paterson and others half a centry ago (1).

As a result of these observations three theories
evolved, each attempting to explain thrombosis in atherosclerotic coronary arteries although none of them was
accompanied by definitive evidence. Briefly stated these
are the theories of stasis, hypercoagulability and capillary
hemorrhages. The <u>stasis theory</u> proposed that it is the
slowing of blood flow proximal to the narrowed atherosclerotic
coronary artery which causes thrombus formation, but this
does not explain the hemorrhages in the plaques underneath
many thrombi. The <u>hypercoagulability theory</u> postulated that
the thrombus forms due to an increased systemic clotting
tendency of some kind (chemical or cellular) in patients
with atherosclerosis. However, like the stasis theory, this

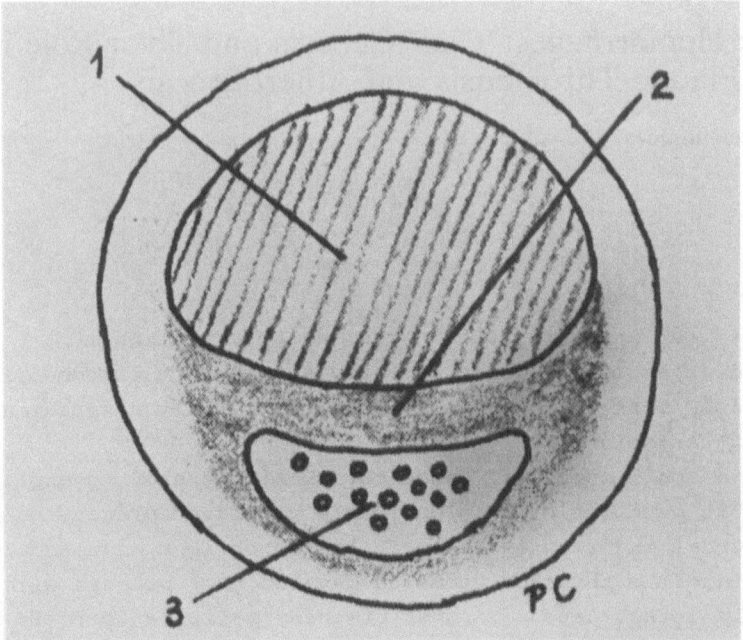

Figure 1. This diagram of a cross-section of a thrombosed
human coronary artery shows a thrombus (the shaded area)
occluding the lumen (1) of the vessel. The thrombus sits
on the fibrous cap (2) of an atheroma whose gruel is
hemorrhagic (3). [Constandinides P (1984) Ultrastructural
Pathology. Amsterdam: Elsevier Publishers]

formulation does not explain the plaque hemorrhages, and
furthermore, when one produces marked systemic hypercoagulability in animals (e.g., by means of intravenous thrombin
or the systemic Schwartzman reaction) many thousands of
little thrombi are observed in the venules and capillaries
of lung, liver and kidney - but not one thrombus over one
hemorrhagic plaque in one coronary artery. Finally, the
capillary hemorrhage theory proposed that the vascular channels which develop in the plaque tend to rupture and, among
other things, the resulting mini-thrombosis which seals the
ruptured vascular ends progresses in a retrograde manner
within those small vessels to reach the artery lumen where
it keeps growing until it occludes the artery (1).

Unfortunately, however, this clever theory (which can explain the hemorrhages) is incompatible with the fact that in the great majority of cases, vascularization of the plaque originates from the adventitial side. The postulated progression of thrombosis from a ruptured capillary inside the plaque to the arterial lumen outside the plaque has never been documented.

Twenty-four years ago, a number of findings led to a different hypothesis, namely that the thrombi are caused by tiny breaks of the caps of plaques, breaks through which blood excavates from the lumen into the plaque interior before they are sealed by thrombi. Furthermore it was postulated that these breaks could occasionally also lead to a plaque hemorrhage without superimposed thrombosis, or to thrombosis before hemorrhage could develop, depending on local and systemic circumstances (depth of break, blood coagulability, etc.). Such breaks, because of their very small size, would usually be missed in one or two random sections through a thrombosed coronary, and would require serial or closely spaced step sections through the length of the thrombosed artery for their detection (Figures 2 and 3).

The experimental findings that led to this "break of the cap" hypothesis can be summarized as follows: In the early sixties highly advanced atherosclerosis of the human type was reproduced in rabbits by means of single wave or intermittent hyperlipemia. This permitted adequate survival times so that the rabbits developed all the features of the human end-stage atheroma including thick collagenous cap, gruel, calcification, capillarization, media destruction and sub-plaque lymphocytic infiltration (2). Many of these animals developed huge thrombi over the plaques. Furthermore these plaques as well as plaques with no thrombi often showed hemorrhages. These intra-plaque hemorrhages were especially frequent in atherosclerotic rabbits injected with a combination of certain vasopressor agents. These included epinephrine, norepinephrine, angiotensin, pitressin, or serotonin and Russel Viper venom (3). The latter was originally

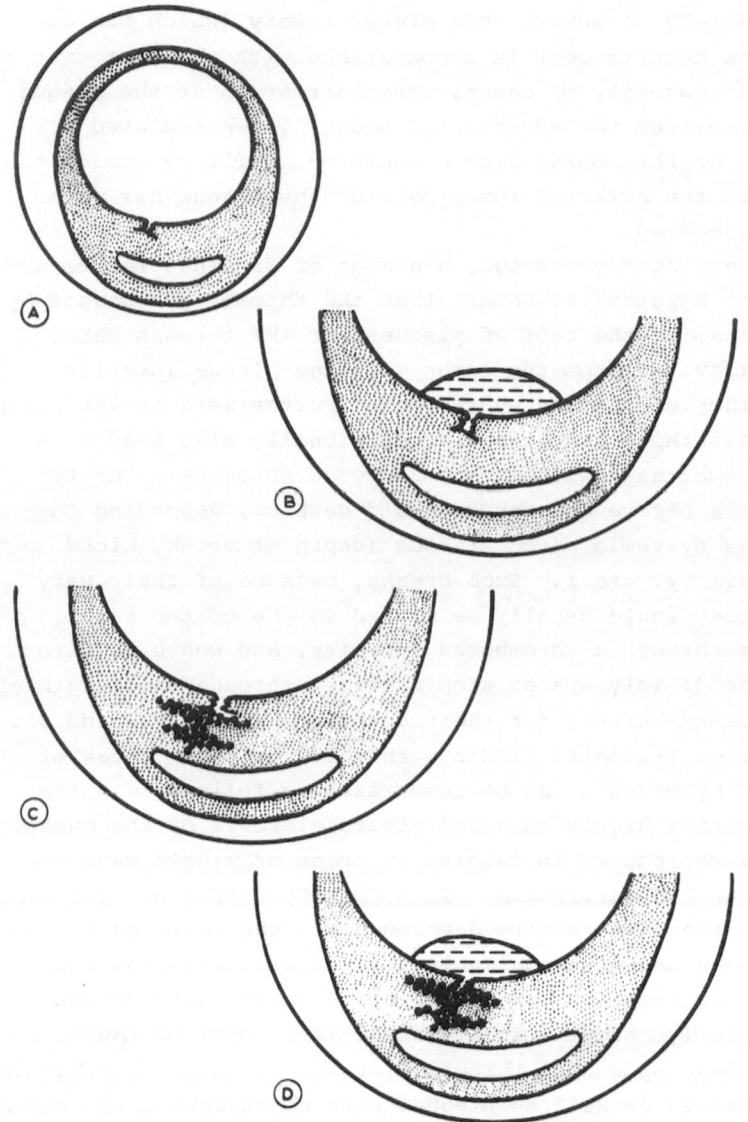

Figure 2. The initiating event is a crack in the surface of a fibrous plaque (A). This crack may be immediately sealed by a thrombus (B), or lead to a dissecting hemorrhage only (C), but usually leads first to a hemorrhage from the lumen into the plaque before it is sealed by a thrombus (D). (Reprinted by permission of Elsevier Publishers, BV).

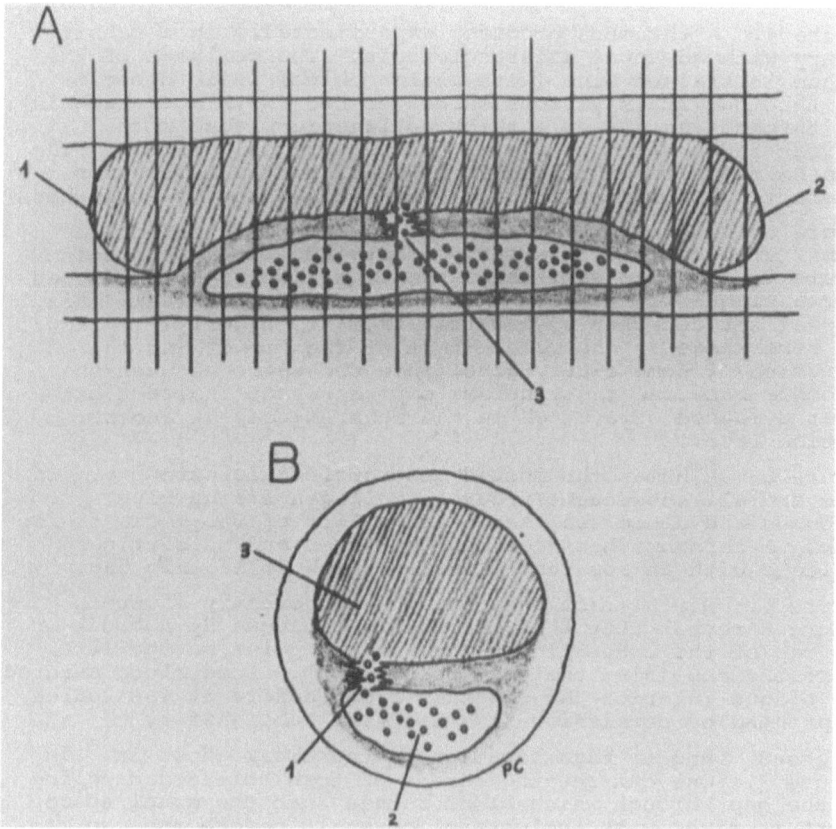

Figure 3. The upper drawing (A) shows a longitudinal section through a thrombosed coronary artery in which a long occlusive thrombus developed over an atheroma with a tiny break of its surface (3) through which blood had poured into the plaque interior spreading both proximal and distal to the site of the break. Only serial sections from one end of the thrombus to the other can reveal the small break that caused both hemorrhage and thrombus (B). [Constantinides P (1984) Ultrastructural Pathobiology. Amsterdam: Elsevier Publishers]

chosen as an inducer of hypercoagulability, but it proved to be highly endotheliotoxic, as was later confirmed with the electron microscope (4). Histologic examination indicated that the intra-plaque hemorrhages had resulted from breaks of plaque surfaces, and that the supra-plaque thrombi had developed as hemostatic seals over those breaks (3) (Figures 4 and 5).

These thrombi and hemorrhages could be produced only in rabbits with advanced atherosclerosis (i.e., with collagenous

Figure 4. A thrombus produced experimentally in a rabbit artery with advanced atherosclerosis. The collagen of the plaque is stained blue (with aniline blue) while blood and thrombus stain various shades of red (with acid fuchsin). The thrombus sits over a thick collagenic plaque with a break-induced hemorrhage in its superficial portion. The detachment of the thrombus from the plaque is a fixation artefact. (Reprinted by permission from Elsevier Publishers).

Figure 5. Another thrombus produced experimentally in a rabbit atherosclerotic artery and stained like the one in Figure 4. In this case the thrombus on the right developed over a plaque with a very thin cap and a large gruel mass, and was not detached by artefact from its underlying plaque. The hemorrhage in the gruel (left of the field) and the extrusion of some fluffy gruel into the space between the thrombus base and the atheroma cap represent indirect but clear evidence of a break in the atheroma cap at another section level.

Figure 6. A human thrombosed atherosclerotic coronary. In this and all subsequent figures, collagen stains blue, thrombus and blood red, and what is left of the media stains pink. A thrombus has occluded the lumen and is sitting on a plaque with an apparently intact thick collagenic cap.

Figure 7. Serial sections through the coronary shown in Figure 6 reveal that this thrombus was caused by a break of the cap of the underlying plaque at the point on the left where the cap joins the rest of the wall. Some blood entered the plaque interior through that break before it was sealed. (Reprinted by permission from Elsevier Publishers).

Figure 8. Higher magnification of the break shown in Figure 7. One can see the shreds of torn collagen dangling in the gap through which blood rushed into the gruel space where it mixed with cholesterol crystals before the cap was sealed by the thrombus. (Reprinted by permission from Elsevier Publishers).

Figure 9. Another thrombosed human atherosclerotic coronary. Here a thrombus developed over a small break in a very thin collagen cap of a plaque with a large gruel space. A discrete hemorrhage can be seen in the gruel. The lower purple granular part of the thrombus that directly overlies the break is the platelet nucleus of the thrombus. (Reprinted by permission of Elsevier Publishers).

Figure 10. A close-up of the break in Figure 9, showing the purple granular platelet masses in direct contact with the torn shreds of cap collagen, and many groups of red cells in the underlying gruel. (Reprinted by permission of Elsevier Publishers).

Figure 11. Thrombosis in a human atherosclerotic coronary, showing how small the thrombogenic break can be. A parietal thrombus developed over a very small break (about 3 red cells, or 20 μ wide) at the point where the thin part joins the thick part of the blue collagenic cap. A round purple mass (the platelet nucleus of the thrombus) is visible directly underneath the microscopic break. (Reprinted by permission of Elsevier Publishers).

Color Plate I

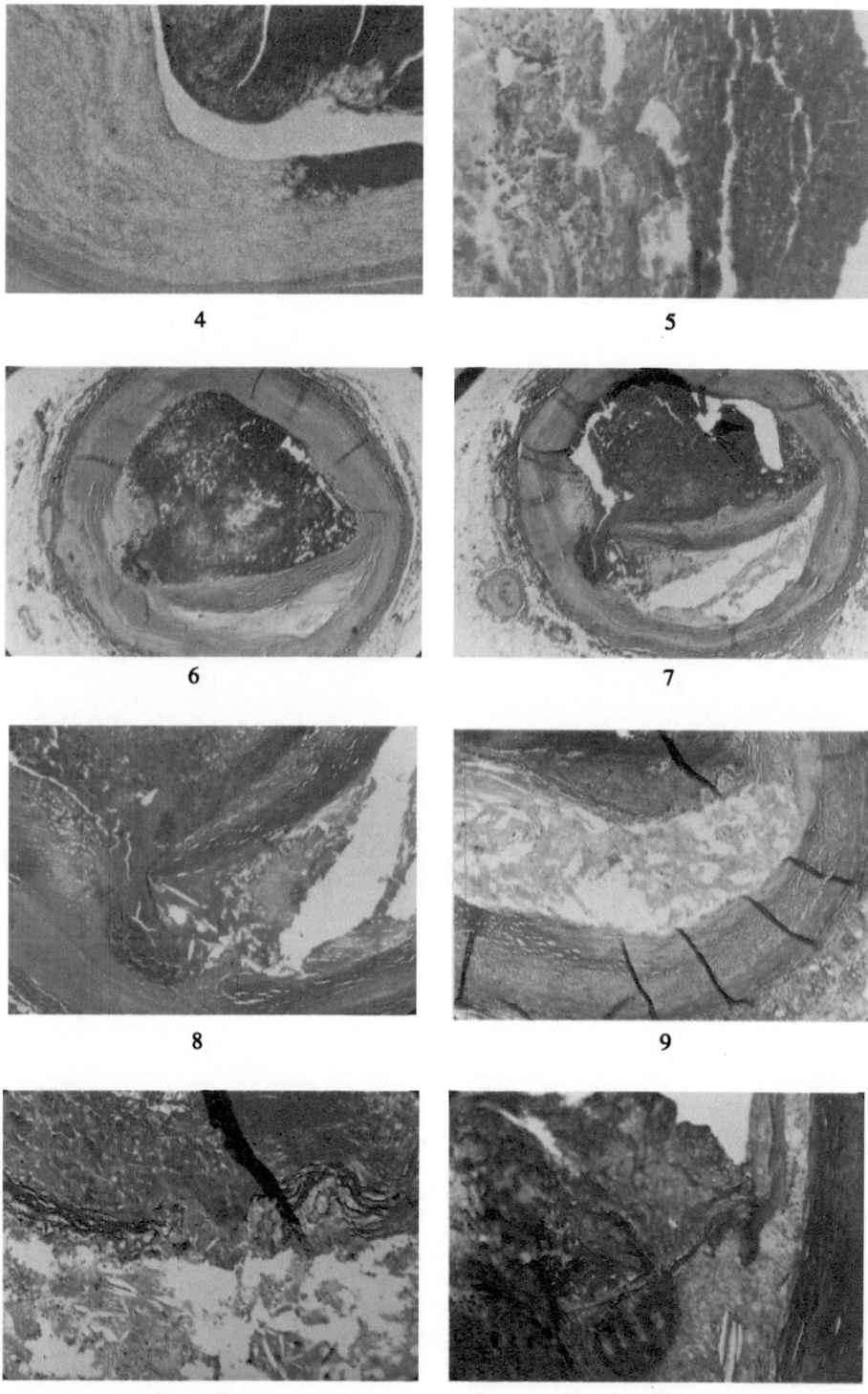

4

5

6

7

8

9

10

11

Color Plate II

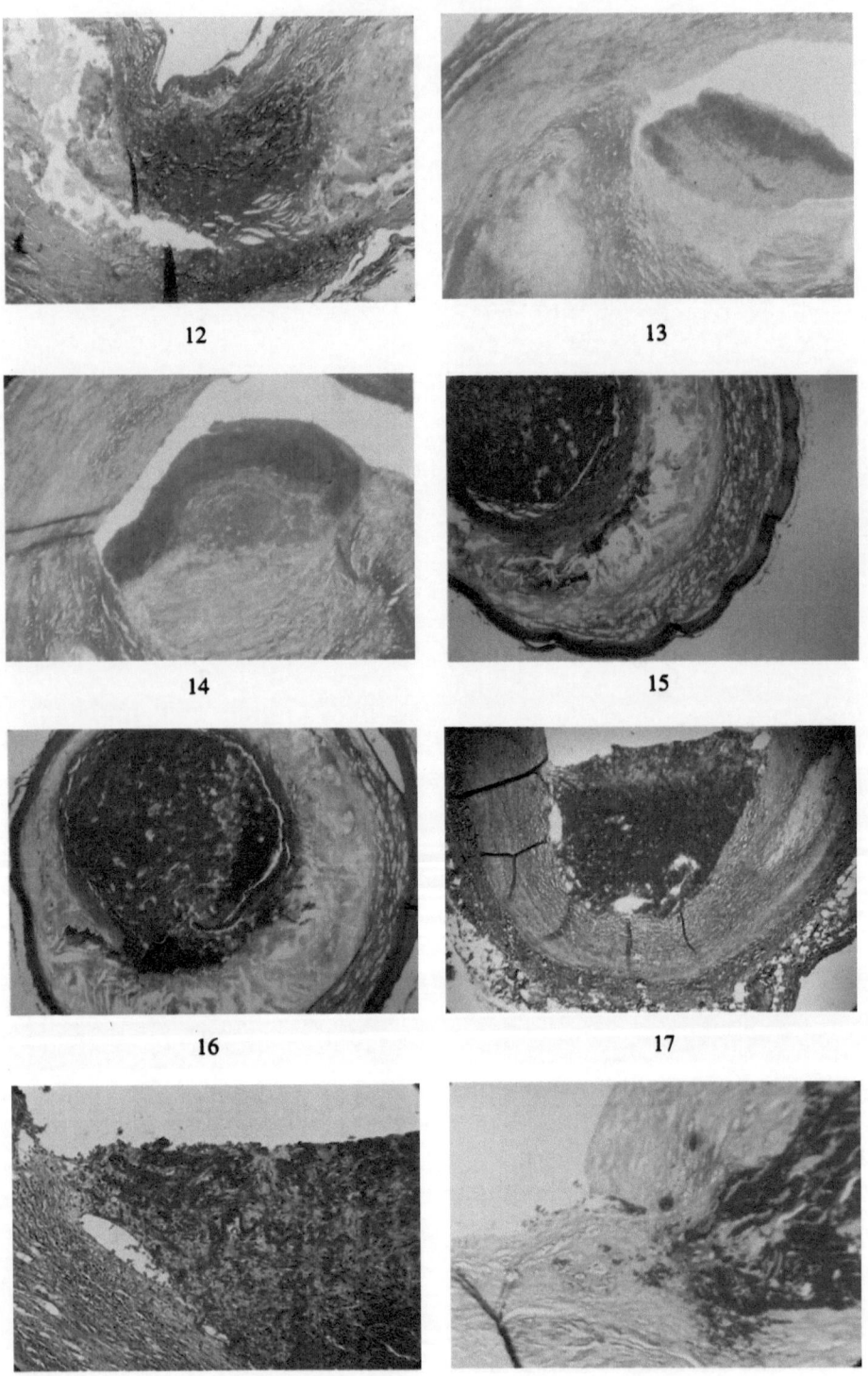

12

13

14

15

16

17

18

19

Figure 12. Thrombosis in a human atherosclerotic coronary
showing how small the thrombus that seals the break can be.
A small break in a collagenic cap has led to a massive
hemorrhage into the gruel and was sealed by a tiny purple
platelet plug that did not mushroom into a large thrombus
(parietal or occlusive) perhaps because of low blood
coagulability at the time of the break. (Reprinted by
permission from Elsevier Publishers).

Figure 13. Thrombosis in a human atherosclerotic coronary.
A mural thrombus sits over a seemingly intact, thick
collagenic cap.

Figure 14. Serial sectioning revealed that the thrombus
shown in Figure 13 developed over multiple fragmentations
of the cap surface through which platelets (the purple
material) infiltrated deep into the cap tissue, separating
its collagen layers. Again the platelet nucleus of the
thrombus is in intimate contact with the cap surface. It
should be noted that four of the 30 cases of this study
revealed thrombosis over cap breaks without hemorrhages,
as in this case.

Figure 15. Thrombosis in a human atherosclerotic cerebral
(basilar) artery. An occlusive thrombus developed over a
seemingly intact collagenic cap of a circular atheroma.
There is a hemorrhage in the gruel under the cap. (Reprinted
by permission of the American Medical Association).

Figure 16. Serial sectioning revealed a break in the cap
that produced both the gruel hemorrhage and the thrombus
shown in Figure 15. (Reprinted by permission of the American
Medical Association).

Figure 17. Mural thrombus in a human atherosclerotic coronary
that was caused by a break at another level. The pale blue-
grey material in the upper part of the thrombus represents
organization, i.e., invasion of the thrombus by collagen-
producing cells that will eventually turn it into a thickening
of the underlying plaque.

Figure 18. Close-up of the left upper edge of the organizing
thrombus shown in Figure 17, at a slightly different level.
The collagen that replaces the thrombus is clearly evident,
as well as an endothelial tube that invades the thrombus
margin from the lumen to vascularize it, representing an
invagination of luminal endothelium.

Figure 19. Upper part of a plaque in a human atherosclerotic
coronary that probably represents an organized mural thrombus
since it is vascularized by a capillary from the lumen on the
left. A capillary hemorrhage has developed deep in the plaque
on the right, but it has not led to any thrombus because
there was no break of the plaque surface. (Reprinted by
permission of Elsevier Publishers).

caps and gruel), never in animals with normal arteries - and
not even in animals with early atherosclerosis (3) (Table).
It was proposed that thrombi could be induced only in arteries with advanced atherosclerosis because their altered
and damaged wall (including the endothelium) broke much more
easily than that of normal vessels. Once broken, the blood
was exposed to powerful platelet-aggregating and coagulation-
promoting materials, such as collagen and gruel lipids, that
do not exist in the normal arterial wall.

Are human thrombi over human hemorrhagic plaques caused
by breaks of atheroma caps, as in the case of atherosclerotic
rabbits? In 1963 complete serial section sets (a section of
7 μ from beginning to end of the thrombosed vascular segments)
were studied from 20 consecutive cases of human thrombosed
coronary arteries in St. Louis. Shortly afterwards 10 consecutive cases of human thrombosed cerebral arteries were
similarly studied in Vancouver. These studies of over
50,000 sections indicated that most plaque hemorrhages were
due to tiny breaks of the atheroma surfaces. It was evident
that virtually all thrombi represented seals over those breaks
(5-8). The majority of the thrombogenic cap fissures occurred
in avascular plaque areas in which the collagenic cap was
mostly acellular (i.e. had lost all the cells that produce
and maintain the collagen) or where the caps were extremely
thin, or exposed to marked circumferential tension (as at
transitions between thick and thin parts of the wall). In
a minority of cases, the cap fissures had developed in
vascularized plaque areas. We should note that while in most
cases the cracks led to hemorrhages before they were sealed
by thrombi, in a few instances they were plugged by thrombi
before any blood escaped into the plaque core (Figures 6-16).

Similar findings have since been published after step-
serial section studies by five other investigators in the
USA, Germany, Britain and Denmark (9-14). Other pathologists
have communicated with us personally. These include A.L.
Liebo (USA), W.A. Harland (Britain) and A. Vichert (Soviet
Union). All these confirmatory results seem to justify the

Table. The Role of Advanced, Fibrous Atherosclerosis in the Induction of Arterial Thrombosis and Hemorrhage[a]

No. of Rabbits per Group	Treatment	State of the Aorta	Aortic Thrombosis (incidence)	Aortic Plaque Hemorrhage (incidence)
16	RVV[b] + serotonine	Advanced fibrous atherosclerosis (with collagenic cap and gruel)	4/16	11/16
16	RVV + serotonine	Normal	0/16	0/16
16	RVV + serotonine	Early, non-fibrous atherosclerosis (only foam cells, no cap or gruel)	0/16	0/16

[a] Constantinides P (1965) Experimental Atherosclerosis. Amsterdam: Elsevier Publishers
[b] RVV = Russel Viper Venom

conclusion that thrombosis in human atherosclerotic arteries
is almost always initiated by breaks in the plaque surfaces.
How big the thrombi become and whether they persist or
disappear probably depends on systemic factors. In other
words, tiny cracks may occur very frequently but in some
persons they may lead to huge occlusive thrombi because of
systemic hypercoagulability at the time of the break, while
in others they may produce only small parietal thrombi - or
only dissecting hemorrhages. This has been demonstrated in
two cases (7) - because anticoagulant or fibrinolytic factors
prevailed at that moment.

The serial section studies in our laboratory have also
confirmed the process postulated by several pathologists
from Rokitansky through Duguid to Morgan (15-17), namely
that parietal thrombi in coronary arteries - if survived -
are overgrown by endothelium, organized and turned into
fibrous atherosclerotic thickenings of the arterial wall.
However, since all the thrombi developed on top of pre-
existing plaques with fissured caps - never over normal
arterial wall - it appears that organized mural thrombi can
be incorporated into the underlying plaques and thus add
substantially to the mass of the plaques over which they
develop. The studies do not provide evidence that mural
thrombi initiate atheromatous plaques. It has also been
demonstrated that such organized thrombi which are transformed into the uppermost layer of certain atheromata are
vascularized from the lumen (through the ingrowth of endothelial tubes from the lumen into the organizing thrombic
masses). When these lumen-derived capillaries rupture in
the absence of cap fissures they can produce intra-plaque
hemorrhages but no supra-plaque thrombi (Figures 17-19).

No one needs to ask - What causes the thrombogenic
breaks?

Although we do not know the answer to this question,
the following six possible mechanisms, which might be involved
alone or in combination, should be explored by careful
investigations.

1. Perhaps breaks can be initiated by <u>physical</u> forces, such as (a) <u>hypertension</u>, which has been shown capable of damaging arterial endothelium (18) - and thus starting a tear - at sufficient intensity and duration, (b) <u>blood turbulence</u>, which is also capable of endothelial injury and which apparently develops to a significant degree when lumen stenosis (due to atherosclerosis) exceeds 50% of the normal diameter (19), (c) the <u>pulsatile circumferential tension</u> (stretching) of the arterial wall which is directly proportional to the intraluminal pressure and radius but inversely proportional to the wall thickness (19) and could therefore undergo a rapid increase in intensity at the transition between thick and thin wall segments, i.e., at the edges of plaques, (d) "<u>suction</u>" of the cap towards the lumen in cases of extreme stenosis, through the operation of Bernoulli's principle (which postulates that as the lumen progressively stenoses, blood flows faster and faster through it, but exerts less and less pressure against the surrounding arterial wall).

2. <u>Many metabolic or nutritional factors and exogeneous chemicals</u> could damage various components of the cap tissue (endothelial lining, myocytes, collagen) and thus increase its fragility or directly cause its fracture. Any of the numerous factors that have been found to injure endothelium, smooth muscle cells, collagen and basement membrane synthesis in arteries or microcirculation may qualify under this heading, e.g., diabetes, ascorbic acid deficiency, copper deficiency, tocopherol deficiency, lathyrus factor, protracted hyperlipemia, carbon monoxide or endotoxin (2).

3. <u>Immune complex injury</u> could produce damage to the endothelium and injure the cap tissue underneath it and promote its disintegration. There is experimental evidence, including ultrastructural observations from this laboratory, that the endothelium which lies over advanced atherosclerotic plaques is much more permeable to big molecules than that which lies over the normal arterial walls. Furthermore the media may also share in this type of injury. We found with

electron microscopic autoradiography that endothelial
junctions are clearly loosened over advanced experimental
plaques. Therefore the entry of labelled lipoproteins and
monocytes into the plaque was greatly increased (21). This
type of increased permeability of supra-plaque endothelium
was previously observed grossly by Anitschkow with dyes (22)
and chemically by Adams with labelled lipids (23). Thus,
antigen-antibody complexes produced elsewhere in the body
may selectively filter into the cap of plaques, activate
complement there and produce substantial arterial wall damage.
Studies should be performed to determine whether advanced
atheromata in animals are more susceptible to fracture of
their fibrous caps and thrombosis when they are subjected to
immune complexes (generated in the same animals or injected
intravenously).

4. Auto-immune injury could also cause necrosis in
atheroma caps through the development of auto-antibodies
against cap myocytes because there are changes in the plaque
smooth muscle cells which could render them antigenically
foreign. Whether these cells, unlike the deeper infra-gruel
myocytes, represent a true somatic mutation, as suggested by
their changes in the type of the enzyme, glucose-6-phosphate
dehydrogenase which has been reported to differ from that of
normal media myocytes in certain human plaques (24). Anti-
plaque auto-antibodies might alternatively be stimulated by
the emergence of bacterial-like lipopolysaccharide antigens
in the plaque from the interaction of immigrating lipoproteins
with resident cap polysaccharides. Regardless of their
origin and/or immunocytes, such auto-antibodies could be
delivered into the plaques from the lumen but also - and
perhaps even more effectively - from the capillaries that
invade the plaque interior in the late, advanced stages of
atherosclerosis.

5. A fifth possibility to explore is that the calcification of the polysaccharide ground substance around the
fibrous cap myocytes buries these cells in stony caves and
kills them, leading to disintegration of the cap tissue which

they produced and maintained - just as the calcification around aging chondrocytes (during endochondral ossification) destroys them and the hyaline cartilage which they produced.

6. A sixth possibility is that, as time goes by, gradual molecular changes of cap collagen make it more and more fragile so that one day it will be broken by the rhythmic movements of the heart, a hypertensive spurt, or even the normal pulse wave; alternately, the gradual dehydration and shrinkage of the collagen fibers could cause them to contract and crack, just as fissures develop in drying mud.

Since it appears that most complex pathological processes can be altered in a given direction by the manipulation of several of their many components and controlling forces, it is likely that cap fissures in advanced atherosclerotic plaques can be caused not only by one, but by several different factors in different patients at different times and at different sites of the arterial tree.

Finally, we must deal with a question raised by certain investigators on purely hemodynamic grounds, namely the possibility that most plaque hemorrhages may result from the rupture of the adventitial-derived capillaries that often vascularize advanced human plaques (19,25).

Unfortunately this proposal is hard to reconcile with the accumulated histological evidence.

The thrombi in all 30 cases which we have studied of thrombosed human atherosclerotic arteries, with complete serial sections so that one has a complete 3-dimensional histologic reconstruction of the entire thrombosed arterial segments, were clearly caused by cracks of the surface of fibrous cap plaques. Furthermore in 4 of these 30 cases there were no hemorrhages under the cracks, evidently because for some reason (superactive thrombogenesis? slow cracking process?) the breaks were sealed by thrombi very quickly, before any bleeding into the plaque could occur. In the great majority of cases, however (i.e., in 26 of the 30 cases) the cracks resulted in a major entry of blood from the lumen into the plaque before they were sealed. The pattern of the hemorrhages clearly indicated a fanning out from the cracks into the plaque interior so that the cap fissures were clearly the "epicenters" of these hemorrhages. Furthermore all of the other studies which are referred to in this paper (9-14, and personal communications of A.L. Liebow, W.A. Harland and A. Vichert) have strengthened this concept that coronary thrombi develop as hemostatic seals over plaque fissures which allow a variable amount of blood to enter from the lumen into the plaques before they are sealed.

However in 4 of our 26 cases with major crack-induced plaque hemorrhages and thrombosis there were, in addition, some minor hemorrhages originating beyong doubt from the rupture of adventitia-derived capillaries in the deep portions of the plaques, and having no physical connection with the major break-induced bleedings in the superficial regions of the atheromata (7). Also, in the few cases of our series in which the breaks tore into vascularized plaque areas, it is quite possible that the ensuing hemorrhages represented a mixed pool of blood coming in from the lumen and blood coming out from broken capillaries in the vascularized area (personal suggestion of R. Beeuwkes III). Furthermore, it is interesting that Davies and Thomas (13), one of the groups that recently re-investigated human thrombosed coronaries with step-serial sections, also reported that in most of their cases, the major lumen-derived hemorrhages were accompanied by minor adventitial capillary-derived hemorrhages in the deep plaque regions which had no connection to the former or to the thrombogenic surface breaks.

Thus histologic observations from a number of studies indicate, that in a variable percentage of thrombosed athero-sclerotic arteries, adventitial capillary-derived hemorrhages coexist with the main lumen-derived hemorrhages. There are a number of possible explanations from this coincidence. Perhaps the same agents that attack the plaque surface also attack the endothelium of adventitial capillaries, or do intra-plaque capillary hemorrhages - particularly when they are extensive, protracted or repeated - damage the cap tissue and thus in-crease its vulnerability to all the physical and non-physical cap-breaking factors we listed earlier? Or is it because

extensive capillarization of a plaque makes it more "spongy"
and therefore more physically fragile? These and other
possibilities could be profitably explored in the intermittent
hyperlipemia rabbit models, in which the majority of the
animals develop (after 4 hyperlipemic waves) extensive
capillarizations from the adventitia within about a year,
including in several cases spontaneous hemorrhages from
adventitial capillaries, in addition to <u>all</u> the other features
of the highly advanced human end-stage atherosclerosis (2).

While capillary hemorrhages result most frequently from
adventitial capillarization there is also <u>less</u> <u>frequent</u>
capillarization of the superficial plaque zones from the
arterial lumen, which can result from the development of a
supra-plaque parietal thrombus that is organized and incorporated into the underlying plaque. The latter capillarization
pattern is observed more rarely than the adventitial type,
probably because it usually develops in the latter, post-
thrombotic stage of advanced atherosclerosis which is frequently not survived long enough for thrombus organization to
occur. And it is hemodynamically interesting that, as observed
by earlier investigators (1) as well as in our own serial
section study (7), such lumen-derived capillaries can rupture
and bleed into the plaque despite the fact that they originate
from a stenosed arterial lumen and are therefore exposed to
very low internal pressure in accordance with Bernoulli's
equation.

As a stimulus for future research it should be kept in
mind that fissure-induced hemorrhages - whether or not they
are accompanied by capillary hemorrhages - are not the prime
movers of the thrombogenic process; they are merely by-products
or markers of the essential thrombus-producing break. For if
there is no break of the plaque surface there rarely is a
thrombus. Thus it would seem that the most useful future
thrust of research in this area should be directed towards
determining the causes of plaque breaks, the real initiators
of thrombosis in atherosclerotic arteries.

No matter what causes we shall ultimately find for the
breaks of plaque surfaces, it seems that the best protection

against them is not to develop advanced atherosclerosis, or to stop the progression of this disease before its plaques reach the advanced, fragile stage.

REFERENCES

1. Paterson JC (1938) Capillary rupture with intimal hemorrhage as a causative factor in coronary thrombosis. AMA Arch Pathol 25:474-479.
2. Constantinides P (1965) Experimental Atherosclerosis. Amsterdam: Elsevier Publishers, pp. 27-34, 41.
3. Constantinides P (1965) Experimental Atherosclerosis. Amsterdam: Elsevier Publishers, pp. 34-39.
4. Constantinides P, Robinson M (1969) Ultrastructural injury of arterial endothelium. III. Effects of enzymes and surfactants. Arch Pathol 88:113-117.
5. Constantinides P (1964) Plaque fissures in human coronary thrombosis. Fed Proc 23:443.
6. Constantinides P (1964) Plaque fissures in human coronary thrombosis. JAMA 188(6):35-37 (Medical News Section).
7. Constantinides P (1966) Plaque fissures in human coronary thrombosis. J Atheroscler Res 6:1-17.
8. Constantinides P (1967) Pathogenesis of cerebral artery thrombosis in man. Arch Pathol 83:422-428.
9. Chapman I (1965) Morphogenesis of occluding coronary artery thrombosis. Arch Pathol 80:256-261.
10. Sinapius D (1965) Uber Wandveranderungen bei Coronar-thrombose. Klin Wschr 43:875-880.
11. Friedman M, Bovenkamp GI (1966) The pathogenesis of a coronary thrombus. Am J Pathol 48:19-39.
12. Davies MJ, Thomas A (1981) The pathological basis and microanatomy of occlusive thrombus formation in human coronary arteries. Philos Trans R Soc London (Biol) 294:225-229.
13. Davies MJ, Thomas A (1984) Thrombosis and acute coronary artery lesions in sudden cardiac ischemic death. N Engl J Med 310:1137-1140.
14. Falk E (1983) Plaque rupture with severe pre-existing stenosis precipitating coronary thrombosis. Brit Heart J 50:127-134.
15. Rokitansky C (1852) A Manual of Pathologic Anatomy. London: The Sydenham Society.
16. Duguid JB (1948) Thrombosis as a factor in the pathogenesis of aortic atherosclerosis. J Pathol Bact 60: 57-69.
17. Morgan AD (1956) The Pathogenesis of Coronary Occlusion. Springfield, IL: CC Thomas.
18. Constantinides P (1984) Atherosclerosis - A general survey and synthesis. Surv Synth Pathol Res 3:477-498.
19. Lusby RJ, Woodcock JP, Machleder HI, et al. (1982) Transient ischaemic attacks: The static and dynamic morphology of the carotid artery bifurcation. Brit J Surg 69(Suppl):S41-S44.

20. Constantinides P (1984) Ultrastructural Pathobiology. Amsterdam: Elsevier Publishers, pp. 78-150.
21. Constantinides P, Wiggers KD (1974) Electron microscopic autoradiographic study of cholesterol passage across arterial and capillary endothelium. Virch Arch A Pathol Anat Histol 326:291-310.
22. Anitschkow N (1933) In: Cowdry EV (ed) Arteriosclerosis - A Survey of the Problem. New York: MacMillan, Chapter 10.
23. Adams CW (1971) Lipids, lipoproteins and atherosclerosis. Proc Roy Soc Med 64:902.
24. Benditt EP, Benditt JM (1973) Evidence for a monoclonal origin of human atherosclerotic plaque. Proc Natl Acad Sci USA 70:1753-1756.
25. Barger AC, Beeuwkes R III, Lainey LL, Silverman KJ (1984) Hypothesis: Vasa vasorum and neovascularization of human coronaries. A possible role in the pathophysiology of atherosclerosis. N Engl J Med 310:175-177.

27
Mechanical Properties of Human Atherosclerotic Lesions

Gustav V.R. Born and Peter D. Richardson

ABSTRACT

Atherosclerosis has a long initial phase in which plaques form within the arterial intima, followed by a second episodic phase in which clinical symptoms occur. We are investigating the events that initiate the second phase. It has been established that a major proportion of the acute episodes are thrombotic and that the trigger is exposure to the blood of thrombogenic constituents of the intima when cracks of fissures develop in the cap of atheromatous plaques.

Why plaque fissuring occurs is not known, but it is reasonable to assume it to be due to yielding of tissue in reaction to mechanical forces acting on the structure of the plaque. We are working on the hypothesis that there is a sub-population of plaques, probably only a minority, in which there is a propensity for fissuring. This may be caused by structural and physical properties of the most superficial layer of the plaque, i.e. the cap; by the presence of lipid-rich pool in the plaque producing a potential space in the intima; or by a combination of

Acknowledgments: We wish to acknowledge essential assistance by Mr. G. Panol who constructed the micromechanical apparatus; Mr. C. Owens, Miss A. Parhazgar, and Miss C. Lendon who made the measurements; and Dr. H. Sasken of the Department of Pathology at Rhode Island Hospital for providing specimens. We wish to express our gratitude to the British Heart Foundation, the Fritz-Thyssen Foundation of Colonge, and the Mirma-James Heineman Foundation of Hanover for financial support.

these and other factors. We describe here some initial
investigations.

INTRODUCTION
    Atherosclerotic disease is an almost inevitable con-
sequence of living in the developed world. Atherosclerosis
has a long initiating phase usually lasting many years
during which plaques form in the intima of some but not all
major arteries including the aorta and coronary and cerebral
arteries. During this phase there are no clinical symptoms.
    The presence of atheromatous plaque is a precondition
for the appearance of the second, symptomatic phase of the
disease in which myocardial infarction, angina and sudden
death are the cardiac, and transient ischemic attacks and
strokes the cerebral manifestations. Transition from the
asymptomatic to the symptomatic phase is commonly sudden
and unexpected.
    Recent evidence has established irrefutably that a
major proportion of these sudden events are associated with
thrombosis occurring on an atheromatous plaque (1-3). The
thrombosis itself is triggered by a process which has been
described as fissuring, cracking or rupture of the plaque
(4-9). When this occurs, blood tracks from the lumen into
the intima to produce a hematoma and an intra-intimal
thrombus within the plaque. This causes considerable increase in size of the plaque and in the extent of arterial
obstruction at the site, followed in some cases by the
formation of additional thrombus in the lumen. The intra-
lumenal thrombus may grow to occlude the vessel. Plaque
fissuring and its consequences have now been linked by both
clinical and pathological evidence to sudden ischemic death,
unstable angina and acute myocardial infarction (10,11).
    The cause of plaque fissuring is completely unknown.
It has been suggested (12) that the process is analogous to
the fatigue failure of metallic structures which develop
fissures under the cumulative effect of continuous but
variable stresses (13). On this hypothesis, fissuring is an
ultimate consequence of the uninterrupted exposure of plaques
to the continuously varying hemodynamic forces, and presumably also to those arising from variable tone of the smooth

muscle in the vessel wall in the vicinity of the plaque. The role of plaque fissuring as a trigger for thrombosis does not detract from the evidence that it can also be initiated by local arterial spasm.

The immediate variable on which these forces act is the biochemical structure of the plaque cap. A major component of the cap is collagen, so one possibility is that susceptibility to fissuring depends on functional characteristics of the collagen, via the different collagen types and the extent and type of cross-linking. In arteries of the cerebral circulation, a low ratio of type III to type I collagen predisposes to rupture of cerebral aneurysms (14). Types I and III are the predominant collagens in normal intima and in plaques (15), but no systematic comparisons of collagens in plaques of different individuals, in different plaques from the same individual, and in plaque cap vs plaque base have yet been published.

It has been suggested that cross-links have evolved in collagen to provide resistance to tensile forces while retaining extensibility so that precipitous fractures do not occur (16). If that is so, the structural effectiveness of collagen could be diminished by either too much or too little cross-linking. Collagen cross-links are formed from peptide-aldehydes derived from hydroxylysine and lysine, which form reducible Schiff bases of aldol condensation products. These are unstable, decrease with age, and are converted into the non-reducible compounds hydroxyaldo-histidine and pyridinoline (16-18). With techniques available at present, it is not possible to quantify such stable cross-links in the components of atherosclerotic lesions.

Another structural variable is the proportion of elastin in plaque caps. Differences in the amount of elastin can be presumed to be associated with measurable heterogenity in the mechanical properties of plaques. Yet another variable is the calcium content of the plaques.

Even from the same aorta, atheromatous plaques differ greatly in their macroscopic or microscopic appearances and in their biochemical make-up. Several classifications of plaques have been proposed (19) but are sufficiently inconsistent to make comparison difficult. For example, the description "white fibrous plaque" could mean one with a lipid pool and a cap sufficiently thick to be opaque or a plaque consisting entirely of fibrous tissue. Variations in the structure of plaques raises the possibility that fissuring depends on plaque having a particular structure or biochemical composition. Almost nothing appears to be known about this.

Fatigue, in engineering terms, refers to the behavior of materials which are subjected repeatedly to oscillating stress less than that required under normal circumstances to cause fracture of the material. With most engineering materials, when the maximum oscillating stress applied is below a certain limit the endurance of the material, i.e. the number of loading reversals which it can endure without failure becomes essentially infinite. For stresses greater than that but less than the single-load ultimate strength, materials endure a finite number of cycles before failure occurs.

Investigations of fatigue are generally done with structures very simple in shape (sometimes with an intentional local defect such as a circular hole, which acts as a predictable stress-raiser) and with single-frequency, single-amplitude cyclic loads. Fatigue failures are the final results of the accumulation of irreversible damage sustained throughout the life of the structure. The loads causing the damage are variable in amplitude and frequency, and often unpredictable over long time scales. Recognition of this had led to the development of probabalistic methods for study of structural failure (20,21). These methods make use of fatigue test results from cohorts of specimens, but the resulting information is more phenomenological and less mechanistic.

MATERIALS AND METHODS

Micromechanical Testing Device

It is evident, of course, that atheromatous plaques are not homogeneous. Different parts of individual plaques can be presumed to have quantitatively different compositions.

We are, therefore, endeavoring to correlate the mechanical properties of plaque components, in the first instance the cap, with their cellular and biochemical composition. For this purpose, we have developed a micromechanical device in which small specimens of tissue are subjected to uniaxial loading, and the elongation of the specimen is measured as a function of the force applied. The tissue samples are about 0.5 mm in cross-section and 3-4 mm long (22). Samples of this size permit determination of the mechanical proper-ties of the different layers of an artery. It is technically possible to use smaller samples of tissue; however, the mechanical properties may then be sufficiently non-uniform to prevent reliable measurements.

In this way we began to investigate, as a base line, the mechanical properties of carotid arteries taken from sheep (23). An early question was how rapidly and to what extent autolytic processes affect the mechanical properties of arterial specimens. Therefore, the effect of time after removal on the mechanical behavior of canine thoracic aorta has been determined. Samples were cut circumferential from the aorta and were tested uniaxially. The results (Figure 1) show that the stress/strain relation remained constant for several hours, suggesting that effects of autolysis are non significant during that period.

Initial Observations with Human Coronary Arteries

Up to the present we have done experiments with specimens taken from 25 autopsies at Rhode Island Hospital; these specimens were obtained according to an established protocol. Unfixed specimens were used for immediate micro-mechanical testing.

To study the relationship between stress and elongation, measurements were made without any preconditioning or pre-straining of the tissue. We have observed that when tissue is elongated considerably and then relaxed and reelongated, fiduciary marks placed on the tissue indicate localized permanent elongations; presumably this is due to local fractures of load-bearing components.

Most measurements were made with a single series of incremental elongations. In some experiments the elongation

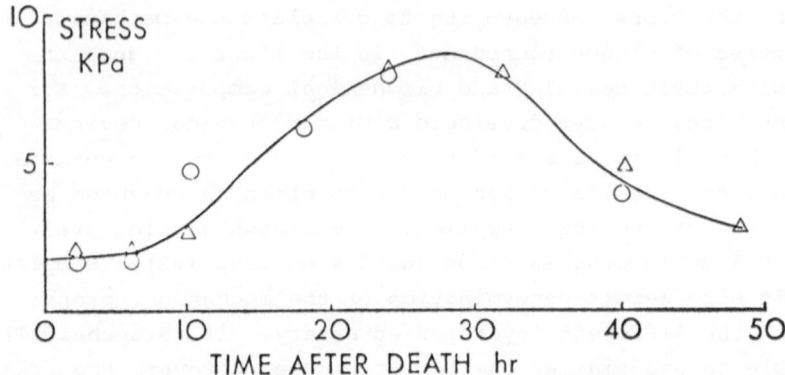

Figure 1. Alterations of arterial tissue mechanics as a function of time post mortem. The stress supported by canine aortic tissue at an elongation of 1.05 followed to 48 hours post mortem.

was increased and decreased in zigzag fashion; this procedure is more appropriate for investigating the fatigue failure behavior of the tissue rather than its simple elastic and ultimate strength. In our continuing experiments both procedures are being used in order to determine fatigue properties as well as ultimate strength. Maximum stress is a controlled parameter in fatigue tests.

Specimens used for mechanical testing are taken from atherosclerotic plaques and from nearby intima not involved in a lesion. Plaques which abut the portion of the vessel taken for histological studies provide us with direct histological evidence of their structure before mechanical testing. Specimens which have been used for mechanical testing are fixed for quantitative histological examinations.

Effect of Sample Orientation

Most samples are taken with their major axis in the longitudinal direction of the vessel. The reason for this is practical: with many plaques it is easier to get a sample of sufficient length in longitudinal orientation. However, we know already (23) that there is some anistropy in the mechanical behavior of arterial wall components. Therefore, when the opportunity presents itself, circumferential samples are taken from both plaque and apparently normal intima nearby.

Effect of Temperature

The micromechanical tester allows us to perfuse the well in which the tissue is supported with physiological media at any desired temperature. At present the experiments are being carried out at 20°C, but the effect of temperature will be systematically investigated. The range from 5°C to 45°C is intended to include effects of surgical hypothermia at one end and or high fever at the other.

Results of Mechanical Testing

Coronary arteries were opened longitudinally with dissecting scissors, exposing the lumen. Regions with well-defined plaques and regions where there were no plaques were identified visually. Specimens were cut from the intimal layer from plaque and from an apparently normal segment. Results of subjecting specimens to uniaxial mechanical testing are shown in Figures 2 and 3. (Not all results are shown because of overlapping of several curves.) Intimal specimens which appeared normal had smooth variation of stress as a function of elongation, whereas the response of plaque material was quite different, i.e., initial elongation with little or no stress followed by a sudden steep rise in stress with little or no increase in elongation. This has been characteristic of all samples of plaques tested so far; it does not appear to have been reported before. The measurements for normal and plaque regions showed considerable variability. However, in all cases examined the elongation of normal intima was greater than that of plaque for stresses which exceeded the stress necessary to overcome the step in the plaque response. In some vessels the normal tissue was up to five times more compliant than the plaque material.

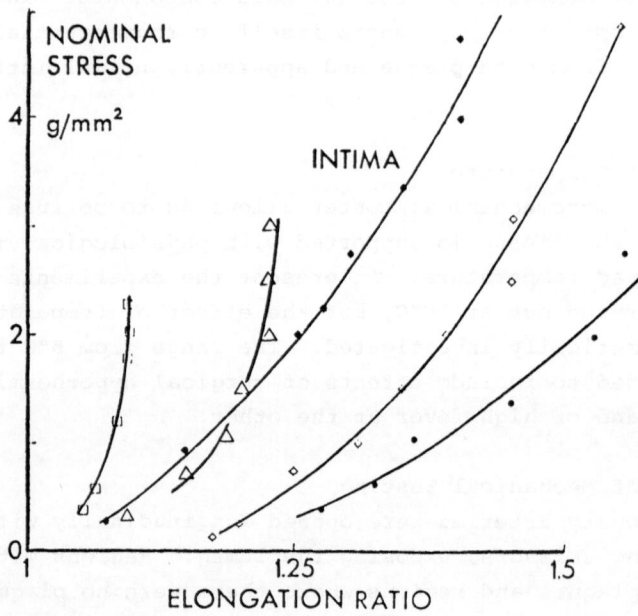

Figure 2. Mechanical behavior of human coronary artery intima
(not locally involved in atherosclerotic plaques). Nominal
stress is the stress calculated from the load divided by. the
original, unloaded specimen cross-section area. Elongation
ratio here is the distance between fiduciary marks in the
direction of the uniaxially applied load divided by the
distance between the same fiduciary marks when no load is
applied. Five different subjects illustrate typical range.

DISCUSSION

Our study has been enlarged to use aortic plaques obtained at post mortem. Aortic plaques are large enough to
carry out multiple biochemical analysis and can be dissected
consistently into a cap, body and base component. In a
further series of 25 deaths from coronary artery disease and
25 non-coronary deaths (excluding patients with known hypertension), every non-ulcerated plaque over 1 cm in length and
more than 2 mm in height is being utilized. In each case the
total numbers of ulcerated and non-ulcerated plaques will be
recorded. This will ultimately permit conclusions about
similarities or otherwise between ulceration of aortic plaques

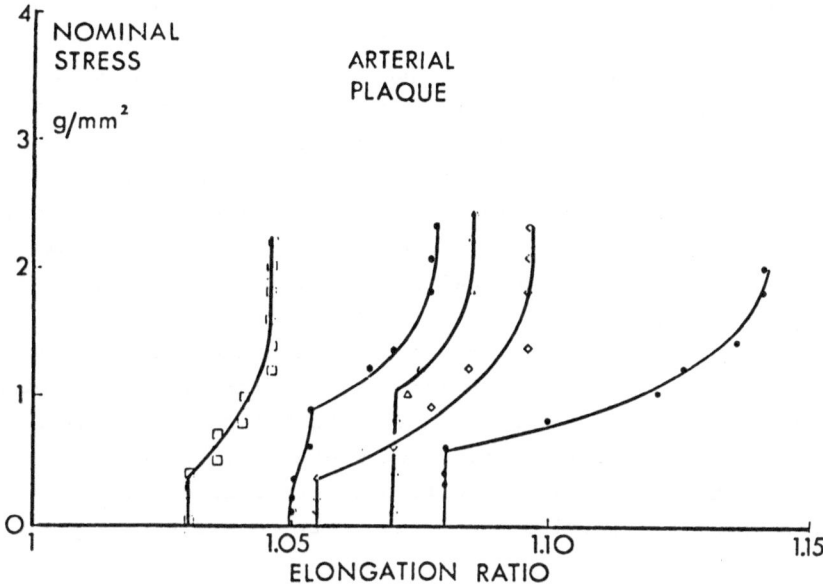

Figure 3. Mechanical behavior of human coronary artery plaque. The tissues tested were taken entirely from the intimal portion of the plaques. Stress and elongation are defined as in Figure 2. Five different subjects illustrate the typical range. At elongation ratios below about 1.05 the stress supported was too small to register reliably on transducers employed. A "plaque gap" appears in the mechanical behavior at these low elongation ratios.

and fissuring of coronary plaques. The main difference between aortic and coronary atheromatous plaques seems to be size. Coronary artery plaques have been and are being tested mechanically but their small size precludes all the biochemical parameters being measured on the same plaques. It is an observed fact (19) that in some patients but not in others a high proportion of aortic plaques are ulcerated. It is possible that in such patients non-ulcerated plaques are predisposed to ulceration. Of particular interest are plaques which have a fissure at one end commonly covered by thrombus, and an intact cap at the other end.

It should be emphasized that the investigation which is outlined here is focused on behavior of tissue and on the corresponding histopathology. Investigation of the overall problem requires study of the ways in which stresses arise locally in the tissue (how is stress affected by the pulse rate, and the pulse pressure width?). Do the local anisotropies in the vessel wall mechanics cause focusing effects for longitudinal waves and consequent local stress intensification? How does tissue structural damage accumulate (the development of pathological changes is much studied already) and how does the structural damage alter the mechanical behavior of the layers of the vessel wall? This is a concern because our present ability to predict the mechanical behavior of tissue from histological information on structure is inadequate (20). However, some new approaches are being developed (24) which may allow better estimation of mechanical behavior from ultrastructural details. We intend to determine the contribution of collagen and its cross-linking (25-27). The ultimate purpose is to find out whether it is possible to affect the mechanical properties of atherosclerotic plaques so as to minimize their liability to fissure.

CONCLUSION

Preliminary determinations of the mechanical properties of plaque cap tissue have shown already that they are different from those of nearby non-involved arterial intima. This begins to provide an explanation for the fissuring of plaque caps as the initiating event in the clinical phase of atherosclerotic disease. Much remains to be done in extending these novel measurements and relating them to the cellular and biochemical properties of plaques.

REFERENCES
1. DeWood MA, Spores J, Notsk ER, et al. (1980) Prevalence of total coronary occlusion during the early hours of transmural myocardial infarction. N Engl J Med 303:897.
2. Davies MJ, Fulton WFM, Robertson WB (1979) The relation of coronary thrombosis to ischaemic myocardial necrosis. J Pathol 127:99.
3. Davies MJ, Woolf N, Robertson WB (1976) Pathology of acute myocardial infarction with particular reference to occlusive coronary thrombi. Brit Heart J 38:659.
4. Horie T, Sekiguchi M, Hirosawa K (1979) Coronary thrombosis in pathogenesis of acute myocardial infarction: Histopathological study of coronary arterial in 108 necropsied cases using serial sections. Brit Heart J 40:153.

5. Friedman M (1971) The coronary thrombus - its origin and fate. Human Pathol 2:81.
6. Ridolfi RL, Hutchins GM (1977) The relation between coronary artery lesions and myocardial infarcts: Ulceration of atherosclerotic plaques precipitating coronary thrombosis. Am Heart J 93:468.
7. Constantides P (1966) Plaque fissures in human coronary thrombosis.   J Atheroscler Res 6:1.
8. Chandler AB (1974) Mechanisms and frequency of thrombosis in the coronary circulation. Thromb Res 4:3.
9. Falk E (1983) Plaque rupture with severe pre-existing stenosis precipitating coronary thrombosis: Characteristics of coronary atherosclerotic plaques underlying fatal occlusive thrombi. Brit Heart J 50:127.
10. Davies MJ, Thomas AC (1985) Plaque fissuring - the cause of acute myocardial infarction, sudden ischaemic death, and crescendo angina. Brit Heart J 53:363.
11. Ambrose JA, Winters SL, Stern A, et al. (1985) Angiographic morphology and the pathogenesis of unstable angina pectoris. JACC 5:609.
12. Born GVR (1979) Coronary thrombosis, fancies and facts. Proc. World Congress Cardiol, Tokyo, Amsterdam: Elsevier.
13. Frost NE, Marsh KJ, Poole LP (1974) Metal Fatigue. Oxford: Clarendon Press.
14. Neil-Dwyer G, Bartlett JR (1983) Collagen deficiency and ruptured cerebral aneurysms. J Neurosurg 59:16.
15. Morton LF, Barnes MJ (1982) Collagen polymorphism in the normal and diseased blood vessel wall. Atheroscler 42:41.
16. Tanzer ML, Waite JH (1982) Collagen cross linking. Collagen Rel Res 2:177.
17. Robins SP (1982) Analysis of cross linking components in collagen and elastin. Methods Biochem Anal 28:329.
18. Robins SP (1982) An enzyme linked immunoassay for collagen cross link pyridioline. Biochem J 207:617.
19. Smith Elspeth, Davies MJ Personal discussion.
20. Madsen HO, Krenk H, Lind NC (1986) Method of Structural Safety. Prentice-Hall.
21. Boganoff JL, Kozin F (1985) Probabilistic Models of Cumulative Damage. J Wiley.
22. Richardson PD, Parhizgar A, Sasken HF, Chiu TH, Aebischer P, Trudell LA, Galletti PM (1986) Tissue characterization by micromechanical testing of growths around bioresorbable implants. In: Nose Y, Kjellstrand C, Ivanovich P (eds) Progress in Artificial Organs - 1985. Cleveland: ISAO Press, pp. 1015-1019.
23. Owens C, Richardson PD (1985) Mechanical properties of carotid artery walls. Proceedings 11th Annual NE Bioengineering Conf, pp. 12-15.
24. Aspden RM (1986) Relation between structure and mechanical behavior of fibre-reinforced composite materials at large strains. Proc Roy Soc A406:287.
25. Laemmli UK (1970) Cleavage of structural proteins during the assembly of the head of Bacteriophage T4. Nature 227: 680.
26. Burleigh MC, Barrett AJ, Lazarus GS (1974) Cathespin B: A lysosomal enzyme that degrades native collagen. Biochem J 137:387.
27. Griffin S, Knox P (1985) Characterization of apolipoprotein B by sodium dodecyl sulphate gel electrophoresis and immunoblotting. Biochem Soc Trans 13:775.

28

Cinemicrographic Studies of the Vasa Vasorum of Human Coronary Arteries

Reinier Beeuwkes III, A. Clifford Barger, Kenneth J. Silverman and
Lewis L. Lainey

INTRODUCTION

The role of the vasa vasorum in the pathophysiology of
atherosclerotic coronary artery disease remains controversial.
There is no doubt that these small vessels of the arterial
wall exist in far greater numbers in regions associated with
plaque. Observations made as early as 1876 and confirmed in
1938 have firmly established this association (1,2). In
recent times, most authors pay little attention to the vasa
vasorum in their focus on the lipid constituents of the
plaque. On the other hand, some have proposed a fundamental
role for the vasa vasorum in the progression of the lesion
(3,4). Within the context of the present symposium, the
issue which seems to call for particular attention is the
contribution of the vasa vasorum to plaque hemorrhage and
the formation of lumenal thrombus.

In order to estimate the potential contribution of blood
from the vasa vasorum to intramural hemorrhage, it is necessary to find the origin and disposition of these small
vessels. From Bernoulli's principle we know that the flow
of blood through a narrowed section of a vessel creates a
region of low pressure centered in the narrowest point. If
the vasa vasorum arose from the lumen at such a location it
would seem unlikely that blood would flow from the lumen into
the vessel wall. On the other hand, if the vasa vasorum were
supplied from regions upstream from the lesion, one might
expect to find higher pressures within these capillaries than

in the adjacent lumen. Study of the vasa vasorum in relation
to atherosclerotic plaque in the human heart is difficult.
The human heart is typically fat covered and requires disruptive dissection before plaques can even be located.
Further, although serial section techniques enable the pathologist to follow these microvessels through short distances,
the dynamics of flow in them and their origin and distribution around the coronary artery are difficult to define.
Accordingly, we have applied an injection technique which
allows direct visualization of flow in vasa vasorum in
cleared tissue. In an earlier published report (5), we
showed the ability of this technique to demonstrate the association of neovascular structures with calcified plaques. In
this presentation, we focus upon the origin of the blood
vessels which supply these capillary networks, and the significance of these new observations in the pathophysiology of
coronary thrombus.

METHODS
      Eighty human hearts were obtained at autopsy from male
and female patients ranging in age from 19 to 96 years. These
were fixed by pressure perfusion with 2% glutaraldehyde in
lactated-Ringer's solution, then dehydrated, whole, in an
ethanol series (25%, 50%, 75%, 95%, absolute alcohol, for
24 hours at each level). The organs were then cleared by
placing them in methyl salicylate. This process rendered the
epicardial fat and blood vessel walls transparent. Myoglobin
in cardiac muscle retained its dark red color, and allowed
the relationship of vessels and myocardium to be clearly
defined. To demonstrate vascular and microvascular structures,
a white silicone polymer (MV 112, Canton Biomedical Products,
Boulder, CO) was injected into the cleared vessels, and the
path of the injectate was filmed using a special optical
system. The basic technique of clearing and injection, is,
of course, not new. The present approach is based upon
improvements developed for study of renal microvasculature (6).
The major improvements include the use of low viscosity silicone materials for injection and the application of micro-
cinematography for documentation of flow patterns in the
microvasculature.

RESULTS

These injection studies showed that dense capillary networks of neovascular appearance were clearly associated with
calcified plaques. In contrast, arteries free of atherosclerosis had walls containing only sparse adventitial
vessels which did not tend to form a capillary plexus.
Studies of the film, combined with histological examination
of tissue taken from the photographed regions, showed that
the vasa vasorum were present in the adventitia, media, and
intima of the injured vessel wall (7). Microvessels within
the thickened intima tended to lie in the shoulder region
or below calcified or necrotic plaque core.

The injection technique, by giving a continuous demonstration of the filling process, clearly defined the origin
of the blood supply to these capillary vessels. In nearly
all instances the plaque-associated vasa vasorum were
supplied with blood from an adventitial vessel extending
from a more proximal branch of the artery; occasionally
some of the supply could be seen deriving from a major
branch lying below the narrowed region. In no case, among
several hundred calcified plaques examined, was there a
direct communication from the lumen of the affected coronary
artery to the local microvascular network. Accordingly, we
conclude that the blood supply to vasa vasorum in the
regions of atherosclerotic injury is derived from sources
of relatively high pressure which generally branch from the
artery above the plaque. These relationships are illustrated
in Figures 1 and 2.

DISCUSSION

The association between atherosclerotic plaque and proliferation of vasa vasorum has many implications. It has
been demonstrated that these vessels provide increased flow
to the media and intima (8). Circulating vasoactive and
chemotactic substances may thus be preferentially delivered
in such a region whether in solution or as carried by
cells (5,9). It is also conceivable that these vessels
could be a local source of lipid (3). During bypass surgery
or angioplasty these vessels may be ablated or may rupture,
leading to bleeding or inflammatory processes in the
operated area.

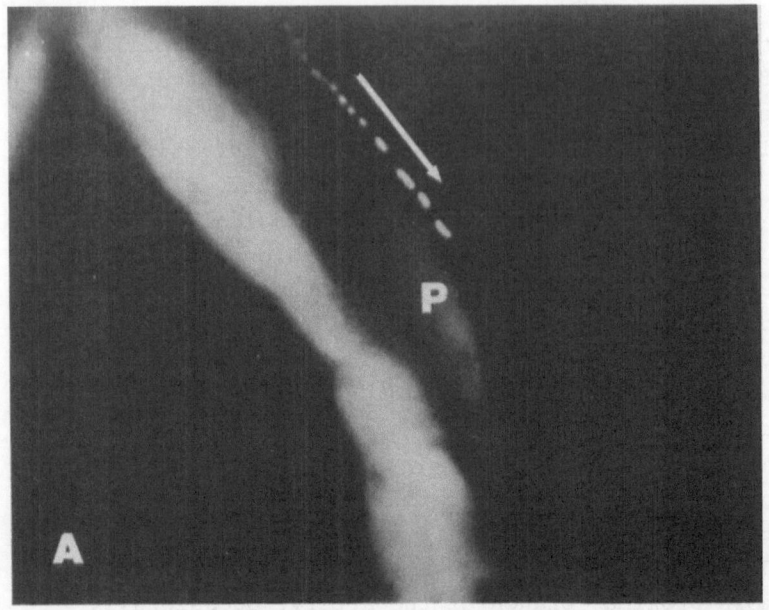

Figure 1. Prints derived from single frames of the film
record the filling of a capillary network associated
with a calcified atherosclerotic plaque in the left anterior descending coronary artery of a 70 year old male.
A. (above) The lumen of the cleared artery has been
filled with white silicone polymer. Deep indentations
in this filling show the presence of severe, localized,
intimal thickening. A deposit of calcium (P) is incorporated in the thickening on one side. An adventitial vessel
descending from above (parallel to arrow) lies somewhat to
the near side of the calcium deposit. B. (opposite page,
top) As injection of the vasa vasorum continues, branches
extend across and around the region of injury and converge
to join with an adventitial vein on the left (arrows). No
communication between the lumen in this area and the
capillary network can be detected. C. (opposite page,
bottom) Continuing injection of the microvasculature
shows that the vasa vasorum are localized in the region of
injury. Also, the microvessels have a blunted and irregular
appearance characteristic of neovascular structures. Such
structures are present in the intima in both the calcified
region and in the relatively less involved intima of the
vessel's opposite side.

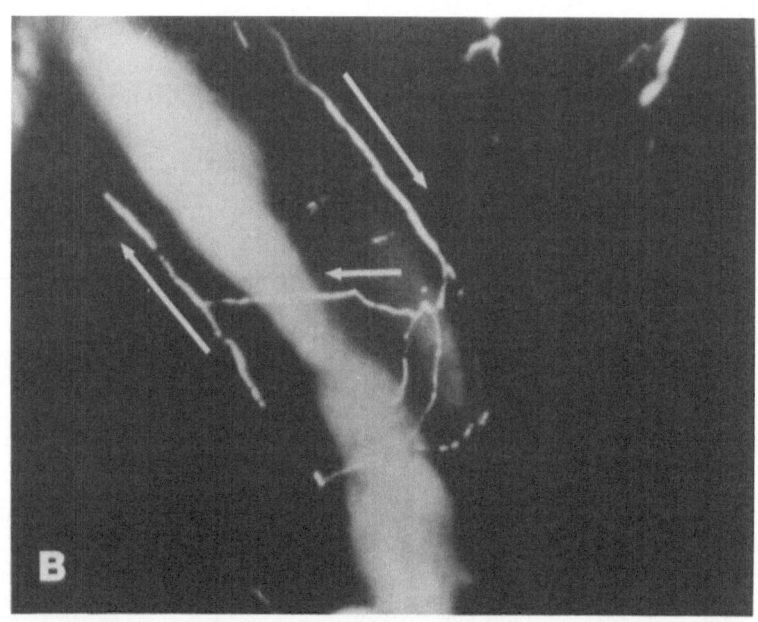

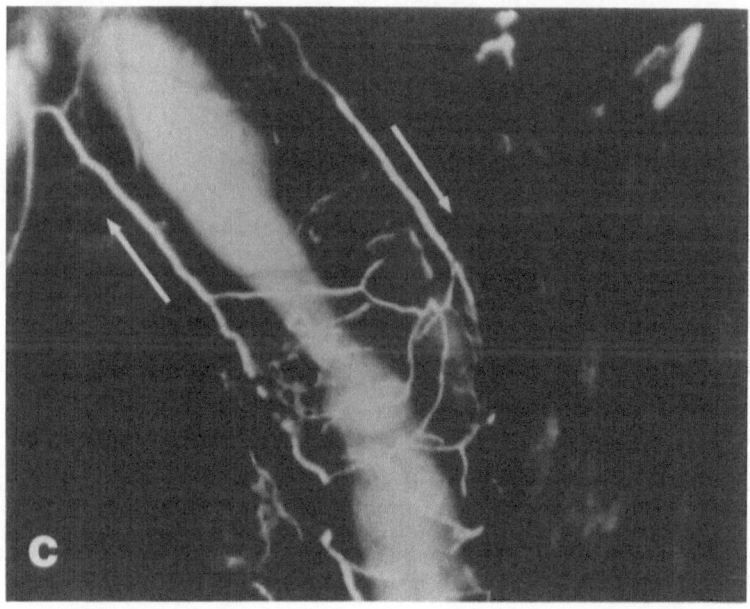

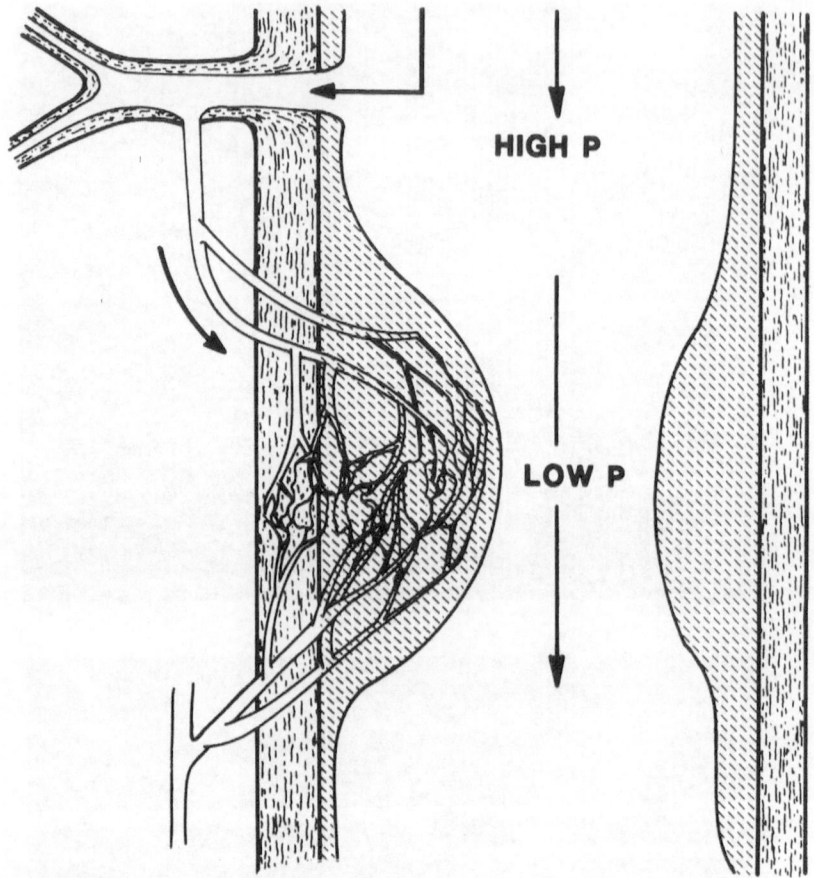

Figure 2.   Illustration of structural and hydrodynamic
relationship in coronary artery lumen and vasa vasorum.
A segment of the lumen is narrowed by atherosclerotic
plaque (diagonal shading).   Due to Bernouilli's principle,
the hydrostatic pressure in the narrow channel will be
lower ("Low P") than in the wide part of the lumen above
("High P").   The blood supply to the profuse vasa vasorum
of the plaque is derived from branches arising from the
"high pressure" region proximal to the plaque (such branches
actually arise much more proximally than illustrated in this
diagram).   These anatomical and hemodynamic factors may
lead to a substantial pressure gradient directed outward
from the plaque capillaries toward the plaque interior and
arterial lumen.

The importance of bleeding from these vessels in the
events leading to ischemic symptoms or thrombotic occlusion
is difficult to evaluate. These vessels are fragile neovascular structures without pericytes, and are prone to
bleed (see 4 for brief review). Indeed, Davies and Thomas
report that vasa vasorum derived hemorrhage was "universal"
in coronary arteries from both cardiac death and non-cardiac
death patients (10). A role for such hemorrhages in plaque
development seems probable, though not proven (11,12).
There is, however, a clear association between lumenal
thrombus, the presence of a fissure or rupture of the plaque
surface and extravascular cells and platelets within the
plaque itself (13,14 Constantinides, this volume).

If mechanical stress ruptures a plaque, then mechanical
motion could move blood from the lumen into the plaque.
This would lead to the presence of the red cells sometimes
observed in avascular regions of the intima. However, it
must be recognized that such flow (i.e., from lumen into
plaque) is against the expected pressure gradient if the
plaque contains blood vessels derived from an upstream
source. Such an upstream source has been clearly demonstrated in the present work. In this case, Bernouilli's
principle would predict lower pressure in the narrowed lumen
than in the adjacent capillary. The pressure gradient could
be large. King (15) has published simple calculations indicating possible capillary-to-lumen gradients of up to 50 mmHg
if flow is increased (due to exercise) and the lumen area is
reduced by three fourths. Such an area reduction is often
asymptomatic, except during exercise. Stenosis of 90% is
not unusual. Such narrowing which would lead to even greater
capillary-to-lumen pressure gradients, seem to be clearly
associated with terminal occlusive thrombus formation (14).

It seems reasonable, therefore, to make two proposals.
First, relatively high pressure in new capillaries can lead
to hemorrhage within the plaque, potentially contributing to
plaque rupture. Second, whenever a rupture or fissure of
whatever origin occurs into a region containing vasa vasorum,
then local pressure relations will lead to hemorrhage from
within the plaque toward the lumen. Such hemorrhage, in
which blood is exposed to activating factors as it passes

out through the tissue, could lead to lumenal thrombosis
and occlusion.

REFERENCES

1. Koster W (1876) Endarteritis and arteritis. Berlin
    Klin Wschr 13:454-455.
2. Winternitz MC, Thomas RM, LeCompte PM (1938) The
    Biology of Arteriosclerosis. Springfield, Illinois:
    Charles C. Thomas.
3. Groszek E, Grundy SM (1980) The possible role of the
    arterial microcirculation in the pathogenesis of
    atherosclerosis. J Chem Dis 33:679-684.
4. Cliff WJ, Schoefl GI (1983) Pathological vasculari-
    zation of the coronary intima. In: Development of
    the Vascular System. London: Pitman Books, pp 207-221.
5. Barger AC, Beeuwkes III R, Lainey LL, Silverman KJ
    (1984) Hypothesis: Vasa vasorum and neovasculari-
    zation of human coronary arteries. N Engl J Med 310:
    175-177.
6. Beeuwkes III R, Bonventre JV (1975) Tubular organi-
    zation and vascular-tubular relations in the dog
    kidney. Am J Physiol 229:695-713.
7. Kamat BR , Galli SJ, Berger AC, Lainey LL, Silverman KJ
    (1987) Neovascularization and coronary atherosclerotic
    plaque: Cinematographic localization and quantitative
    histologic analysis. Human Pathol 18:1036-1042.
8. Heistad DD, Armstrong ML (1986) Blood flow through
    vasa vasorum of coronary arteries in atherosclerotic
    monkeys. Atherosclerosis 6:326:331.
9. Forman MB, Oates JA, Robertson D, Robertson RM, Roberts
    LJ, Virmani R (1985) Increased adventitial mast cells
    in a patient with coronary spasm. N Engl J Med
    313:1138-1141.
10. Davies MJ, Thomas A (1984) Thrombosis and acute coronary-
    artery lesions in sudden cardiac ischemic death. N Engl
    J Med 310:1137-1140.
11. Paterson JC (1938) Capillary rupture with intimal
    hemorrhage as a causative factor in coronary thrombosis.
    Arch Pathol Lab Med 25:474-487.
12. Lusby RJ, Ferrell LD, Ehrenfeld WK, Stoney RJ, Wiley EJ
    (1982) Carotid plaque hemmorhage, its role in pro-
    duction of cerebral ischemia. Arch Surg 117:1479-1488.
13. Constantinides P (1966) Plaque fissures in human
    coronary thrombosis. J Athero Res 6:1-117.
14. Falk E (1983) Plaque rupture with severe pre-existing
    stenosis precipitating coronary thrombisis, character-
    istics of coronary atherosclerotic plaques underlying
    fatal occlusive thrombi. Br Heart J 50:127-134.
15. King ESJ (1952) The haemodynamics of subintimal haemo-
    rrhage. Australasian Ann Med 1:18-25.

29
Atherosclerosis Regression and Arterial Repair

M.R. Malinow

INTRODUCTION

In view of the overwhelming amount of anatomical data
on progression of atherosclerosis, any discussion of its
possible regression must address first the question of whether
atherosclerosis is a relentlessly advancing process. Many
authors have concluded on morphological grounds that atherosclerosis progression is not inevitable; only a few representative reports will be quoted here. Roberts depicted the
evolution of lesions in his extensive studies on coronary
atherosclerosis and clearly interpreted certain cases as
compatible with regression (1). Glagov and Zarins commented
that (human atherosclerotic) "lesions have shown evidence of
healing and organization, implying that obstruction...changes
...over time are not necessarily progressive" (2). Blankenhorn
expressed that, "the histologic picture...suggests...(that)
...the growth of coronary lesions is probably episodic, with
periods of growth alternating with stationary periods or
periods of regression" (3). And Harlan and Landis indicated,
"It is possible that...atherosclerosis lesions may progress,
remain unchanged, or regress without specific therapy...and
that these changes may occur in a 'stuttering' or rapid-slow
fashion rather than linearly" (4). This "stuttering" progress,
previously referred to as waxing and waning of atherosclerotic
lesions (5), usually results in advanced lesions over the
course of years, apparently because plaque progression exceeds
regression for most individuals (3). However, the occurrence

of transitory episodes of regression cannot be documented in postmortem examinations, except by inference, because there are no criteria to identify regression.

The question of atherosclerosis regression will be addressed based on studies performed with postmortem patho-logical or *in vivo* arteriographic techniques. Information is necessarily incomplete and will be mostly confined to the aorta and the coronary arteries, but a few examples of other arterial territories will be presented. However, it is recognized that mechanisms may not similarly apply to different arterial territories. Aspects of regression have been reviewed by different investigators (6-14). Previous reviews (5,15-17) will be quoted freely here.

A.   The Evolution of Atherosclerotic Plaques

This brief review will emphasize what we need to learn and how the missing knowledge might be generated. Current evidence indicates that an orderly sequence of events may lead to fibrous plaques and complicated plaques with thrombosis superimposed on fissured or ulcerated plaques, as diagrammed in Figure 1. This may begin with a fatty streak or with other hypothetical lesions (18-21). As aptly expressed by Woolf (22), "since the histopathologist must, perforce, view any lesion at one moment in its natural history, ideas of the events leading up to that point can at best be the result of a more or less imaginative reconstruction". Accordingly, the relationships between those discrete lesions is surmised using "imaginative reconstruction", but the "sequence" needs yet to be demonstrated in humans.

B.   Definition of Regression

A hypothetical sequence implied in progression of athero-sclerosis is shown in the upper panel of Figure 1. Vectors denote transformation of a lesion into another lesion. One postulate is that in plaque transformations, an interplay of of injury and repair mechanisms results in changes in the size (S) (19), composition (C) (23), or severity (Se) (2) of plaques. Tissue and cellular injury and repair mechanisms are authoritatively discussed by Constantinides (24). In the evolution of a plaque, positive values of the slopes

HYPOTHETICAL SEQUENCE IN ATHEROGENESIS

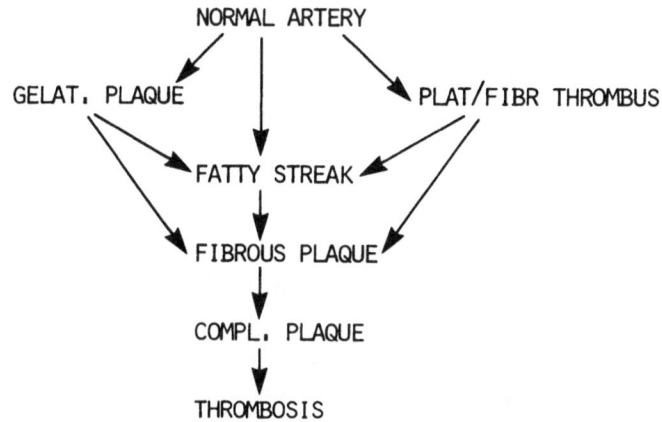

HYPOTHETICAL SEQUENCE IN REGRESSION

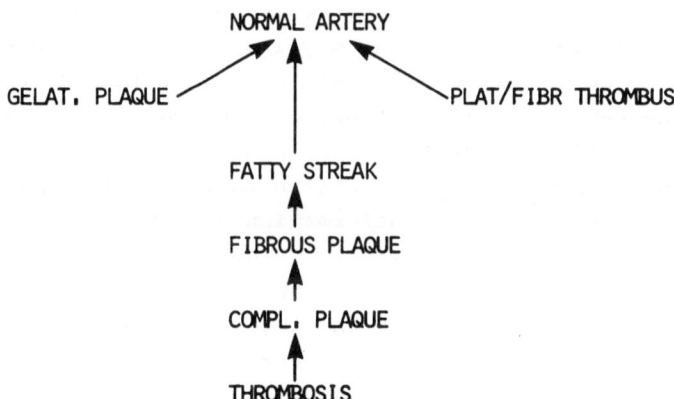

Figure 1. A hypothetical sequence in the evolution of atherosclerotic plaques. (Upper) Vectors suggesting transformation of discrete lesions during progression of atherosclerosis are derived from the interpretation of numerous literature sources. See reviews in 18-21. Platelet fibrin microthrombi are further discussed in M.D. Haust, in Bond *et al*, Eds., <u>Clinical</u> <u>Diagnosis</u> <u>of</u> <u>Atherosclerosis</u>, Springer-Verlag, 1983, pg. 513. Thrombosis in ulcerated or fissured plaques is discussed in 23, 46, 47, and 139; for early references see 140, 141. (Lower) Vectors representing a reversal of the stated transformations are postulated in regression of atherosclerosis; certain of those transformations are discussed in this review.

Gelat. = gelatinous; plat/fibr = platelet/fibrin; compl. = complicated.

dS/dt, dC/dt or dSe/dt would indicate progression, (*i.e.*, injury>repair); zero values of the slopes would indicate stabilization (*i.e.*, injury=repair), and negative values would indicate regression (*i.e.* injury<repair). These slopes need yet to be defined quantitatively. Moreover, changes occurring in plaques often modify simultaneously their size, composition and severity, and it is only for convenience that these different parameters are expressed separately.

In a similar way as in progression, regression (Figure 1, lower panel) could then be defined as those lesion transformations that result in a decrease in the size of plaques, in certain changes in plaque composition, or in diminished severity, involving repair processes that overcome injury mechanisms. It is likely, though, that not all progression changes are reversible; thus, the lower panel of Figure 1 should be considered as a postulated progression that still needs demonstration.

Although plaque size and composition seem to be amenable to quantitative measurements, the concept of severity is often a value of judgment; thus a reduction in blood flow by a progressively larger plaque may indicate increased severity of the process, and its reverse, *i.e.*, an enlarged lumen with a consequent increase in flow, may indicate regression. Furthermore, a fibrous plaque may be considered a more severe lesion than a fatty streak, but a less severe lesion than a complicated plaque; thus, transformation of fibrous plaques to fatty streaks, and of complicated plaques to fibrous plaques, respectively, may represent regression. Moreover, a thrombo-atherosclerotic plaque in which the thrombus is reduced in size, or a calcified plaque which reverts to a fibrous non-calcified plaque, may also be considered instances of regression. Most of these examples require confirmation.

Evidence on the Occurrence of Regression
A. Anatomical Evidence
   1. Regression of fatty streaks
Early anatomical observations (reviewed by Hueper, 25) indicated that fatty streaks in the aorta and large elastic arteries increase in frequency and extent during the first two decades of life, and tend to disappear thereafter. The

fate of the fatty streak has been extensively studied more recently (18-20, 26-28), suggesting that fatty streaks may progress to fibrous plaques, may regress toward a normal intima, or may remain unchanged. Data supporting regression of fatty streaks (29) are shown in Figure 2. It depicts the average percent intimal surface involved with fatty streaks in the thoracic and the abdominal aorta in different age groups. The wide scatter presumably present in the 975 individual cases is not indicated. The mean extent of fatty streak involvement increased initially but decreased after 25-34 years of age. Such decrease was not observed in the mean extent of aortic raised lesions in the same vessels, nor in fatty streaks of the coronary arteries of the same individuals (Figure 3). Interpretation of the fatty streak changes in the aorta suggests that "regression" may be due to any of three different mechanisms, or a combination thereof, i.e., (1) transformation of fatty streaks into a normal artery (true regression), (2) transformation of fatty streaks into fibrous plaques (probable progression of severity), or (3) no change in the extent of fatty streaks, associated with an enlarged aortic surface (stabilization of plaques). This last mechanism is illustrated in Figure 4 (30) with data obtained by tracing and planimetry in the postmortem examinations of 195 men (31). The area of the aorta (panel A) increased with age whereas the area affected with fatty streaks (panel B) did not. Panel C depicts an "eye view" estimate of percent area affected with fatty streaks, showing that the apparent "regression" was mainly due to the increase in aortic area and not to a decrease in fatty streaks area. Additionally, since the extent of fibrous plaques increased in spite of the aortic enlargement (not shown), transformation of fatty streaks into fibrous plaques may have also played a role. The authors clearly recognized the artifact associated with interpretation of the findings (31).

Aschoff (32) was probably the first investigator to observe that atherosclerosis in humans might be reversible through exogenous factors. He stated, "With the increasing duration of war (World War I), the atheromatous spots on the aorta were observed less frequently." Other pathologists confirmed his findings but no quantitative data were presented

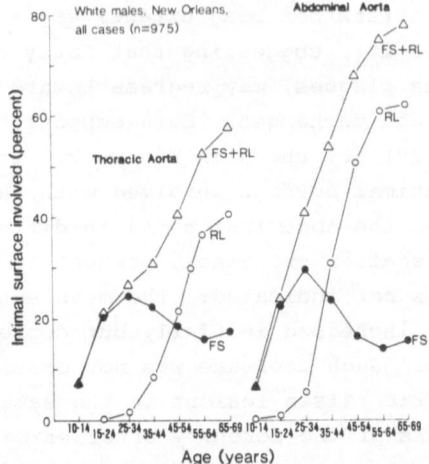

Figure 2. Average percent intimal surface involvement in the thoracic aorta and abdominal aorta by age groups. Data adapted from reference tables 2 and 3, p 131 in The Geographic Pathology of Atherosclerosis, H.C. McGill, Jr., Ed., Williams and Wilkins Co., Baltimore, 1968. FS = fatty streaks; RL = raised lesions.

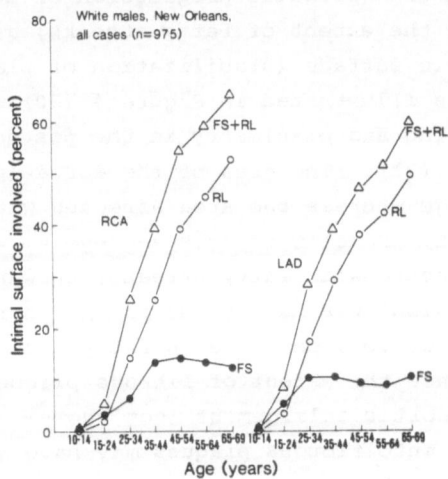

Figure 3. Average percent intimal surface involvement in the coronary arteries by age groups. Data adapted from reference tables 6 and 7, p. 183 in The Geographic Pathology of Atherosclerosis, H.C. McGill, Jr., Ed., Williams and Wilkins Co., Baltimore, 1968. RCA = right coronary artery; LAD = left anterior descending coronary artery; FS = fatty streaks; RL = raised lesions.

(33). Data on patients with terminal weight loss also suggest
that arterial lipid deposits may be removed (34), but selection
bias may have influenced the results (5). And age-stratified
data on 1456 postmortem aortic examinations in Finland showed
less tissue necrosis and complicated arterial plaques in the
"lean years" of World War II (1939-45) than from 1933 to 1938,
but no differences were seen in fatty streaks (35).

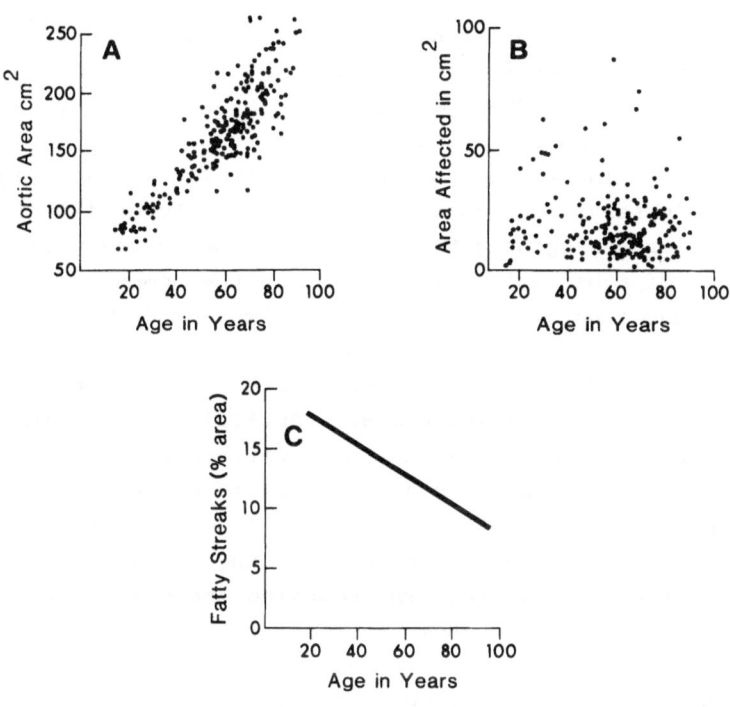

Adapted from Mitchell et al; 1964

Figure 4. "Regression" of aortic fatty streaks in humans.
A. Area of standard aortic segment as measured by tracing and
planimetry in 195 men. B. Area affected by flat sudanophilic
plaques in these 195 men. C. Decrease in the ratio (A/B) X
100, $i.e.$, percentage of aorta surface covered by fatty streaks
--calculated by "eye view" approximation--was mainly due to the
increase in aortic area and not to a decrease in sudanophilic
plaques. The data from A and B were taken from ref. 31. Each
point represents a patient. This figure is taken from ref.
30.

2.   Regression of Complicated Plaques

Data on patients with anorexia nervosa demonstrate
a lower frequency of advanced coronary lesions than in control
cases (36). Whether this represents regression or lack of progression cannot be determined. Studies in cancer patients
also suggest that regression of advanced lesions may be
observed. While a number of investigators (37-39) have demonstrated that patients with malignant diseases have less severe
atherosclerosis than non-cancer patients, this phenomenon has
not been observed in other series (40-43). An extensive
review of the literature was conducted by Restrepo *et al* (40);
in seven series, no effect of cancer on atherosclerosis was
demonstrated, whereas the extent of atherosclerosis was reduced
in 13 series. The reason for these disparities is not known.
Postmortem observations conducted earlier by Lober (44) in
cancer patients suggested that, "There might actually be some
regression of atherosclerotic lesions in the human."

From one study involving 1,835 postmortem examinations
performed and graded by a single pathologist in Denmark (37),
we have analyzed data showing less severe atherosclerosis in
cancer patients (30,45) (Figure 5). Sufficient data points
allowed adequate statistical tests at different age intervals,
and the study was probably conducted before antitumoral agents
were widely available; thus, a potentially confounding effect
was avoided. Another important confounding variable was also
avoided by the investigators who compiled these data; that is,
they excluded persons in whom atherosclerosis or its effects
were of primary importance as a cause of death. Except in
younger persons, cancer patients of all ages had less atherosclerosis than non-cancer patients (37); the difference was
equivalent to a 16.9 year span (95% confidence limits:13.1 and
20.8 years, respectively) (30). Interpretation of these
findings suggested that even if progression had been arrested
during a terminal period, the difference in the atherosclerotic involvement between cancer and non-cancer patients would
still have been too large, and it was probably partly due to
regression of atherosclerosis in the cancer patients (30).
Based on the grading system used by the authors (37), regression would, in the older individuals, indicate transformation
of intimal ulcerations and extensive calcifications into

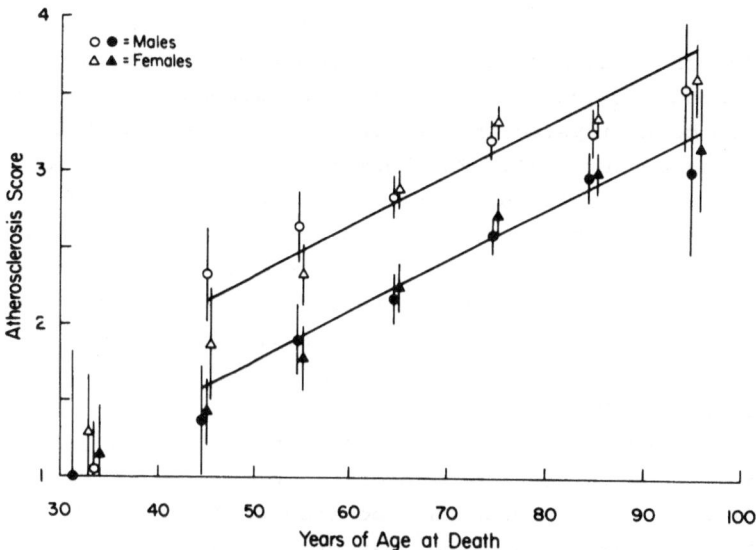

Figure 5. Best fitting lines showing the relationship between age and the extent of atherosclerosis. Key: White symbols, non-cancer patients; black symbols, cancer patients; vertical bars, 95% confidence limits. Data taken from ref. 37; the figure is taken from ref. 30.

non-ulcerated and patchy calcified lesions. Mechanisms involved in the possible regression of atherosclerosis in cancer patients are unknown. Further anatomical evidence suggestive of thrombus incorporation into atherosclerotic plaques and its organization and retraction--likely to be associated with an enlarged stenotic diameter--are discussed by Roberts (1), Davies and Thomas (46), and Fuster *et al* (47).

3. Advantages and Limitations of Pathological Studies

Pathological studies allow anatomical and biochemical characterization of plaques (48,49). However, there is large intra- and interobserver variability, especially when comparative methods are used to assess the extent of coronary stenosis (50). Moreover, there are limitations when trying to construct an "imaginary moving picture" (22) on the basis of

single view in time (5). Important biases also exist in
selection of cases subjected to postmortem examinations (19);
e.g., deaths assigned to cardiovascular diseases are least
likely to be necropsied in the U.S. (51), except perhaps in
specialized centers (1). Furthermore, averages obtained from
groups of individuals in a series of autopsies may not necessarily apply to subgroups, as discussed previously (5), and
it is even possible that in certain subsets, lesions could
regress or progress at rates different from the mean estimates
without altering the overall group results (5).

4. Future Needs

Paraphrasing Insull's scholarly exposition (52), it
seems important to develop methods to define regression in
terms of changes in number and location of lesions; the length,
width, bulk, size and surface characteristics of plaques; the
histological and chemical composition; the length and diameter
of stenosis; the extent of complicating features such as
mineralization, necrosis, hemorrhage, organization, vascularity, ulceration and thrombosis; as well as the characteristics
of the disease-free wall and their relation to the degree of
obstruction (53). The methods should obtain time-related
information of these parameters and the criteria for serial
studies must be defined in terms of intra- and interobserver
reproducibility, as well as on accuracy, sensitivity, and
specificity of measurements. The measurements should allow
observations with simultaneous controls in well-defined time
intervals. Finally, the measurements should determine changes
related to the natural history of the disease, to therapeutic
interventions, or to perturbations introduced by other factors,
such as conflicting secular effects (54,55).

B. Radiological Evidence of Atherosclerotic Regression

1. Regression of Localized Coronary Stenoses

There is evidence demonstrating by serial contrast
angiography that coronary arterial stenoses, presumably
secondary to atherosclerotic plaques, may improve; these
changes are compatible with atherosclerotic regression. But
since contrast angiograms, in the absence of calcifications,
do not visualize the arterial walls, interpretations derived
from luminal images are only inferential.

a.   Retrospective Studies

Table 1 shows several retrospective series in
which regression was observed when two angiographic studies
were repeated months to years apart in the same patients.
The criteria for interval change were not different from those
in other series negative for regression (56-61) and the reasons
for this discrepancy are not apparent.   Gensini *et al* (62)
were probably the first to document regression of well-defined
coronary atherosclerosis in 4 of their 174 patients.   Bruschke
et al (63), who saw regression in 12 (4.7%) patients, felt
that in one patient it was due to spasm.   In five patients
100% stenosis reverted to significant narrowings; in four
patients subtotal narrowings regressed to >50% stenosis; and
in two patients significant obstructions reverted to less than
50% narrowing.   In five of the patients progression was seen
simultaneously in other coronary arteries.   Shub *et al* (64)
indicated that regression occurring in 13 of 405 lesions was
not related to the presence of the usual risk factors; two
complete occlusions regressed.   Kramer *et al* (65) analyzed
317 cases and they observed regression in 15 (4.7%), also not
related to the usual risk factors; in 13 patients an initial
occlusion was recanalized.   VanHaecke *et al* (66) reviewed the
clinical records and angiograms of 100 consecutive patients.
They observed regression in 7; in 4 of these progression of
the disease occurred simultaneously in other vessels.   Moise
et al (67) studied 313 consecutive medically treated patients;
they observed regression in 12 patients, 3 of whom showed
revascularization of an occluded artery.   Singh (68) reviewed
52 non-operated coronary artery disease (CAD) patients undergoing two arteriograms; 3 lesions that originally showed 50
to 99% stenosis, regressed.

b.   Prospective Studies

Table 2 shows the results of nine series of
coronary patients.   Here, the performance of the repeated
angiogram was based on a prospective study design, not on
increased symptoms.   Although regression was not observed
in one series, in which successful management of hypercholesterolemia was associated with a lack of progression of

Table 1. Reports of Arteriographic Progression or Regression of Coronary Disease Based on Retrospective Patient Selection and Subjective Visual Assessment of Disease (Patients with Stable Lesions Not Shown)

Reference	Number of Patients	Study Average Interval (mo)	Progression (% of patients)	Regression (% of patients)
62	174	13 and 26	73	2.3
63	256	(<12-76)[a]	56	4.7[b]
64	65	24	78	13 of 405
65	317	(2-182)[a]	47	4.7
66	100	35	60	7
67	313	39	44	4
68	52	51	(34)[c]	(3)[c]
Totals	(n)1125		668 55	>4 >50

n = number of patients

a = range, months

b = changes in one patient thought to be caused by spasm (ref. 63).

c = number of lesions

Modified from MR Malinow, Am Heart J, 108;1523-1537, 1984 by permission of the author and the publisher, C.V. Mosby Company.

Table 2. Reports of Arteriographic Progression or Regression of Coronary Artery Disease Based on Prospective Study Design (Patients with Stable Lesions Not Shown)

Reference	Number of Patients	Study Interval (months)	Progression (% of Patients)	Regression (% of Patients)
70	22	24	23	14
71	25	12	44	20
69	12	36-48	33	0
72	1	9[a]	0	100
73	114	46	27	17
74	47	18	77	38
75	1	120	0	100
76	143	60	T25[b]	3.4
			P35	1.8
77	39	24	43	18
Total	(n) 290		44	20
			129	57

n = number of patients

a = Clinical indications for restudy

b = T, treated with cholestyramine and diet; P, placebo and diet

Modified from MR Malinow, Am Heart J, 108;1523-1537, 1984 by permission of the author and the publisher, C.V. Mosby Company.

coronary atherosclerosis (69), regression was recognized
in 57 instances, *i.e.*, in about 20% of the remaining patients.
Buchwald *et al* (70) reported regression in 3 of 24 hypercholesterolemic patients who underwent partial intestinal bypass
operations; plaques decreased in size or disappeared, and a
totally occluded left anterior descending coronary artery
(LAD) became patent. Raffenbeul *et al* (71) studied 25 patients
treated medically for unstable angina. In five patients,
stenosis regressed from an average of 82% to 55% in one year.
Roth and Kostuk (72) documented regression in a 46-year-old
man with recent onset of angina; angiography demonstrated
significant stenosis of the LAD. A repeat angiogram about
9 months after the first one showed a much smaller LAD lesion
and collateral circulation was no longer present. The authors
interpreted the changes as compatible with resorption of
thrombus superimposed on an atherosclerotic plaque.

Gohlke *et al* (73) described 114 patients under the age
of 40, who had coronary angiograms within 10 months of a
myocardial infarction and again around 4 years later. Progression was seen in 27% of the patients and regression in
17%. Brown *et al* studied practically all lesions observed
in clinically indicated coronary angiograms of 47 patients,
establishing variability of lesion analysis by computer-
assisted measurements. The method constitutes one of the
best procedures for quantifying coronary lesions; results
showed regression in 18 patients when they were studied prospectively 18 months after the initial angiogram.

The extent of regression was marked in the hypercholesterolemic patient of Buchwald *et al* (75), who underwent a
partial ileal bypass operation and was restudied 10 years
later; from 70% to 20% stenosis in the left circumflex artery,
from 45% to 20% stenosis in the middle segment of the right
coronary artery, and from 80% to 50% stenosis in the distal
right coronary artery.

One hundred forty-three patients with coronary artery
disease were randomized into cholestyramine-treated (n=72)
and placebo-treated (n=71) groups in the study reported by
Brensike *et al* (76). Regression was observed in both groups
but the incidence was twice as great in the treated as in the
placebo group (p not significant).

Arntzenius *et al* (77) studied 39 patients with angina
pectoris who had at least one coronary artery showing >50%
lumen diameter stenosis; they received a vegetarian diet with
a P:S ratio >2.0 and they were advised to stop smoking. The
angiogram was repeated 2 years later. The lesions were assessed
visually as well as by computer-assisted analysis. Progression,
no change, or regression were defined when the average stenosis
of all lesions measured in a patient changed in one direction.
From their Figure 2 (77), and using the criteria of average
diameter change of >0.2 mm (*i.e.*, 2 times the standard deviation of the differences between repeated measurements), progression was observed in 17 patients, no change in 15, and
regression in 7. At a recent symposium (78), the authors also
reported results on 163 individual lesions in these patients:
90 lesions progressed, 13 did not change, and 60 regressed;
progression and regression occurred simultaneously in 30 of
39 patients.

   c. Comparison of Retrospective and Prospective
     Studies

     The prevalence of regression seems very different
in patients studied retrospectively (≈4%, Table 1) and prospectively (20%, Table 2). However, the series showed marked
differences in clinical indications, study design, characteristic of patients, interval between angiographic studies,
methods of lesion assessment, and criteria for progression
and regression. Thus, drawing conclusions from such diverse
studies is not justified. A report from a single clinic (65)
provides more adequate information. Although the observation
was not designed to compare the results of serial angiograms
in patients studied electively or after clinical indications,
Table 3 suggests that regression is more common in the former
than in the latter patients.

  2. Regression in Other Arteries

     Regression has also been documented angiographically
in peripheral arteries of 91 patients (5). Results indicate
that progression occurred in more than 31 patients, and
regression in more than 21 patients; stable lesions were
observed in the remaining patients.

Table 3. Regression in Elective and Clinically-Indicated
Repeated Coronary Angiograms (Adapted from ref.
65)

Reevaluation	No. of Patients	Regression (n)	(%)
Elective	20	8	40.0*
Clinically-indicated	297	7	2.4*
Total	317	15	4.7

* $p(x^2) < 0.001$

3. Importance of Local Factors

As indicated above, progression and regression may
occur simultaneously in different plaques of certain individuals (63,65,76-78). The independent evolution of lesions
underlies the importance of local arterial factors in atherogenesis and hence in regression; local factors in human as
well as in experimental atherosclerosis were discussed
previously (5). Further illustration is provided in Figure
6, showing five main coronary lesions in a patient initially
studied because of angina pectoris (79); percent stenosis
was calculated from data kindly provided by Dr. D. G. Brown
(personal communication) assuming that lesions and arteries
were circular. Fifteen months later the severity of symptoms
increased. Repeated angiography revealed that one artery
(#1) became occluded. Two lesions (#2,3) became more stenotic
and two lesions (#4,5) may have shown progression and
regression, respectively, but the changes are small and might
be below methodological resolution. The figure also shows
that the average changes, *i.e.*, from 29 to 54% stenosis,
indicated by the horizontal bars, occurring in 15 months, or
1.7%/month, do not reflect the evolution of individual lesions
and thus fail to depict the clinically important occlusion of
artery #1, and the possible regressive changes of artery #5.

4. Examples of Angiographic Regression

Angiograms suggestive of regression of atherosclerosis in the coronary arteries have been published (5,16,17,66,

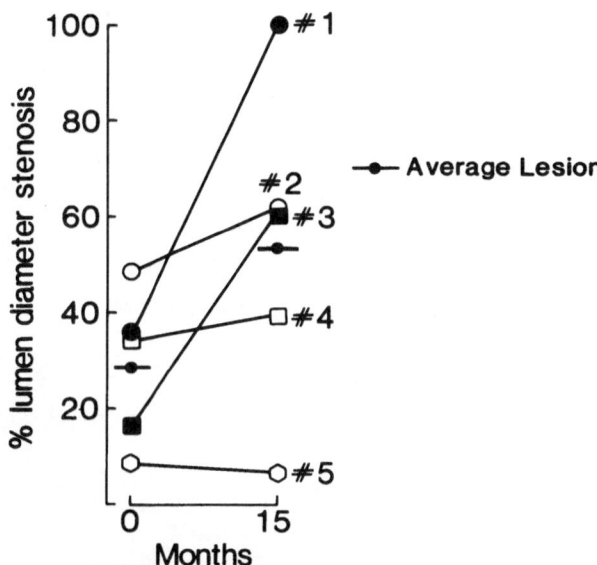

Figure 6. Percent lumen diameter stenosis in coronary artery lesions. Angiograms were performed in a patient with angina pectoris at 0 and 15 months because of clinical indication. Data derived from ref. 79 (see text).

68,72,73,80). The examples selected here have been kindly provided by the investigators mentioned below. The angiogram of one of the 7 patients with regression reported by VanHaecke et al(66) is shown in Figure 7. The patient had an acute anterior myocardial infarction 3 months prior to the angiogram (Figure 7, upper panel); a marked stenosis of the LAD (arrows) had disappeared. Figure 8 shows marked narrowing in the LAD 8 weeks after acute anteroseptal myocardial infarction (arrow, Panel A). Panel B shows an elective angiogram performed 4 years later; the stenosis is now less severe. Dr. H. Gohlke (personal communication) interpreted the changes as being compatible with resorption of a thrombus superimposed on an atherosclerotic plaque.

Figure 9 shows a remarkable disappearance of vascular calcifications in a 42-year-old man with chronic renal failure (81). The extensive calcification of vessels in the hand (arrow heads, panel A) have nearly disappeared 7 months later (panel B). Initially elevated blood calcium levels were maintained within normal range by hemodialysis, and

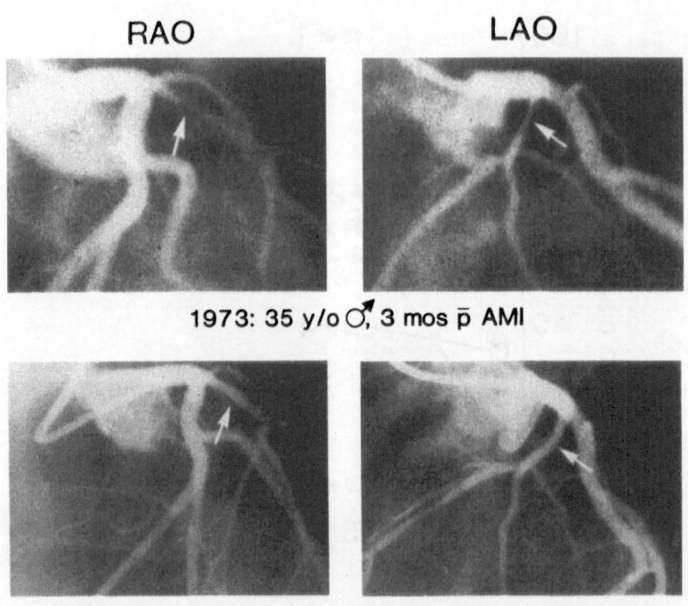

RAO LAO

1973: 35 y/o ♂, 3 mos p̄ AMI

1977

Figure 7. Angiograms of coronary arteries in a 35-year-old man, 3 months after an acute myocardial infarction. The arrows point to a tight stenosis in the proximal segment of the left anterior descending coronary artery, that had disappeared 4 years later. RAO, right anterior oblique; LAO, left anterior obliques. Reprinted with permission of Dr. J VanHaecke *et al* and Academic Press, European Heart Journal 4:547 (1983).

intake of vitamin D_3 and aluminum hydroxide. The angiocardiographic calcifications probably do not correspond to classical atherosclerosis but to medial calcification (82); the case demonstrates the potential for marked pathological vascular changes to decrease in a relatively short time interval.

  5. Advantages and Limitations of Angiographic Methods

    Sequential contrast angiography is at present the method of choice to establish the evolution of atherosclerotic plaques; newer methods under development may extend the invasive angiographic techniques (83,84). Moreover, comparison of arteriograms obtained at different times must rely on methodology that assumes that the following are identical at each examination: (1) magnification and positioning; (2) ratio of film density of background tissue to that of the

contrast medium in the vessel; (3) completeness of filling
by the contrast material in the vessel; (4) timing in relation
to the cardiac cycle or to the pulse wave; (5) arterial blood
pressure; (6) vascular tone; and (7) heart rate. Moreover,
the usual expression of results as percent stenosis related
to a supposedly uninvolved segment, greatly limits interpretation of angiographic findings. Finally due to the acknow-
ledged intra- and interobserver measurement variabilities,
it is common to accept as valid only large sequential changes
when coronary lesions are classified as grades, for instance,

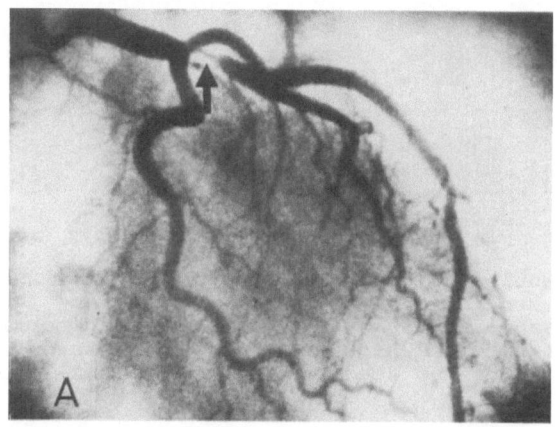

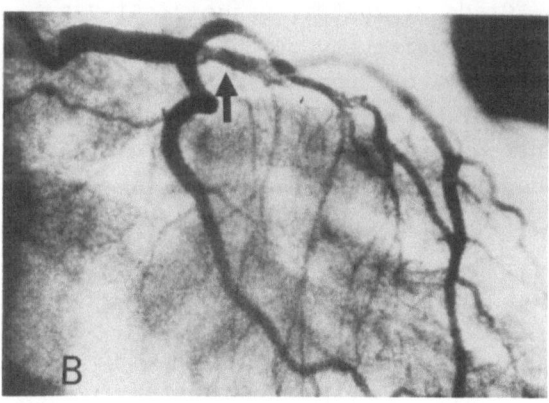

Figure 8. Coronary angiograms in the right anterior oblique
projection of a 40-year-old man, 8 weeks after an acute anteroseptal myocardial infarction. The tight stenosis in the
proximal segment of the left anterior descending coronary
artery (panel A, arrow) has almost disappeared 4 years later
(panel B, arrow). Angiograms kindly provided by Dr. H.
Gohlke from ref. 73.

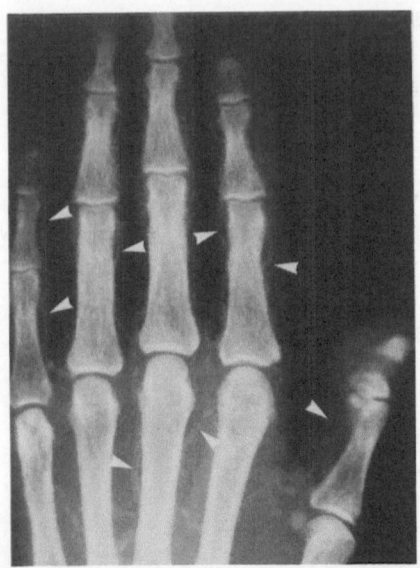 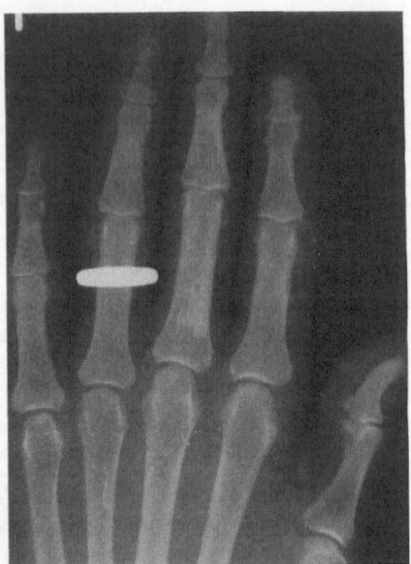

Nov. 1972   Sept. 1973

Figure 9.   Vascular calcification in the hand of a 42-year-
old man with chronic renal failure (arrow heads) (top panel)
had almost disappeared 8 months later after appropriate
therapy (lower panel).   Reproduced with permission of
Dr. R. Verberckmoes and Academic Press from Ann Intern Med.
1975; 82:529.

grade 1: 0-25%; Grade 2: 26-50%; Grade 3: 51-75%, etc.

Because of the low sensitivity of the grading methods, a

change from 45% to 30% or from 20% to 0% stenosis is usually

disregarded, but more precise methods of measurement might

reveal those changes as indicative of regression.   Methodologic

factors have been lucidly discussed by Blankenhorn and Sanmarco

(85), by Brown *et al* (74), and by Gould (86).

Although angiographic and postmortem findings have been compared in patients with CAD (87-92), there is lack of histologic data on angiographic regression. Thus, the enlargement of stenotic arterial segments revealed by sequential angiography could be due to different mechanisms which cannot always be accurately identified:

(1) plaque shrinkage, that is, depletion of lipids and reduction in cell numbers and in extracellular material (seen in animal experiments, 93-98);

(2) lysis or retraction of thrombi superimposed on atherosclerotic plaques;

(3) incorporation of thrombi into the arterial wall followed by organization, condensation and contraction, or channel formation;

(4) release of spasm;

(5) arterial ectasia or dilatation;

(6) medial thinning with outward bulging of the plaque; or

(7) plaque ulceration.

As a final consideration, it is recognized that "the angiographic analysis of...(atherogenesis) is immensely complicated by the number of biases involved" (99). Selection bias operates in patients initially studied usually because of the presence of angina; repeated angiography is generally carried out because of persistence of symptoms or unfavorable clinical situation. Thus, retrospective series are probably biased in favor of the most severe cases. An opposite bias of patient selection occurs with the natural evolution of disease leading, in certain cases, to early death. And, patients or doctors may refuse to submit to a potentially dangerous or expensive procedure, unless certain treatments, *i.e.* bypass surgery or angioplasty, are contemplated.

6. Future Needs

Analyses of the angiographic quantification of

coronary lesions have been published (74,85,86). Moreover, methods able to quantitate lesions *in vivo* in a similar way as outlined under A. Anatomical evidence (pg 436) is needed. This obviously will require the availability of sensitive non-invasive or minimally invasive methods that could be applied without risk to asymptomatic patients or at specified intervals to patients with CAD. In addition, the functional significance of arterial stenoses, and of non-obstructive atherosclerotic lesions (100), at rest or under increased metabolic requirements (86), needs to be established. The methods should provide data preferably "on-line", during the catheterization procedure. Finally, the correspondence of angiographic evolutionary changes with the pathological nature of lesions needs yet to be determined.

Pathogenesis of Regression

Since the anatomic basis for regression in humans is unknown, a discussion of its genesis must be conjectural. Experimental studies where variables can be controlled may be better suited, though, to provide the basis for its inter-pretation (101-104).

A. Role of Plasma Lipids in Angiographic Regression

Regression of cholesterol-induced atherosclerosis in nonhuman primates is observed when hypercholesterolemia is reduced to around 200 mg/dl for prolonged periods (95). This reduction is usually accomplished through removal of added cholesterol from the diet (93-98,101,102). Whether one could achieve such regression in humans by simply removing choles-terol from the diet needs to be tested. However, in view of the difficulties encountered when control of hypercholesterol-emia is attempted by diet modification alone (105), regression under these circumstances seems unlikely. In animals, regress-ion has also been induced by the addition of cholestyramine (106,107), alfalfa meal (95), or alfalfa saponins (108), to a cholesterol-containing diet. These substances interfered with the intestinal absorption of cholesterol (109-111). However, the relevance of regression data on animals to regression in humans depends heavily on the etiologic correspondence of experimentally induced and "spontaneous" human atherosclerosis (112).

Most retrospective series in humans were not designed to
permit analysis of risk factor intervention, and the role
of plasma lipids in regression could not be ascertained. Prospective studies were better suited to such an analysis. Factors probably involved in regression are reduced plasma cholesterol and LDL levels, and increased HDL levels (80,113,114).
Although this review deals only with plasma total cholesterol,
the conclusions probably are applicable to LDL levels. In
several studies, regression was observed much more frequently
when plasma cholesterol levels decreased, (75,80,113-116),
and when the ratio total cholesterol/HDL-C was changed favorably (77). However, it was not necessary to attain normal
levels for regression to occur. Thus, of the nine patients
reported to have regression of femoral atherosclerosis by
Barndt *et al* (114), four had cholesterolemia above 260 mg/dl.
In patients reported by Brensike *et al* (76) to have a favorable
evolution of coronary atherosclerosis, the average plasma
cholesterol level was reduced from 310 to 256 mg/dl; the
last average values are still indicative of elevated risk
(117). In the patient described by Buchwald *et al* (75),
remarkable regression was observed with cholesterolemia that
changed from 757 mg/dl (preoperatively) to between 450 and
608 mg/dl during the 10-year study. These observations
suggest that when plaques attain a certain size at a given
plasma cholesterol level, sustained reduction from that
level can be associated with regression, even if normal
cholesterolemia is not reached.

The mechanisms for removal of arterial lipids when
cholesterolemia is partially reduced are not completely
understood; it could entail removal by fat-laden macrophages
(118-119). Alternatively, since even cholesterol in advanced
atherosclerotic plaques is in dynamic equilibrium with plasma
cholesterol (120), arterial cholesterol removal may involve
[1] availability of an appropriate acceptor, such as HDL
particles (121); [2] hydrolysis of cholesterol esters (122),
which would provide free cholesterol for participation in
[1]; and [3]inhibition of cholesterol esterifying reactions
(122), which would increase the mass of free cholesterol
available for removal. How the reduced arterial cholesterol
content might affect the concentration of other lipids as

well as cellular proliferation---and secretion or
reabsorption of interstitial material---needs investigation.

Finally, regression probably not associated with
thrombus resolution seems to involve only minor changes in
the diameter of coronary stenotic lesions, likely to be in
the order of a fraction of a mm (77). These small diameter
changes, though, as earlier speculated by Roberts (1), may
have an important bearing on flow characteristics, since flow
is related to the fourth power of radius (86,100). As an
illustration, Table 4 shows that in a coronary artery with
70% lumen diameter stenosis, an increase in diameter of
0.2 mm would increase blood flow by 19%. Moreover, the
incidence of angina changed in an inverse way to the occurrence of regression, defined as an average enlarged stenosis
of 0.2 mm or more (78) in patients receiving dietary intervention for 2 years; whether the favorable clinical findings
were related to ensuing coronary hemodynamics or to other
independent factors needs to be investigated.

B. Regression Without Normalization of Blood Lipid
   Levels; Thrombus Resolution

Several investigators have hypothesized that
regression occurs independently of plasma lipid changes
(64,65,73). For instance, 15% of femoral artery lesions
with changes compatible with regression occurred in patients

Table 4. Hypothetical Coronary Flow Changes Brought by
         Regression in an Artery with 0.2 mm Increase in
         Lumen Diameter Stenosis (Initial Diameter = 3.0 mm)

	Before Regression	After Regression
Diameter (mm)	0.9	1.1
Lumen diameter stenosis (%)	70	63
% of Control Flow (a)	57	68
Δ Flow (%)		19

(a) Based on equation for low resistance distal vascular
    bed (86).

Table 5. Regression in Coronary Arteries Probably due to Resolution of Thrombus

References	No. of Cases	Type of Study	Cases with Regression (No. of Patients)	Probable Resolution of Thrombi (No. of Patients)	(%)
63	256	R	11	5	45
64	65	R	(11)[a]	(2)[a]	(18)[a]
65	317	R	15	13	87
67	313	R	12	3	25
70	22	P	3	1	33
72	1	P	1	1	100
74	47	P	18	4	22
77	39	P	7	0[b]	0
Totals	1062		67	27	40

R = retrospective

P = prospective

a = number of segments

b = 3/163 lesions not included in the data analysis, showed possible recanalization with sustained cholesterolemia around 290 mg/dl (115), and definitive angiographic regression was also observed in CAD patients with cholesterolemia around 290 mg/dl (76). If the arterial content of lipids did not change in the presence of elevated levels of plasma cholesterol, the most likely explanation is that one or more of the following occurred: retraction and lysis of thrombi, incorporation of thrombi into the arterial wall with subsequent condensation and contraction, and channel formation or other undefined factors (see Section C, below). These processes have been postulated in the resolution of coronary occlusive lesions in patients with myocardial infarction (123-127), as well as in the numerous patients studied in clinical trials of thrombolytic therapy (128,129). Thrombus resolution was probably thus involved in 43 of the 91 patients reviewed by Stary (130), in which decrease in coronary artery occlusion followed closely the infusion of streptokinase (see reviews in 131, 132). A detailed angiographic study of the sequence of events involved in the lysis of thrombi superimposed on ulcerated plaques is reported by Brown *et al* (133).

In the series reviewed on Tables 1 and 2, certain angiographic characteristics suggestive of the presence of thrombus were reported, and thrombus resolution was also suspected when total arterial occlusions changed to partial obstruction. These criteria were used in the construction of Table 5, indicating that in about 40% of reported cases of regression, resolution of thrombus may have been present. The relative proportion of the putative thrombus resolution seems variable among series of patients.

It seems likely that there might be a continuum from resolution, that is, retraction and lysis of thrombi, to incorporation of thrombi into the arterial wall and subsequent condensation and contraction (5). Only the latter could possibly be named regression of atherosclerosis, but both processes may occur simultaneously. It is tempting to speculate that---probably superimposed upon injured endothelium or a fissured plaque---thrombi incorporated into the arterial wall with subsequent condensation and contraction might be involved in progression and regression of atherosclerosis; the process could also include deposition and

resorption of lipids. Repetition of such cycles---causing
waxing and waning of atherosclerotic plaques (5)---might
restrict the lumen above a symptomatic threshold or, conversely, might render symptom-free a patient experiencing
ischemic episodes (72). The role that channel formation
within organized thrombi might play in restoring flow needs
to be evaluated.

C. Miscellaneous Mechanisms in Regression Not Primarily
   Involving Intimal Changes

   Arterial growth, ectasia, and medial thinning may
be associated with decreased luminal stenosis. Anatomic
descriptions of such phenomena, based on the interpretation
of postmortem findings, have been provided by Osborn (134),
Roberts (1), and Mann *et al* (135), and the phenomena have
been recently demonstrated in a series of pressure-fixed
coronary arteries by Glagov *et al* (136). Vasomotor activity, that is, relaxation of contracted smooth muscle cells,
can also enlarge luminal stenosis, especially when occurring
in less involved segments of coronary arteries having eccentric plaques (53). Any of the changes could be interpreted
as regression; their role in patients with reported regression
is unknown.

Conclusions

   From the voluminous anatomical data on human atherosclerotic lesions, it is possible---using imaginative reconstruction (22)---to describe how plaques may change during
life span. Interpretation of available pathologic data in
groups of individuals suggests that although atherosclerosis
usually progresses with age, it may stabilize or even
regress in certain subjects with metabolic abnormalities
associated with body weight reduction (34,36), with cancer
(37), or with other undefined mechanisms (25,136). However,
bias in the selection of cases and other methodological
limitations make interpretation of anatomical data on regression inferential at best.

The evolution of atherosclerotic plaques can also be inferred from serial angiographic studies. Regression of atherosclerosis, $i.e.$, enlargement of a previously stenotic arterial segment, has been documented in over 100 cases by serial angiography, but possible mechanisms involved need investigation. Lipid depletion, other changes in plaque composition, thrombus resolution and certain undefined factors may be implicated. Methods performed without risk to living individuals need to be developed in order to obtain sequential, accurate measurements of the size and composition of plaques. A dynamic view of atherogenesis suggests that injury and repair occurring in the same artery, or in other arterial territories, may lead to simultaneous progression, stabilization and regression of atherosclerotic plaques. Anatomical data correlated to the angiographic evolution of plaques is sorely needed.

Although a series of patients who underwent dietary modification for 2 years apparent regression was associated with decrease in angina severity (78), questions still remain about the clinical implications of atherosclerosis regression (5). How common is it? What are the hemodynamic consequences? How can we influence its course? Certain of these questions may be addressed in nine clinical trials in progress (137), involving almost 1,500 patients allocated to placebo and treated groups, in which major changes in blood lipid levels are expected after dietary intervention, medication, or partial ileal bypass operations. Sequential angiograms of the coronary, carotid, pelvic and femoral arteries will probably permit elimination of many uncertainties concerning regression. However, it seems likely that until atherosclerosis regression can be consistently induced, a more easily attainable goal will be to use interventions that prevent progression of the disease (138).

REFERENCES
1. Roberts WC (1975) The coronary arteries in coronary heart disease. Morphologic observations. Pathobiol Ann 5:249-282.

2. Glagov S and Zarins CK (1982) Natural history of human
    atherosclerotic lesions: changes in luminal configura-
    tion. In: Noninvasive techniques for assessment of
    atherosclerosis in peripheral, carotid and coronary
    arteries. Budinger et al Eds. Raven Press, New York
    pgs 15-19

3. Blankenhorn DH (1981) Will atheroma regress with diet
    and exercise? Am J Surg 141:644-645

4. Harlan WR and Landis JR (1982) What the epidemiologist
    and clinical interventionist expect and need for studies
    of atherosclerotic disease. In: Noninvasive techniques
    for assessment of atherosclerosis in peripheral, carotid,
    and coronary arteries. Budinger et al, Eds. Raven
    Press, New York, pgs 41-47

5. Malinow MR (1984) Atherosclerosis: Progression, regres-
    sion and resolution. Am Heart J 108:1523-1537

6. Crawford DW and Blankenhorn DH (1979) Regression of
    atherosclerosis (review). Ann Rev Med 30:289-300

7. Gotto AM (1981) Regression of atherosclerosis. Am J
    Med 70:989-991

8. Blankenhorn DH (1985) Noninvasive atherosclerosis
    assessment for controlled clinical trials. In: Drugs
    affecting lipid metabolism. VIII. Kritchevsky et al,
    Eds. Plenum Press, New York

9. Kuo PT (1982) Regression, retardation of atherosclero-
    sis progression, and collateral circulation. Their
    functional importance. Chest 81:3-4

10. Malinow MR (1984) Regression of atherosclerotic lesions.
    Experimental studies and observations in humans. MR
    Malinow and VH Blaton, Eds, Plenum Press, New York

11. Blankenhorn DH (1978) Reversibility of latent athero-
    sclerosis. Studies by femoral angiography in humans.
    Mod Concepts in Cardiovasc Dis 47:79-84

12. Mustard J, Fraser KR, Raelene L, et al (1983) Vessel
    injury, thrombosis and the progression and regression
    of atherosclerotic lesions. In: Clinical Diagnosis of
    Atherosclerosis. MG Bond et al, Eds., Springer Verlag,
    New York

13. Barth JD (1986) Progression and Regression of Coronary
    Atherosclerosis. Role of Diet, Lipoproteins and Lipases.
    Nijmegen

14. Wissler RW and Vesselinovitch D (1977) Regression of
    atherosclerosis in experimental animals and man. Mod
    Concepts of Cardiovasc Dis 46:27-32

15. Malinow RM (1981) Regression of atherosclerosis in
    humans: Fact or myth? Circ 64:1-3

16. Malinow RM and Connor WE (1985) Regression of atheroscler-
    osis: what is the evidence? In: Coronary Heart Disease:
    prevention, complications and treatment. WE Connor and
    JD Bristow, Eds., JB Lippincott, Philadelphia, pgs
    215-230

17. Malinow MR (1984) Regression of atherosclerosis in humans:
    the evidence. In: Recent Advances in Cardiology, Vol 9
    D Rowlands, Ed, Churchill Livingstone, London, pgs 227-
    239

18. Geer JC and Haust MD (1972) Smooth muscle cells in
    atherosclerosis. Monographs on Atherosclerosis, Vol 2,
    OJ Pollak, HS Simms, and JE Kirk, Eds, S. Karger,
    Basel, pgs 1-140

19. McGill Jr, HC, Geer JC, and Strong JP (1963) Natural history of human atherosclerotic lesions. In: Atherosclerosis and its origins. M Sanders, Ed., Academics, New York, pgs 39-65

20. Holman RL, McGill Jr, HC, Strong JP *et al* (1958) The early aortic lesions as seen in New Orleans in the middle of the 20th century. Am J Pathol 34:209-229

21. Robertson Jr AL (1977) Section II. The pathogenesis of human atherosclerosis. In: Scope monograph. Atherosclerosis, AM Gotto Ed., Upjohn Company, Kalamazoo, pgs 38-54

22. Woolf N (1982) Pathology of Atherosclerosis. T Crawford, Ed., Butterworth Scientific, London

23. Smith E (1965) The influence of age and atherosclerosis on chemistry of aortic intima. Part 1. The lipid. J Atheroscler Res 5:224-240

24. Constantinides P (1984) Ultrastructural Pathobiology, Elsevier, New York

25. Hueper WC (1945) Arteriosclerosis. The anoxemia Theory. Arch Pathol 39:187-205

26. Geer JC (1945) Fine structure of human aortic intimal thickening and fatty streaks. Lab Invest 14:1764-1783

27. Geer JC, McGill Jr HC, Robertson WB *et al* (1968) Histologic characteristics of coronary artery fatty streaks. In: The geographic pathology of atherosclerosis, HC McGill Jr, Ed. Williams and Wilkins Co., Baltimore, pgs 565-570

28. Strong JP and McGill Jr HC (1963) The natural history of aortic atherosclerosis: relationship to race, sex and coronary lesions in New Orleans. Exp Mol Pathol 1:15-27

29. McGill Jr HC (1968) Fatty streaks in the coronary arteries and aorta. In: The geographic pathology of atherosclerosis, HC McGill Jr, Ed., Williams and Wilkins Co, Baltimore, pgs 560-564

30. Malinow MR (1984) Regression of atherosclerosis in humans: anatomical evidence from postmortem studies. In: Regression of atherosclerotic lesions, MR Malinow and VH Blaton, Eds., Plenum Press, New York, pgs 329-337

31. Mitchell JRA, Schwartz CJ and Zinger A (1964) Relationship between aortic plaques and age, sex and blood pressure. Br Med J 1:205-209

32. Aschoff L (1924) Lectures of pathology (delivered in the U.S., 1924), Hoeber Medical Division, Harper and Row Publishers, Inc., New York, pgs 131-153

33. Beitske H (1928) Zur entstehung der atherosklerose. Virchows Arch (Pathol Anat) 267:625-647

34. Wilens SL (1947) Reabsorption of arterial atheromatous deposits in wasting disease. Am J Pathol 23:793-804

35. Vartianen I, Kanerva K (1947) Arteriosclerosis and war-time. Ann Med Internae Fenniae 36:748-758

36. Waller BF, Brosius FC, and Roberts WC (1981) Massive obesity (greater than 160 kg) not an accelerator of coronary atherosclerosis. Comparison of amounts of coronary narrowing in massive obesity, cachexia and normal weight individuals. Lab Invest 44:A72-A73

37. Wanscher O, Clemmesen J, Nielson A (1951) Negative correlation between atherosclerosis and carcinoma. Br J Cancer 5:172-181

38. Eakins D (1965) Atherosclerosis and malignant disease. Br J Cancer 19:9-14

39. Klassen AC, Loewensen RB and Resch JA (1973) Cerebral atherosclerosis in selected chronic disease states. Atherosclerosis 18:321-336

40. Restrepo C, Montenegro MR, Solberg LA (1968) Athero-sclerosis in persons with selected diseases. Lab Invest 18:552-559

41. Parrish HM (1961) Epidemiology of ischemic heart disease among white males. Part I. Relationship between coronary atherosclerosis and cancer of various sites. J Chron Dis 14:311-325

42. Parrish HM, Goldner JC, Silberg SL (1966) Coronary atherosclerosis and cancer in women. Arch Intern Med 117:639-642

43. Vihert AM, Zhadanov S, Matova EE (1969) Atherosclerosis of the aorta and coronary vessels of the heart in cases of various diseases. J Atheroscler Res 9:179-192

44. Lober PH (1953) Pathogenesis of coronary sclerosis. Arch Pathol 55:357-383

45. Malinow MR, Senner JW (1983) Arterial pathology in cancer patients suggests atherosclerosis regression. Med Hypotheses 11:253-257

46. Davies MJ and Thomas AC (1985) Plaque fissuring--the cause of acute myocardial infarction, sudden ischemic death, and crescendo angina. Br Heart J 53:363-373

47. Fuster V, Steel PM, Chesebro JH (1985) Role of plate-lets and thrombosis in coronary atherosclerotic disease and sudden death. A Am Coll Cardiol Suppl 5:175B-184B

48. Cornhill JF and Bond MG (1983) Morphology: morphometric analysis of pathology specimens. In: Clinical diagnosis of atherosclerosis: quantitative methods of evaluation. MG Bond et al, Eds., Springer-Verlag, New York, pgs 67-68

49. Thomas AC and Davies MJ (1985) Post-mortem investigation and quantification of coronary artery disease. Histopathology 9:959-976

50. Robbins SL and Rodriguez FL (1966) Problems in the quanti-tation of coronary arteriosclerosis. Am J Cardiol 18:153-159

51. McMahan CA (1961) Paper presented at the International Population Conference, New York University, Sept 11-16 quoted by McGill et al in ref 19

52. Insull Jr W (1983) Universal reference standards for measuring atherosclerotic lesions: the quest for the gold standard. In: Clinical Diagnosis of Atherosclerosis, MG Bond et al, Eds., Springer-Verlag, New York

53. Saner H, Gobel F, and Salomonowitz E (1985) The disease-free wall in coronary atherosclerosis: its relation to degree of obstruction. JACC 6:1096-1099

54. Strong JP and Guzman MA (1980) Decrease in coronary atherosclerosis in New Orleans. Lab Invest 43:297-301

55. Elveback L and Lie JT (1984) Continued high incidence of coronary artery disease at autopsy in Olmsted County, Minnesota, 1950 to 1979. Circ 70:345-349

56. Bemis CE, Gorlin R, Kemp HG et al (1973) Progression of coronary artery disease. A clinical arteriographic study. Circ 47:455

57. Kimbiris D, Lavine P, VenDen Broek H et al (1974) Devolutionary pattern of coronary atherosclerosis in patients with angina pectoris. Am J Cardiol 33:7-11

58. Marchandise B, Bourassa MG, Chaitman RB *et al* (1978)
    Angiographic evaluation of natural history of normal
    arteries and mild coronary atherosclerosis. Am J
    Cardiol 41:216-220
59. Moise A, Therous P, Taeymans Y *et al* (1983) Unstable
    angina and progression of coronary atherosclerosis.
    N Engl J Med 309:685-689
60. Nash DT, Caldwell N, Ancona D (1974) Accelerated
    coronary artery disease arteriographically proved.
    NY State J Med 74:947-950
61. Rosch J, Antonovic R, Trenouth RS *et al* (1976) The
    natural history of coronary artery stenosis. Radiol
    119:513-520
62. Gensini GF, Esente P, Kelly A (1974) A natural history
    of coronary disease in patients with and without coronary
    bypass graft surgery. Circ 49 and 50 (Suppl II):II-98
    to II-102
63. Bruschke AVG, Wijers TS, Kolsters W *et al* (1981) The
    anatomic evolution of coronary artery disease demonstrated
    by coronary arteriography in 256 nonoperated patients.
    Circ 63:527-536
64. Shub C, Vliestra RE, Smith HC *et al* (1981) The unpredic-
    table progression of symptomatic coronary artery disease.
    A serial clinical-angiographic analysis. Mayo Clin Proc
    56:155-160
65. Kramer JR, Kitazume H, Proudfit WL *et al* (1983) Progression
    and regression of coronary atherosclerosis: relation to
    risk factors. Am Heart J 105:134-144
66. VanHaecke J, Piessens J, Van de Werf F *et al* (1983)
    Angiographic evolution of coronary atherosclerosis in
    nonoperated patients. Eur Heart J 4:547-556
67. Moise A, Theroux P, Taeymans Y *et al* (1984) Clinical and
    angiographic factors associated with progression of cor-
    onary artery disease. J Amer Coll Cardiol 3:659-667
68. Singh RN (1984) Progression of coronary atherosclerosis-
    clues to pathogenesis from serial coronary arterio-
    graphy. Br Heart J 52:451-461
69. Kuo PT, Hayase K, Kostis JB *et al* (1979) Use of combined
    diet and colestipol in long-term (7-7 1/2 years) treat-
    ment of patients with type II hyperlipoproteinemia.
    Circ 59:199-211
70. Buchwald H, Moore RB, Varco RL (1974) Surgical treatment
    of hyperlipidemia. Circ 49: (Suppl 1) 1-1 to 1-37
71. Raffenbeul W, Smith, LR, Rogers WJ *et al* (1979)
    Quantitative coronary arteriography. Coronary anatomy
    of patients with unstable angina pectoris reexamined
    1 year after optimal medical therapy. Am J Cardiol
    43:699-707
72. Roth D, Kostuk WJ (1980) Noninvasive and invasive
    demonstration of spontaneous regression of coronary
    artery disease. Circ 62:888-896
73. Gohlke H, Stürzenhofecker P, Görnandt L *et al*. (1980)
    Progression und Regression der koronaren Herzerkrankung
    im chronischen Infarktstadium bei Patienten unter 40.
    Jahre. Schweiz Med Wochenschr 110:1663-1665
74. Brown BG, Bolson EL, Dodge HT (1982) Arteriographic
    assessment of coronary atherosclerosis. Review of cur-
    rent methods, their limitations, and clinical appli-
    cations. Arteriosclerosis 2:2-15

75. Buchwald H, Moore RB, Rucker Jr, RD, *et al* (1983) POSCH Arteriography Review Panel: Clinical angiographic regression of atherosclerosis after partial ileal bypass. Atherosclerosis 16:117-128

76. Brensike JF, Levy RI, Kelsey SF, *et al* (1984) Effects of therapy with cholestyramine on progression of coronary arteriosclerosis: Results of the NHLBI Type II Coronary Intervention Study. Circ 69:313-324

77. Arntzenius AC, Kromhout D, Barth J, *et al* (1985) Diet, lipoproteins and the progression of coronary atherosclerosis. The Leiden Intervention Trial. N Engl J Med 312:805-811

78. Barth JD and Arntzenius AC (1985) Regression of human atherosclerosis: an update on clinical, angiographic and pathological aspects. In: Regression of Atherosclerosis, Buenos Aires

79. Brown BG, Bolson E, Frimer M *et al* (1977) Quantitative coronary arteriography: estimation of dimensions, hemodynamic resistance, and atheroma mass of coronary artery lesions using the arteriogram and digital computation. Circ 55:329-37

80. Olsson AG, Carlson LA, Erikson U, *et al* (1982) Regression of computer estimated femoral atherosclerosis after pronounced serum lipid lowering in patients with asymptomatic hyperlipidaemia. Lancet 1:1311

81. Verberckmoes R, Bouillon R, Krempien B (1975) Disappearance of vascular calcifications during treatment of renal osteodystrophy. Two patients treated with high doses of vitamin D and aluminum hydroxide. Ann Intern Med 82:529-533

82. Massry S, Gordon A, and Coburn J (1970) Vascular calcification and peripheral necrosis in a transplant recipient. Am J of Med 49:416

83. Selzer RH (1983) Atherosclerosis quantitation by computer image analysis. In: Clinical Diagnosis of Atherosclerosis: quantitative methods of evaluation. MG Bond *et al*, Eds., Springer-Verlag, New York, pgs 43-64

84. Budinger TF, Berson AS, Ringqvist I, *et al*, Eds. (1982) Noninvasive techniques for assessment of atherosclerosis in peripheral, carotid, and coronary arteries. Raven Press, New York

85. Blankenhorn DH and Sanmarco ME (1979) Editorial: angiography for study of lipid-lowering therapy. Circ 59:212-214

86. Gould KL (1985) Quantification of coronary artery stenosis *in vivo*. Circ Res 57:342-353

87. Vlodaver Z, Frech R, Van Tassel RA, *et al* (1973) Correlation of the antemortem coronary arteriogram and the postmortem specimen. Circ 47:162-169

88. Grondin CM, Dyrda I, Pasternac A *et al* (1974) Discrepancies between cineangiographic and postmortem findings in patients with coronary artery disease and recent myocardial revascularzation. Circ 49:703-708

89. Schwartz JN, Kong Y, Hackel DB *et al* (1975) Comparison of angiographic and postmortem findings in patients with coronary artery disease. Am J Cardiol 36:174-178

90. Levin DC and Fallon JT (1982) Significance of the angiographic morphology of localized coronary stenoses. Histopathologic correlations. Circ 66:316-320

91. Fisher CM (1983) Correlation of antemortem angiography with pathology. In: Clinical Diagnosis of Atherosclerosis, MG Bond *et al* Eds., Springer-Verlag, pgs 265-282

92. Zarins CK, Zatina MA, and Glagov S (1983) Correlation of postmortem angiography with pathologic anatomy. In: Clinical Diagnosis of Atherosclerosis, MG Bond *et al*, Eds., Springer-Verlag, New York, pgs 282-303

93. Wissler RW and Vellelinovitch D (1976) Studies of regression of advanced atherosclerosis in experimental animals and man. Ann NY Acad Sci 275:363-378

94. St Clair, RW (1983) Atherosclerosis regression in animal models: current concepts of cellular and biochemical mechanisms. Prog Cardiovasc Dis 26:109-132

95. Malinow MR, McLaughlin P, Naito HK, *et al* (1978) Effect of alfalfa meal on shrinkage (regression) of atherosclerotic plaques during cholesterol feeding in monkeys. Atherosclerosis 30:27-43

96. Clarkson TB, Lehner NDM, Wagner WD *et al* (1979) Study of atherosclerosis regression in *Macaca mulatta*. 1. Design of experiment and lesion induction. Exp Mol Pathol 30:360-385

97. Eggen DA, Strong JP, Newman III WP, *et al* (1974) Regression of diet-induced fatty streaks in rhesus monkeys. Lab Invest 31:294-301

98. Stary HC (1977) Ultrastructural changes in the lipid inclusion of arterial smooth muscle cells after reduction of high serum cholesterol levels. Prog Biochem Pharmacol 13:46-51

99. Kramer JR, Kitazume H, Proudfit WL *et al* (1983) Segmental analysis of the rate of progression in patients with progressive coronary atherosclerosis. Am Heart J 106:1427-1431

100. Sumner DS (1983) Correlation of lesion configuration with functional significance. In: Clinical Diagnosis of Atherosclerosis. MG Bond *et al*, Eds., Springer-Verlag, New York, pgs 227-258

101. Stary HC, Eggen DA, and Strong JP (1977) The mechanism of atherosclerosis regression, In: Atherosclerosis IV, G Schettler, Y Goto, Y Hata, *et al*, Eds., Springer-Verlag, Berlin, pgs 394-404

102. Stary HC (1979) Regression of atherosclerosis in primates. Virchows Arch (Anat Pathol) 383:117-134

103. Malinow MR (1980) Atherosclerosis: regression in non-human primates. Circ Res 46:311-320

104. Armstrong ML (1976) Regression of atherosclerosis. Atherosclerosis Reviews 1:137-182

105. Havel RJ and Kane JP (1982) Therapy of hyperlipidemic states. Annu Rev Med 33:417-433

106. Wissler RW, Vesselinovtich D, Borensztajin J *et al* (1975) Regression of severe atherosclerosis in cholestyramine-treated rhesus monkeys with or without a low-fat, low-cholesterol diet (abstr). Circ 52: (Suppl II) 16

107. Malinow MR, McLaughlin P, McNulty WP *et al* (1978) Treatment of established atherosclerosis during cholesterol feeding in monkeys. Atheroscler 31:185-193

108. Malinow MR, McLaughlin P, Stafford C *et al*, (1983) Effects of alfalfa saponins on regression of atherosclerosis. In: Rheinisch-Westfalische Academie der

Wissenschaften, Abhandlung Band 70. Second Munster International Arteriosclerosis Symposium: Clinical implications of recent research results in arterio- sclerosis. WH Hauss and RW Wissler, Eds., Opladen, West Germany,West Deutscher Verlag, pgs 241-254

109. Malinow MR, McLaughlin P, Papworth L *et al* (1977) Effect of alfalfa saponins on intestinal cholesterol absorption in rats. Am J Clin Nutr 30:2061-2067

110. Malinow MR, McLaughlin P, Stafford C, *et al* (1979) Comparative effects of alfalfa saponins and alfalfa fiber on cholesterol absorption in rats. Am J Clin Nutr 32:1810-1812

111. Malinow MR, Connor WE, McLaughlin P, *et al* (1981) Cholesterol and bile acid balance in *Macaca fascicularis*: Effects of alfalfa saponins. J Clin Invest 67:156-162

112. Malinow MR (1983) Experimental models of atherosclero- sis regression. Atherosclerosis 48:105-118

113. Olsson AG, Erikson U, Helmius G, *et al* (1984) Regression of femoral atherosclerosis in humans: Methodological and clinical problems associated with studies on femoral atherosclerosis development as assessed by angiograms. In: Regression of Atherosclerotic Lesions. Plenum Press, New York, pgs 311-328

114. Brandt R, Blankenhorn DH, Crawford DW, *et al* (1979) Regression and progression of early femoral atherosclero- sis in treated hyperlipoproteinemic patients. Ann Intern Med 86:139-146

115. Duffield RGM, Lewis B, Millar NE, *et al* (1983) Treatment of hyperlipidaemia retards progression of symptomatic femoral atherosclerosis. A randomized controlled trial. Lancet 2:639-641

116. DePalma RG, Insull W, Bellon EM, *et al* (1972) Animal models for the study of progression and regression of atherosclerosis. Surgery 72:268-278

117. Castelli WP and Moran RF (1971) Lipid studies for assess- ing the risk of cardiovascular disease and hyperlipidemia. Human Pathol 2:153-164

118. Gerrity RG and Naito HK (1980) Lipid clearance from fatty streak lesions by foam cell migration. Artery 8:215-219

119. Faggiotto A, Ross R, and Harker L (1984) Studies of hypercholesterolemia in the nonhuman primate. I. Changes that lead to fatty streak formation. Arteriosclerosis 4:323-340

120. Jagannathan SN, Connor WE, Baker WH, *et al* (1974) The turnover of cholesterol in human atherosclerotic arteries. J Clin Invest 54:366-377

121. Stein O, Vanderhoek J, and Stein Y (1976) Cholesterol content and sterol synthesis in human skin fibroblasts and rat aortic smooth muscle cells exposed to lipoprotein- depleted serum and high density apolipoprotein/phospho- lipid mixtures. Biochim Biophys Acta 431:347-358

122. Brown MS, Goldstein JL (1973) Recanalization in a coronary artery Thrombus. JAMA 224:1152-1155

123. Spring DA, Thomsen JH (1973) Recanalization in a coronary artery thrombus. JAMA 224:1152-1155

124. Henderson RR, Hansing CE, Razavi M, *et al* (1983) Resolution of an obstructive coronary lesion as demon- strated by selective angiography in a patient with transmural myocardial infarction. Am J Cardiol 31:785-788

468

125. Kavanagh-Gray D (1974) Angiographic evidence of coronary occlusion and resolution. Can Med Assoc J 110:945-946

126. Smith ND and De Mots H (1979) Spontaneous return of patency in a completely occluded artery. Chest 76:705

127. DeWood MA, Spores J, Notske R, *et al* (1980) Prevalence of total coronary occlusion during the early hours of transmural myocardial infarction. N Engl J Med 303:897-902

128. Rentrop KP, Feit F, Blanke H, *et al* (1984) Effects of intracoronary streptokinase and intra coronary nitroglycerin infusion on coronary angiographic patterns and mortality in patients with acute myocardial infarction. N Engl J Med 311:1457-1463

129. Smalling RW (1983) Sustained improvement in left ventricular function and mortality by intracoronary streptokinase administration during evolving myocardial infarction. Circ 68:131-138

130. Stary HC (1984) Comparison of the morphology of atherosclerotic lesions in the coronary arteries of man with morphology of lesions produced and regressed in experimental primates. In: Regression of Athero-sclerotic Lesions. MR Malinow and VH Blaton, Eds., Plenum Press, New York, pgs 235-254

131. Rentrop KP (1985) Thrombolytic therapy in patients with acute myocardial infarction. Circ 71:627-631

132. Furberg CD (1984) Clinical value of intracoronary streptokinase. Am J Cardiol 53:626-627

133. Brown BG, Gallery CA, Badger RS, *et al* (1986) Incomplete lysis of thrombus in the moderate underlying atherosclerotic lesions during intracoronary infusion of streptokinase for acute myocardial infarction: Quantitative angiographic observations. Circ 73:653-661

134. Osborn GR (1963) The incubation period of coronary thrombosis. Butterworth and Co., Ltd., London, Pg 190

135. Mann GV, Spoerry A, Gray M *et al* (1972) Atherosclerosis in the Masai. Am J Epidemiol 95:26-37

136. Glagov S, Weisenberg E, Kolletis G, *et al* (1986) Compensatory enlargement of human atherosclerotic coronary arteries prevents narrowing of the lumen. Fed Proceed 45:583

137. Azen S, Blankenhorn DH, Nessim S (1984) Status of con-trolled clinical trials in peripheral vessel athero-sclerosis. In: Regression of Atherosclerotic Lesions. MR Malinow and VH Blaton, Eds., Plenum Press, New York, pgs 263-275

138. Lipid Research Clinics Program (1984) The Lipid Research Clinics coronary prevention trial results. I. Reduction in incidence of coronary heart disease. JAMA 252:351-364

139. Falk E (1983) Plaque rupture with severe preexisting stenosis precipitating coronary thrombosis. Br Heart J 50:127-134

140. Benson RL (1926) Present status of coronary arterial disease. Arch Pathol Lab Med 2:876-916

141. Saphir O, Priest WS, Hamburger WM, *et al* (1935) Coronary arteriosclerosis, coronary thrombosis and the resulting myocardial changes. Am Heart J 10:567-595

30
Adaptive Responses of the Artery Wall as Human Atherosclerosis Develops

Mark L. Armstrong, Marjorie B. Megan, and Donald D. Heistad

When we think of atherosclerosis as a morphologic
process, several images come to mind. We see an angiopathy
that affects the intimal coat of certain arteries, chiefly
the aorta and the first three orders of its branches (1,2).
We see an intimal process that is hyperplastic as well as
infiltrative, that starts from inconspicuous precursor
lesions (3) and progresses to a predominantly fibrous plaque
stage (4). With plaque growth, we see narrowing of the
vascular lumen. Finally, we see progression of luminal
narrowing to the point of hemodynamic compromise, causing
tissue ischemia or necrosis with ensuing symptoms or death.

It is the early phase of this familiar story of lesion
progression that we wish to re-examine, in order to see how
it fits currently available morphologic data on human
atherosclerosis. We will present evidence that the early
phase of plaque formation in atherosclerosis may be accompanied
by adaptive responses of the involved arterial wall, and that
a process of remodeling of the wall may attenuate lesion
encroachment on the lumen and forestall narrowing of the
luminal channel until continuing plaque growth and evolution
reach a stage at which the adaptive responses fail.

Research was supported by the National Institutes of Health
under Arteriosclerosis Specialized Center of Research Grant
HL 14230 and Research Grant HL 16066.

We will show data that suggest two aspects of arterial
remodeling in atherosclerosis: 1) adaptive enlargement of the
transverse area of arteries subjected to development of
atherosclerotic plaques, and 2) medial thinning that is in
part an adaptive response rather than pure atrophy. If
such remodeling is the rule in the early phases of human
plaque growth, it will modify our understanding of this phase
of atherogenesis.

Previous Views of Artery Size in Atherosclerosis
     The atherosclerotic plaque is most commonly viewed as
a lesion of increasing size in the vessel of unchanging transverse area. Yet even in adult life the transverse area of
arteries is potentially susceptible to change. For example,
the transverse area increases markedly with the diffuse
ectasia of extreme age and the cross-sectional area enlarges
greatly in aneurysm formation as part of atherosclerosis.
     Aside from such obvious causes of enlargement, there
is a less well understood kind of arterial enlargement that
has been described in adults who are not aged. Because of
this change the aortic lumen may increase 40% during the
presenile adult years (9). Cross-sectional area is described
as increasing both without reference to (5), and in the
presence of (6), atherosclerotic plaques. Thus, a relationship of this dilated condition to atherosclerotic plaques
has been uncertain. The histologic picture is an apparent
change in elastic tissue with no special medial cell abnormalities. When atherosclerosis was present in this condition
it was termed "wide atherosclerosis" (6) (referring to the
wide lumen), in contrast to "narrow atherosclerosis" seen
in younger persons. The conclusion from these and similar
observations (7,8) is that in the adult years there may be
an increase in the transverse area of arteries related to
presenile changes in elastic properties of the vessel that
could alter the consequences of atherosclerotic plaques.
     Young and associates described a more consistent rela-
tionship between the transverse area of arteries and lesion
size (10-12). They found highly significant correlations
in both coronary and cerebral arteries between the amount of
plaque and the transverse area of the artery. The relationship,

however, seemed to be that of arterial size determining lesion
size, and these investigators concluded that the outer diameter of the vessel wall was not increased by atherosclerotic
plaques (11). In their view, increasing lesion size was
equivalent to increasing encroachment on the lumen.

A Re-Examination of Transverse Arterial Area and Atherosclerotic Plaques

Thus, these older observations seem to be simple
glosses on the prevailing view that atherosclerotic plaques
characteristically lead directly to luminal stenosis.
Recently, Bond and associates proposed a different effect
of plaques in studies of experimental primate atherosclerosis
(13). They found that diet-induced atherosclerosis in nonhuman primates caused consistent changes in size of the
portion of the artery enclosed by the internal elastic lamina:
intimal thickening occurred, as expected, but there was also
an enlargement of the cross-sectional area bounded by the
internal elastic lamina. The lumen remained large because
the area within the internal elastic lamina was enlarged to
contain both lesion and a lumen of normal size (Table 1).

Table 1. Transverse Area of Coronary Arteries in
         Experimental Atherosclerosis

Artery	Intimal Area	ILEL Area[1]	Lumen Area
Normal	0.02 ± 0.03	0.71 ± 0.12	0.70 ± 0.12
Athero-sclerotic	0.93 ± 0.45	1.59 ± 0.66	0.66 ± 0.01

[1] Area within internal elastic lamina.
   (Adapted from Bond *et al.*, 1981)

The surprise in this and subsequent studies (14-17) lay
in the fairly consistent outward displacement of the media.
Some of these experimental lesions were large and they bulged
into the lumen in immersion-fixed specimens, but in specimens
fixed at physiologic distending pressures there was little
bulge inward and the lumen was quite normal. Thus, the total
cross-sectional size of the vessel along an arterial segment

tended to correlate with the size of the lesion at a given site and the lumen area in diseased segments remained essentially equal to the lumen area of normal arteries.

These are experimental studies. We cite them because we believe that they are potentially relevant to the evolution of the human atherosclerotic plaque. We should note that in studies of nonhuman primates an increase in transverse area of the artery with preservation of lumen size is now recognized as the most common response to experimental atherosclerosis. It is seen within several species of the macaque genus and among several genera of Old World monkeys. Comparable information under experimentally controlled conditions is not available in humans. What is the likelihood that human atherosclerotic arteries follow this model?

Evidence has been obtained that a similar increase in transverse artery area may also occur in human atherosclerosis. We will note what has been found in three laboratories. At the University of Iowa, high frequency echoarteriograms have been obtained intraoperatively during heart surgery (Figure 1). Substantial increases in wall thickness caused by plaques are associated, in some vessels, with lumen sizes equal to those of anatomically comparable normal, thin-walled coronary arteries (unpublished studies, D.D. McPherson *et al.*).

At the University of Chicago, Glagov *et al.* have studied human coronary arteries at autopsy after pressure-fixation (18). These workers evaluated changes in the left main coronary artery. They found that the cross-sectional area bounded by the internal elastic lamina enlarged as the plaque enlarged. They found that the arterial lumen did not decrease until the degree of stenosis exceeded 40%. In absolute terms, the original lumen size thus tended to be maintained until plaque size was almost as great as lumen size.

At Albany Medical Center, Daoud *et al.* also studied the human epicardial coronary bed at autopsy after pressure-fixation. They found changes in cross-sectional artery size that were compatible with outward displacement of media by plaque, but changes suggestive of encroachment of plaque on lumen size were more common when stenosis exceeded 50% (A.S.

Daoud *et al.*, unpublished studies). Thus, current human studies suggest that dilatation of atherosclerotic arteries occurs that tends to maintain lumen size.

There are other well-known observations that may fit the idea that outward displacement of atherosclerotic plaques is a common occurrence. One observation is the apparent character of atherosclerosis in young adults. The atherosclerotic lesions in young adults who had traumatic deaths include a significant fraction of fibrous plaques (19-21). About 10% of the intimal surface area of the coronary arteries in these persons consists of raised lesions and 27% show fibrous plaques in the left anterior descending coronary artery (21), yet the coronary angiographic picture that we expect in healthy persons in this age group shows no plaques and a normal lumen. We suggest that raised lesions in young adults may be compatible with normal coronary arteriograms because, in part, the lesions are displaced outwardly.

A second related observation is the frequently cited discrepancy between the lesion the pathologist sees and the lesion the angiographer identifies. It is often said that angiography underestimates atherosclerosis. There are two ways in which systematic underestimation may occur. One is simply an artifact of procedure: the degree of stenosis as defined by the pathologist in immersion-fixed material may not agree with the frequently lesser degree of stenosis noted at angiography. Pressure-fixed pathologic material, however, tends to give lumen measurements quite similar to those found at angiography. We believe that the second, important cause of underestimation occurs when findings in pressure-fixed material are compared with angiographic results. The angiographer measures lesions in relation to encroachment on the lumen, and the morphologist measures the total plaque. We postulate that underestimation of lesions by angiography in this setting becomes an instructive truism: The extent of underestimation is the extent of outward displacement of the lesions.

Reconsideration of Medical Changes in Atherosclerosis

In advanced atherosclerosis, thinning of the media occurs which is clearly atrophy. Moderate degrees of plaque formation also are associated with medial thinning. This finding suggests that a plaque formation may cause atrophy as an early effect. If there is early loss of muscle mass, it implies reduction of vasoactive function in atherosclerotic arteries. One problem with this view is that there is evidence of preserved, and even exaggerated, vascular responses in both human and experimental atherosclerosis. Thus, one wonders whether the thinned media under atherosclerotic plaques retains vasoactive function despite the appearance of atrophy, and even whether a significant degree of atrophy is present.

Systematic studies of this question are probably not feasible in man. Detailed measurements would be required concerning the degree of wall involvement and of segmental vascular responsiveness, in order to know to what extent hemodynamic responses persist in the face of atherosclerosis-induced medial change. In studies of both structure and function (17), we evaluated three aspects of medial structure in primate atherosclerosis: 1) the degree of overall medial loss, as a measure of diffuse atrophy; 2) the extent of focal medial loss, as a measure of localized atrophic change; and 3) medial distensibility under plaques. The primate groups cited for this discussion had been on a highly atherogenic diet for an average of 5 years, and moderately severe atherosclerotic plaques were present (17), with total lesion mass exceeding total medial mass.

To determine whether there is a decrease in medial mass in atherosclerosis, we studied the ileofemoral arterial bed, in which most of the vascular media lay under lesioned intima. Surprisingly, the medial mass in normal monkeys and the diffusely thinned appearance of media in atherosclerosis was caused by outward displacement of media, so that the media formed a large thin ring around an enlarged intimal mass, but with no decrease in mass.

To answer the question of how much focal medial loss occurs under plaques, we measured focal thinning of media in atherosclerotic arteries and compared it to focal thinning in

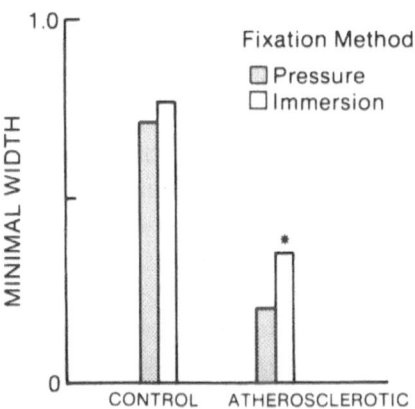

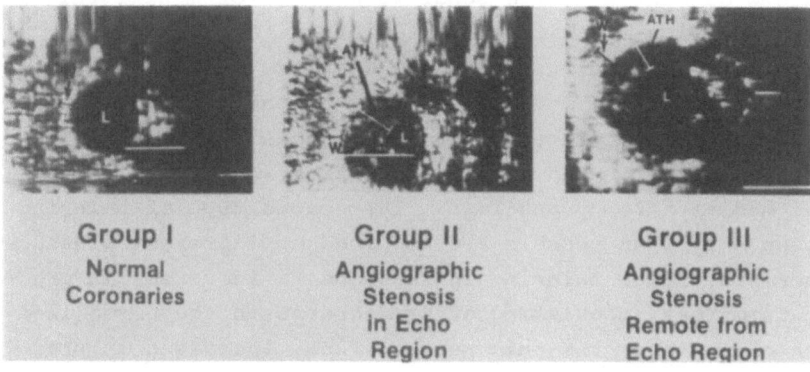

Figure 1. The effect of pressure fixation on the normalized minimal medial width of ileofemoral artery segments in monkeys. The bars are median values in pressure-fixed (stippled) and immersion-fixed (open) vessels. *P <0.05, pressure-fixation vs immersion-fixation, by the rank-sum test. Reprinted from Armstrong *et al* , Arteriosclerosis, 5;336-345, 1985, by permission of the American Heart Association, Inc.

Figure 2. High frequency echo arteriograms of coronary arteries obtained intraoperatively. Three groups of arteries were seen: those with a thin wall and normal lumen (Group I), those with a thick wall (because of lesion) and a lumen that was near-normal (Group III). Abbreviations: ATH, atherosclerotic artery; L, lumen; W, wall. Horizontal bar, 3 mm. (Reprinted by permission of McPherson *et al*, and the New England Journal of Medicine 316:304-309, 1987).

normal arteries. The difference between focal thinning in atherosclerosis, and the amount of thinning in normal media (*i.e.*, the normal variance) was an index of the extent of focal medial loss in atherosclerosis. Focal medial loss was clearly greater in atherosclerosis. The focal decrease in media represented media lost to atrophy, replacement fibrosis and lipogranulomatous arteritic invasion of media. The focal effect of atherosclerosis on media is thus a localized loss of media under plaques.

To answer the question of whether there is increased medial distensibility under plaques, we compared focal narrowing in undistended arteries and in response to physiologic pressure in atherosclerotic and normal arteries (17). Figure 2 demonstrates two separate aspects of medial thinning after immersion-fixation and after pressure-fixation at physiologic distending pressure. One form of thinning is focal atrophy. The media is focally thinner in atherosclerotic than in normal arteries. This thinning is seen after both immersion-fixation and pressure-fixation and simply illustrates focal medial atrophy and loss. The second type of thinning is seen only when vessels are compared at different pressures. In normals, focal thinning in response to increases in pressure is modest, consisting of 6% decrease in the normalized width of media at the thin point. Thus, increases in pressure cause greater distension of media under plaques -- a change that would favor outward displacement of plaques.

Thus, structural changes in the media in experimental atherosclerosis include preservation of overall medial mass despite diffuse thinning. The diffuse medial thinning reflects a change in shape rather than an atrophic change. There is marked focal thinning under plaques, however, caused by a real but localized loss of media. Finally, there is increased distensibility of media under plaques, which suggests a change in the elastic properties of media.

Possible Causes of Artery Remodeling in Atherosclerosis

We have presented evidence that lumen preservation may occur in atherosclerosis despite considerable plaque formation. We have shown preservation of total medial mass despite focal medial loss. This tends to exclude diffuse atrophy as a cause of artery enlargement. There are several other hypotheses that have been offered concerning mechanisms of remodeling of arteries.

We have suggested that the interaction of lesion, wall, and pressure defines whether outward displacement is likely (17). For example, as enlargement of atherosclerotic intima occurs, distensibility of the media may increase and early plaques may be displaced outwardly at physiologic distending pressures. We have shown increased distensibility of media in the atherosclerotic iliofemoral vessels of primates, and this has also been shown in iliac arteries in man (22). Lesion shape must also be considered. If lesions are concentric, as in primates, lesions as well as media must be distensible in response to distending pressure to allow outward displacement of lesions.

Glagov and associates have described atrophic media under the eccentric lesions of human coronary arteries, and suggested that this favors outward displacement of the lesions (18). This agrees with part of our formulation. They also have suggested that another mechanism occurs with eccentric lesions: encroachment on the lumen by an eccentric lesion tends to increase flow velocity, and the spared sector of the artery opposite the plaque may dilate in response to increased flow rates until the previous normal level of wall shear stress and diameter are restored.

The Limits to Remodeling

The adaptation which we have described can accommodate a significant degree of atherosclerotic change in the wall, but disease eventually triumphs over adaptation and luminal narrowing occurs.

What are the limits to adaptive remodeling? The recent studies of changes in lumen size in human coronary atherosclerosis that we have cited show, in sum, that the lumen of coronary arteries tends to be preserved until the plaque area is about equal to the size of the lumen; beyond this limit, plaque growth causes luminal narrowing. Evidences of a limit defined by lesion size are particularly appropriate for eccentric lesions, because the size of the eccentric lesion and the extent of the sector of spared artery wall are key morphologic representations of the vectors involved in remodelling. When lesions are concentric, outward displacement is not possible unless part of the _lesion_ is distensible. When a concentric lesion is fibrous and outward displacement occurs, the connective tissue matrix of the lesion must still have some extensibility. With further plaque evolution this property is lost, plaque growth may be uncompensated, and lumen stenosis may occur at such sites.

It is possible that other factors become dominant as lesions evolve. For example, it has been postulated that stenosis occurs then thrombosis becomes a factor in the evolution of atherosclerotic lesions (23). Thrombosis intensifies fibrosis of the lesion (24), and stenosis may well be a consequence of increased scarring caused by ongoing thrombotic events during atherogenesis.

SUMMARY AND CONCLUSIONS

1. Conclusive studies in nonhuman primates and initial studies in man point to an important remodeling of the artery as atherosclerotic plaques develop. The remodeling attenuates lumen stenosis, as outward displacement of plaques allows maintenance of a normal lumen in an artery of expanded transverse size. This adaptation may continue to accommodate an enlarging intima as long as media and intima can yield to hydraulic forces. Thus, a lumen of normal size may be preserved despite moderately severe wall changes.

2. Total mass of the media, which is responsible for vascular responses, tends to be maintained in experimental studies, despite diffuse thinning and quite marked focal atrophy. Comparable data in humans are not available. Maintenance of medial mass explains the preservation of vasoconstrictor capacity in atherosclerotic arteries.

3. Factors that permit adaptation of the wall, and factors that limit continued adaptation, are poorly understood. Clarification of these factors may eventually help to avert some of the consequences of plaque growth.

REFERENCES

1. Adams CWM (1967) Vascular Histochemistry. Chicago:
    Year Book, 35-82
2. Armstrong ML (1976) Regression of atherosclerosis In:
    Paoletti R and Gotto AM Jr (eds) Atherosclerosis
    Reviews, Vol 1. Raven, New York, pp 137-182
3. Minkowski WL (1947) The coronary arteries of infants.
    Amer J Med Sci 214:623-629
4. Gore I, Tejada C (1957) The quantitative appraisal of
    atherosclerosis. Amer J Path 33:875-885
5. Ophuls W (1933) The pathogenesis of arteriosclerosis.
    In: Cowdry EV (ed) Arteriosclerosis. A survey of the
    problem. Macmillan, New York, pp 249-270
6. Von Albertini A (1955) General aspects. In: GEW
    Wolstenholme and MP Cameron (eds) Ciba Foundation Colloquia
    on Ageing. Vol 1. Little Brown, Boston, pp 56-66
7. White NK, Edwards JE, Dry TJ (1950) The relationship
    of the degree of coronary atherosclerosis with age in
    men. Circulation 1:645-654
8. Lober PH (1953) Pathogenesis of coronary sclerosis.
    Arch Pathol 55:357-383
9. Aschoff L (1933) Introduction. In: Crowdry EV (ed)
    Arteriosclerosis. A survey of the problem. MacMillan,
    New York, pp 1-18
10. Young W, Gofman JW, Tandy R (1960) The quantitation
    of atherosclerosis. I. Relationship to artery size.
    Amer J Cardiol 6:288-293
11. Young W, Gofman JW, Tandy R (1960 The quantitation of
    atherosclerosis. II Quantitative aspects of the
    relationship of blood pressure and atherosclerosis.
    Amer J Cardiol 6:294-299
12. Young W, Gofman JW, Tandy R (1960) The quantitation
    of atherosclerosis. III The extent of correlation
    of degrees of sclerosis within and between the coronary
    and cerebral vascular beds. Amer J Cardiol 6:300-308
13. Bond MG, Adams MR, Bullock BC (1981) Complicating
    factors in evaluating coronary artery atherosclerosis.
    Artery 9: 21-29
14. Armstrong ML, Heistad DD, Marcus ML, Piegors DJ, Abboud
    FM (1983) Hemodynamic sequelae of regression of experi-
    mental atherosclerosis. J Clin Invest 71:104-113
15. Glagov S, Zarins CK (1983) Quantitating atherosclero-
    sis, problems of definition. In: Bond MG, Insull W Jr,
    Glagov S, Chandler AB, Cornhill JF (eds) Clinical
    Diagnosis of Atherosclerosis. Springer-Verlag, New
    York, pp 11-35
16. Hollander W, Prusty S, Nagraj S, Paddock J, Colombo M
    (1981) Morphometric changes in the coronary arteries
    during the induction and "regression" of atherosclerosis.
    Circulation 64:IV, 45
17. Armstrong ML, Heistad DD, Marcus ML, Megan MB, Piegors
    DJ (1985) Structural and hemodynamic responses of
    peripheral arteries of macaque monkeys to atherogenic
    diet. Arteriosclerosis 5:336-345
18. Glagov S, Weisenberg E, Zarins CK, Stankunavicius R,
    Kolletis G (1987) Compensatory enlargement of human
    atherosclerotic coronary arteries. N Eng J Med 316:371-
    375

19. Enos WF, Holmes RH, Beyer JC (1953) Coronary disease among United States soldiers killed in action in Korea, JAMA 152:1090-1093

20. Enos WF, Beyer JC, Holmes RH (1955) Pathogenesis of coronary disease in American soldiers killed in Korea. JAMA 158:912-914

21. Tejada C et al. (1968) Distribution of coronary and aortic atherosclerosis by geographic location, race and sex. In: McGill HC Jr (ed) Geographic Pathology of Atherosclerosis. Wilkins & Wilkins, Baltimore pp 49-66

22. Crawford T, Levene CI (1953) Medial thinning in atheroma. J Pathol Bacteriol 66:19-23

23. Solberg LA et al. (1985) Stenosis in the coronary arteries: Relation to atherosclerotic lesions, coronary heart disease and risk factors. The Oslo Study. Lab Invest 53:648-655

24. Stary HC (1989) Changes in the cells of atherosclerotic lesions as advanced lesions evolve in coronary arteries of children and young adults. In: Glagov S, Newman WP, Schaffer S (eds) Pathobiology of the Human Atherosclerotic Plaque. New York: Springer-Verlag, pp 93-106

31

Hemodynamic Consequences of Changes in the Artery Wall During Atherogenesis

J. Antonio Lopez, David G. Harrison, Mark L. Armstrong, and Donald D. Heistad

The pathogenesis of coronary vasospasm has been of interest since originally proposed by Latham in 1845 (1). Prinzmetal et al.(2) described a "variant" form of angina pectoris and reintroduced the concept of coronary spasm as an important factor in some instances of rest angina. Gensini et al (3) used coronary angiography to document for the first time appearance of spontaneous vasospasm associated with angina, in a patient with mild atherosclerotic coronary artery disease, as well as the resolution of this vasoconstriction and chest pain with administration of nitrates. Later, Guazzi et al. (4) and Maseri et al. (5) demonstrated that in "variant" angina, in contrast to typical angina, there is no increase in myocardial metabolic demand before the episodes of chest pain. Additional studies have suggested that spasm-induced decreases in myocardial perfusion are not only responsible for "variant" angina, but also lead to unstable angina, myocardial infarction and sudden death (6-7).

Investigations into the pathogenesis of vasospasm have centered on dysfunction of the autonomic nervous system (8), enhanced platelet activation with subsequent release of

———————
Acknowledgement. We thank Joanne Henderson for typing the manuscript. Original studies by the authors were supported by a Medical Investigatorship and research funds from the Veterans Administration and by National Institutes of Health ASCOR HL 14230, Program Project Grant HL 14388, and research grant HL 16066.

vasoconstrictor agents (9) and deficiency of endogenous
vasodilators (10). Recent efforts to understand the pathophysiology of vasospasm have focused on changes in vascular
responses produced by the atherosclerotic process of the
vessel wall (11-16).

Recent observations in patients (11), experimental
animals *in vitro* (12-13), and in animals *in vivo* (14-15)
suggest that vasospasm is most likely to develop when atherosclerosis is present. Spasm often occurs at sites with modest
lesions as defined angiographically (16). Moreover, although
the coronary arteriogram may not reveal segmental narrowing
due to atherosclerosis, there may be evidence at autopsy of
minimal atherosclerosis in the segment of vessel at which
spasm occurred.

In this review we will consider the role of altered
vascular responses to endothelium-dependent agonists in the
pathogenesis of vasospasm. Specifically, we will suggest that
atherosclerosis potentiates vasoconstrictor responses and
thereby predisposes to vasospasm.

Importance of Endothelium in the Normal Vessel
Furchgott proposed that endothelium is necessary for
vascular relaxation in response to several agonists (17).
Studies *in vitro* indicate the relaxation in response to a
variety of agonists, including acetylcholine (17), ATP and
ADP, histamine, thrombine (18), platelet activating factor,
and the calcium ionophore A23187 (19) only occurs when the
endothelium is present. There is strong evidence that these
agonists release a labile endothelium-derived relaxing factor
(EDRF) which has an inhibitory effect on contraction of
vascular smooth muscle (20). Removal of endothelium in these
preparations abolishes vasodilator responses to endothelium-
dependent agonists (21) or unmasks contraction in response
to other agonists (22-24). Agents such as adenosine, prostacyclin, nitroprusside and nitroglycerin act directly on
vascular muscle and are not endothelium-dependent dilators
in most vessels (21).

Endothelium and Vascular Responses in Atherosclerosis

Recent evidence suggests that atherosclerosis may contribute to increased responsiveness to vasoconstrictor stimuli by producing a functional defect in the endothelium (15,25-27) (Figure 1). This defect is not produced by a diffuse alteration in the endothelium caused by hypercholesterolemia (15,27) because vessels from hypercholesterolemic animals without atherosclerotic lesions relax normally in response to endothelium-dependent agonists (27) (Figure 2).

Iliac Artery Acetylcholine Response

Normal Monkey
Unrubbed

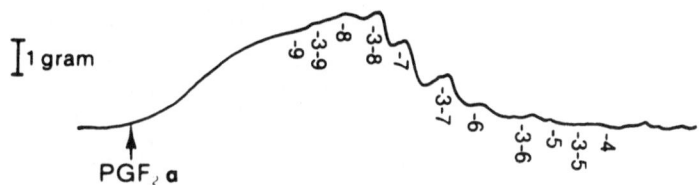

Atherosclerotic Monkey
Unrubbed

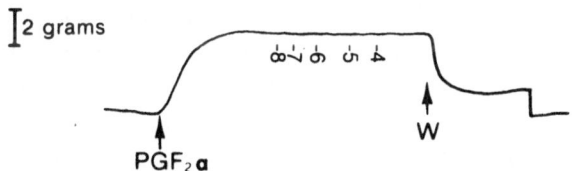

Figure 1. Response to acetylcholine in preconstricted normal and atherosclerotic monkey iliac arteries. Vessels were preconstricted with prostaglandin $F_2\alpha$ and then subjected to serial increasing doses of acetylcholine. Responses were measured in normal (above) and atherosclerotic (below) iliac arteries. Reprinted from Freiman *et al*, Circ. Res., 58:783-789, 1986 by permission of the American Heart Association, Inc.

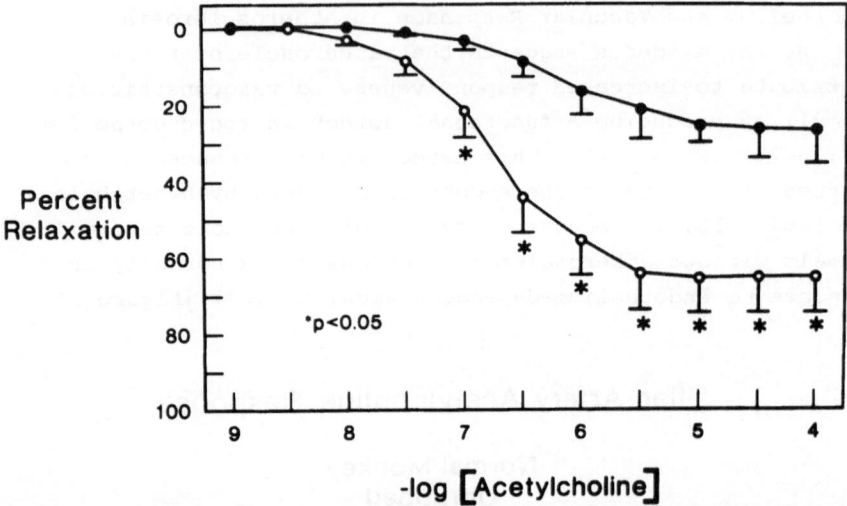

Figure 2. Relaxation in response to acetylcholine in iliac arteries from normal (0) and atherosclerotic (●) monkeys. Cumulative doses of acetylcholine are shown along the abscissa, and percent relaxation is shown along the ordinate. Acetylcholine produced less relaxation in atherosclerotic iliac arteries than in normal vessels * P < 0.05 compared to normal arteries. Reprinted from Freiman *et al*, Circ. Res., 58:783-789, 1986 by permission of the American Heart Association, Inc.

Atherosclerosis produces morphological alterations of the endothelium (28). There are several mechanisms by which atherosclerosis may alter endothelium-dependent responses. First, atherosclerosis may impair synthesis of endothelium-derived relaxing factor (EDRF). Second, the atherosclerotic process may produce a barrier between endothelium and vascular smooth muscle so that EDRF may not reach its site of action. Because EDRF has a half-life of a few seconds (20), intimal thickening and increased diffusion distance in atherosclerotic vessels may result in decreased magnitude of the EDRF-mediated response. Increased lipids in the vessel wall may also provide a functional barrier to diffusion of EDRF if this factor is a lipophilic substance. It also is possible that cellular elements in the intima-media of atherosclerotic vessels destroy or inactivate EDRF as it diffuses toward the media. Third, alteration of vascular responses could be related to changes in membrane lipid composition and fluidity (29), which might alter affinity of vascular

muscle for EDRF, or alter EDRF release. This possibility
is not likely because vascular responses are not impaired
by hypercholesterolemia (27). There may also be concomitant
impairment in endothelial prostacyclin or monoamine oxidase
production by atherosclerosis with subsequent hyperresponsiveness to vasoactive agents. This possibility is unlikely
because inhibition of monoamine oxidase or cyclooxygenase
does not alter responses to an endothelium-dependent agent
such as serotonin in isolated ring preparations with and without endothelium (34). Lastly, the endothelium in atherosclerosis might produce a vasoconstrictor agent (30). Recent work
in hypertensive rats has shown that the endothelium produces
a constrictor substance (31-32). Atherosclerosis may increase
synthesis of an endothelium-derived vasoconstrictor factor.

Cholesterol, Atherosclerosis and Receptors

Changes in membrane lipids of endothelial cells may
change receptor number or affinity. Preliminary studies
suggest that the density of histamine H_1 receptors and
serotonin S_2 receptors (33) is increased in atherosclerotic
rabbit aorta after eight to ten weeks of a high cholesterol
diet. Increased receptor density in these studies may have
been due to hypercholesterolemia, since lipoprotein concentration affects receptor density in other tissues (35). A
recent preliminary report by Bossaller *et al.* (36) suggested
that endothelium-dependent responses to the calcium ionophore
A23187, which are not receptor mediated, were not impaired in
cholesterol fed rabbits. This is in contrast to studies in
our laboratory in rabbits and monkeys where non-receptor
mediated responses (37) as well as responses to acetylcholine
and thrombin which are receptor-mediated, are impaired by
atherosclerosis (27,36). Thus, impairment of endothelium-
dependent relaxation in atherosclerotic vessels either involves
impairment of EDRF production and/or transfer.

Importance of Blood-Borne Elements

Platelet aggregation occurs periodically at or just
distal to sites of experimental narrowing of coronary
arteries (38-39). Aggregation of platelets induces a gradual

decrease of coronary blood flow that is often followed by
a spontaneous, sudden return to the initial level. Reductions
in flow are abolished by agents which inhibit platelet aggregation (38,40). If endothelial injury is present, platelets
adhere to the intima and release serotonin and thromboxane
A_2 (43) contract coronary vessels and may contribute to
platelet-induced contractions that occur in denuded coronary
arteries (22,34). Recently, epidermal growth factor and
platelet derived growth factor, which are vascular smooth
muscle mitogens that are present in platelets, were shown to
produce vasoconstriction in isolated vessels (45-46). Thus,
the acute effects of platelets on vessel tone have been well
documented *in vitro*.

In an animal model, intact endothelium prevented platelet-
induced coronary vasospasm (47). The role of platelets in
clinical vasospasm, however, is not well defined. It is of
interest that studies of human coronary arteries often reveal
platelet aggregates in the myocardial and intramyocardial
arteries of patients with coronary artery disease who die
suddenly (48).

Macrophages produce leukotrienes, which are potent
vasoconstrictors of coronary arteries (49) and thus may be
implicated in vasospasm. The mast cell is another blood-
formed element which may be involved in the pathogenesis of
vasospasm, because mast cells are a rich source of histamine
and leukotrienes. Histamine can induce coronary vasospasm
in patients with variant angina (50). Postmortem studies
in humans have shown the presence of mast cells around atherosclerotic lesions (51) and in segments of vessels that are
implicated in acute coronary occlusion (52).

Studies of Vascular Responses in Atherosclerosis *In Vivo*

Limb Circulation. We have examined effects of diet-
induced atherosclerosis on vasoconstrictor responses to serotonin in the limb *in vivo* (15). Responses were compared in
normal cynomolgus monkeys and in monkeys that were fed an
atherogenic diet for three to five years.

In normal monkeys, serotonin produced modest constriction of large arteries in the limb but, because small vessels
dilated, the net response to serotonin in the hindlimb was

vasodilatation. In atherosclerotic monkeys there was a ten-
fold increase in constrictor responses of large arteries to
serotonin in the hindlimb (Figure 3). Responses to norepinephrine were not increased in atherosclerotic monkeys. This
binding suggests that there is some specificity in potentiation of constrictor responses to serotonin by atherosclerosis.

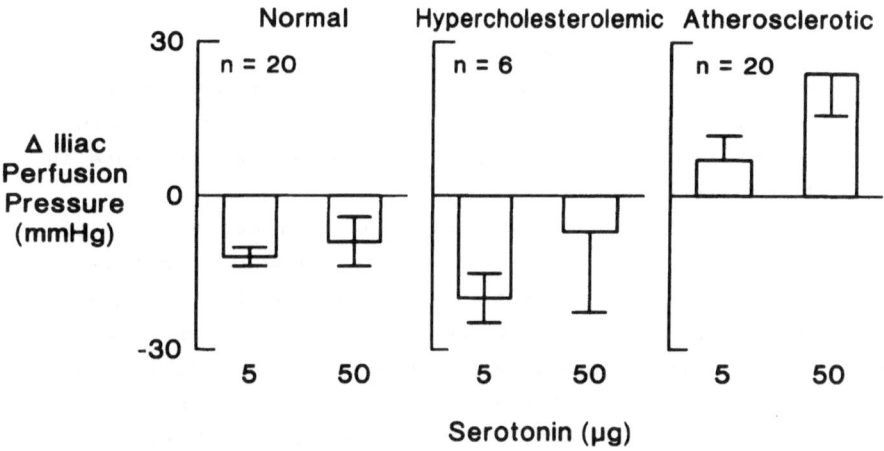

Figure 3. Vascular responses to intra-arterial injections
of serotonin (5 and 50 µg) in the perfused hindlimb of normal (N), atherosclerotic (AS), and hypercholesterolemic (HC)
cynomolgus monkeys. Values are changes in total hind limb
(iliac) perfusion pressure. Increases in total limb perfusion pressure in response to serotonin were augmented in
atherosclerotic monkeys (P <0.05, As vs N and CH). Serotonin produced more constriction of large arteries in atherosclerotic than in normal or hypercholesterolemic monkeys
(P <0.05). Reprinted from Heistad et al, Circ. Res., 54:711-718,
1984 by permission of the American Heart Association, Inc.

Responses to serotonin were examined in hypercholesterolemic monkeys that were fed an atherogenic diet for four to
five months. The monkeys did not yet have atherosclerotic
lesions in the limb. Vasoconstrictor responses to serotonin
were normal in hypercholesterolemic monkeys (Figure 3). Thus,
potentiation of responses to serotonin is associated with the
presence of atherosclerotic lesions, and is not the result
of hypercholesterolemia per se.

Cerebral Circulation. Recently we have examined
responses to serotonin in the cerebral circulation of atherosclerotic monkeys and suggested that vasoconstriction is an
additional mechanism that may contribute to transient ischemic
attacks (TIAs) (54).

Serotonin was infused into the carotid arteries to
stimulate local release of serotonin from platelet aggregates.
Intracarotid infusion of serotonin reduced pressure in cerebral arterioles, which indicates constriction of large arteries
upstream, but cerebral blood flow did not decrease because
small vessels dilated (Figure 4). Serotonin produced a two-
fold greater reduction in cerebral microvascular pressure in
atherosclerotic monkeys.

It is thought that TIAs are produced by aggregation of
platelets in the carotid arteries, with subsequent embolic
occlusion of cerebral arteries or arterioles (53). We suggest
that the release of serotonin during aggregation of platelets
may produce cerebral vasoconstriction. It is possible that
constriction of large arteries by serotonin reduces cerebral
microvascular pressure and, in the presence of subcritical
distal stenosis, may contribute to focal cerebral ischemia.

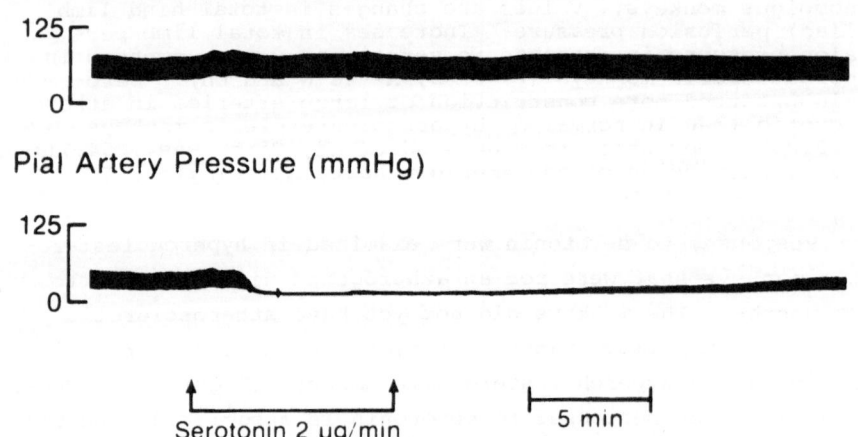

Aortic Pressure (mmHg)

125

0

Pial Artery Pressure (mmHg)

125

0

Serotonin 2 µg/min

5 min

Figure 4. Recording of aortic and pial artery pressure in
an atherosclerotic monkey during infusion of serotonin into
the carotid arteries. Serotonin produced a profound reduction
in cerebral microvascular pressure by constricting large
arteries upstream. (Reprinted from Tamaki *et al*, Stroke 17;
1209-1214, 1986 by permission of the American Heart Assocation,
Inc.).

Mesenteric Circulation. Responses to serotonin were studied by measuring blood flow to the mucosa and submucosa of the gastrointestinal tract with microspheres (55). In normal monkeys, infusion of serotonin did not affect blood flow to the small bowel or colon. In atherosclerotic monkeys, serotonin reduced flow to the small bowel or colon. In atherosclerotic monkeys, serotonin reduced flow to the small bowel by about 50% and produced a greater than 90% reduction in blood flow to the colon.

Thus, atherosclerosis greatly potentiates vasoconstrictor responses to serotonin, particularly in the distal bowel. We speculate that aggregation of platelets at atherosclerotic lesions, coupled with augmented vasoconstrictor responses to serotonin, may play a role in the pathogenesis of non-occlusive splanchnic ischemia (56).

Clinical Investigations. Role of Thromboxane A_2. In a recent study the role of thromboxane A_2 as a mediator of coronary vasospasm was examined (57). Thromboxane A_2 production was inhibited with aspirin. Peripheral venous levels of thromboxane B_2, the stable metabolite of thromboxane A_2, were reduced by aspirin to less than 3% of control values. The duration, severity and incidence of symptomatic episodes of vasospasm were not significantly reduced by inhibition of thromboxane A_2 production. This study suggests that thromboxane A_2 is not responsible for initiation of coronary vasospasm.

Role of Serotonin. Two recent studies examined effects of antagonism of serotonergic receptors with ketanserin, a selective serotonin-2 (S_2) antagonist in patients with documented coronary vasospasm (58-59). Efficacy of receptor blockade was evaluated by examining constrictor responses of hand veins to serotonin before and after ketanserin (58) or by examining platelet aggregation in vitro with serotonin (59). Ketanserin did not reduce episodes of variant angina, which suggests that serotonin does not mediate vasospastic angina.

An important limitation of these studies is that the doses of antagonists that were used may not have been adequate. Aggregation of platelets produces very high levels of serotonin in the vessel wall (42). It is possible that doses of

ketanserin that attenuate vasoconstrictor responses of hand
veins and aggregation of platelets in response to exogenous
serotonin that may be achieved within the arterial wall (42).

It is also possible that there are redundant mediators
of vasospasm. For example, both serotonin and thromboxane
A_2 may be able to produce pronounced basospasm. If there are
redundant mechanisms, it may be necessary to block both
mediators to prevent episodes of vasospasm.

Regression of Atherosclerosis

There is extensive morphological evidence that experimental atherosclerosis in primates regresses when the atherogenic stimulus is removed (60-62). Regression is characterized
by reduction in intimal lipids and decrease in lesion size (63).
Vasodilator responses fail to improve in several vascular
beds, especially in the limb, despite clear morphological
evidence of regression (64) (Figure 5). It is likely that
vascular fibrosis, which occurs during regression of atherosclerosis (65-67), limits hemodynamic improvement.

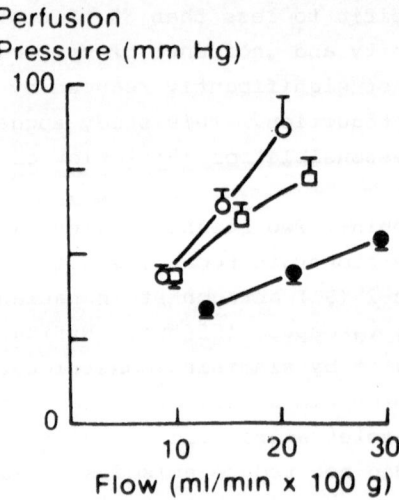

Perfusion
Pressure (mm Hg)

Flow (ml/min x 100 g)

Figure 5. Pressure-flow curves in the perfused limb bed
during maximal vasodilatation with papaverine. Data points
are group means ± SD. Resistance was greater in atherosclerotic and regression monkeys than in normal monkeys
(p < 0.05). At high flow rates, resistance was greater
(p < 0.05) in regression monkeys than in atherosclerotic
monkeys. (Reprinted from Armstrong *et al*, J Clin Invest
71;104-113, 1983 by copyright permission of the American
Society for Clinical Investigation, Inc.).

Recently we examined effects of dietary treatment of atherosclerosis on vascular responses to serotonin (68). As in a previous study (15), vasocontrictor responses to serotonin in the limb were greatly exaggerated in a group of atherosclerotic monkeys. A striking finding was that dietary treatment for 18 months completely abolished the hyperresponsiveness to serotonin. Furthermore, endothelium-dependent relaxation in response to acetylcholine and thrombin was restored to normal (68). It is possible that treatment of atherosclerosis may be effective in reduction of susceptibility to vasospasm, even when treatment is not successful in improving maximal dilator responses.

We are aware of only one study evaluating hemodynamic effects of regression of atherosclerosis in humans. Patients with Type III hyperlipoproteinemia were studied before and after three to six months of treatment with a therapeutic diet and clofibrate (70). Peak reactive hyperemic blood flow in the most severely affected extremity increased markedly. This finding suggests that patients with Type III hyperlipoproteinemia may have improvement of their peripheral vascular disease after treatment of this disorder.

SUMMARY

We have described studies which are compatible with the hypothesis that the endothelium is dysfunctional in atherosclerosis. We speculate that vasospasm, which is an important complication of atherosclerosis, may be a result of vascular responses to the products of blood-borne formed elements. Vasoconstrictor responses to serotonin are augmented by atherosclerosis, and we suggest that serotonin may play a critical role in the pathogenesis of vasospasm. Finally, the experimental findings suggest that treatment of atherosclerosis may be effective in reduction of susceptibility to vasospasm since regression of atherosclerosis abolishes the hyperresponsiveness to serotonin and restores endothelium-dependent vascular responses to normal.

REFERENCES

1. Latham PM (1876) Lecture XXXVII and XXXVIII. In: Martin R (ed) The collected works of Dr. P. M. Latham with memoir by Thomas Watson. London, The New Sydenham Society, pp 445-480

2. Prinzmetal M, Kennamer R, Merliss R, Wada T, Bor N (1957) Angina pectoris I. Variant form of angina pectoris. Preliminary report. Am J Med 27:375-388

3. Gensini GG, DiGiorgi S, Murad-Netto S, Black A (1962) Arteriographic demonstration of coronary artery spasm and its release after the use of a vasodilator in a case of angina pectoris and in the experimental animal. Angiology 13:550-553

4. Guazzi M, Polese A, Florentini C, Magrini F, Bartorelli C (1971) Left ventricular performance and related haemodynamic changes in Prinzmetal's variant angina pectoris. Br Heart J 33:84-94

5. Maseri A, Parodi O, Severi S, Pesola A (1976) Transient transmural reduction of myocardial blood flow, demonstrated by thallium-201 scintigraphy, as a cause of variant angina. Circulation 54:280-288

6. Oliva PB, Breckenridge JC (1977) Arteriographic evidence of coronary arterial spasm in acute myocardial infarction. Circulation 56:366-374

7. Maseri A, L'Abbate A, Baroldi G, et al. (1978) Coronary vasospasm as a possible cause of myocardial infarction. A conclusion derived from the study of "Preinfarction" angina. N Eng J Med 299:1271-1277

8. Yasue H, Touyama M, Shimamoto M, Kato H, Tanaka S, Akiyama F (1974) Role of autonomic nervous system in the pathogenesis of Prinzmetal's variant form of angina. Circulation 50:534-539

9. Mehta J, Mehta P, Pepine CJ (1978) Platelet aggregation in aortic and coronary venous blood in patients with and without coronary disease. Role of tachycardia, stress, and propranolol. Circulation 58:881-886

10. Chierchia S, Patróno C, Crea F, et al. (1982) Effects of intravenous prostacyclin in variant angina. Circulation 65:470-477

11. Waters DD, Szlachcic J, Bonan R, Miller DD, Duawe F, Theroux P (1983) Comparative sensitivity of exercise, cold pressor and ergonovine testing in provoking attacks of variant angina in patients with active disease. Circulation 67:310-315

12. Henry PD, Yokoyama M (1980) Supersensitivity of atherosclerotic rabbit aorta to ergonovine. Mediation by a serotonergic mechanism. J Clin Invest 66:306-313

13. Yokoyama M, Akita H, Mizutani T, Fukuzaki H, Wantanabe Y (1983) Hyperreactivity of coronary arterial smooth muscles in response to ergonovine from rabbits with hereditary hyperlipidemia. Circ Res 53:63-71

14. Shimokawa H, Tomoike H, Nabeyama S et al. (1983) Coronary artery spasm induced in atherosclerotic minature swine. Science 221:560-562

15. Heistad DD, Armstrong ML, Marcus ML, Piegors DJ, Mark AL (1984) Augmented responses to vasoconstrictor stimuli in hypercholesterolemic and atherosclerotic monkeys. Circ Res 54:711-718

16. MacAlpin RN (1980) Relation of coronary arterial spasm to sites of organic stenosis. Am J Cardiol 46:143-153

17. Furchgott FR, Zawadzki JV (1980) The obligatory role of endothelial cells in the relaxation of arterial smooth muscle by acetylcholine. Nature 288:373-376

18. DeMey JG, Claeys M, Vanhoutte PM (1982) Endothelium-dependent inhibitory effects of acetylcholine, adenosine triphosphate, thrombin and arachidonic acid in the canine femoral artery. J Pharmacol Exp Ther 222:166-173
19. Singer HA, Peach MJ (1982) Calcium- and endothelial-mediated vascular smooth muscle relaxation in rabbit aorta. Hypertension 4:II-19-25
20. Rubanyi GM, Lorenz RR, Vanhoutte PM (1985) Bioassay of endothelium-derived relaxing factor(s): Inactivation by catecholamines. Am J Physiol (Heart Circ Physiol 18) 349:H95-101
21. Furchgott RF (1983) Role of the endothelium in responses of vascular smooth muscle. Circ Res 53:557-573
22. Cohen RA, Shepherd JT, Vanhoutte PM (1983) Inhibitory role of the endothelium in the response of isolated coronary arteries to platelets. Science 221:273-274
23. Martin W, Furchgott RF, Villani GM, Jothanianandan D (1986) Depression of contractile responses in rat aorta by spontaneously released endothelium-derived relaxing factor. J Pharmacol Exp Ther 237:529-538
24. Lamping KG, Marcus ML, Dole WP (1985) Removal of the endothelium potentiates canine large coronary artery constrictor responses of 5-hydroxytryptamine in $vivo$. Circ Res 57:46-54
25. Habib JB, Bossaller C, Wells S, Williams C, Morrisett JD, Henry PD (1986) Preservation of endothelium-dependent vascular relaxation in cholesterol-fed rabbit by treatment with the calcium blocker PN 200110. Circ Res 58:305-309
26. Verbeuren TJ, Jordaens FH, Zonnekeyn LL, Van Hove CE, Coene M-C, Herman AG (1986) Effect of hypercholesterolemia on vascular reactivity in the rabbit. I. Endothelium-dependent and endothelium-independent contractions and relaxations in isolated arteries of control and hypercholesterolemic rabbits. Circ Res 58:552-564
27. Freiman PC, Mitchell GG, Heistad DD, Armstrong ML, Harrison DG (1986) Atherosclerosis impairs endothelium-dependent vascular relaxation to acetylcholine and thrombin in primates. Circ Res 58:783-789
28. Trillo AA, Prichard RW (1979) Early endothelial changes in experimental primate atherosclerosis. Lab Invest 41:294-302
29. Lurie KG, Chin JH, Hoffman BB (1985) Decreased membrane fluidity and β-adrenergic responsiveness in atherosclerotic quail. Am J Physiol 249 (Heart Circ Physiol 18):H380-385
30. DeMey JG, Vanhoutte PM (1982) Heterogenous behavior of the canine arterial and venous wall. Importance of endothelium. Circ Res 51:439-447
31. Rubanyi GM, Vanhoutte PM (1985) Hypoxia releases a vasoconstrictor substance from the canine vascular endothelium. J Physiol 364:45-56
32. Luscher TF, Vanhoutte PM (1986) Endothelium-dependent contractions to acetylcholine in the aorta of the spontaneously hypertensive rat. Hypertension 8:344-348
33. Nanda V, Henry PD (1982) Increased serotonergic and alpha adrenergic receptors in aortas from rabbits fed a high cholesterol diet (abstr). Clin Res 30:209A

34. Cohen RA, Shepherd JT, Vanhoutte PM (1983) 5-Hydroxy-tryptamine can mediate endothelium-dependent relaxation of coronary arteries. Am J Physiol 245 (Heart Circ Physiol 14):H1077-1080

35. Renaud JF, Scanu AM, Kazazoglou T, Lombet A, Romey G, Lazounski M (1982) Normal serum and lipoprotein-deficient serum give different expressions of excitability, corresponding to different stages of differentiation, in chicken cardiac cells in culture. Proc Natl Acad Sci USA 79:7768-7772

36. Bossaller C, Habib JB, Wells S, Henry PD (1985) Dissociation between muscarinic and Ca-ionophore induced endothelium-dependent relaxation in atherosclerotic rabbit aorta and human coronary artery (abstr). Circulation 72:35

37. Harrison DG, Freiman PC, Armstrong ML, Heistad DD (1986) The effect of atherosclerosis regression on endothelium dependent vascular relaxation (abstr). Clin Res 34:895A

38. Folts JD, Crowell EB Jr, Rowe GC (1976) Platelet aggregation in partially obstructed vessels and its elimination with aspriin. Circulation 54:365-370

39. Uchida Y, Yoshimoto N, Murao S (1978) Effects of anti-anginal agents on cyclical reductions of coronary blood flow. Jpn Heart J 19:904-912

40. Bush LR, Campbell WB, Kern K, Tilton BD, Aprill P, Ashton J, et al (1984) The effects of α_2-adrenergic and serotonergic receptor antagonists on cyclic blood flow alterations in stenosed canine coronary arteries. Circ Res 55:642-652

41. Zucker MB, Nachmias VT (1985) Platelet activation. Arteriosclerosis 5:2-18

42. Benedict CR, Mathew B, Rex KA, Cartwright J Jr, Sordahl LA (1986) Correlation of plasma serotonin changes with platelet aggregation in an in vivo dog model of spontaneous occlusive coronary thrombus formation. Circ Res 58:58-67

43. Ellis EF, Oelez O, Roberts LJ II et al (1976) Coronary arterial smooth muscle contraction by a substance released from platelets: Evidence that it is thromboxane A_2. Science 193:1135-1137

44. Houston DS, Shepherd JT, Vanhoutte PM (1986) Aggregating human platelets cause direct contraction and endothelium-dependent relaxation of isolated canine coronary arteries. Role of serotonin, thromboxane A_2, and adenine nucleotides. J Clin Invest 78:539-544

45. Berk BC, Brock TA, Webb RC et al (1985) Epidermal growth factor, a vascular smooth muscle mitogen, induces rat aortic contraction. J Clin Invest 75:1083-1086

46. Berk BC, Alexander RW, Brock TA, Gimbrone MA Jr, Webb RC (1986) Vasoconstriction: A new activity for platelet-derived growth factor. Science 232:87-90

47. Bing RJ, Burger W, Chemnitius JM, Saeed M, Metz MZ (1985) Effect of intact endothelium against platelet-induced coronary artery spasm in isolated rabbit hearts. Am J Cardiol 55:1596-1600

48. Haerem JW (1972) Platelet aggregates in intramyocardial vessels of patients dying suddenly and unexpectedly of coronary artery disease. Atherosclerosis 15:199-213

49. Piper PJ (1984) Formation and actions of leukotrienes. Physiol Rev 64:744-761
50. Ginsburg R, Bristow MR, Kantrowitz N, Baim DS, Harrison DC (1981) Histamine provocation of clinical coronary artery spasm: Implications concerning pathogenesis of variant angina pectoris. Am Heart J 102:819-822
51. Pollak OJ (1957) Mast cells in the circulatory system of man. Circulation 16:1084-1089
52. Pomerance A (1958) Peri-arterial mast cells in coronary atheroma and thrombosis. J Path Bact 76:55-79
53. Barnett HJM (1980) Progress towards stroke prevention: Robert Wartenberg Lecture. Neurology 30:1212-1225
54. Tamaki K, Armstrong M, Heistad D (1986) Effects of atherosclerosis on cerebral vessels: Hemodynamic and morphometric studies. Stroke 17:1209-1214
55. Brown BP, Armstrong ML, Piegors DJ, Heistad DD (1986) Response of the mesenteric circulation to serotonin in normal and atherosclerotic monkeys (abstr). Gastroenterology 90:1359
56. Clark RA, Gallant TE (1984) Acute mesenteric ischemia: Angiographic spectrum. AJR 142:555-562
57. Chierchia S, De Caterina R, Crea F, Patrono C, Maseri A (1982) Failure of thromboxane A_2 blockade to prevent attacks of vasospastic angina. Circulation 66:702-705
58. Freedman SB, Chierchia S, Rodriquez-Plaza L, Bugiardina R, Smith G, Maseri A (1984) Ergonovine-induced myocardial ischemia: No role for serotonergic receptors? Circulation 70:178-183
59. De Caterina R, Carpeggiani C, L'Abbate A (1984) A double-blind, placebo-controlled study of ketanserin in patients with Prinzmetal's angina. Evidence against a role for serotonin in the genesis of coronary vasospasm. Circulation 69:889-894
60. Armstrong ML, Warner ED, Connor WE (1970) Regression of coronary atheromatosis in rhesus monkeys. Circ Res 27:59-67
61. Malinow MR, McLaughlin P, Papworth L, Naito HK, Lewis L, McNulty WP (1976) A model for therapeutic intervention on established coronary atherosclerosis in a nonhuman primate. Adv Exp Med Biol 67:3-31
62. Clarkson TB, Bond MG, Bullock BC, Marzetta CA (1981) A study of atherosclerosis regression in macaca mulatta IV. Changes in coronary arteries from animals with atherosclerosis induced for 19 months then regressed for 24 or 48 months at plasma cholesterol concentration of 300 or 200 mg/dl. Exp Mol Path 34:345-368
63. Armstrong ML, Megan MB (1972) Lipid depletion in atheromatous coronary arteries in rhesus monkeys after regression diets. Circ Res 30:675-680
64. Armstrong ML, Heistad DD, Marcus ML, Piegors DJ, Abboud FM (1983) Hemodynamic sequelae of regression of experimental atherosclerosis. J Clin Invest 71:104-113
65. Armstrong ML, Megan MB (1973) Responses of two macaque species to atherogenic diet and its withdrawal. In: Schettler G and Weizel A (eds). Atherosclerosis III. Springer-Verlag, New York, pp 336-338

66. Malinow MR, McLaughlin P, McNulty WP, Naito HK, Lewis LA (1978) Treatment of established atherosclerosis during cholesterol feeding in monkeys. Atherosclerosis 31:185-193

67. Vesselinovitch D, Wissler RW (1980) Reversal of atherosclerosis: Comparison of Nonhuman Primate Models. In: Gotto AM Jr, Smith LC, and Allen B (eds). Atherosclerosis V. Springer-Verlag, New York, pp 369-374

68. Heistad DD, Piegors DJ, Mark AL, Armstrong ML (1986) Dietary treatment of atherosclerosis abolishes hyperresponsiveness to serotonin: implications for vasospasm (abstr). Circulation 74:III-286

69. Freiman PC, Mitchell GG, Gagnon NJ, Armstrong ML, Heistad DD, Harrison DG (1986) Regression of atherosclerosis restores endothelium dependent vascular relaxation in primates (abstr). Fed Proc 45:767

70. Zelis R, Mason DT, Braunwald E, Levy RI (1986) Effects of hyperlipoproteinemias and their treatment on the peripheral circulation. J Clin Invest 232:87-90

32
Lipoproteins and Pathogenesis of Atherosclerosis

Daniel Steinberg

INTRODUCTION

Let us start with the assumption that we all agree,
along with the NIH Consensus Panel on Lowering Blood
Cholesterol (1), that hypercholesterolemia in some way
contributes importantly to the progress of human atherosclerosis. The question that remains to be answered is:
How? Most investigators have assumed that hypercholesterolemia does its damage as a consequence of a high rate of
delivery of cholesterol and other lipids into the artery
wall. This is really just a restatement of the Virchow
lipid infiltration hypothesis put forward about 100 years
ago. However, even a casual look at a complicated human
atherosclerotic lesion makes it clear that much more goes
on than just the deposition of lipids. There are crucially
important elements of cellular proliferation and accumulation
of connective tissue matrix materials that contribute significantly to the ultimate stenosis of the vessel. Any
complete theory of the pathogenesis of the disease must
account not only for the accumulation of lipid but also the
overgrowth of cells, the deposition of collagen and glycosaminoglycans, and, in the later lesions, the erosion of
endothelial surface.

In the best and simplest of all possible worlds there
would be a single primary cause of atherosclerosis and
primary cause would initiate a linear series of events
culminating in the atheroma. Probably the closest that we

ever come to this "ideal" of a linear pathogenesis is in the case of familial hypercholesterolemia. There we know that the primary defect is a failure of normal LDL receptor function, leading in turn to a slow removal of LDL from the plasma and thus a higher plasma level of LDL. In this instance, because the disease is a single-gene disease, we can say with confidence that the primary cause of the atherogenesis is the hypercholesterolemia. But even here we are not yet in the position to describe the detailed pathogenetic sequence beyond the hyperbetalipoproteinemia.

Before going further it should be noted that there are two general categories of mechanisms that should be considered when we talk about the mechanisms by which hyperbetalipoproteinemia causes atherosclerosis. The first, as put forward in the lipid infiltration hypothesis, is that the atherogenesis results, in a direct or indirect fashion, from an increased rate of LDL penetration into the artery wall. However, it is also possible that it does something more than simply increase the rate of lipid penetration and uptake. In other words, hyperbetalipoproteinemia could trigger other things highly relevant to the atherogenic process. For example, LDL is capable of damaging endothelial cells, at least *in vitro* (2,3). If a similar phenomenon occurs *in vivo*, endothelial damage might be an immediate consequence of hypercholesterolemia and contribute, along with increased lipid uptake, to the progression of the lesions. Another example: hyperlipoproteinemia has been reported to favor platelet aggregation (4) and thus patients with hypercholesterolemia may be more likely to have microthrombi that could initiate lesion formation and they may be more likely to suffer a major fatal thrombus.

It seems to this investigator that none of the various initiating causes that have been proposed is an exclusive cause. I believe it's more likely that there are several different potential initiating factors, each capable in itself of starting the trouble and all sharing a final common path, as discussed elsewhere (5). After all, what we designate as atherosclerosis embraces a heterogeneous collection of lesions and we are still not totally certain how they relate to each other in terms of pathogenesis or

in the time sequence of their development. We must keep an
open mind regarding the relatedness or unrelatedness of
these lesions and be on the alert to recognize and evaluate
factors that initiate or accelerate lesion progression,
unprejudiced by any particular theory dogmatically held.
In the remainder of this presentation I would like to
elaborate on three major points:

1. Recent studies on the receptor-deficient (WHHL)
rabbit increase our confidence that the basic reaction of
the artery wall to hypercholesterolemia is qualitatively
similar in the animal model and in man.

2. A new hypothesis regarding the role of oxidatively
modified LDL or of other modified forms of LDL in the
pathogenesis of atheroscleorsis has been put forward based
on recent studies indicating that foam cells are mostly
derived from monocytes and that unusual receptors are
expressed in the monocyte/macrophage.

3. Neither in animal models nor in man are we totally
confident about the sequence of events leading to the late
lesion; while studies of cells in culture promise to be of
enormous importance, the relevance of these *in vitro* phenomena to changes *in vivo* remains to be established; thus, our
best chance of reconstructing the detailed sequence of
events in pathogenesis may lie in combining *in vivo* and
in vitro approaches.

Homyzygous Familial Hypercholesterolemia in Man and in the
WHHL Rabbit

For many years of the cholesterol-fed and/or fat-fed
rabbit model was the most widely used of animal models.
However, the relevance of this model to human disease was
by no means universally accepted. The skeptics correctly
pointed out that rabbits are normally herbivorous and that
feeding them animal fat and cholesterol was, in a sense,
"agin nature." Others pointed out ways in which the
apparent natural history of the rabbit lesion differed
from that of the human lesion. Even though the severity of
the lesions was roughly in proportion to the degree of
elevation of the plasma cholesterol level (strongly implying
that the hypercholesterolemia <u>was</u> the relevant antecedent

cause) it could be argued -- and <u>was</u> -- that the "abnormal" diet might be inducing <u>other</u> metabolic changes that made the study of this model irrelevant to the study of human atherosclerosis.

With the discovery by Watanabe and his coworkers of the LDL receptor-deficient (WHHL) rabbit (6), it was now possible to develop atherosclerosis in a rabbit <u>on</u> <u>a</u> <u>normal</u> <u>vegetarian</u> <u>diet</u>. Here it cannot be argued that the animals are being subjected to a grossly abnormal regimen; in fact, they develop their atherosclerosis on a perfectly normal chow diet in no way different from that of wild-type animals.

The basic defect in the WHHL rabbit is almost exactly the same as that in some forms of human homozygous familial hypercholesterolemia. The exact defect in the LDL receptor has been identified in the WHHL rabbit as a deletion of several amino acids from the ligand-binding domain (7). This is very similar to the genetic error in some kindreds with classical familial hypercholesterolemia (8). Thus we have an animal model in which there is a single gene defect and that defect is almost precisely the same as that in the "human model". Moreover, the earliest lesions in both models are fatty streaks characterized by lipid-laden foam cells. And in both models many or most of those foam cells have been shown to derive from circulating monocytes (9,10). To me this constitutes a very strong case for proceeding on the assumption that, at least in a qualitative sense, the reactivity of the rabbit artery wall to hypercholesterolemia is like that of the human artery wall. To be sure, there are differences but they are probably less important than the similarities. One would expect in fact to find some differences because of the different hemodynamics (blood pressure and blood flow patterns) and the very different metabolic rates and life spans of the two species. If the investigator is concerned that fine points in the patho-genesis are determined in "microenvironments" or by "micro-metabolic differences" he will be wise to exert caution in transferring information from one model to the other. If, however, he is concerned with the initiating event -- as I believe he should be -- he would appear to be on safe ground in assuming that the pathogenesis is similar or identical in the two species when they are confronted with hyperbetalipoproteinemia.

Before leaving this issue it should be stressed that we are not at all certain about the relative atherogenicity of different lipoprotein fractions. Nor are we certain that the pathogenesis will turn out to be the same independent of which lipoprotein fraction is elevated. For example, the cholesterol-fed rabbit shows an elevation predominantly in the beta-VLDL rather than in the LDL fraction (11). As a result, the metabolic and cellular responses of the artery wall may be different in the cholesterol-fed rabbit (in response to beta-VLDL) than in the receptor-deficient rabbit or receptor-deficient patient (in response predominantly to LDL). But even here the differences may turn out to be less important than the similarities. The monocyte/macrophage expresses a receptor for the efficient uptake of beta-VLDL (12) as well as the scavenger receptor that takes up LDL of modified structure (13). If the development of foam cells is truly the first step and all the subsequent evolution follows, then it may not matter too much whether the initial loading of the cells occurs by way of one or another macrophage receptor.

The Generation of Foam Cells, a Hallmark of the Fatty Streak Lesion

The fatty streak is widely (although not universally) accepted as the first stage in a process that culminates in the fibrous plaque and the complicated atherosclerotic lesion. This early lesion is characterized by a large number of cytoplasmic lipid droplets containing primarily cholesterol esters. For many years these cells were believed to derive from smooth muscle cells that had migrated into the subendothelial space but it is now generally accepted that many or most of them are derived from circulating monocytes. Indeed, one of the earliest events after an animal is placed on a cholesterol-rich diet is an increase in the adherence of monocytes to the endothelial lining of large vessels. This was first described in the laboratory of Colin Schwartz by Gerrity et al. (14). Within a few weeks

of starting pigs on a cholesterol-rich diet they were able
to demonstrate large numbers of monocytes adhering, particularly to areas known to be most susceptible to the development of atherosclerosis. Similar findings have been made by
Fagiotto and Ross in cholesterol-fed monkeys (15). Exactly
how the cholesterol feeding induces adherence is not clear.
Gerrity has presented evidence that both the monocyte and
the vessel wall are affected (16). Bevilacqua and coworkers
(17) have shown that treatment of cultured endothelial cells
with Interleukin-1 incudes them to express a specific
membrane protein to which monocytes adhere. It remains to
develop the link between the feeding of cholesterol and
stimuli that evoke the expression of such adhesion proteins
in endothelial cells, on monocytes, or both.

What can we say about how these foam cells become so
heavily loaded with lipids? Goldstein et al. (13) tackled
this problem and found to their surprise that incubation of
resident peritoneal macrophages with LDL, even very high
concentrations of LDL, failed to convert them to foam cells.
These cells do express the LDL receptor but the number expressed is small. Moreover those receptors are downregulated
in the presence of LDL. Consequently the cells can evidently
protect themselves against accumulation of cholesterol if it
is presented in the form of normal LDL. That presents a
paradox. Animals with primarily an elevation of LDL (e.g.,
the Watanabe rabbit or the patient with familial hypercholesterolemia) develop foam cells and presumably the
sterol comes, as it does in atherosclerosis generally, from
deposition of lipoprotein cholesterol.

A similar paradox presents itself with respect to total
body catabolism of LDL in the animal without receptors. The
net flux of LDL is not only normal but greater than normal
in the Watanabe rabbit and in the patient with homozygous
familial hypercholesterolemia (18,19). We considered the
possibility that modification of LDL might be necessary in
order to explain these phenomena and attempted to modify LDL
by enzymatic methods (20). Trypsin-treated LDL was taken up
somewhat more rapidly than native LDL by receptor-deficient
cells but the effect in normal cells was questionable.
Goldstein et al. showed that chemical modification of LDL --

by treatment with acetic anhydride -- generated a form of LDL that was then taken up much more rapidly than native LDL by the macrophage and that that uptake was by way of an alternative receptor termed the "scavenger receptor" or acetyl LDL receptor (13). Other chemical modifications of an analogous type have been shown to do the same thing (21,22). However, these chemical modifications are not known to occur *in vivo*.

A biological modification that generates a lipoprotein recognized by the acetyl LDL receptor was described by Henriksen and coworkers in our laboratory in 1981 (23). Simply incubating LDL with cultured endothelial cells over-night altered it in such a way that it was taken up five to ten times more rapidly than native LDL by mouse resident peritoneal macrophages. Most important, this uptake occurred by way of the same receptor that recognized acetylated LDL. LDL incubated in the absence of cells or incubated with human skin fibroblasts or rat hepatocytes was not altered in this way. The endothelial cell-modified LDL, while taken up much more rapidly by the macrophage, is actually recognized less well by the B/E receptor. Subsequent studies showed that smooth muscle cells and macrophages themselves can effect a similar modification of LDL (24,25).

Without taking time to go into detail, we can summarize what we know about this modification by reference to the scheme in Figure 1. It depends upon the generation of free radical oxygen, either by the cells or as a result of incubation in the presence of added copper ions even in the absence of cells. The changes induced by endothelial cells or by macrophages can be mimicked in a cell-free system as long as metal ions, sulfhydryl compounds and perhaps other conditions necessary for generation of free radicals are present. We know that the lipids undergo extensive peroxidation, that the lecithin is extensively degraded to lyso-lecithin and that the apoprotein B is fragmented in the course of the oxidative modification (26-28). Exactly how these various aspects of the oxidative damage are linked is under investigation. We do know that the whole process can be arrested either by the addition of an antioxidant to the medium (e.g., butylated hydroxytoluene or vitamin E) or

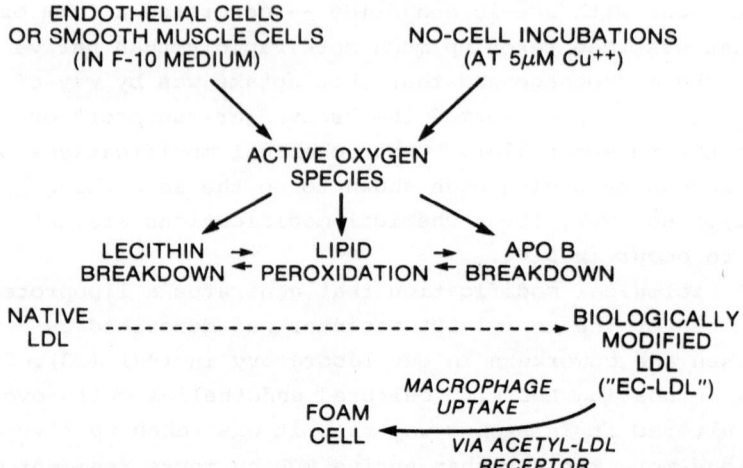

Figure 1. Schematic representation of the events involved in the biological modification of LDL to a form recognized by the acetyl LDL receptor of the macrophage.

by the addition of a specific inhibitor of phospholipase A_2. Recent studies established that the partially degraded polypeptides from oxidatively modified LDL can be resolubilized with the use of octylglucoside and demonstrated to compete with acetyl LDL for uptake by the macrophage and to be themselves taken up at a rate comparable to the rate of uptake of oxidatively modified holo LDL (29).

We postulate, then, that LDL *in vivo* may undergo an analogous modification and that the oxidatively modified form is what is really taken up by resident macrophages in the artery wall and leads to foam cell formation. It should be stressed, however, that there is still only minimal evidence for the occurrence of such oxidative modification *in vivo*. Studies by Goldstein, Brown, Hoff and their coworkers (30) shows that there is some kind of modified LDL in arterial lesions and that this is taken up more readily by macrophages. Further studies by Hoff, however, suggest that the uptake is not by way of the acetyl LDL receptor (31). Raymond and his coworkers (32) have isolated a modified form of LDL from inflammatory fluid that is taken up more avidly by the macrophage but it is not yet clear whether this modified form corresponds to oxidatively modified LDL generated by endothelial cells.

Recruitment and Retention of Macrophages

The first step in the recruitment of monocytes, as discussed above, must be the adhesion of them to the endothelial surface. Next there must be chemotactic factors that induce the migration through the endothelial layer into the intima. The list of chemotactic factors for the monocyte is a long one and undoubtedly more remain to be discovered. Which are relevant *in vivo* remains to be determined. Recently Mr. Mark Quinn and Dr. Sampath Parthasarathy in our laboratory tested the possibility that LDL itself might be chemotactic since that would nicely explain why more white cells penetrate into developing lesions that are rich in LDL. Native LDL itself turned out to have no activity al all -- neither chemotactic nor inhibitory. However, endothelial cell-modified LDL (or LDL oxidized in other ways) was a potent <u>inhibitor</u> of macrophage motility (33). We suggested that if there were some normal, steady state rate of movement of monocytes into and out of the intima, then the presence of oxidized LDL might arrest their exit and cause them to accumulate at sites containing high levels of oxidatively modified LDL. This phenomenon would be analogous to what is seen in inflammatory sites where MIF (macrophage inhibitory factor) helps insure that macrophages arriving on the scene stay there to "do their job."

More recently Mr. Quinn and Dr. Parthasarathy have made the intriguing observation that oxidized LDL does <u>not</u> inhibit the motility of the normal circulating human monocyte. In fact it actually <u>enhances</u> its motility (34). So now we can propose a scenario in which the presence of oxidatively modified LDL in the intima would act as a chemoattractant to bring monocytes in and then, after they have altered their phenotypic properties to those of resident macrophages, this same oxidatively modified LDL would inhibit their exit. We would have a kind of baited lobster trap that draws them in and then clobbers them to prevent their getting out again (Figure 2).

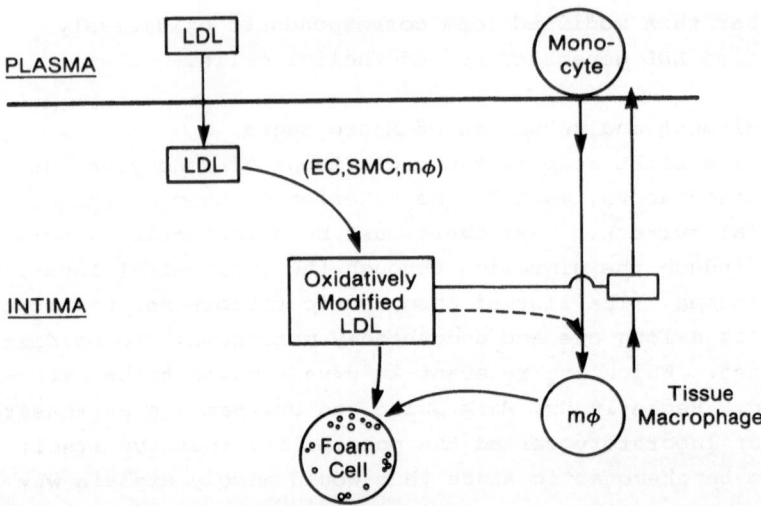

Figure 2. Schematic representation of how oxidatively modified LDL may play a role in the recruitment of circulating monocytes, on the one hand, and retention of tissue macrophages, on the other hand (see text for discussion).

Endothelial Damage Induced by Oxitatively Modified LDL

There is a third way in which oxidatively modified LDL may contribute to atherogenesis. Some years ago Henriksen and coworkers in Oslo (2) and Morel and coworkers in Cleveland (3) observed that LDL was toxic to endothelial cells in culture. Further studies by Morel, Chisolm and coworkers in Cleveland (35) established that this toxicity depended upon prior oxidative damage to the LDL molecule and that native LDL was in fact <u>not</u> toxic. Thus, if there is sufficient oxidative modification of LDL *in vivo*, and especially if the LDL concentrations in a given location are high, this might lead to endothelial cell damage and give us one more way to indict oxidative modification of LDL as contributing to atherogenesis.

Studies in a number of laboratories over the last decade have altered our view of the primary role of endothelial injury in atherosclerosis. It is now widely accepted that endothelial denudation is <u>not</u> a necessary first step in atherogenesis. Instead, the fatty streak is believed to develop under an <u>intact</u> endothelial lining.

Gerrity called attention to the lifting off of sectors of endothelial cells overlying fatty streaks later in lesion development (16) and similar observations have been reported by Fagiotto and Ross (15). When one looks at the fatty streak lesion, one is struck by the very close approximation of the abluminal surface of the endothelial cell and the membrane of the underlying fat-loaded macrophage. It is easy to visualize, then, how the many potentially toxic substances released by the macrophage (lytic enzymes, active oxygen) might eventually cause the endothelial cell bridges to weaken and cause a patch of cells to lift off (36).

SUMMARY AND CONCLUSIONS

The four elements of our new hypothesis regarding the role of oxidatively modified low density lipoproteins in atherogenesis are indicated in the scheme of Figure 3. Reconstructing the sequence of events that leads to the clinically significant atherosclerotic lesion is difficult indeed. The pathologist tries to reconstruct the process by looking at snapshots taken at different stages during the progress of the disease. One difficulty, however, is that

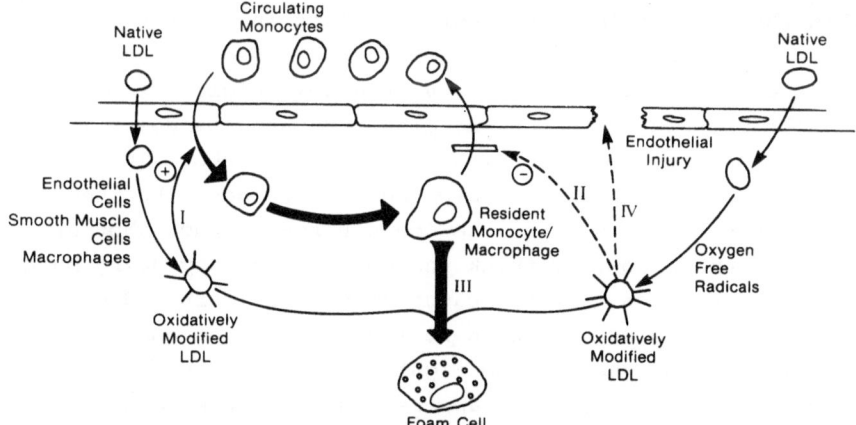

Figure 3. Schematic representation of four separate processes influenced by oxidatively modified LDL that could contribute to the atherogenic process.

he's not always sure in which sequences those snapshots
should be placed. Further, he rarely has enough snapshots
to satisfy himself and he's not sure that he has all of the
stages captured. You will recall that many years ago
Eadweard Muybridge applied his then revolutionary system
for fast-motion photography to try to settle a bet that
Leland Stanford had made. The railroad magnate contented
that a trotting horse had all four legs off the ground at
the same time. So Muybridge developed a shutter with an
exposure time of 2/1000 second and set up a battery of 24
cameras equipped with his special shutter and triggered by
threads pulled across the path of the trotting horse. He
got the classic set of photographs shown in Figure 4 and
Leland Stanford won his bet. But suppose he had only a
few snapshots and wasn't sure about their sequence, as in
Figure 5. That is in a way the difficult position of the
pathologist. Eventually we hope he will have a complete
reconstruction with assurance about the sequence much as
Muybridge had in his historic series of pictures. In a way,
Muybridge managed to slow down rapid motion through the use
of multiple cameras. What the pathologist might prefer to
do is to be able to speed up the agonizingly slow process
of atherosclerosis so that he might better understand the
various stages and how they relate to one another.

The cell biologist is in some ways in a better position
than the pathologist; in other ways he's in a worse position.
Because it's so difficult to get the full sequence of pictures of the real thing in vivo, the cell biologist decides
to take pictures of something else. He studies cells in
culture or enzymatic phenomena in the test tube. These he
can follow with great precision and he can describe them
in great detail. However, he doesn't really know whether
they happen or not. I think the hope is that by going back
and forth between what the pathologist can learn and what
the cell biologist can learn we may finally get enough
pictures to put them in the right sequence and satisfy ourselves about exactly what happens. Right now we can't do
that.

Whatever the mechanism may be it is already clear that
there is a horse out there and that he is running, and that

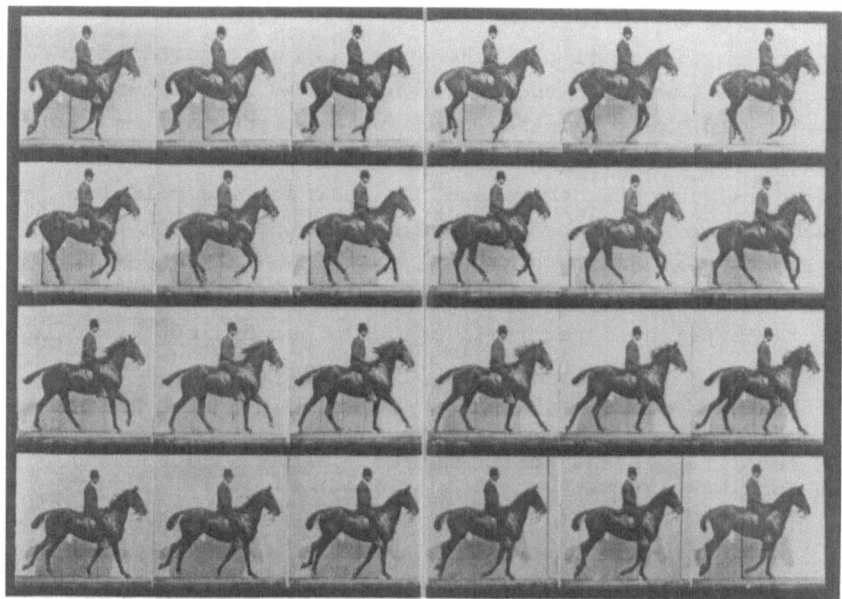

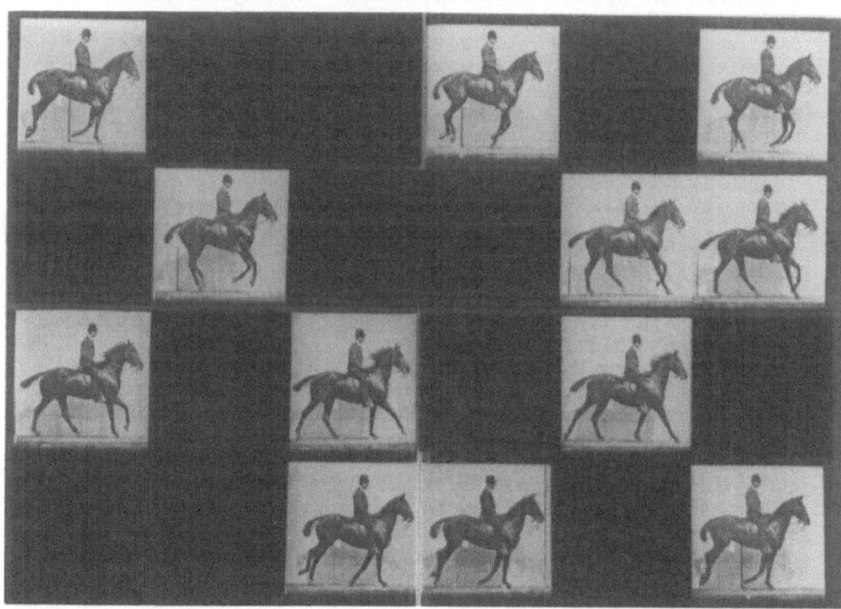

Figure 4. Complete reconstruction, "step"-by-"step", of how a horse trots (Eadweard Muybridge, 1878).
Figure 5. The incomplete set of "steps" (with uncertainty about the sequence) generally available to the pathologist.

a high level of cholesterol in the blood makes him run faster. So, if we simply take away his cholesterol we will slow things down even though we don't know exactly what it is we're slowing. In other words we can forestall coronary heart disease without necessarily knowing the cellular mechanisms. On the other hand, by learning the cellular mechanisms we may uncover new ways to intervene, ways to intervene by affecting cell wall reactions to hypercholesterolemia and other noxious stimuli, even if we can't control the hypercholesterolemia or the other noxious stimuli.

REFERENCES

1. Consensus Conference (1985) Lowering blood cholesterol to prevent heart disease. JAMA 253:2080-2090.
2. Henriksen T, Evensen SA, Carlander B (1979) Injury to human endothelial cells in culture induced by low density lipoproteins. Scand J Clin Lab Invest 39: 361-368.
3. Hessler JR, Morel DW, Lewis LJ, Chisolm GM (1983) Lipoprotein oxidation and lipoprotein-induced cytotoxicity. Arteriosclerosis 3:215-222.
4. Carvalho A-C, Colman RW, Lees RS (1974) Platelet function in hyperlipoproteinemia. N Engl J Med 290:434-438.
5. Steinberg D (1983) Lipoproteins and atherosclerosis. A look back and a look ahead. Arteriosclerosis 3:283-301.
6. Watanabe Y (1980) Serial inbreeding of rabbits with hereditary hyperlipemia (WHHL-rabbit). Incidence and development of atherosclerosis. Atherosclerosis 36: 261-268.
7. Yamamoto T, Bishop RW, Brown MS, Goldstein J, Russell DW (1986) Deletion in cysteine-rich region of LDL receptor impedes transport to cell surface in WHHL rabbit. Science 232:1230-1237.
8. Goldstein JL, Brown MS, Anderson RGW, Russell DW, Schneider WJ (1985) Receptor-mediated endocytosis. Annual Rev Cell Biol 1:1-39.
9. Fowler S, Shio H, Haley WJ (1979) Characterization of lipid-laden aortic cells from cholesterol-fed rabbits. IV. Investigation of macrophage-like properties of aortic cell populations. Lab Invest 41:372-378.
10. Tsukuda T, Rosenfeld M, Ross R, Gown WM (1986) Immunocyte chemical analysis of cellular components in atherosclerotic lesions. Arteriosclerosis 6:601-613.
11. Mahley RW (1979) Dietary fat, cholesterol, and accelerated atherosclerosis. Atherosclerosis Rev 5:1-34.
12. Mahley RW, Innerarity TL, Rall Jr SC, Weisgraber KH (1985) Lipoproteins of special significance in atherosclerosis. Insights provided by studies of Type III hyperlipoproteinemias. Ann NY Acad Sci 454:209-221.

13. Goldstein J, Ho YK, Basu SK, Brown MS (1979) Binding site on macrophages that mediates uptake and degradation of acetylated low density lipoprotein, producing massive cholesterol deposition. Proc Natl Acad Sci USA 76:333-377.

14. Gerrity RG, Naito HK, Richardson M, Schwartz CJ (1979) Dietary induced atherogenesis in swine. Am J Pathol 95:775-793.

15. Fagiotto A, Ross R, Harker L (1984) Studies of hypercholesterolemia in the nonhuman primate. I. Changes that lead to fatty streak formation. Arteriosclerosis 4:323-340.

16. Gerrity RG (1981) The role of the monocyte in atherogenesis. I. Transition of blood-born monocytes into foam cells in fatty lesions. Am J Pathol 103:181-190.

17. Bevilacqua MP, Pober JS, Wheeler ME, Cotran RS, Gimbrone Jr MA (1985) Interleukin 1 acts on cultured human vascular endothelium to increase the adhesion of polymorphonuclear leukocytes, monocytes, and related leukocyte cell lines. J Cell Invest 76:2003-2011.

18. Pittman RC, Carew TE, Attie AD, Witztum JL, Watanabe Y, Steinberg D (1982) Receptor-dependent and receptor-independent degradation of low density lipoprotein in normal rabbits and in receptor-deficient mutant rabbits. J Biol Chem 257:7994-8000.

19. Simons LA, Reichl D, Myant NB, Mancini M (1975) The metabolism of the apoprotein of plasma low density lipoprotein in familial hyperbetalipoproteinemia in the homozygous form. Atherosclerosis 21:283-298.

20. Carew TE, Chapman MJ, Goldstein S, Steinberg D (1980) Enhanced degradation of trypsin-treated low density lipoprotein by fibroblasts from a patient with familial hypercholesterolemia. Biochim Biophys Acta 529:171-175.

21. Mahley RW, Innearity TL, Weisgraber KH, Oh SY (1979) Altered metabolism (in vivo and vitro) of plasma lipoprotein after selective chemical modification of lysine residues of the apoproteins. J Clin Invest 64:743-750.

22. Fogelman AM, Schechter JS, Hokom M, Child JS, Edwards PA (1980) Malondialdehyde alteration of low density lipoprotein leads to cholesterol accumulation in human monocyte-macrophages. Proc Natl Acad Sci USA 77:2214-2218.

23. Henriksen T, Mahoney EM, Steinberg D (1981) Enhanced macrophage degradation of low density lipoprotein previously incubated with cultured endothelial cells: recognition by receptors for acetylated low density lipoproteins. Proc Natl Acad Sci USA 78:6499-6503.

24. Henriksen T, Mahoney EM, Steinberg D (1982) Enhanced macrophage degradation of biologically modified low density lipoprotein. Arteriosclerosis 3:149-159.

25. Parthasarathy S, Printz DJ, Boyd D, Joy L, Steinberg D (1986) Macrophage oxidation of low density lipoprotein generates a modified form recognized by the scavenger receptor. Arteriosclerosis 6:505-510.

26. Steinbrecher UP, Parthasarathy S, Leake DS, Witztum JL, Steinberg D (1984) Modification of low density lipoprotein by endothelial cells involves lipid peroxidation and degradation of low density lipoprotein phospholipids. Proc Natl Acad Sci USA 81:3883-3887.

27. Parthasarathy S, Steinbrecher UP, Barnett J, Witztum JL, Steinberg D (1985) Essential role of phospholipase A_2 activity in endothelial cell-induced modification of low density lipoprotein. Proc Natl Acad Sci USA 82: 3000-3004.

28. Fong LG, Parthasarathy S, Witztum JL, Steinberg D (1986) Nonenzymatic degradation of aproprotein B-100 during the oxidative modification of low density lipoprotein (submitted to J Biol Chem).

29. Parthasarathy S, Fong SG, Otero D, Steinberg D (1987) Recognition of resolubilized apoproteins from delipidated, oxidatively-modified low density lipoprotein (LDL) by the acetyl-LDL receptor. Proc Natl Acad Sci USA 84:537-540.

30. Goldstein JL, Hoff JH, Ho YK, Basu SK, Brown MS (1981) Stimulation of cholesteryl ester synthesis in macrophages by extracts of atherosclerotic human aortas and complexes of albumin/cholesteryl ester. Arteriosclerosis 1:210-226.

31. Hoff HF, Morton RE (1985) Lipoproteins containing apo B extracted from human aortas: Structure and function. Ann NY Acad Sci 454:183-194.

32. Raymond TL, Reynolds SA, Swanson JA (1985) Lipoproteins of the extravascular space: Enhances macrophage degradation of low density lipoproteins from interstitial inflammatory fluid. J Lipid Res 26:1356:1362.

33. Quinn MT, Parthasarathy S, Steinberg D (1985) Endothelial cell-derived chemotactic activity for mouse peritoneal macrophages and the effects of modified forms of low density lipoprotein. Proc Natl Acad Sci USA 82:5949-5953.

34. Quinn MT, Parthasarathy S, Fong LG, Steinberg D (1987) Oxidatively modified low density lipoproteins: A potential role in recruitment and retention of monocyte/macrophages during atherogenesis. Proc Natl Acad Sci 84:2995-2998.

35. Morel DW, DiCorleto PE, Chisolm GM (1984) Endothelial and smooth muscle cells alter low density lipoprotein *in vitro* by free radical oxication. Arteriosclerosis 4:357-364.

36. Steinberg D (1986) Lipoproteins and atherogenesis: Current concepts. In: Hallgren B, Levin O, Rossner S, Vessby B (eds) Diet and Prevention of Coronary Heart Disease and Cancer. New York: Raven Press, pp. 95-112.

33
A Cellular Basis for the Potential Atherogenicity of Triglyceride-Rich Lipoproteins

Sandra H. Gianturco and William A. Bradley

Initiating Events in Atherosclerosis

Two potential intiating events in atherosclerosis are endothelial injury and the accumulation of lipid-filled foam cells in the arterial intima. Ross and Glomset suggested that atherosclerosis may be a response to some form of endothelial injury (1). By this mechanism, changes in endothelial permeability could expose the arterial intima, the site of plaque initiation, to all blood components, including monocytes, lipoproteins, platelets, and coagulation factors with ensuing lipid accumulation and fibrin deposition. A second important initiating event in atherosclerosis is the accumulation of foam cells in the intima of the arterial wall (2-4). Many arterial foam cells are monocyte-derived macrophages that are engorged with cholesteryl ester (5). LDL are the major carriers of cholesterol in the blood and have long been considered to be the primary atherogenic lipoprotein. This represents a paradox in terms of the initiation of atherosclerosis, however, since native, unmodified LDL are not toxic in endothelial cells and do not produce foam cells *in vitro* when incubated with macrophages. Endothelial cell-modified LDL (6) and malondialdehyde-modified LDL (7), however, can produce macrophage lipid engorgement and conceivably these could be formed *in vivo*. Likewise, oxidized LDL are toxic to endothelial cells *in vitro* (8).

These modified LDL have not been found in plasma. There are, however, two types of native human plasma lipoproteins known to produce lipid engorgement in macrophages *in vitro*: the triglyceride-rich lipoproteins, chylomicrons and their remanants and very low density lipoproteins (VLDL) (9-12).

Triglyceride-Rich Lipoproteins

Chylomicrons are synthesized in the intestine and are normally converted into remnants that are quickly taken up by the liver. Chylomicrons can, however, rapidly convert macrophages into foam cells after receptor-mediated uptake *in vitro* (9,10) and *in vivo* (13).

Very low density lipoproteins are synthesized in the liver and are normally converted to remnants, intermediate density lipoproteins, and low density lipoproteins. Large VLDL are triglyceride-rich particles ($\sim$ 66% triglyceride by mass) and it is often overlooked that, per particle, VLDL actually carry more total cholesterol than do LDL. VLDL are much larger than LDL, with diameters ranging from 50-80 nm compared with an average diameter of 22 nm for LDL. The VLDL surface contains cholesterol, phospholipid, and apoprotein (apo) B, apoC peptides, and apoE. ApoB and apoE are the only apoproteins known to bind to the LDL receptor, and both apoproteins are present in VLDL. VLDL have cores composed of both triglyceride and cholesteryl ester, the neutral lipids. Normally, the triglycerides of large VLDL are hydrolyzed by lipoprotein lipase. During lipolysis many VLDL surface components (including phospholipid and cholesterol as well as all of the transferable apoproteins, the C peptides and apoE) are lost, forming LDL. LDL retain apoB as the only apoprotein, cholesterol, and phospholipid in the surface; the core of LDL contains cholesteryl ester and a small amount of triglyceride.

Chylomicrons and VLDL are correctly considered to be triglyceride-rich particles, and on a mass percentage basis they contain seemingly small amounts of cholesterol and cholesteryl ester (5 to 15% total cholesterol versus > 65% triglyceride). Their large size, however, translates to much more cholesterol carried per triglyceride-rich particle than is carried by one cholesteryl ester-rich LDL. As Table 1 illustrates, each low density lipoprotein carries approximately 2,000 molecules of total cholesterol, that is cholesterol plus cholesteryl ester (14). By contrast, each chylomicron carries about thirty times the amount of total cholesterol, or about 60,000 molecules of total cholesterol (cholesterol plus cholesteryl ester) per particle. Of course these are triglyceride-rich lipoproteins; chylomicrons also carry approximately 500,000 molecules of triglyceride, in contrast to the 300 carried by LDL. Each large VLDL (S_f100-400) contains at least five times as much total cholesterol as does one LDL particle. In addition, VLDL contain about ten times as much triglyceride. The VLDL data are representative of normolipidemic subjects (14). VLDL from subjects with hypertriglyceridemia, however, are enriched in cholesteryl esters relative to normal VLDL, so that the values shown in this table are minima (15). Considering the large number of molecules of cholesterol and triglycerides carried by the various lipoprotein particles, it is apparent that when particles such as large VLDL or chylomicrons enter via receptors, they can potentially cause massive lipid engorgement.

Normally, however, large VLDL do not interact with cell surface receptors (9,16-19). Certain abnormal VLDL are taken up by cells via specific receptors, such as the β-VLDL that accumulate in the plasma in response to cholesterol feeding (4) and VLDL from hypertriglyceridemic humans (9,10,16-20).

Interaction of Triglyceride-Rich Lipoproteins with Cell Surface Receptors

Large VLDL from normal subjects (S_f60-400) do not interact with cell surface receptors and are not normally catabolized by these receptor pathways. More specifically, normal VLDL do not bind to the LDL receptor (16-20). Large VLDL are converted into smaller VLDL remnants (S_f20-60), intermediate density lipoproteins (IDL), and LDL. These smaller, triglyceride-poor particles then can bind to LDL receptors via apoB (20-22) and be removed from the plasma compartment, primarily in the liver. LDL receptors are

Table 1: Molecules of Components per Particle

Lipoprotein	Lipoprotein M_r x 10^6	Lipoprotein Radius (nm)	Cholesterol	Cholesteryl Ester	Triglycerides
Chylomicrons	504	60.0	25,840	27,000	507,000
VLDL Sf100-400	31.1	23.3	4,160	5,630	23,530
LDL	2.3	9.6	475	1,310	298

Adapted from: Shen BW, Scanu AM, Kezdy FJ (1977) Proc Natl Acad Sci USA 74:837-841

present, however, on virtually every cell of the body (23).
Of particular relevance to atherogenesis is their presence
on arterial smooth muscle cells, monocyte-macrophages, and
endothelial cells as well as fibroblasts. In contrast to
normal VLDL S_f60-400, VLDL S_f60-400 from hypertriglyceridemic humans (HTG-VLDL), are taken up by receptors on
cultured fibroblasts (7-11,16-18,20), lymphocytes (19),
macrophages (9,10,12), and endothelial cells (24). In
hypertriglyceridemia, there is redistribution of apoE into
VLDL (25) producing particles which have the abnormal
ability to bind to the LDL receptor due to the presence of
additional apoE that is of a conformation that permits binding (21). Normal VLDL S_f60-400 do not bind to LDL receptors
because the apoE present is of an inappropriate conformation (22). Likewise, the apoB of large VLDL is in an
inappropirate conformation for binding to the LDL receptor
(20,26).

Receptor-mediated uptake of HTG-VLDL is deleterious
to some cell types, such as cultured endothelial cells (24).
Hypertriglyceridemic VLDL from certain subjects also have
the abnormal ability to rapidly convert macrophages into
foam cells via receptors (9,12). From these observations
we hypothesize that the abnormal receptor-mediated cellular
uptake of hypertriglyceridemic VLDL may be involved in
atherogenesis by inducing endothelial cell injury and by
promoting foam cell formation.

Endothelial Injury Induced by Hypertriglyceridemic VLDL

Hypertriglyceridemic VLDL S_f100-400 are toxic to
cultured bovine aortic endothelial cells (24). After 48
hours of exposure to low levels of hypertriglyceridemic
VLDL (28 µg protein/ml), the number of viable cells was
reduced by approximately 60% (24). This toxicity persisted
for 72 hours in culture without refeeding the cells. The
same concentration of normal VLDL or LDL had no significant
effect on viability of the endothelial cells. The levels
of HTG-VLDL found to be injurious to the cells were those
that are present in normal humans in the fasting state,
far lower than the levels present in hypertriglyceridemic
subjects. Thus, it is conceivable that circulating levels

of VLDL in hypertriglyceridemic subjects could perturb the endothelium *in vivo*.

Foam Cell Formation by Abnormal Triglyceride-Rich Lipoproteins

Macrophages develop large numbers of visible lipid inclusions when incubated with human chylomicrons (9,12). Similar lipid inclusions are produced when the cells are incubated with cholesteryl ester-rich β-VLDL from cholesterol-fed animals (4). Likewise, large VLDL from certain hypertriglyceridemic subjects rapidly induce visible lipid engorgement (9,12). By contrast, normal VLDL and normal LDL fail to induce appreciable lipid accumulation even after prolonged incubation (4,9,12).

Binding studies in murine macrophages (9,12) and human monocyte-derived macrophages (11) indicate that HTG-VLDL and chylomicrons but not normal VLDL from fasting subjects bind to distinct receptors on macrophages. As shown in Table 2, the lipid that accumulates in macrophages after receptor-mediated uptake of a lipoprotein initially reflects the lipid composition of the lipoprotein (4,9,12). Macrophages incubated *in vitro* in the absence of lipoproteins contain only a small amount of triglyceride and cholesterol, with virtually no cholesterol ester. Macrophages incubated with normal LDL or with normal VLDL do not accumulate appreciable lipid. As mentioned, the only native human lipoproteins known to induce massive lipid accumulation in macrophages *in vitro* are VLDL from hypertriglyceridemic subjects (lipoprotein profiles of type 4, 5, 2b, and 3) and chylomicrons from type 5 subjects. These lipoproteins induce massive triglyceride accumulation (up to forty-fold over control), as expected, since these are triglyceride-rich lipoproteins. Chylomicrons and HTG-VLDL can also induce increased cellular cholesterol and cholesterol-ester, as shown in Table 2 (12). β-VLDL from cholesterol-fed rabbits cause the accumulation of cholesterol and cholesteryl ester primarily, again reflecting the composition of these particular VLDL. Acetyl LDL, which is a modified LDL that enters the cell through a distinct receptor pathway, induce cholesteryl ester accumulation (4).

Table 2.   Effects of Lipoproteins on the Lipid Composition of P338D$_1$ Macrophages

Lipo-protein	Pro-tein	TG	CHOL	CE	TG	CHOL	CE
	Concentration in Medium (µg/ml)				Cellular Lipid Content µg Lipid/mg Cell Protein[b]		
None	--	--	--	--	15.4	16.3	0.6
LDL	10	2	11.4	22	11.2	10.7	1.0
	40	8	45.6	86	8.0	9.9	3.9
HTG-VLDL$_1$	10	120	10.0	4	45.6	19.6	0
	40	481	40.0	18	96.1	19.1	6.5
Chylo-microns[a]	02.8	127	9.7	6	45.7	26.1	1.4
	11	510	39.0	21	102.0	30.0	16.0
β-VLDL	40	13	191.6	351	14.1	32.0	16.4
Acetyl LDL	10	2	11.6	26	6.5	20.6	20.1
	40	10	46.4	105	5.5	27.0	36.3

[a] Chylomicron protein content estimation from average composition reported (38) using a TG/Prot = 45. TG was assayed enzymatically.

[b] Cells were grown as described in the legend to Fig. 1 of ref. 20. Each dish received 2 ml of complete medium containing the indicated lipoproteins and was incubated at 37°C for 4 hr. The lipoprotein concentrations are given in terms of micrograms lipoprotein protein, triglyceride (TG), cholesterol (Chol), and cholesteryl ester (CE) per milliliter. The LDL preparation was from a normal donor. The HTG-VLDL$_1$ and chylomicron preparations were from a patient with type 5 hypertriglyceridemia. Acetyl LDL were prepared from normal LDL. β-VLDL were isolated from cholesterol-fed rabbits and tested in a separate experiment. Intracellular lipid concentrations are expressed as micrograms lipid per milligram cell protein, and each value is the average of values from duplicate dishes, which varied by < 9%.

Adapted from: Gianturco SH, Brown SA, Via DP, and Bradley WA (1986) J Lipid Res 27:412-420

In vivo Implications

Certain observations made in human subjects with hypertriglyceridemia suggest that these potentially athero-genic events observed *in vitro* may occur *in vivo*. First, the catabolism of VLDL in subjects with hypertriglyceridemia is abnormal. In contrast to VLDL catabolism in normal individuals, much of the VLDL S_f60-400 in hypertriglyceri-demic subjects disappears directly from the plasma without being converted to small VLDL, IDL, or LDL (27). This direct disappearance could be due to the removal of HTG-VLDL, S_f60-400 via LDL receptors. Second, premature athero-sclerosis is common in certain types of hypertriglyceridemic subjects, particularly diabetic subjects (28). Third, foam cells accumulate in xanthomas, the spleen, and bone marrow in subjects with hypertriglyceridemia types 1, 3, and 5 (28). Further, foam cells accumulate in eruptive xanthomas in hypertriglyceridemic diabetics under poor control (13). These foam cells are initially filled primarily with tri-glyceride and with some cholesteryl ester, as noted *in vitro* (Table 2). Insulin treatment of these subjects results in a lowering of plasma triglyceride levels; concomitantly, the xanthoma triglyceride is hydrolyzed, leaving cholesterol behind in the foam cells; this too can be resolved with time (13). We suggest that a similar sequence could occur in hypertriglyceridemic subjects producing arterial foam cells initially engorged with both triglyceride and cho-lesteryl ester. With time and the action of neutral tri-glyceride lipase, the triglyceride could be removed, leav-ing cholesteryl ester. Indeed, the neutral triglyceride lipase of macrophages is catalytically far more active than is the cholesteryl ester hydrolase activity, a ratio which would promote triglyceride hydrolysis and permit cholesteryl ester accumulation (29).

SUMMARY

Structurally and functionally abnormal VLDL exist in fasting hypertriglyceridemic humans. These large abnormal VLDL, in contrast to large normal VLDL, interact with cell surface receptors. One large VLDL particle carries far more total cholesterol than one LDL particle. Receptor-mediated uptake of abnormal VLDL is injurious to endothelial cells and converts macrophages into foam cells *in vitro*. These observations lead to the hypothesis that if similar phenomena occur *in vitro*, abnormal VLDL, which have prolonged residence times and increased opportunity to interact with peripheral cells, are atherogenic by promoting endothelial injury and initiating foam cell formation. Since premature atherosclerosis is associated with some forms of hypertriglyceridemia and foam cells accumulate in certain hypertriglyceridemic subjects, similar events may indeed occur *in vivo*.

REFERENCES

1. Ross R, Glomset JA (1973) Atherosclerosis and the arterial smooth muscle cell. Science 180:1332-1339
2. Gerrity, RG (1981) The role of monocyte in atherogenesis: I. Transition of blood-borne monocytes into foam cells in fatty lesions. Am J Clin Pathol 103(2):181-190
3. Faggiotto A and Ross R (1984) Studies of hypercholesterolemia in the nonhuman primate. Arterosclerosis 4:323-340
4. Brown MS, Goldstein JL (1983) Lipoprotein metabolism in the macrophage: implications for cholesterol deposition in atherosclerosis. Am Rev Biochem 52:223-261
5. Fowler S, Shio H and Haley NJ (1979) Characterization of lipid-laden aortic cells from cholesterol-fed rabbits. Laboratory Investigation 41(4):372-378
6. Steinbrecher UP, Parthasarathy S, Leake DS, Witztum JL, Steinberg D (1984) Modification of low density lipoprotein by endothelial cells involves lipid peroxidation and degradation of low density. Proc Natl Acad Sci USA 81:3883-3887
7. Fogelman AM, Shechter I, Seager J, Hokom M, Child JS, Edwards, PA (1980) Malondialdehyde alteration of low density lipoproteins leads to cholesteryl ester accumulation in human monocyte-macrophages. Proc Natl Acad Sci USA 77:2214-2218
8. Hessler JR, Morel DW, Lewis LJ, Chisolm, GM (1983) Lipoprotein oxidation and lipoprotein-induced cytotoxicity. Arteriosclerosis 3:215-222
9. Gianturco SH, Bradley WA, Gotto AM Jr, Morrisett JD, Peavy DL (1982) Hypertriglyceridemic very low density lipoproteins induce triglyceride synthesis and accumulation in mouse peritoneal macrophages. J Clin Invest 70:168-178
10. Nestel PJ, Billington T, Bazelmans J (1985) Metabolism of human plasma triacylglycerol-rich lipoproteins in rodent macrophages: capacity for interaction at β-VLDL receptor. Biochim Biophys Acta 837:314-324
11. Van Lenten BJ, Fegelman AM, Hokom MM, Benson L, Haberland ME, Edwards PA (1983) Regulation of the

uptake and degradation of β-very low density lipoprotein in human monocyte-macrophages. J Biol Chem
258:5151-5157.

12. Gianturco SH, Brown SA, Via DP, Bradley WL (1986) The
β-VLDL receptor pathway of murine P388D₁ macrophages.
J Lipid Res 27:412-420

13. Parker F, Bagdade JD, Odland GF, Bierman EL (1970)
Evidence for the chylomicron origin of lipids accumulating in diabetic eruptive xanthomas: a correlative
lipid biochemical, histochemical, and electron microscopic study. J Clin Invest 49:2172-2187

14. Shen BW, Scanu AM, Kezdy FJ (1977) Structure of human
serum lipoproteins inferred from compositional analysis.
Proc Natl Acad Sci USA 74:837-841

15. Eisenberg S, Gavish D, Oschry Y, Fainaru M, Deckelbaum
RJ (1984) Abnormalities in very low, low, and high
density lipoproteins in hypertriglyceridemia. Reversal toward normal with bezafibrate treatment. J Clin
Invest 74:470-482

16. Gianturco SH, Gotto AM Jr, Jackson RL, Patsch JR,
Sybers HD, Taunton OD, Yeshurun DL, Smith LC (1978)
Control of 3-hydroxy-3-methylglutaryl-CoA reductase
activity in cultured human fibroblasts by very low
denisty lipoproteins of subjects with hypertriglyceridemia. J Clin Invest 61:320-328

17. Gianturco SH, Packard CJ, Shepherd J, Smith LC,
Catapano AL, Sybers HD, Gotto AM Jr (1980) Abnormal
suppression of 3-hydroxy-3-methylglutaryl-CoA
reductase activity in cultured human fibroblasts by
hypertriglyceridemic very low density lipoprotein sub-
classes. Lipids 15:456-463

18. Gianturco SH, Brown FB, Gotto AM Jr, Bradley WA (1982)
Receptor-mediated uptake of hypertriglyceridemic very
low density lipoproteins by normal human fibroblasts.
J Lipid Res 23:984-993

19. Poyser A, Nestel PJ (1979) Metabolism of very low
density lipoproteins by human mononuclear cells.
Artery 6:122-143

20. Krul ES, Tikkanen MJ, Cole TG, Davie JM, Schonfeld G
(1985) Roles of apolipoproteins B and E in the cellular binding of very low density lipoproteins. J
Clin Invest 75:361-369

21. Gianturco SH, Gotto AM Jr, Hwang S-LC, Karlin JB, Lin
AHY, Prasad SC, Bradley WA (1983) Apolipoprotein E
mediates uptake of S_f100-400 hypertriglyceridemic very
low density lipoproteins by the low density lipoprotein receptor pathway in normal human fibroblasts. J
Biol Chem 258:4526-4533

22. Bradley WA, Hwang S-LC, Karlin JB, Lin AHY, Prasad SC,
Gotto AM Jr, Gianturco SH (1984) Low-density lipoprotein receptor binding determinants switch from
apolipoprotein B during conversion of hypertriglyceridemic very-low-density lipoportein to low-density lipoproteins. J Biol Chem 259:14728-14735

23. Brown MS, Goldstein JL (1986) A receptor-mediated
pathway for cholesterol homeostasis. Science 232
(4746):34-47

24. Gianturco SH, Eskin SG, Navarro LT, Lahart CJ, Smith
LC, Gotto AM Jr (1980) Abnormal effects of hypertri-
acylglycerolemic very low-density lipoproteins on

3-hydroxy-3-methylglutaryl-CoA reductase activity and viability of cultured bovine aortic endothelial cells. Biochim Biophys Acta 618:143-152

25. Glum CB, Aron L, Sciacca R (1980) Radioimmunoassay studies of human apolipoprotein E. J Clin Invest 66:1240-1250

26. Schonfeld G, Patsch W, Pfleger B, Witztum JL, Weidman SW (1979) Lipolysis produces changes in the immuno-reactivity and cell reactivity of very low density lipoproteins. J Clin Invest 64:1288-1297

27. Reardon MF, Fridge NH, Nestel PJ (1978) Catabolism of very low density lipoprotein B apoprotein in man. J Clin Invest 61:850-860

28. Fredrickson DS, Goldstein JL, Brown MS (1978) The familial hyperlipoproteinemias. In: Stanbury JG, Syngaarden MF, Fredrickson DS (eds) The Metabolic Basis of Inherited Diseases, 4th edition. McGraw-Hill, New York, pp 604-655

29. Khoo, JC, Vance JE, Mahoney, EM, Jensen D, Wancewicz E, Steinberg D (1984) Neutral triglyceride lipase in macrophages. Arteriosclerosis 4:34-40

Response of Human Lesions to Direct Intervention and Risk Factor Control

34
Strategies for Statistical Analysis of Angiographic Data: Individual Lesions Versus Individual Patients

Sheryl F. Kelsey

INTRODUCTION

Since angiography enabled visualization of individual lesions, clinical study results can be analyzed lesion by lesion. In contrast with earlier studies that used clinical endpoints such as myocardial infarction (MI) or coronary heart disease (CHD) death, a new generation of studies underway uses angiographically measured outcome of change in atherosclerotic lesions. Current randomized clinical trials to test the effect of lipid lowering therapy on atherosclerosis include those by Alderman, Blankenhorn, Brown, Buchwald and Havel (1).

Strategies for the statistical analysis of angiographically measured outcome is the subject of this report, which is organized around the question: Should the patient or the lesion by the primary unit of analysis? Angiographic evaluation focuses on lesions which suggest that information about individual lesions is most relevant. One perceived advantage of using lesions is the studies would require fewer patients, since a single patient typically has more than one lesion. Of course smaller sample sizes imply lower costs.

On the other hand, evaluation of therapy is important on a patient basis. Lipid lowering treatment is not directed at specific lesions, but rather administered on a patient

basis. In randomized trials, it is the patient not the
lesion assigned to treatment. The protection of randomization is lost if patients are not considered as the primary
units of analysis.

Standard statistical methods are based on the assumption that units of analysis are independent. While this
assumption is reasonable for patients it may not be reasonable for lesions. Do lesions behave independently? Lesions
in an individual patient are exposed to the same risks in
terms of serum lipid levels, smoking, blood pressure. However, lesions may also be exposed to different risks according to their location and morphology and therapy, such as
coronary angioplasty, is direct to specific lesions.

The National Heart, Lung, and Blood Institute (NHLBI)
Type II Coronary Intervention Study (The Type II Study) was
the first study to use coronary angiographic change as a
measure of outcome (2). Data from the Type II Study will
be used to illustrate the issues of patient vs. lesion
analysis. Briefly, the Type II Study was a randomized,
double-blind clinical trial designed to determine whether
reducing LDL cholesterol in patients with Type II hyperlipidemia and coronary artery disease (CAD) would retard
progression of CAD. Patients who had elevated LDL cholesterol after one month of diet therapy and who had presump-
tive evidence of coronary disease underwent coronary
angiography. Eligible patients were assigned at random to a
daily dosage of 24 grams of cholestyramine or to placebo.
The Type II diet was prescribed for all patients. After
5-years of therapy, patients were hospitalized and coronary
angiography was performed in the same manner it had been
carried out prior to the start of treatment. The results
of the Type II Study provided strong evidence that cholestyramine is effective in retarding progression and that reduction in the ratio of HDL/total cholesterol is the mechanism by which this is accomplished.

Use of an appropriate unit for analyses is not unique
to analysis of change in atherosclerotic lesions. Our
clinical and biostatistical counterparts in ophthalamologic
research wrestled with a similar problem as evidenced by the
1973 editorial by Fred Ederer, "Shall we count the numbers

of eyes or the numbers of subjects?" (3) Since it had been
demonstrated that ocular measures generally were correlated
between right and left eyes of patients, the answer was to
count both eyes and subjects. This answer implies that a
distinction is made between two paired eyes of a single
subject and between (unpaired) eyes of different subjects.

Intrapatient Correlation of Lesions

Do lesions within an individual patient change
independently? Analyses which disregard the patient and
focus only on lesions as the unit of analysis have the
underlying assumption that lesions for a given individual
change independently. Such an assumption is not reasonable
from a conceptual or empirical viewpoint.

Conceptually, it is unlikely that change is independent
since treatment as well as many risk factors are patient
specific i.e., within a patient, lesions are "exposed" to
the same specific dosage of drug, lipid levels, and
blood pressure.

Empirically, evidence show that lesions do not behave
independently has been derived from the Type II Study.
Shown in Table 1 is the distribution of lesion changes per
patient in the Type II Study. There are six patients who
had both lesion progression and lesion regression so that
it is clear that changes are not completely dependent. On
the other hand, note, one patient had 7 changes, three patients had 6 changes. This clustering of changes in some
patients suggests that there may be intrapatient correlation of lesion changes.

Lesion data, disregarding the patient, are presented
in Table 2. If we assume independence, then we would
expect for example, in the placebo group 42 progressions
and 5 regressions would be distributed without regard to
patient among 354 existing lesions. We would expect 16
new lesions distributed without regard to patient among 771
normal segments. A simulation was carried out in which
lesion changes were assigned at random without regard to
patient among the lesions and normal segments in the
placebo group. After these changes were assigned, we
reconsidered patients. The distribution of changes among

patients in the placebo group were tallied. The same procedure was carried out with changes in the cholestyramine group and then the two treatment groups were combined. This was repeated 500 times.

Table 1. Coronary Lesion Changes per Patients in the Type II Coronary Intervention Study

Patients with:	Number of Patients		
	Placebo	Choles-tyramine	Total
2 regressions and no progression	0	1	1
1 regression and no progression	4	3	7
No change	24	31	55
Progression and regression	1	5	6
1 progression and no regression	15	11	26
2 progressions and no regression	8	2	10
3 progressions and no regression	1	3	4
4 progressions and no regression	1	2	3
5 progressions and no regression	0	0	0
6 progressions and no regression	2	1	3
7 progressions and no regression	1	0	1

Table 2. Number of Coronary Artery Lesions and Lesion Changes by Treatment in the Type II Study

	Placebo (57 pts)	Cholestyramine (59 pts)	Total (116 pts)
Normal segments	771	818	1589
Lesions	354	322	676
New lesions	16	12	28
Progressions	42	35	77
Regressions	5	10	15

Table 3 presents a comparison of the actual observed Type II results with the 500 simulations. In the Type II Study, there were 55 patients among both treatment groups with no change. Among the simulated studies, the number of patients with no changes ranged from 33 to 51. On the average, there were only 42.8 patients with no change. Changed lesions clustered among certain patients in the actual study while changes were more spread out among patients according to the simulated studies. Based on the assumption of independence of lesion change, the probability that as many as 55 patients would be without a lesion change is only 1 in 10,000. Since the observed distribution of lesion changes among patients is so unlikely if lesions were to behave independently, we take this as evidence that lesions indeed do not change independently.

Table 3. Comparison of Observed and Simulated Data

Patient Category	Number of Patients Observed	Mean Number of Patients from 500 Simulations	P
Placebo			
No change	24	19.5	.004
Regression	4	1.5	.026
Mixed Response	1	3.3	.046
Progression	28	32.7	.034
Cholestyramine			
No change	31	23.3	.002
Regression	4	3.4	--
Mixed Response	5	5.8	--
Progression	19	26.5	.004
Total			
No change	55	42.8	.0001
Regression	8	4.9	.06
Mixed Response	6	9.1	.07
Progression	47	59.2	.0001

P = Estimated probability that observed result or more extreme would occur under the assumption that lesion changes are independent.

Analysis Strategies

How then should we analyze these angiographically measured atherosclerotic changes? Four methods will be discussed.

1. Treat each lesion as an independent unit of analysis. As demonstrated above the assumption of independence is not appropriate so that statistical analyses such as chi-square tests, t-tests and regression would be invalid.

2. Use a ratio statistic methodology that measures secondary units of analysis, i.e., lesions, while maintaining the patient as the primary unit of analysis.

For example, in the Type II Study, we wish to compare groups by number of lesions progressed. Among patients in the placebo group there were 42 lesion progressions among 354 initial lesions and among cholestyramine patients there were 35 lesion progressions among 322 initial lesions.

To test the difference in the average ratios between treatments, we need to calculate standard errors of these ratios which take into account that the numerator (changes) may vary from patient to patient and the denominator (initial lesions) may vary from patient to patient. This can be accomplished using methodology described by Cochran (4). Results are illustrated with data from the Type II Study in Table 4. For all lesions there was no treatment effect. However, if we restrict our attention to only significant lesions, that is, those 50% or greater luminal diameter reduction at baseline, then there are significantly fewer lesion progressions among the cholestyramine patients.

This method does have limitations. It does not take into account the size of lesion changes but rather uses a dichotomous outcome, progression yes or no. Thus, while valid this method does not make most efficient use of available data.

3. Develop a patient summary measure that incorporates lesion changes.

This was the strategy for presenting the primary results of the Type II Study. Ultimate patient outcome was classified as a dichotomy, progression, yes or no.

Many steps were taken along the way to reach this outcome classification and these methods have been previously reported (1,5). Briefly, each lesion was classified as a probable or definite change or as not changed based on agreement of at least two out of three independent panel readings.

Table 4. Comparison of Ratios of Lesion Changes by Treatment for Patients in the Type II Study

	Placebo N = 57		Cholestyamine N = 59		
	Ratio	Std. Error	Ratio	Std. Error	Z-value
Progressions / Initial lesions	.121	.027	.109	.025	.33
Progressions / Initial lesions ≥50%	.143	.030	.054	.022	2.43**

** p <.01 for one-sided test

Then, based on lesion classification patients were classified as exhibiting definite progression, probable progression, no change, definite regression, probable regression, or mixed response. Mixed response were patients who exhibited both lesion progression and lesion regression. Finally, four different dichotomous definitions of progression were formed: 1) definite lesion progression and no lesion regression, 2) definite lesion progression with or without lesion regression, 3) definite or probable lesion progression and no lesion regression, and 4) definite or probable lesion progression with or without lesion regression. Primary treatment results of the Type II were reported for each of these four outcome definitions. In further analysis, the outcome variables were based in logistic regression analysis which enabled examination of the effect of lipid change, as well as treatment, on progression.

4. Use a multivariate model that uses lesion change as the outcome variable but takes into account intra-patient correlation among lesions.

Such a model must allow for the number of lesions to vary from patient to patient. Ideally, we would like to use as explanatory variables both patient specific characteristics such as treatment, lipid levels, and age as well as lesion specific characteristics such as location, morphology, and calcification.

Prompted by needs to properly analyze eyes and patients, statisticians working with researchers in ophthalmology developed methodology which accounted for intra patient correlation between eyes (6,7). While the number of eyes per patient is limited to two, unfortunately such a limit does not apply to number of atherosclerotic lesions per person. Fortunately, the methodology can be extended to analyze a variable number of subunits within a patient. There are methods for outcome variables that are dichotomous as would be the case if we classified lesions as progressed or not. There are also methods for outcome variables that are normally distributed as might be the case with change in luminal diameter reduction or with an appropriate transformation of such a measure. In this analysis a positive number would represent a progression and a negative number a regression. Software is available to carry out these analyses. Analyses are underway which use this model to examine lesion and patient characteristics which are predictors of lesion progression based on the panel readings in the Type II Study patients.

Sample Size Issues

The use of angiographic measured outcome in clinical trials does require fewer patients than do clinical trials that use mortality or morbidity as outcome measures. The reason is not, entirely, because the count of lesions is greater than the count of patients. An advantage comes about because of the rate of change. For example, in the Type II Study for the placebo group, the 5-year mortality rate was about 10% while the rate of progression at least one lesion per patient was 50%. Suppose we had 200 patients and wished to design a clinical trial with 80% power for one-sided hypothesis test with a alpha = .05. If we were to test a therapeutic agent to reduce the mortality rate, the study has power to detect a significant effect if the rate of mortality with the therapeutic agent were 2% versus 10% in the placebo group. By comparison, the study could, with the same probability, detect as significant an effect if the progression rate were 33% versus 50% in the placebo group, it would seem that reduction of progression by such an amount is much more likely than reduction of mortality by the amount mentioned.

CONCLUSION

The answer to "Shall we count the numbers of lesions or the numbers of patients?" is neither patient or lesions but both.

Valid analysis of lesion changes must take into account intrapatient correlation. Multivariate models that do take into account intrapatient correlation and that allow for both lesion specific and patient specific explanatory variables are recommended for analysis of angiographic data.

REFERENCES

1. Detre KM (1986) Effect of resins on atheroma progression. In: Pharmacological Control of Hyperlipidaemia. Barcelona, Spain: JR Prous Science Publishers, SA, pp 35-53
2. Brensike JF, Levy RI, Kelsey SF, *et al* (1984) Effects of therapy with cholestyramine on progression of coronary arteriosclerosis: Results of the NHLBI type II Coronary Intervention study. Circulation 69(2):313-324
3. Ederer F (1973) Shall we count number of eyes or numbers of subjects? Arch Ophthalmo 89:1-2
4. Cochran WB (1980) Sampling Techniques. New York, John Wiley and Sons, pp 30-31
5. Detre KM, Kelsey SK (1986) Interpretation of sequential angiography: The Type II Coronary Intervention Study. In: Fridge NH, Nestel PJ (eds) Atherosclerosis VII. Amsterdam: Elsevier Science Publishers, pp 99-102
6. Rosner B (1982) Statistical Methods in Ophthalmology: An adjustment for the intraclass correlation between eyes. Biometrics 38:105-114
7. Rosner B (1984) Multivariate methods in ophthalmology with application to other paired - data situations. Biometrics 40:1025-1035

35

Quantitative Arteriography in Coronary Intervention Trials: Rationale, Study Design, and Lipid Response in the University of Washington Familial Atherosclerosis Treatment Study (FATS)

B. Greg Brown, Wendy A. Adams, John A. Albers, Jiin Lin, Edward L. Bolson, and Harold T. Dodge

SUMMARY

The current technology with greatest precision and statistical efficiency for studying the natural course and the therapy of coronary atherosclerosis is the quantitative analysis of lesion change from serial arteriograms. This approach was used in 47 patients who were electively recatheterized 18 months after the clinically indicated arteriograms, in whom 642 disease coronary segments were identified, representing the entire spectrum of minimal-to-severe atherosclerosis. The frequency distribution of <u>change</u> in the "percent stenosis" (%S) parameter was a bell-shaped curve centered at + 1.6% (average increase in percent stenosis in all lesions in 18 months), with a standard deviation of $\pm$ 8%. Using three standard deviations of the short-term variability of the Poiseuille flow resistance estimate as a criterion for "true" lesion change, we found that 13.4% of all lesions progressed in 18 months. On average, 16% of all lesions progressed in patients with hyperlipidemia, as compared with 9.9% of lesions in normolipidemic patients (p = 0.036).

Supported in part by USPHS Grants P01-HL 30086, HL 19451, HL 18805, in part by VA Merit Review No. 1102-01, in part by a grant from the R.J. Reynolds Foundation, in part by NIDDKD No. DK-35816-02 for the Clinical Nutrition Unit, and by the University of Washington Clinical Research Center Grant (NIH, RR-37).

Based on these observations, we have enrolled 150 patients in a study designed to test the hypothesis that drug therapies which normalize the plasma lipoprotein levels will, at the least, reduce atherosclerosis progression rate to that seen in normolipidemic individuals. Patients with angiographic coronary disease and plasma apolipoprotein B exceeding 135 mg/dL and with a family history of premature CAD are counseled in diet and are randomly assigned to one of three treatment groups: a) conventional therapy (placebo or colestipol, depending upon LDL_C level); b) niacin plus colestipol; or c) mevinolin plus colestipol. Arteriograms are electively repeated at two and one-half years.

Statistically, this is to be treated as an observational trial studying lesion change among patients randomly assigned to therapy. Independent variables include patient-specific, lesion-specific, and therapy variables. The dependent variable will be the Poiseuille flow resistance parameter. Results will be strengthened by a parallel analysis of percent stenosis (%S), a fundamentally different index of lesion severity, as a second dependent variable. Univariate regression analysis is to serve as a screen to identify predictors of progression in these two indices of coronary disease. Variables predictive ($p < 0.1$) of progression are then included in a multivariate analysis to determine which are independently predictive of progression (or regression). Although the statistical analysis of this data is a subject of on-going controversy and theoretical development, we believe that the chosen patient sample size is sufficient to resolve a 40% treatment benefit at an alpha (significance) level of 0.05 and beta level of 0.10 (power of 0.90), with a comfortable cushion for patient drop-out and certain statistical concerns.

Enrollment for this study is now complete; the response to conventional therapy has been a modest favorable alteration in lipids; the response to the combination therapies has been striking. Analysis of the progression indices in each group relative to therapy (intention to treat) and to various lipid responses should be complete by December, 1989.

INTRODUCTION

Because hard clinical events (myocardial infarction and death) are relatively infrequent and because there is not necessarily a direct association between clinical events and atherosclerosis progression, arteriographic follow-up has been proposed as an alternative to the purely clinical evaluation of the natural course and therapy of coronary artery disease. Unfortunately, the subjective visual estimate of the location and severity of arterial narrowing, as seen on the coronary arteriogram, has considerable intra- and interobserver variability. For example, a group of qualified angiographers would have a standard deviation of about 10% in group estimates of the severity of a specified coronary lesion (1,2). Such variability in estimating stenosis is unacceptable for research in disease progression. Because of this, we developed a computer-assisted lesion measurement technique in 1975 (3) which provides substantially improved precision and accuracy.

Quantitative Coronary Arteriography

In this method, routine coronary cineangiograms are projected at approximately five-fold magnification in a darkened room. The image borders of the diseased segment are traced manually from the "normal" proximal portion, through the stenosis, to the "normal" distal portion. The catheter is used as a scaling factor. This border information is digitized into a computer that converts the lesion image to true scale by compensating for the forms of image distortion inherent to cineangiograms. Figure 1 illustrates the hard-copy computer printout of this analysis. Two images from perpendicular angiographic projections are combined in a three-dimensional characterization of the diseased segment. Absolute dimensions and percent diameter and area reduction are estimated, as well as lesion length, atheroma mass, and stenosis flow resistance. With this technique, absolute dimensional measurements are accurate to $\pm$ 0.1 mm; the variability averages $\pm$ 3% in multiple estimates of "percent stenosis" (%S). Such precision reflects a substantial improvement over visual evaluation (1,2) and permits objective assessment of atherosclerosis progression.

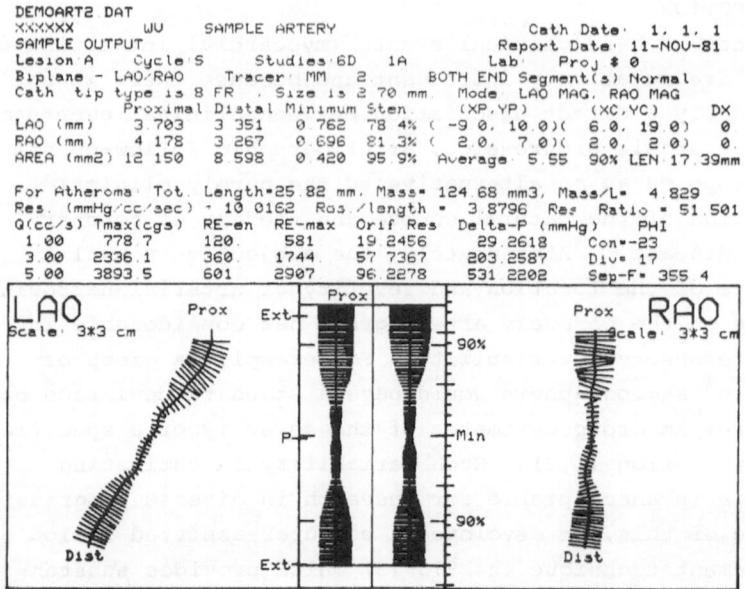

```
DEMOART2 DAT
XXXXXX        WU     SAMPLE ARTERY                    Cath Date  1. 1. 1
SAMPLE OUTPUT                                     Report Date  11-NOV-81
Lesion A    Cycle S     Studies 6D    1A        Lab   Proj $ 0
Biplane - LAO/RAO    Tracer  MM   2      BOTH END Segment(s) Normal
Cath  tip type is 8 FR  . Size is 2 70 mm   Mode  LAO MAG. RAO MAG
          Proximal Distal Minimum Sten    (XP,YP)      (XC,YC)      DX
LAO (mm)    3.703   3 351   0 762  78 4% ( -9 0, 10.0)(  6.0, 19.0)    0
RAO (mm)    4 178   3 267   0.696  81.3% (  2.0,  7.0)(  2.0,  2.0)    0.
AREA (mm2) 12 150   8.598   0 420  95.9% Average  5.55  90% LEN 17.39mm

For Atheroma  Tot. Length=25.82 mm, Mass= 124.68 mm3, Mass/L=  4.829
Res. (mmHg/cc/sec) - 10 0162  Res./length =  3.8796  Res Ratio = 51.501
Q(cc/s) Tmax(cgs)  RE-en  RE-max  Orif Res  Delta-P (mmHg)    PHI
 1.00     778.7    120.    581    19 2456      29.2618    Con=-23
 3.00    2336.1    360.   1744    57 7367     203.2587    Div= 17
 5.00    3893 5    601    2907    96.2278     531 2202    Sep-F= 355 4
```

Figure 1. Hard copy print-out of the computer analysis of a coronary stenosis.

Natural History of Coronary Lesion Change

In our laboratories, serial computer-assisted measurements have been made of virtually all atherosclerotic lesions in 47 patients (4-6). These males were prospectively enrolled and electively recatherized 18 months after the initial clinically indicated arteriogram. Six hundred forty-two coronary segments were analyzed, including 13 segments from of the two arteriograms that were totally occluded in one of the two studies; about 50 segments appeared normal on the initial angiogram and the rest were involved with the complete spectrum of mild-to-severe atherosclerosis. All segments with ≥ 15% stenosis were measured if technically possible. As summarized in the histogram of Figure 2, interval changes in %S were usually small, although some lesions became considerably worse and some actually appeared to improve. In

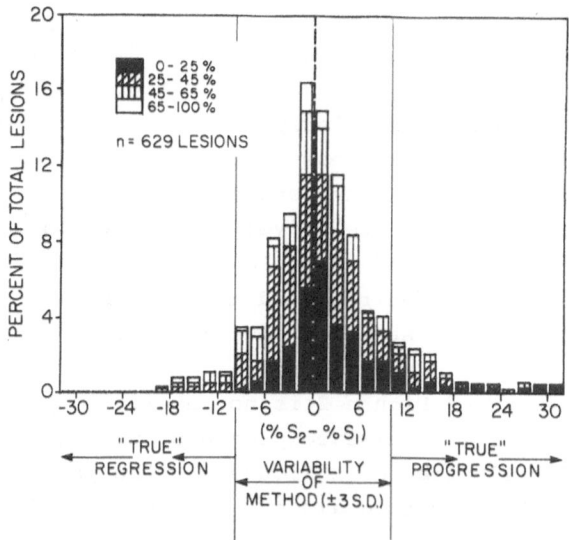

Figure 2. Internal changes in %S over 1.5 years in the
629 lesions found open in each of the two arteriograms.
Three standard deviations of the short-term variability of
the method for measurement of %S amounted to 10.2%. When
this cutoff is used to define "true" change (99.5% confidence), 12% of all lesions progressed and 4% regressed.

order to determine what should be considered a significant
interval change in a measured parameter, we analyzed 39
lesions from two projection pairs separated by an average
of 21 minutes during the catheterization. Interval change
between these two measurements reflects only changes in
vasomotor tone, small variations in patient position, and
the intrinsic variability of lesion analysis by this method.
The mean change was virtually zero; the SD of this short-
term change distribution was called "short-term variability".
For the %S parameter, one SD was 3.4%; for the Poiseuille
resistance ratio: $R_{P(max)}/R_{P(min)}$, it was 0.24. Thus,
using 3 SD of the short-term change distribution as a 99%
confidence criterion for "true" disease change, a lesion
was considered to have changed significantly (in either

direction) if its "percent stenosis" changed by $\pm$ 10.2%, or
if the above resistance ratio exceeded 1.72. Applying this
criterion to the %S change histogram of figure 2, 12% of the
642 lesions progressed; similarly, using 3 SD of the resistance parameter, 13.4% progressed. These two parameters have
been selected from among many potential measures of stenosis
severity because they are relatively sensitive to lesion
change, are clinically and physiologically relevant, and
have a low variability on repeated measurement that is
independent of initial stenosis severity (Brown BG, unpublished data).

The histogram of Figure 2 is not easily adapted to the
statistical analysis of disease progression. An alternative
data format is illustrated in Figure 3. The probabilities
of progression by specified amounts in either the %S parameter or the R_p ratio are plotted over the range of initial
stenosis severity. Normal segments almost never (< 2%) progressed by + 10.2% stenosis. The frequency and magnitude of
progression were greatest for lesions of 60% to 80% diameter
stenosis. Lesions exceeding 80% are usually proximal to a
previous transmural myocardial infarction (7) and commonly
represent previously thrombosed and recanalized segments now
serving a diminished distal flow requirement. Thus, the
reduced progression probability for these very severe lesions
appears to reflect their somewhat different morphologic and
hemodynamic characteristics. The similarity of the two
families of progression probability curves in Figure 3 adds
confidence in the robustness of this approach to analysis of
disease progression. "Percent stenosis" and "Poiseuille
resistance" are fundamentally different indices of disease
severity; and yet at comparable criterion levels they provide
comparable progression frequencies over the complete range
of initial lesion severity.

Hyperlipidemia significantly increased the overall risk
of progression; 9.9% of all lesions progressed in patients
with normal cholesterol and triglycerides compared with 16.0%
(p = 0.036) in those with serum cholesterol greater than
260 mg/dL or triglycerides greater than 200 mg/dL. Figure 4
illustrates the interactions among progression (by R_p),
regression, initial stenosis severity, and hyperlipidemia.

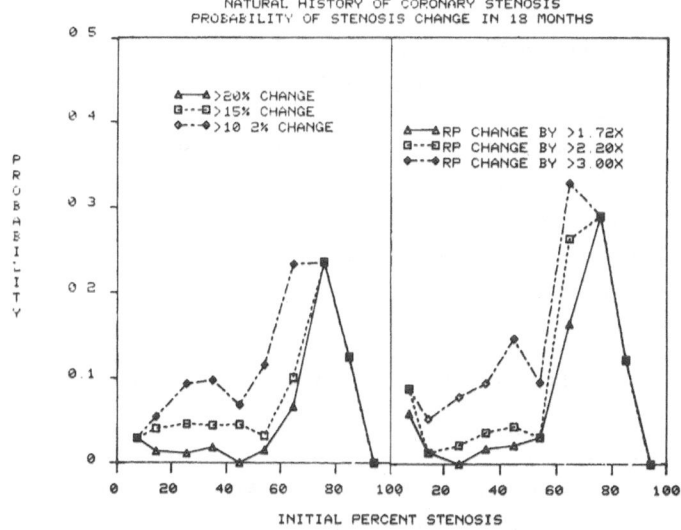

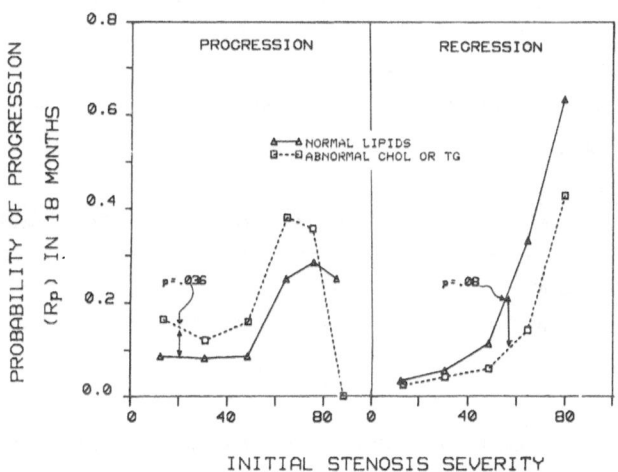

Figure 3. Probabilities of coronary stenosis progression by different amounts (or to complete occlusion) as assessed by two different criteria. Left panel shows the probability of %S progression by 10.2% (3 SD), 15%, and 20%. Right panel shows probability of R_p progression by x 1.72 (3 SD), x 2.2, and x 3. Probabilities are strongly dependent on initial stenosis severity.

Figure 4. Probabilities of coronary stenosis <u>progression</u> and regression (by 3 SD of R_p) in normolipidemic and hyperlipidemic patients. Statistical comparison of curves is by Cochran's test (8).

Abnormal lipids also significantly increased the risk
that <u>two lesions</u> would progress in a given patient (65% vs
35%; p < 0.05). This <u>patient-specific</u> index of accelarated
lesion progression is proposed as an alternative dependent
variable that is patient-based and thus avoids the statistical concerns discussed below. Table 1 summarizes the lesion-
specific and patient-specific data that form the basis of
sample-size estimates for coronary intervention trials with
lipid-lowering therapy.

Table 1. Effect of Lipids on Coronary Stenosis Progression (Wadsworth VA/UCLA Data; 47
patients)

	# of lesions with progression of R_p by 3 SD in 18 months	# of patients with progression of at least <u>one</u> lesion in 18 months	# of patients with progression of at least <u>two</u> lesions in 18 months
Normolipidemia	27/273 (9.9%)	15/21 (71%)	7/21 (33%)
Hyperlipidemia (chol ≥ 260 or TG ≥ 200)	59/369 (16.0%*)	23/26 (88%)	17/26 (65%*)

Apo B > 135 mg/dl

Apo B ≤ 135 mg/dl

Rationale for Familial Atherosclerosis Treatment Study (FATS)

The observation that hyperlipidemia in patients with
clinically manifest coronary disease predicts a significantly
increased rate of lesion progression generates the following
testable hypothesis:

In patients with hyperlipidemia and thus a predict-
ably increased rate of coronary lesion progression,
therapy which brings lipids into the normal range
will reduce the rate of disease progression to that
expected among normolipidemic patients.

The study design is presented below. Estimates of the patient sample size necessary to test this may be made using binomial probability theory for discrete variables, by the following formula (8):

$$N = \frac{(z + Z)^2 [P_2(1 - P_2) + P_1(1 - P_1)]}{n(P_2 - P_1)^2}$$

<u>where</u> N = the number of subjects in each treatment group in the intervention trial; z = 1.65 for p = 0.05; Z = 1.28 for p = 0.1; P_2 is progression probability over 2.5 years in the hyperlipidemic (untreated) state; P_1 is progression probability in the normolipidemic (treated) state. n is 1 for the patient-based analysis and is approximately 9 (lesions per patient) for the lesion-based analysis. Progression probabilities are not presently available for the 2.5-year time interval, but may be extrapolated (see Table 2) from the 18-month data provided in Table 1, assuming that a constant fraction of the non-progressed lesions will progress during each succeeding 18-month period. Table 3 provides ample size estimates based on these probabilities.

By comparison, the probability of myocaridal infarction and that of death are each about 4% per year in patients with angina. By the above formula, a <u>clinical</u> intervention trial designed to demonstrate a comparable 38% reduction in the combined frequency of these events would require a patient sample of 400 per treatment group to achieve a comparable level of statistical confidence with 2.5 years' follow-up.

Trial Design

Figure 5 is the study flow diagram. Patients are referred from three potential sources; in practice the principal sources (> 70%) are the various University of Washington catheterization laboratories, in which about 1400 men are studied annually. The majority of these patients undergo detailed risk-factor assessment at the time of catheterization, including lipid and apolipoprotein B determinations and a detailed interview to determine smoking, blood pressure, and family history. Patients are eligible for randomization for therapy if aged 60 or younger, with

Table 2. Probabilities of Lesion-Based and Patient-Based Progression Projected to 2.5 Years

	Mean probability of any lesion progression in 2.5 years	Mean probability of within-patient progression of at least 1 lesion in 2.5 years	Mean probability of within-patient progression of at least 2 lesions in 2.5 years
P_1 Normolipidemic (treated)	0.16	0.87	0.49
P_2 Hyperlipidemic (untreated)	0.25	0.97	0.83

Table 3. Sample-Size Estimates for Test of Hypothesis for = 0.05 and = 0.01

Unit of Observation	Lesion	Patient	
		R_p increase by	R_p increase by
Criterion for "Progression"	R_p increase by 3 SD	3 SD in at least 1 of all lesions	3 SD in at least 2 of all lesions
Subjects required per treatment group	38	122	29

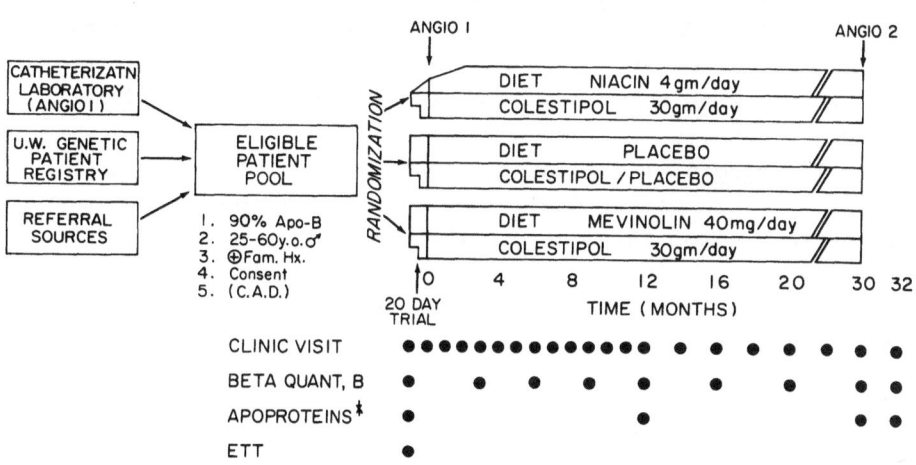

U.W. FAMILIAL ATHEROSCLEROSIS TREATMENT STUDY
(FATS)

Figure 5. Flow diagram of University of Washington Familial Atherosclerosis Treatment Study (FATS). One hundred fifty-five patients are randomized to three different treatment regimens.

plasma apolipoprotein B exceeding 135 mg/dL (approximately 90th percentile for population-based sample), with a significant positive family history of premature vascular disease (objectively defined) on at least one side of the family, and if they have at least moderate CAD on the initial angiogram. Criteria for exclusion include significant intercurrent renal, hepatic or myocardial failure, diabetes, drug intolerance, or high-risk coronary anatomy.

Those consenting to participate in the trial all receive continued AHA level I-to-II dietary counseling and are randomly assigned to:

1. "Conventional Therapy": avicel capsule (mevinolin) placebo plus colestipol placebo. Of patients randomized to this arm of the study the 40% having LDL-cholesterol above the age-adjusted 90th percentile were given colestipol in accordance with the findings of the Lipid Research Clinics Coronary Primary Prevention Trial (9).

2. Niacin, 1 gm qid, plus colestipol, 10 gm tid with meals. Niacin was gradually increased to maximum dose in order to develop tolerance to the flushing side effect. If LDL-cholesterol is not reduced below 120 mg/dL by 4 months with this regimen, niacin is increased to 1.5 gm qid, but no further after that.

3. Mevinolin, 20 mg bid plus colestipol, 10 gm tid. If LDL-cholesterol is not reduced below 120 mg/dL by 4 months with this regimen, mevinolin is increased to 40 mg bid, but no further.

Clinic follow-up occurs at the Northwest Lipid Clinic, Harborview Medical Center, on a monthly basis for the first ten months and every two months thereafter. The approximately 25% of patients who enter without prior angiography are catheterized after a 20-day drug trial. Lipid and lipoprotein determinations and liver, renal, and hematologic function are assessed at intervals specified in Figure 5. A repeat coronary arteriogram is performed electively 2.5 years after the initial study.

Current Status: Enrollment

Enrollment began January 15, 1984 and was completed at 155 active patients on November 15, 1986. Dropout rate averaged 12% of those enrolled to this point. Dropout, usually for lack of interest or drug intolerance, most commonly occurred in the first three months and very seldom thereafter.

Current Status: Lipid Response

Figure 6 documents the plasma lipid and apo-B responses to each of the three treatment regimens among the first 47 patients to complete 16 months of therapy. Cholesterol, initially averaging 275 mg/dL in all patients, fell roughly

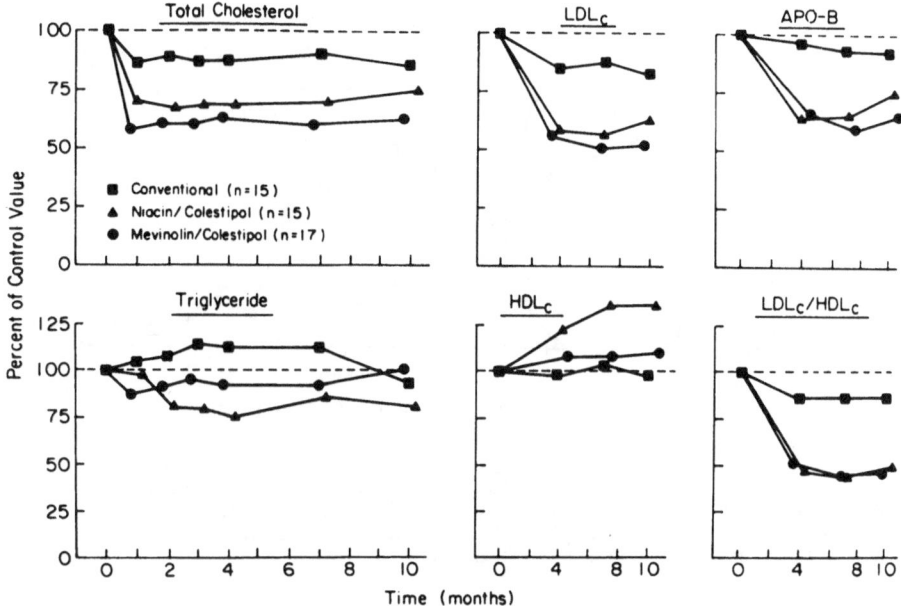

Figure 6. Plasma lipid and lipoprotein responses in the first 47 patients to complete 16 months of therapy follow-up in the U.W. FATS program.

10% with CON, 30% with N + C, and 40% with M + C. Triglycerides averaged 189 mg/dL initially, and rose transiently with CON, fell transiently with N + C, and were unaltered by M + C. LDL cholesterol, averaging 203 mg/dL initially, fell 15% with CON, 40% with N + C, and 50% with M + C. HDL cholesterol was initially 40 mg/dL; it was unaltered by CON, rose 10% with M + C, and 40% over six months with N + C. Apo-B averaging 158 initially, fell 5% with CON, 35% with N + C, and 40% with M + C. The ratio LDL_C/HDL_C was 5.8 initially; it fell 15% with CON and 55% with each of the other two regimens.

Apo-B response is further documented in Figure 7, in which its frequency distribution is plotted for 66 patients with entirely smooth, normal coronary arteries, for the 74 patients enrolled in FATS at the time the data were compiled,

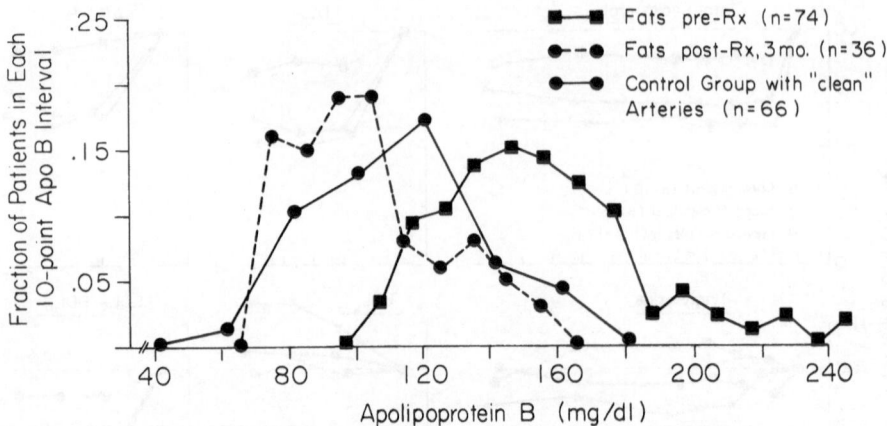

Figure 7. Distribution of apo-B among 66 patients with angiographically smooth, <u>normal</u> arteries, 74 patients enrolled in FATS at the time these data were compiled, and all 36 patients who at that time had been treated for at least four months with M + C or N + C.

and for 36 patients randomized to N + C or to M + C and having completed the first four months of the study at that time. Relative to patients without disease, candidates for FATS have a strikingly abnormal apo-B distribution. Following four months of therapy, a randomly selected large subgroup of these patients has an apo-B distribution which compares favorably to those without disease.

FATS - Planned Statistical Analysis
The data can be analyzed by the one-way analysis of variance implied by the above sample size estimations. However, statisticians object, in principle, to the approach which treats each lesion as a dependent variable because of the implicit assumption that each lesion behaves independently of its sister lesions in a given patient. Indeed we have found that certain patient-specific variables, such as serum cholesterol, are significantly correlated with progression

on multivariate regression analysis. Conversely, an analysis that uses the patient as the observational unit of interest (e.g., percentage of patient's lesions that progress) is inappropriate because it ignores the fact that certain lesion-specific variables (e.g., stenosis severity) are important determinants of progression; also, patient-based analysis reduces the effective sample size considerably.

Presently, pending further statistical modeling of this problem, we believe that a multivariate regression analysis which incorporates patient-specific, lesion-specific, and therapy variables will optimize the potential statistical efficiency of quantitative arteriographic analysis while maintaining statistical rigor. An example of such an analysis is one applied to data on coronary bypass graft occlusion (10). The use of multivariate linear regression analysis, or its nonlinear analog, ligistic regression, is necessary because the fundamental unit of interest in the <u>study</u> <u>of</u> <u>athero-sclerosis</u> is the progression or regression of disease in a defined segmental lesion; yet it is not possible to randomize individual lesions to therapy. The multivariate regression models use the lesion as the observational unit and allow for adjustment for imbalances in patient- and lesion-specific variables in assessing the impact of therapy. The analysis is then "observational" in nature, since the lesions were not randomized. Use of these models avoids the assumption of independent behavior of two lesions in the same patient by assuming that any dependence of two such lesions can be modeled by including appropriate patient- and lesion-specific variables.

An intensive study of the appropriate statistical methods for such and analysis is now underway in collaboration with faculty in the Biostatistical Division of the University of Washington School of Public Health. We anticipate that an efficient and statistically defensible model will be confirmed in time for the planned FATS data analysis in the fall of 1989.

REFERENCES

1. Koh D, Mitten S, Stewart D, Bolson E, Hodge HT (1979)
    Comparison between computerized quantitative coronary
    arteriography and clinical interpretation (abstract).
    Circulation 60(Suppl II):II-160.
2. Scoblionko DP, Brown BG, Mitten S, Caldwell JH,
    Kennedy JW, Bolson EL, Dodge HT (1984) A new digital
    electronic caliper for measurement of coronary arterial
    stenosis: Comparison with visual estimates and
    computer-assisted measurements. Am J Cardiol 53:689-693.
3. Brown BG, Bolson E, Frimer M, Dodge HT (1977) Quanti-
    tative coronary arteriography: Estimation of dimensions,
    hemodynamic resistance, and atheroma mass of coronary
    artery lesions using the arteriogram and digital
    computation. Circulation 55:329-337.
4. Brown BG, Bolson EL, Dodge HT (1986) Quantitative
    computer techniques for analyzing coronary arteriograms.
    Prog Cardiovasc Dis 28:403-418.
5. Brown BG (1983) Coronary atherosclerosis: Understanding
    its progression and regression. Univ Washington Med 9:
    14-18.
6. Brown BG, Bolson EL, Pierce CD, Peterson RB, Dodge HT
    (1984) Regression of atherosclerosis in man: Current
    data and their methodologic limitations. In: Malinow
    MR, Blaton VH (eds) Regression of Atherosclerotic
    Lesions. Plenum Publishing Corp, pp. 289-310.
7. McMahon M, Brown BG, Rolett EL, Bolson EL, Frimer M,
    Dodge HT (1977) Quantitative link between the
    severity of coronary stenosis and clinical syndromes
    of coronary disease (abstract). Circulation 56
    (Suppl III):III-924.
8. Snedecor GW, Cochran WG. Statistical Methods. Ames,
    Iowa: Iowa State University Press.
9. The Lipid Research Clinics Coronary Primary Prevention
    Trial Results (1984) I. Reduction in incidence of
    coronary heart disease. JAMA 251:351-364.
10. Brown BG, Cukingnan RA, DeRouen T, Goede LV, Wong M,
    Fee HJ, Roth JA, Carey JS (1985) Improved graft
    patency in patients treated with platelet-inhibiting
    therapy after coronary bypass surgery. Circulation 72:
    138-146.

36

Measured Coronary Lesion Change in Relation to Blood Lipid Levels in the Leiden Intervention Trial and a View of the Atherosclerotic Process

A.C. Arntzenius, D. Kromhout, and J.D. Barth

Research Into the Atherosclerotic Process in Perspective

Atherosclerosis has long been studied in both animals and man by post mortem examinations. Virchow proposed, in 1862, that progression of plaque is caused mainly by accumulation of cholesterol from lumen into the wall by way of "insudation" (1). In 1913 Anitschkow published results of experiments in which he fed rabbits pure cholesterol which resulted in experimental atherosclerosis (2). Aschoff noted in 1914 that overstretching of the ground substance of the intima produced a reactive proliferation of elastic tissue which permitted increased permeation of lipid from the lumen into the intima (3). As early as 1933, Anitschkow evoked regression of atherosclerotic lesions following cessation of the atherogenic diet (4). Our insight into pathogenesis of atherosclerotic plaque growth has been advanced by the endothelial injury and repair theory which emphasizes the importance of platelets (5). The prerequisite for the atherosclerotic process has been elucidated by Brown and Goldstein when they demonstrated the function of LDH receptors and regulation of cholesterol metabolism (6). LDL-cholesterol is now well established as atherogenic and HDL-cholesterol as probably anti-atherogenic. Recently at the 10th World Congress of Cardiology Barth stressed that Hepatic Lipase may play an important role with regard to the regression of atherosclerosis (7).

Epidemiologists in the past 30 to 40 years have demonstrated the widespread impact that atherosclerosis has on the population: half of all deaths, in industrialized countries, are caused by atherosclerosis. They introduced the practical risk factor concept. In the same period, arteriography had enabled clinicians to visualize the narrowing of coronary arteries, which has been a major step forward in quantification of the disease. When serial angiography was introduced for the first time, progression and occasionally regression of the human atherosclerotic lesions was seen to occur. Arteriography, however, does not visualize the surroundings of the arterial lumen and we are, thus, as yet unable to study the evolution of the plaque itself. To achieve this will be another leap forward; if this technical feature can be achieved in man non-invasively, we then will be able to follow closely the sometimes, slow, sometimes fast processes of progression and regression of atherosclerosis. This ultimately will provide us with measurements which are necessary to find the optimal intervention for primary and secondary prevention of the disease, with the ultimate goal being its eradication.

We do not necessarily need to wait till we have this non-invasive plaque analysis but can now put a few cornerstones together for prevention and treatment of the disease. One of these is constructed from the views of the fundamental researchers that we have cited previously and illustrated in Figure 1. It shows what emanates from their work: coronary narrowing is not caused by one process only, but instead is influenced by two processes. The second of these, the rapid ones are superimposed on the first one, which is slow and usually progressive in nature.

The Leiden Intervention Trial

The trial was conducted between 1978 and 1982 (8); patients with stable angina, in whom coronary arteriography had demonstrated severe narrowing of the diameter (> 50%) of one of the nine major coronary segments, were selected for the trial. The coronary segments analyzed were the right coronary artery: proximal, mid and distal portion;

Theory on the process of coronary obstruction

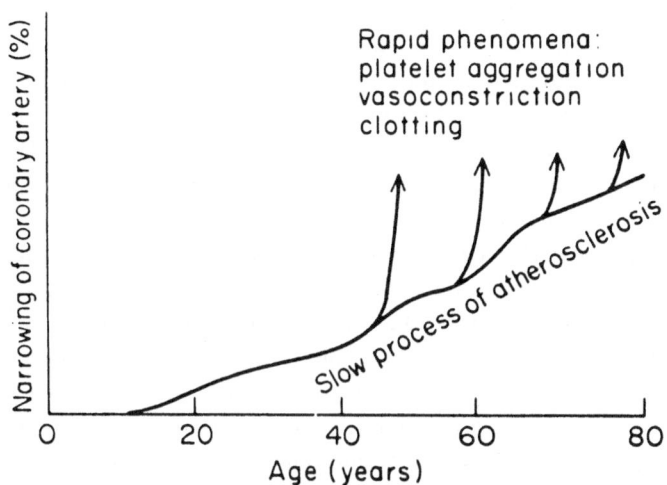

Figure 1. An illustration of the theory of the two processes which cause luminal narrowing of coronary arteries:
(1) Slow process of atheromatous growth, particularly
related to serum cholesterol levels. (2) Fast phenomena
on top of the slow process which at any point may cause the
vessel to become obstructed completely: vasoconstriction,
platelet aggregation, clotting of blood. Smoking and blood
pressure seem to play a role both in the slow process and
in the rapid phenomena.

left circumflex artery: proximal and distal portion, and
the main stem.

Each patient followed a diet for two years, during which
the usual, appropriate individual therapy was also given for
angina pectoris, elevated blood pressure, cardiac arrhythmias,
and symptoms of heart failure, e.g., beta-blockers, diuretics,
digitalis, nitroglycerin and anticoagulants. Complete
information was available for 39 patients. The 35 men and
4 women were between 35 and 59 years of age (average 48.9).

Diet

Intervention consisted of a vegetarian diet with a P/S
(polyunsaturated/saturated fat) ratio of 2 and a dietary

cholesterol intake of less than 100 mg per day. Much
emphasis was placed on continuous supervision and dietary
instruction of the patients and their spouses. Instruction
was individualized and based on 24-hour recall of food
intake, which was recorded before intervention. To evaluate
adherence one year after the trial had begun, information on
food intake was collected by seven-day record under supervision of a dietitian.

At baseline, the diet contained on average 1988 Kcal
per day, had a P/S ratio of 0.73 and had a cholesterol
content of 97.8 mg/1000 Kcal. In the Dutch population in
general, the P/S ratio is 0.57 and dietary cholesterol is
140 mg/1000 Kcal. These data suggest that the participating
patients were already following some type of a cholesterol-
lowering diet before they entered the study. Subjects were
placed on the intervention diet at entry. Polyunsaturated
fat rich oils and margarines were used. Meat and meat
products were exchanged for specially prepared vegetable
protein-rich substitutes. The total fat content of the diet
amounted to 34% of energy before and during intervention.
The P/S ratio increased however from 0.73 to 1.92. The
increase in polyunsaturated fat conformed by a significant
increase (from 52.4 to 60/8 percent in the linoleic acid
content of plasma cholesteryl esters). The intervention
diet also contained more vegetable protein, polysaccharides
and dietary fiber due to a higher intake of cereals, vegetarian meat substitutes, raw vegetables, and fruits, than
did the baseline diet.

On the basis of changes in the fatty acid and cholesterol content of the diet, the expected decrease in average
plasma total cholesterol level could be calculated according
to Keys' equation. The expected average decrease did not
differ from the observed -30.2 versus -31.7 mg per deciliter.

During the intervention period, risk factors of the 39
patients changed; serum total cholesterol decreased significantly by 11% during the intervention period; HDL cholesterol decreased by 3% but this difference was not statistically
significant. The serum total/HDL cholesterol decreased significantly with 9% during the intervention period (Table 1).

Table 1. Change in Values for Risk Factors in the 39 Patients Over 2 Years[a]

Risk Factor	At Baseline	At 2 Years	Change
Bodyweight (kg)	74.5 ± 11.4	73.5 ± 11.3	-1.2 ± 3.6[b]
Quetelet index (kg/m^2)	24.0 ± 2.4	23.7 ± 2.6	-0.4 ± 1.1[b]
Serum total cholesterol (mmol/L)[c]	6.9 ± 1.4	6.2 ± 1.3	-0.7 ± 0.7[d]
HDL cholesterol (mmol/L)[c]	1.01 ± 0.21	0.98 ± 0.16	-0.03 ± 0.14
Total/HDL cholesterol	7.1 ± 1.8	6.4 ± 1.6	-0.6 ± 1.2[e]
Blood pressure (mmHg)			
systolic	130.4 ± 17.4	126.3 ± 14.2	-4.2 ± 11.2[b]
diastolic	84.4 ± 11.1	82.1 ± 7.6	-2.4 ± 8.5
Smoking (No. of patients)	18	18[f]	0

[a]Values are means ± SD
[b]Significant difference (p < 0.05)
[c]To convert to milligrams per deciliter, multiply by 38.7
[d]Significant difference (p < 0.001)
[e]Significant difference (p < 0.01)
[f]Includes 4 patients who stopped smoking during the second year of intervention.

Body weight decreased slightly (1.5%); systolic blood pressure dropped a mean of 4.2 mmHg and diastolic pressure with a mean of 2.4 mmHg; changes in body weight were significantly inversely related to changes in HDL cholesterol and positively to total/HDL cholesterol. Changes in alcohol intake were positively related to both total and HDL cholesterol but unreleated to the ratio of total/HDL cholesterol. From the results of this long-term study, it can be concluded that total cholesterol can be lowered effectively without affecting HDL cholesterol. This study stresses the great importance of body weight in regulating total, HDL and total/HDL cholesterol.

Coronary Artery Lesions

Coronary arteriography was performed on all patients immediately before entering the study. Patients with at least one obstruction of 50% or more in a major coronary artery were asked to participate. The examination was repeated after two years of dietary intervention.

Films were assessed visually by two experienced observers who had no knowledge of the lipid values, could not distinguish between the first and second angiogram since identical techniques had been used, and since pertinent data was not provided to the evaluators. Computer-assisted analysis was performed with the computer-based Coronary Angiography Analysis System (CAAS, Thorax Center, Rotterdam) (9). This system permits the accurate delineation of the contours of user-selected coronary arterial segments by means of automated edge-detection algorithms. With this system, the variability defined as the standard deviation of the differences between repeated measurements, was found to be 0.10 mm. According to computer assessment, a total of 166 lesions were detected in the 9 major epicardial coronary segments. On average, the patients 4.26 $\pm$ 1.52 lesions. Seven patients had one-vessel disease, 11 had two-vessel disease, and 21 had three-vessel disease.

The mean diameter of vessels at the 166 sites of obstruction was 2.12 $\pm$ 0.99 mm on the first arteriogram and 1.99 $\pm$ 0.01 mm on the second, illustrating that on average, the

coronary lesions of the 39 patients progressed during the
two years of observation (p < 0.01). Similar results were
found using visual assessment of the lesions. Change of the
coronary arteries diameter at the site of the lesions was
determined as follows. For each individual the mean was
taken of the computer-measured 2 to 8 coronary lesions,
both at the baseline and at the final exam. The change was
defined as the baseline score minus the final exam result.
Thus, every change with a plus (+) sign will mean that on
average the vessel diameters have diminished (worsened).
Any change with a minus (-) sign will mean that on average
the vessel diameters have increased a little.

Coronary Lesion Growth and Serum Lipid (Lipoprotein) Values

The association analyzed between serum lipid (lipoprotein) values and computer-measured coronary lesion growth
as defined previously gave following results (see Table 2).

Table 2.   Leiden Intervention Trial. Association Between
           Serum Lipids (Lipoproteins) and Computer-Measured
           Lesion Growth

		r	p
Serum Total Cholesterol	0	0.27	0.10
Serum Total Cholesterol	$\bar{2}$	0.13	0.42
Serum HDL Cholesterol	0	−0.46	0.003
Serum HDL Cholesterol	$\bar{2}$	−0.37	0.02
Total/HDL Cholesterol	0	0.55	0.001
Total/HDL Cholesterol	$\bar{2}$	0.39	0.01

Values at baseline are denoted by 0 and mean values
at two years by $\bar{2}$.

A significant inverse correlation was found to exist between
mean two-year serum HDL cholesterol levels of the 39 participants and computer measured lesion growth (Figure 2). However, no significant correlation was found between mean two-
year serum total cholesterol levels and lesion growth. The
mean two-year total/HDL cholesterol again did correlate
significantly and positively with lesion growth (r = 0.39,
p = 0.01) (Figure 3). Correlation between the same ratio

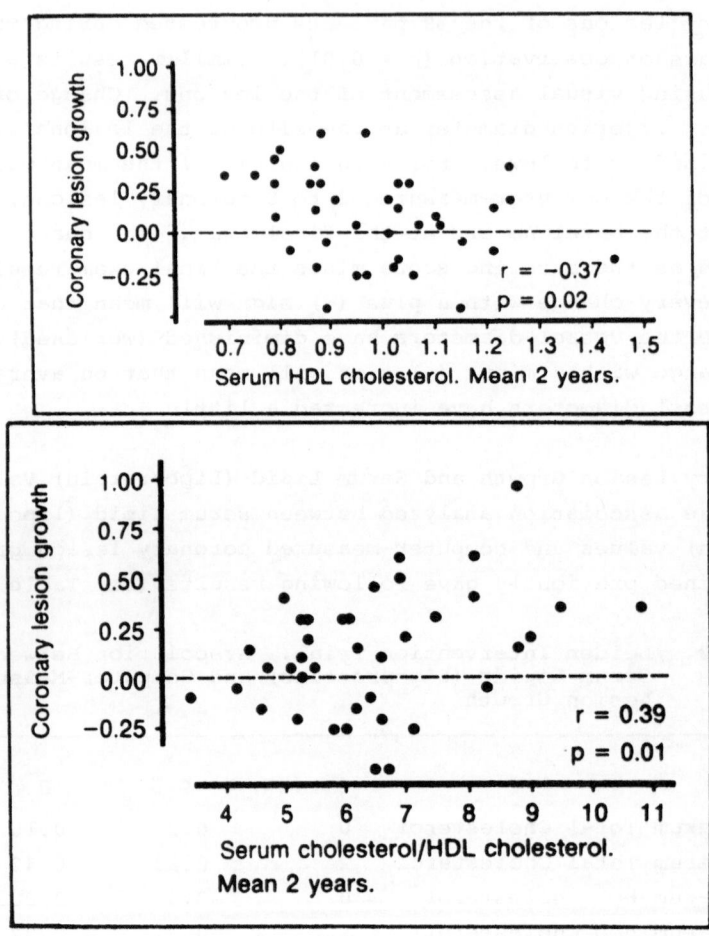

Figure 2. Correlation between coronary lesion growth and HDL cholesterol - computer measurement.
Figure 3. Correlation between coronary lesion growth and cholesterol/HDL ratio - computer measurement. (Reprinted from Drugs 31 (Suppl 1):61-65, 1986 by permission of ADIS Press Limited.

and human eye measurement of lesion growth proved to be of the same magnitude (r = 0.38, p = 0.02) (Figure 4). The correlation became stronger if the baseline values of the means were included rather than the mean two-year values of the serum lipids (lipoproteins). The mean of HDL choles- terol at baseline and two-year values correlated with computer-measured coronary lesion growth significantly (r = 0.45, p = 0.03) and the mean of baseline and two-year total/HDL cholesterol values demonstrated the strongest correlation with coronary lesion growth (r = 0.50, p = 0.001) (Figure 5). Since the baseline values of the serum lipids

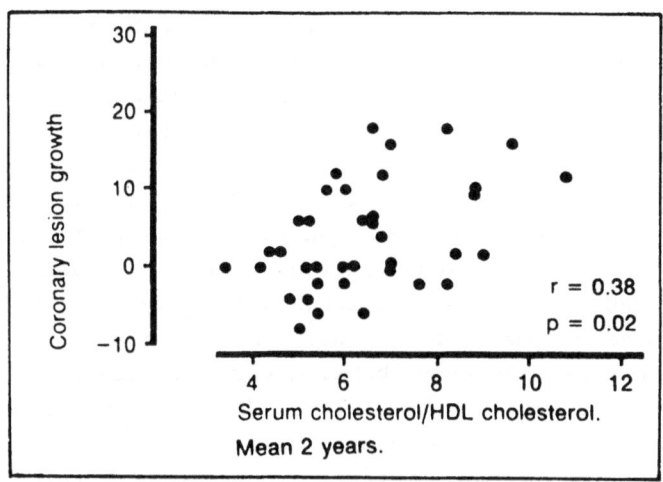

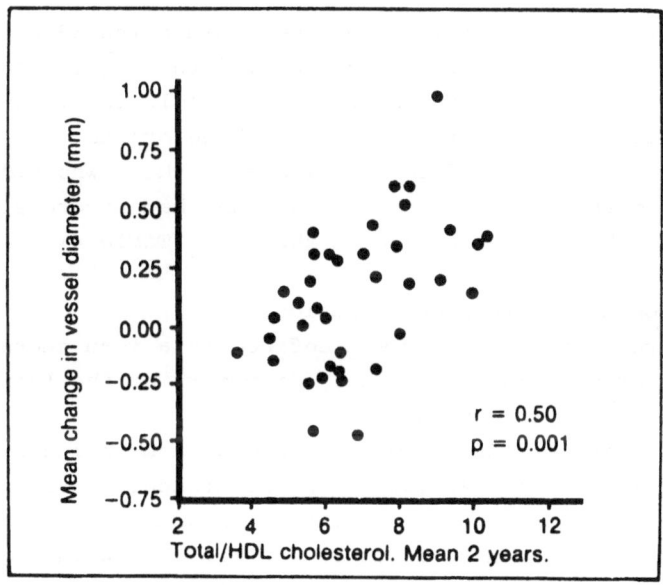

Figure 4.   Correlation between coronary lesion growth and cholesterol/HDL ratio - human eye measurement.   (Reprinted from Drugs 31 (Suppl 1):61-65, 1986 by permission of ADIS Press Limited.
Figure 5.   Association between mean changes (mm) in coronary luminal diameters as measured by a computer-assisted program versus total/HDL cholesterol ratio values, which are the averages of baseline and mean values during the two years of intervention.   It can be seen that progression of lesion growth (values above 0.00 mm) is associated with relatively high values of total/HDL cholesterol ratio, whereas no progression occurs in patients with relatively low values of total/HDL cholesterol ratios.   (Reprinted from Drugs 31 (Suppl 1):61-65, 1986 by permission of ADIS Press Limited.

influenced the associations with lesion growth, we looked at
the baseline differences between those individuals whose
total/HDL cholesterol was lower than the median 6.9 level
and those who had higher levels (> 6.9). However, the groups
did not differ in fatty acid content of the diet, blood
pressure, weight, or smoking status. There was also no
difference at baseline between the two groups in terms of
numbers of coronary lesions, whether assessed visually or by
computer (Table 3). They had roughly the same vessel diameters and same number of lesions. The lesions in the
ensuing two years, however, behaved very differently. In
the individuals with levels of total/HDL cholesterol below
6.9, there was on average no progression of disease but in
those with levels above 6.9 there proved to be severe progression.

We also analyzed the difference between the 18 patients
who showed no lesion growth and the 21 with progression of
disease. Cholesterol and the total/HDL cholesterol ratio
were significantly lower in the 18 with no growth. In
addition, HDL was significantly higher in those who had no
lesions growth compared with the ones who had progression of
lesions, both at baseline and at the mean (Table 4).

Progression and Regression of Lesions

Progression of lesions was defined as a mean decrease
of 0.1 mm or more in the coronary diameters at the lesion
sites (computer assessment).

Regression of lesions was defined as a mean increase of
0.2 mm or more, which is two times the standard deviation of
the differences between the repeated measurements. This
definition was chosen so as to be certain that with regression
a significant deviation from the natural progression course
has occurred. As regards progression, only one standard
deviation was considered sufficient. Using the above
criteria, progression of coronary atherosclerosis occurred
in 21 of the 39 patients and regression in 7 patients. In
all of the 39 patients, neither progression nor regression
was observed; we called this situation stable (Figure 6).

Table 3. Relation Between Serum Total/HDL-C at Baseline and Coronary Lesions at Baseline and After 2 Years of Intervention

Coronary Lesions	Total/HDL-Cholesterol at Baseline			
	< 6.9		> 6.9	
	n = 19		n = 20	
	m ± SD		m ± SD	
Number/person:				
Visual	7.74 ± 2.80		8.15 ± 2.76	
Computer	4.37 ± 1.74		4.15 ± 1.31	
Caliber diameter:				
Computer (mm) Baseline	2.15 ± 0.58		2.30 ± 0.47	
After 2 years	2.15 ± 0.61		2.07 ± 0.45	
Caliber Diameter Change (mm) (baseline minus 2 year value)	-0.002 ± 0.23		+0.237 ± 0.32[xx]	

[xx] $p < 0.01$

(Reprinted by permission of the New England Journal of Medicine, 312:805-811, 1985).

Table 4.   Relation Between Coronary Lesion Growth (Computer
           Assessment) and Total Cholesterol, HDL Cholesterol,
           and Total/HDL Cholesterol at Baseline and After 2
           Years of Intervention[a]

	No growth (18 patients)	Lesion growth (21 patients)
Total cholesterol (mmol/L)[b]		
at baseline	6.4 + 1.1	7.4 + 1.5[c]
at 2 years	5.8 + 0.9	6.5 + 1.5[c]
HDL Cholesterol (mmol/L)[b]		
at baseline	1.1 + 0.2	0.9 + 0.2[c]
at 2 years	1.0 + 0.1	0.9 + 0.2[c]
Total/HDL cholesterol		
at baseline	5.8 + 1.2	8.1 + 1.7[d]
at 2 years	5.7 + 1.2	7.1 + 1.7[d]

(Reprinted by permission of the New England Journal of
Medicine, 312:805-811, 1985.

[a] Values are means + SD

[b] To convert to milligrams per deciliter, multiply by 38.7

[c] Significantly different from value for patients with no
lesion growth ($p < 0.01$).

[d] Significantly different from value for patients with no
lesion growth ($p < 0.001$).

     Of interest is the finding that when severe obstructions
(more than 50%) are compared with less severe obstructions,
the severe obstructions on average showed slight regression.
In contrast, less severe obstructions (less than 50%), on
average, showed slight progression of disease.

     An important question to each practicing physician is
the following: Does regression influence the clinical
course of coronary atherosclerotic disease in patients? To
try and answer this question, we examined two clinical aspects
of the disease, namely persistent angina pectoris and total
mortality. After 24 months of dietary intervention, 23 of
the 39 patients still had angina pectoris on exertion.
Persistent angina was present in 17 of the 21 patients with
progression of disease, in 5 of 11 patients with stable
lesions, and in 1 of 7 patients with regression. Statistical

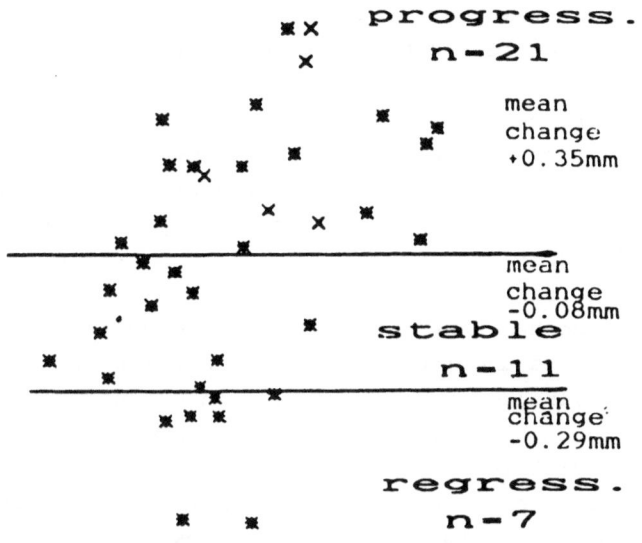

progress.
n=21

mean
change
+0.35mm

mean
change
-0.08mm

stable
n=11

mean
change
-0.29mm

regress.
n=7

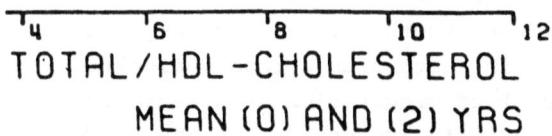

TOTAL/HDL-CHOLESTEROL
MEAN (0) AND (2) YRS

Figure 6. Association between change in lesions (computer measurement) and the mean value of the baseline (0) and mean 2 years (2) ratios of total cholesterol and HDL cholesterol. The 39 dots are the same as those of Figure 5. In the plot is shown the division lines between the 21 patients with progression, the 11 with stable lesions and the 7 with regression. The 5 patients that have died in the three and one half years of follow-up are marked. For significance see text.

analysis showed that persistent angina pectoris was significantly correlated (p = 0.005) with progression of coronary
lesions (Table 5).

An inquiry conducted three and one half years after the
final examination of the Leiden Trial showed that 5 patients
had died and 34 were alive. The five deaths all had occurred
in the group of the 21 patients with progression of disease
(p = 0.05) (Figure 6).

The fact that all five deaths occurred in the group of
21 patients who had shown progression of coronary atherosclerotic disease underscores the clinical importance of the
angiographic finding of small changes in coronary diameters.

Blankenhorn has pointed out that in American men who
die of myocardial infarction at the age of 40, the lesions
must have spread over endothelial coronary surface with a
rate of 3% per year (10). By the same token, men who die
of myocardial infarction at 80 years of age will have had
lesions that grew to cover 1% more of the endothelial coronary surface each year. The implication is that a small
reduction in the growth rate of coronary lesions may produce
a major delay in death from coronary disease.

The arrest of progression of disease in 18/39 patients
(including 7/39 with regression) of the Leiden Trial may
have thus important implications.

DISCUSSION

Atherosclerotic lesions have a tendency to progress,
with a growth rate that is greatly variable. A number of
recent observations, however, strongly support the view
that human atherosclerosis may be reversible (11-13).
Repeated angiographic examinations are often carried out
in patients with increasing symptoms, yet even in those
regression of the luminal narrowing has been observed.
Gensini, for example, noted in 1974 that in 4 of 174 persons examined, the coronary vessels at the site of obstruction had increased in diameter 1 to 2 years after the first
examination (14). Buchwald performed a prospective study
in 1974 with 24 patients with hypercholesterolemia in whom
partial ileal bypass surgery was performed: 3 of them later

Table 5.   Relation Between Computer Assessed Changes in
Coronary Diameters and Exertional Angina Pectoris

	Progression	Stable	Regression
	n = 21	n = 11	n = 7
Mean change (mm)*			
in obstruction size	+ 0.35	− 0.08	− 0.29
Angina after study	17	5	1 (p = 0.005)

n = number of patients
*   a change with a + sign means that vessel diameters have
     diminished (worsened), any change with a − sign means
     that vessel diameters on average have increased

showed regression (15). Blankenhorn (1978) observed in 25
patients with femoral artery lesions, low lipid values
correlated with regression which occurred in 9/25 patients
(16). Rafflenbeul (1979) measured coronary diameters in
25 patients who received optimal treatment and in five he
noticed regression had occurred (17). Gohlke (1980)
applied angiography to 144 young (< 40 years) patients with
myocardial infarction and found upon repeating the coronary
arteriographies 4 years later, there was progression in 30
patients and regression in 19 patients (18). Bruschke
(1981) observed regression in 12 of the 256 patients who
had been on the waiting list for a long time for coronary
bypass surgery, requiring re-examination (19). Brensike
(1984) repeated coronary angiograms on 83 patients with
severe coronary sclerotic lesions; the tests were read
independently by three radiologists and they noted regression
in 9 of the 83 patients (20). Finally, in the Leiden Intervention Trial, as outlined previously regression occurred in
7/39 patients (8). There is no doubt, therefore, that
atherosclerosis can occasionally be reversible. In the
studies reported, repeated angiography showed regression to
occur in 4/174; 3/24; 7/25; 5/25; 19/114; 12/256; 9/83; and
7/39 patients. These figures cannot be added up to arrive
at a percentage: the groups of patients, the methods and

the definition of regression applied, differ far too much.
Also, it is of importance to observe here that repeat
angiograms are not exactly the proper way to measure
regression of atherosclerotic disease: as yet we cannot
analyze the contents of the plaques not can we readily
distinguish between atheroma and spasms. We should therefore develop newer techniques so as to obtain information
on plaque growth.

Two Hypotheses on the Atherosclerotic Process
    Regression does not necessarily follow the exact
opposite pathway of progression. Of interest is the finding
of Vartiainen that during the war 1940-45, when there was a
famine in Finland, the elevated atheromatous aortic plaques
at autopsy had diminished by 20-40% when compared to the 1933-
38 findings (21). The incidence of fatty streaks (the early
stages of atherosclerosis) however had not decreased.
Vartiainen's observations is in keeping with Strøm and
Jensen's data which show that in Norway in 1940 and 1941,
soon after beginning of World War II the death rate from
circulatory diseases decreased abruptly and considerably, a
finding which seems to point towards regresion particularly
of advanced plaques (22). The same was seen to occur in the
Leiden Intervention Trial. The two-year-application of the
cholesterol lowering diet had significantly more effect on
the severe (stenosis > 50%) lesions than the lesser ones
(< 50%) (p = 0.02). It is unlikely that the different
behavior of the severe lesions versus the lesser lesions can
be ascribed to the phenomenon of the "regression to the mean",
since the time interval between the two measurements was two
years: too long a period for "regression to the mean." On
the basis of the Vartiainen and Strøm and Jensen studies and
the findings of the Leiden Intervention Trial, we submit that
there is evidence that with dietary intervention, atherosclerotic lesions in the advanced stage are more likely to
regress than the early ones. This hypothesis clearly needs
further confirmation but it raises the possibility for prevention of clinical sequelae of coronary artery disease in
angina pectoria patients, most of whom will have advanced
atherosclerotic plaques.

As a second hypothesis we would like to discuss very briefly the possibility that progression of the plaque is influenced strongly by the level of serum total cholesterol, while serum HDL cholesterol levels possibly contribute more to regression of the plaque. The hypothesis finds a basis in the evidence given by pathologists that HDL cholesterol clears cholesterol from the arterial wall, the reversed cholesterol transport, as described by Miller and Miller, a basic requirement surely for regression to occur (23). Also, in at least three angiographic trials carried out in patients with angina pectoris, a closer correlation was found between extent of coronary artery disease and HDL cholesterol than with total cholesterol (24-26). In the Leiden Intervention Trial the same finding was noticed: the coronary lesions correlated significantly with mean two-year HDL cholesterol levels but not with total cholesterol (Table 2).

On closer analysis of the three groups of patients with progression (n = 21), stable lesions (n = 11), and regression (n = 7), again it was seen that the mean two-year total cholesterol levels of the 21 patients with pro-gression was not significantly different from those of the stable group, not from those with regression. The mean two-year values of HDL cholesterol, however, was signifi-cantly lower in the patients that showed progression (0.93 mmol/L) than in those that had stable lesions (1.07 mmol/L). But the ratio of total/HDL cholesterol had a wider discrimination between the three groups (Table 6). The fact that HDL level was a better predictor of coronary artery changes than total cholesterol may well have implica-tions for secondary preventive measures for those persons who already have angina pectoris. These data suggest that diets for lowering serum total cholesterol should not lower HDL cholesterol.

The Leiden Intervention Trial shows that a two-year vegetarian linoleic acid enriched, fat modified diet lowers cholesterol effectively without affective HDL cholesterol.

Table 6. Mean Serum Lipids and Lipoproteins at Baseline (0) and Two Years ($\bar{2}$) for the Three Groups of Patients with Progression, Stable Lesions and Regression, Respectively

	n = 21 Prog.	n = 11 Stable	n = 7 Regr.	P
Mean Change Diameter	+0.35mm	-0.08mm	-0.29mm	
Total cholesterol 0	7.41	6.08	6.78	0.03
Total cholesterol $\bar{2}$	6.46	5.62	6.18	0.23
HDL cholesterol 0	0.93	1.12	1.10	0.02
HDL cholesterol $\bar{2}$	0.93	1.07	0.99	0.06
Total/HDL cholesterol 0	8.12	5.57	6.28	0.001
Total/HDL cholesterol $\bar{2}$	7.06	5.37	6.27	0.01

Values at baseline are denoted by 0 and mean values at two years by $\bar{2}$.

CONCLUSIONS

A low ratio of total cholesterol to HDL cholesterol reduces the likelihood of progression of coronary lesions even in patients who have severe obstructions.

The Leiden Intervention Trial, the one intervention study that used diet alone as mode of intervention, suggests that a diet with a P.S ratio of 2 may reduce the rate of coronary lesion growth.

Progression of coronary atherosclerotic lesions was significantly correlated with persistent angina pectoris and total mortality after three and one half years of follow-up.

REFERENCES
1. Virchow R (1862) Gesammelte Abhandlungen zur wissenschaftlichen Medizin. Berlin.
2. Anitschkow N, Chalatow S (1913) Zentralbl Allg Pathol 24:1.
3. Aschoff L (1924) Arteriosclerosis. In: Lectures in Pathology (delivered in the United States, 1924). New York: Hoeber, p. 131.

4. Anitschkow N (1933) Experimental arteriosclerosis in animals. In: Cowdry EV (ed) Arteriosclerosis: A Survey of the Problem. New York: Macmillan, pp. 271-322.

5. Ross R, Glomset JA (1976) The pathogenesis of atherosclerosis. New Engl J Med 295:369-428.

6. Brown MS, Goldstein JL (1984) How LDL receptors influence cholesterol and atherosclerosis. Sci Am 251:52-60.

7. Barth JD (1986) Diet and postheparin lipoprotein lipases in regression of coronary atherosclerosis. Washington, D.C.: World Congress of Cardiology, Sept. 18.

8. Arntzenius AC, Kromhout D, Barth JD et al. (1985) Diet, lipoproteins and the progression of coronary atherosclerosis. The Leiden Intervention Trial. New Engl J Med 321:805-811.

9. Reiber JHC, Serruys PW, Koopman CE et al. (1985) Assessment of short-, medium-, and long term variations in arterial dimensions from computer-assisted quantitation of coronary cineangiograms. Circulation 71:280-288.

10. Blankenhorn DH (1985) Two new Diet-heart studies. Editorial. New Engl J Med 321-851-852.

11. Nikkila EA (1981) Is human atherosclerosis reversible? In: Miller NE, Lewis B (eds) Lipoproteins, Atherosclerosis and Coronary Heart Disease. Elsevier/North Holland

12. Gotto AM (1981) Regression of atherosclerosis. Am J Med 170:989-991.

13. Manilow MR (1984) Regression of atherosclerosis in humans: The evidence. In: Rowlands DJ (ed) Recent Advances in Cardiology 9. Edinburgh: Churchill Livingston, pp. 227-239.

14. Gensini GR, Esente P, Kelly A (1974) Natural history of coronary disease in patients with and without coronary bypass graft surgery. Circulation 49,50 (Suppl. II):98-102.

15. Buchwald H, Moore RB, Varco RL (1974) Surgical treatment of hyperlipidemia. Circulation 49(Suppl. I): 1-37.

16. Blankenhorn DH, Brooks SH, Selzer RH, Barndt R (1978) The rate of atherosclerosis change during treatment of hyperlipoproteinemia. Circulation 57:355-361.

17. Rafflenbeul W, Smith LR, Rogers WJ et al. (1979) Quantitative coronary arteriography. Coronary anatomy of patients with unstable angina pectoris re-examined one year after optimal medical therapy. Am J Cardiol 43:699-707.

18. Gohlke H, Stürzenhofecker P, Görnandt L et al. (1980)· Progression und Regression der koronaren Herzerkrankung im chronischen Infarktstadium bei Patienten unter 40 Jahre. Schweiz Med Wochenschr 110:1663-1665.

19. Bruschke AVG, Wijers TS, Kosters W, Landman J (1981) The anatomic evolution of coronary artery disease demonstrated by coronary arteriography in 256 non-operated patients. Circulation 63:527-536.

20. Brensike JF, Levy RI, Kelsey SP et al. (1984) Effects
    of therapy with cholestyramine on progression of
    coronary: Results of the NHLBI Type II coronary
    intervention study. Circulation 63:527-536.
21. Vartiainen I, Kanerva K (1957) Arteriosclerosis and
    wartime. Ann Med Intern Fenn 36:748-758.
22. Strøm A, Jensen RA (1951) Mortality from circulatory
    disease in Norway 1940-1945. Lancet 1:126-129.
23. Miller GJ, Miller NE (1975) Plasma-high-density
    lipoprotein concentration and development of ischemia
    heart-disease. Lancet 1:16-19.
24. Jenkins PJ, Harper RW, Nestel PJ (1978) Severity of
    coronary artery atherosclerosis related to lipoprotein
    concentration. Br Med J 2:388-391.
25. Zampogna A, Luria MH, Manuben SJ, Luria MA (1980)
    Relationship between lipids and occlusive coronary
    artery disease. Arch Intern Med 140:1067-1069.
26. Campeau L, Enjalbert M, Lesperance J et al. (1984)
    The relation of risk factors to the development of
    atherosclerosis in saphenous-vein bypass grafts and
    the progression of disease in the native circulation.
    New Engl J Med 311:1329-1332.

37

The Repetitive Plasma Exchange/Drug Trial in Familial Hypercholesterolemia: Very Early Results from Two-year Coronary Angiograms

Evan A. Stein, Richard L. Kirkeeide, Lance Gould, Akira Nishikawa, and Glenn Lamkin

INTRODUCTION

Familial hypercholesterolemia (FH) is a dominantly inherited defect of low density lipoprotein (LDL) catabolism due to a defect in the LDL receptor activity. The disorder affects approximately one in 200 to one in 500 persons in North America (1). Thus, between 500,000 and 1,000,000 Americans are likely to be affected. The great majority of affected subjects are heterozygotes in whom the disorder is characterized by elevated LDL cholesterol, frequent appearance of xanthomata in early adult life, and the premature onset of coronary heart disease. In some studies, the risks of developing clinically evident coronary artery disease (CAD) in men with FH were 5% by age 30, while 80% of men were symptomatic by age 60 (2). The risks for CAD in females with the disorder is less but still very much higher than in the non-affected population.

The atheromatous lesions found in the heterozygous FH are indistinguishable from atherosclerotic lesions in non-FH subjucts with CAD, both histologically and in the distribution through the coronary arteries. It is thus generally accepted that evidence of a beneficial effect of rigorous and sustained plasma total and LDL cholesterol reduction on the atheromatous lesions in patients with heterozygous FH and CAD may be

Supported by NIH grant R01-HL28356

extended to subjects with CAD and elevated plasma LDL
cholesterol concentrations on a non-familial (primary or
secondary) basis.

Although a number of studies (3,4) have achieved
dramatic reductions in LDL cholesterol with combined drug
therapy consisting of bile acid binding resins and nicotinic
acid, they have also demonstrated significant long-term
problems in patient compliance. In the study by Kane et al.
(3), only 22 of 50 patients (44%) complied with drug therapy
sufficiently to lower LDL cholesterols into the desired range
of the study. In the study by Kuo et al. (4), approximately
one-third of the group were poor responders to treatment.
More recent studies using HMG CoA reductase inhibitors (5,6)
have indicated more dramatic cholesterol reductions are
attainable with these drugs and that patient compliance, at
least in the short term, is significantly improved. However,
in patients with FH, significant reduction in LDL cholesterol
is still probably attainable only by combinations of these
newer agents with existing lipid-lowering drugs (6-8).

A different approach to control of hyperlipidemia was
initiated by Thompson et al. (9) in 1975 and utilized mechanical removal of LDL through repetitive plasma exchange. Since
that time, the procedure has been adopted by a number of
investigators (10-12) for the long-term control of LDL cholesterol levels in FH. These procedures have become more selective than total plasma exchange and now involve selective
removal of LDL from plasma by a number of varying techniques
(13-15). The advantage of repetitive plasma exchange or LDL
apheresis combined with existing drug therapy over just drug
therapy alone is that it offers tight control of patient
compliance and assessment of therapy in terms of lipid-
lowering effect. The reduction in plasma lipid levels is
obligatory with plasma exchange as long as the patient maintains the program. Thus, the ability to assess the effect
of long-term and substantial lipid lowering on the atherosclerotic lesion in FH subjects is now feasible.

Previous studies to determine progression, non-progression,
or regression of coronary atherosclerotic lesions have suffered

from significant variability in methodology. Numerous
studies (16-24) have indicated that visual interpretation
of coronary arteriography is sufficiently variable that its
as an objective standard for measuring severity of coronary
stenosis is very limited. Furthermore, the effect of a
stenosis on hemodynamic flow depends not only on the relative
stenosis in the artery, but also the absolute reduction in
diameter and the length of the stenosis. Brown et al. (25,
26) develop and refined a method for quantitative coronary
arteriography using x-ray measurements of the stenosis
geometry to predict the pressure gradient flow characteristics of an arterial stenosis. These techniques have also
been applied to patient studies by McMahon et al. (26) and
other groups who are also using computerized quantitative
coronary arteriography for clinical studies. These enhance-
ments, in addition to the use of high quality orthogonal
arteriograms and the use of automatic border recognition
techniques as described by Gould and Kelly (27), have improved
the ability to monitor alterations in atherosclerosis in the
coronary arteries during longitudinal studies with increased
accuracy.

This study in patients with heterozygous FH is designed
to assess whether the aggressive, rigorous, massive, and
consistent reduction in plasma total and LDL cholesterol
achieved by plasma exchange combined with drug therapy can
induce regression or prevent progression of atheromatous CAD.
The study is designed to assess changes over a four-year treatment period and involved 34 subjects in the two treatment
groups. Very early results from 21 subjects at the two-year
phase of the study are presented.

METHODOLOGY

Patients
Male and female patients, aged 25 to 60 years at the time
of screening were eligible for the study. For the diagnosis
of familial hypercholesterolemia, the following criteria were
met: a) plasma LDL cholesterol >225 mg/dL despite good

compliance with AHA Phase I or better diet, plus exclusion
of other disorders known to produce elevated LDL cholesterol;
b) demonstration of a primary elevation of plasma LDL
cholesterol in two of either a sibling, progeny, or parent.
Subjects with severe and persistent hypertension despite
conventional antihypertensive therapy, history of persistent
or recurrent life-threatening cardiac arrhythmias, cardiac
failure defined as an ejection fraction <40% determined on
left ventriculography at the time of cardiac catheterization,
and/or any other disease process which could shorten the
expected life span were excluded from the study. In addition,
subjects maintained an LDL cholesterol >200 mg/dL after
extensive period of maximal <u>tolerable</u> conventional drug
therapy consisting of a bile acid binding resin and/or
niacin.

Final selection of subjects was based on the demonstration of significant and quantitatable coronary artery atherosclerotic lesions. Initial screening included a history for
stable angina, graded exercise electrocardiogram, thallium
exercise test, exercise ventriculogram, and fluoroscopy for
coronary calcification. Subjects meeting the lipid and
history criteria were drawn from the patient population under
treatment at the Cholesterol Treatment Center (EAS) and the
subset meeting the clinical and non-invasive cardiovascular
criteria were flown to the University of Texas for computerized quantitative coronary angiography. Those subjects
meeting the quantitative coronary angiographic criteria for
continued participation in the study were then placed in the
two treatment groups. The first treatment group ("drug only")
continued with a bile acid binding resin (Colestid - colestipol
hydrochloride, Upjohn Company, Kalamazoo, MI) at a maximal
tolerable dose varying between 5 and 30 mg/day. They were
also treated with a slow release nicotinic acid preparation
(Nicobid, USV Pharmaceuticals, New Jersey) at a dose varying
from 1-3 gm/day depending on the ability of the subject to
tolerate the medication. Although no other lipid-lowering
medications were recommended, two patients intermittently took
the clofibrate analog, Gemfibrozil (Lopid). The second

treatment group was placed on identical maximal tolerable drug therapy consisting of the bile acid binding resin and nicotinic acid. In addition, the subjects were treated with three liter plasma exchange every two weeks. This was carried out using continuous flow total apheresis (Fenwall PS400). In addition, both groups maintained an AHA Phase I or better lipid-lowering diet consisting of <200 mg/day cholesterol, a low saturate polyunsaturate enriched diet (P/S 1:1), and a total fat intake of <35% of total calories.

No restrictions were placed on other medications, such as beta blockers, calcium channel blockers, long-acting nitrites, antihypertensives, etc. Subjects, if they were smoking, were encouraged to stop smoking, irrespective of their treatment group, and all subjects were encouraged to maintain optimal body weight and a regular aerobic exercise program. However, no formal intervention strategies were implemented for these other risk factors.

Lipid and apolipoprotein levels were measured at the two-monthly visits for the drug only group and immediately pre- and post-plasma exchange for the plasma exchange group. In addition, daily lipid measurements were obtained in a third of the subjects every two years to monitor the rebound effect of lipid levels post-plasmapheresis. Safety biochemical and hematological testing was carried out at each clinic and plasma exchange visit. These focused predominantly on liver function tests in view of the potential toxicity with niacin, and the complete blood count (CBC), prothrombin time (PT), and partial thromboplastin time (PTT), in view of the repeated plasmapheresis and bile acid binding resin.

Laboratory Methodology

Subjects were always seen fasting (12-14 hours overnight; water only). Blood was collected in EDTA 1 mg/Ml and plasma separated within four hours at 4°C. Plasma total, HDL cholesterol, and triglycerides were measured on a Hitachi 705 instrument with enzymatic procedures, standardized by the CDC according to the Lipid Research Clinic's program (28). HDL was isolated using heparin-2 molar manganese chloride to

precipitate VLDL and LDL (29). LDL cholesterol was calculated by the formula of Friedewald et al. (30). Apolipoproteins Al and B were run by electroimmunoassay and apoA2
by monoclonal ELISA as described previously (31,32).

Cardiovascular Studies

All subjects underwent a symptom-limited graded exercise electrocardiogram with intravenous thallium-201
administration to evaluate myocardial perfusion. The procedure and its interpretation were carried out according to
the method of Watson et al. (33-35). These tests were
carried out at baseline and again at two years into treatment.
Coronary angiography was carried out at the University of
Texas, and quantitative computerized coronary angiography
performed using a modification of the method described by
Brown et al. (25).

RESULTS

Patient Recruitment

Subjects were first evaluated beginning in the summer
of 1983. Initial coronary angiograms after cardiovascular
screening commenced in the fall of 1983, and total recruitment was completed in 18 months, involving 34 subjects.
Eighty patients with severe FH meeting the study criteria
underwent cardiovascular screening. Fifty-three of these
patients were found to meet the non-invasive cardiovascular
criteria, warranting coronary angiography. Of these 53
subjects, 40 had coronary artery disease severe enough to
continue in the study. Two subjects refused further participation, and four patients were deemed to have such severe
disease that they warranted immediate coronary artery bypass
surgery. Of the 17 subjects in each group, there were equal
numbers of males (11) and females (6) and similar numbers of
caucasians (16) and blacks (1). The subjects in the plasma
exchange group were slightly younger (43 $\pm$ 9 vs. 51 $\pm$ 7 years)
and had moderately higher initial LDL cholesterol levels on
diet alone compared to the drug only group (Table 1). The

Table 1. Baseline (Diet Only) and Two Year Lipid (mg/dL) and Lipoprotein Values and Changes (%) on Treatment

| | Baseline | | | Drug Only | | | PE + Drug (Mean Pre and Post) | | |
	Chol	LDLC	HDLC	Chol (%)	LDLC (%)	HDLC (%)	Chol	LDLC	HDLC
PE + Drug	431	356	47	320 (26%)	247 (31%)	49 (+ 4%)	206	155	34
Drug Only	391	312	46	282 (28%)	200 (36%)	56 (+22%)			

response to drug (resin plus niacin) was similar in both
groups at approximately 100 mg LDL cholesterol reduction
compared to diet alone (Table 1). The additional reduction
in cholesterol and LDL cholesterol achieved by plasmapheresis
every two weeks in addition to maintenance of drug therapy
resulted in a mean LDL cholesterol for the plasma exchange
group 23% lower compared to the drug only group (Table 1).
The overall reduction in LDL cholesterol in the plasma
exchange group was 56% compared to diet alone, and approximately 36% additional reduction compared to drug alone.
The drug only group experienced a 36% reduction in LDL
cholesterol compared to diet alone.

As of September 1986, 21 subjects had undergone repeat
coronary angiography. This consisted of 12 subjects in the
drug only group and nine patients in the plasma exchange
group. The distribution of segments analyzed and the lesion
severity at first catheterization in terms of percent diameter
reduction are shown in Table 2. No statistical difference

Table 2. Plasma Exchange Study Population - Preliminary
          Results (September, 1986)

	Control			Experimental		
Number of Patients	12			9		
Segments Analyzed	58			41		
	33% LAD	34% LCX	33% RCA	34% LAD	32% LCX	34% RCA
Lesion Severity at First Cath (% Diameter Reduction)						
0 - 24	30%			12%		
25 - 49	33%			47%		
50 - 74	33%			41%		
75 - 100	4%			0%		

between the two groups was noted. Evaluation in lesion changes at two years compared to baseline are shown in Table 3. Within-group analysis showed significant progression (reduction in lumen size) in terms of absolute minimum diameter and in absolute minimum area in both groups. These results were statistically significant at the $p < 0.01$ level for the drug only group and at the $p < 0.05$ level for the plasma exchange group. The statistically significant ($p < 0.05$) reductions in percent diameter were also noted for both groups and in terms of percent area reduction for the drug only group. Although a reduction in percent area was noted for the plasma exchange group, it did not reach statistically significant levels. No significant difference between the two groups in these parameters was noted. When all lesions were considered independently and progression or regression of lesions determined by an alteration in parameter exceeding two standard deviations (i.e., 95% confidence limits), no significant difference was seen between the two treatment groups (Table 4).

In Table 5, when patient progression was defined as a significant progression of one or more lesions in a patient regardless of changes in other lesions, and no progression was defined as no significant progression in any patient lesions, or alternatively regression only, the results were slightly different. The plasma exchange group showed a tendency toward less progression in all of the four parameters evaluated (Table 5) when compared to the drug only group. In addition, there was correspondingly a greater percentage of the plasma exchange subjects, who showed no progression or regression only in these same four parameters when compared to the drug only group. The differences did not, however, reach statistical significance.

DISCUSSION

The initial and very early results at two years of the plasma exchange/drug study in 21 of 34 heterozygous FH subjects are consistent with the initial objectives of the study. Firstly, significant massive and long-term LDL

Table 3. Net Changes in Coronary Lesions at Two Years (Preliminary Results)

Change Parameter	I Drug Only Group	II Drug + Plasma Exchange Group	I vs II
Minimum Diameter (mm)	-0.16 ± 0.45*	-0.14 ± 0.38*	NS
Minimum Area (mm^2)	-0.56 ± 1.26*	-0.31 ± 0.86*	NS
Diameter Reduction (%)	3.5 ± 13**	4.8 ± 12**	NS
Area Reduction (%)	5.7 ± 12*	4.3 ± 14	NS

Results shown as mean ± standard deviation

* p <0.01
** p <0.05

Table 4. Progression/Regression of Coronary Lesions (Percent of All Lesions in Treatment Subgroups that Significantly Changed)*

Parameter	Progression		Regression	
	Drugs	Drugs + PE	Drugs	Drugs + PE
Minimum Diameter 0.3 mm	41%	42%	16%	12%
Miminum Area 0.8 mm^2	33%	24%	7%	10%
Diameter Reduction 10%	34%	37%	12%	10%
Area Reduction 10%	39%	29%	7%	12%

* Change criteria threshold = $\pm$ 2 S.D.

Table 5. Patient Progression Versus Treatment - Preliminary Results

Parameter*	Progression[a]		Regression[b]	
	Drugs	Drugs + PE	Drugs	Drugs + PE
Minimum Diameter	92%	78%	8%	22%
Minimum Area	75%	56%	25%	44%
Diameter Reduction	75%	67%	25%	33%
Area Reduction	83%	67%	17%	33%

[a] Progression = Significant progression of one or more
[b] lesions in patient regardless of changes in other lesions
No Progression = No significant progression in any
* patient's lesions; regresison only
Criteria = $\pm$ 2 S.D.

cholesterol reductions in the order of 60% compared to diet alone are being achieved and maintained in the plasma exchange group. Patient compliance to plasma exchange during the first two years has been exceptionally good, averaging approximately 95% of all scheduled procedures. At this point in the study, only one subject is no longer actively involved in the protocol in the plasma exchange group due to the fact that she suffered a severe dense hemiplegia one month into the study as a result of a cerebrovascular accident unreleated to the treatment program. Complesion of the two year angiographic studies in all active subjects is expected in early 1987.

Twenty-one subjects who have undergone repeated quantitative coronary angiography at two years have, for the most part, shown continued progression of atherosclerosis associated with their underlying lipid disorder. The plasma exchange group is demonstrating a tendency toward less progression in patients as a whole; however, there is no significant difference when individual coronary artery segments are analyzed independently. These early results have clearly demonstrated that, despite massive lipid lowering, regression of atherosclerosis is not a rapid or frequent phenomenon in patients with severe heterozygous familial hypercholesterolemia.

While the study is meeting its objectives in terms of lipid lowering and the computerized quantitative coronary angiography is sufficiently accurate and precise to measure extremely small changes in lesion size, it is probable that certain subjects with severe FH will require considerably longer lipid lowering than two years to effectively halt progression and possibly induce regression of atherosclerotic lesions. Furthermore, progression, non-progression and regression of lesions may be related to absolute LDL cholesterol levels than degree of reduction.

REFERENCES

1. Fredrickson DS, Levy RI (1972) Familial hyperlipo-
    proteineima. In: Stanbury JB, Wyngaarden JB,
    Fredrickson DS (eds) The Metatolic Basis of Inheri-
    ted Disease. 3rd Ed. New York: Mc-Graw-Hill, p. 546.
2. Slack J (1969) Risks of ischemic heart disease in
    familial hyperlipoproteinemic states. Lancet 2:1380.
3. Kane JP, Malloy MJ, Tun P, Phillips NR, Freedman DD,
    Williams ML, Rowe JS, Havel RJ (1981) Normalization
    of low density lipoprotein levels in heterozygous
    familial hypercholesterolemia with combined drug
    regimen. N Engl J Med 304:251.
4. Kuo PT, Kostis JB, Moreyra AE, Hayes JA (1981)
    Familial Type II hyperlipoproteinemia with coronary
    heart disease, effect of diet-colestipol-nicotinic
    acid treatment. Chest 79:286-291.
5. The Lovastatin Study Group II (1986) Therapeutic
    response to Lovastatin (mevinolin) in non-familial
    hypercholesterolemia: A multicenter study. JAMA
    256:2829-2834.
6. Vega GL, Grundy SM (1987) Treatment of primary mode-
    rate hypercholesterolemia with Lovastatin (mevinolin)
    and colestipol. JAMA 257:33-38.
7. Lees AM, Stein SW, Lees RS (1986) Therapy of hyper-
    cholesterolemia with mevinolin and other lipid lowering
    drugs. Arteriosclerosis 6:544a.
8. East CA, Bilheimer DW, Grundy (1986) Combination drug
    therapy for treatment of patients with familial combined
    hypertriglyceridemia and hypercholesterolemia.
    Arteriosclerosis 6:544a.
9. Thompson GR, Lowenthal R. Myant NB (1975) Plasma
    exchange in the management of homozygous familial
    hypercholesterolemia. Lancet 1:1208.
10. Stein EA, Glueck CJ, Wesselman A, Owens ER, Nichols S,
    Vink P (1981) Repatitive intermittent flow plasma
    exchange in patients with severe hypercholesterolemia.
    Atherosclerosis 38:149.
11. Lupien PJ, Moorjani S, Awad J (1976) A new approach to
    the management of familail hypercholesterolemia;
    Removal of plasma cholesterol based on the principle
    of affinity chromatography. Lancet 1:1261.
12. Burgstaler EA, Pineda AA, Ellefson RD (1980) Removal
    of plasma lipoproteins from circulating blood with a
    heparin-agarome column. Mayo Clin Proc 55:180-184.
13. Yokoyama S, Hayashi R, Satani M, Yamamoto A (1985)
    Selective removal of low-density lipoprotein by plasma-
    pheresis in familial hypercholesterolemia. Arterio-
    sclerosis 5:613-622.
14. Leitman SF, Gregg RE, Adde MA, Smith JW (1986) Selective
    removal of low density lipoprotein (LDL) cholesterol by
    secondary membrane filtration. Transfusion 26:579.
15. Odaka M, Kobayashi H, Soeda K, et al. (1986) Adsorption
    of lipoprotein containing apolipoprotein B through
    plasma separation for treatment of familial hyper-
    cholesterolemia. Int J Artif 9:343-348.

584

16. Bjork L, Spindola-Franco H, VanHouten FX, Cohn FP, Adams DF (1975) Comparison of observer performance with 16 mm cineflorography and 70 mm camera fluorography in coronary arteriography. Am J Cardiol 36: 473-478.

17. Detre KM, Wright PH, Murphy ML, Takaro T (1975) Observer agreement in evaluating coronary angiograms. Circulation 52:979-986.

18. Zir LM, Miller SW, Dinsmore RE, Gilbert JP, Harthorne JW (1976) Interobserver variability in coronary angiography. Circulation 53:627-632.

19. DeRouen TA, Murray JA, Owen W (1977) Variability in the analysis of coronary angiograms. Circulation 55:324-328.

20. Vlodaver Z, Frech R, Van Tassel RA, Edwards JE (1973) Correlation of the antemortem coronary arteriogram and the postmortem specimen. Circulation 47:162-169.

21. Grondin CM, Dryda I, Pasternac A, Campeau L, Bourassa MG, Lesperance J (1974) Discrepancies between cineangiographic and postmortem findings in patients with coronary disease and recent myocardial revascularization. Circulation 49:703-708.

22. Gallagher KP, Folts JD, Rowe GG (1978) Comparison of coronary arteriograms with direct measurements of stenosed coronary arteries in dogs. Am Heart J 95:338-347.

23. Hutchins GM, Bulkley BH, Ridolfe RL, Griffith LSC, Cohr FT, Piasio MA (1977) Correlation of coronary arteriograms and left ventriculograms with postmortem studies. Circulation 56:32-37.

24. Myers MG, Shulman HS, Saibil EA, Nagri SZ (1978) Variations in measurement of coronary lesions on 35 and 70 mm angiograms. Am J Roentgenol 130:913-915.

25. Brown BG, Bolson E, Frimer M, Dodge HT (1977) Quantitative coronary arteriography: Estimation of dimensions, hemodynamic resistance, and atheroma mass of coronary artery lesions using the arteriogram and digital computation. Circulation 55:337.

26. McMahon MM, Brown BG, Cukingram R, Rolett EL, Bolson E, Frimir M, Dodge HT (1979) Quantitative coronary angiography: Measurement of the critical stenosis in patients with unstable angina and single vessel disease without collaterals. Circulation 60:106-113.

27. Gould KL, Kelley KO, Bolson EL (1982) Experimental validation of quantitative coronary arteriography for determining pressure flow characteristics of coronary stenosis. Circulation 66:930-937.

28. Manual of Laboratory Operations, Lipid Research Clinics Program. Lipid and Lipoprotein Analysis. DHEW Publication No. (NIH) 1874:75-628.

29. Warnick GR, Albers JJ (1978) A comprehensive evaluation of the heparin-manganese precipitation procedure for estimating high-density lipoprotein cholesterol. J Lipid Res 19:65-73.

30. Friedewald WT, Levy RI, Fredrickson DS (1972) Estimation of the concentration of low density lipoprotein cholesterol without the use of the preparative ultracentrifuge. Clin Chem 18:499-502.

31. Mendoza SG, Zerpa A, Carrasco H, et al. (1983)
     Estradiol, testosterone, apolipoproteins, lipoprotein
     cholesterol and lipolytic enzymes in men with premature
     myocardial infarction and angiographically assessed
     coronary occlusion. Artery 12:1-23.
32. Stein EA, DiPersio L, Pesce AJ, et al. (1986) Enzyme-
     linked immunosorbant assay of apolipoproteins AII
     in plasma, with use of a monoclonal antibody. Clin
     Chem 32:967-971.
33. Watson DD, Campbell NP, Read EK, Gibson RS, Teates CD,
     Beller GA (1981) Spatial and temporal quantitation of
     plane thallium myocardial images. J Nuclear Med
     22:577-584.
34. Berger BC, Watson DD, Taylor GJ, Craddock GB, Martin RP,
     Teates CD, Beller GA (1981) Quantitative thallium-102
     exercise scintigraphy for detection of coronary artery
     disease. J Nuclear Med 22:585-593.
35. Beller GA, Watson DD, Ackell P, et al. (1980) Time
     course and mechanism of thallium-201 redistribution
     after transient myocardial ischemia. Circulation 61:
     791-796.

38

Histologic and Functional Basis for Ameliorating Plaques by Percutaneous Transluminal Angioplasty

Christopher K. Zarins

INTRODUCTION

Percutaneous transluminal angioplasty using a balloon catheter has been widely used in the treatment of obstructing lesions in the coronary, visceral and peripheral arteries. While the clinical usefulness of this procedure is well established, the precise mechanism by which enlargement of the arterial lumen is achieved has been poorly understood. In their original description of transluminal angioplasty using a rigid coaxial catheter system, Dotter and Judkins attributed the effectiveness of their procedure to compression of the atheromatous plaque against a relatively unyield-artery wall (1). This mechanism was subsequently endorsed by Andreas Gruntzig, the developer of the balloon catheter technique of angioplasty (2) and accepted by most clinicians utilizing the procedure. However, the concept of plaque compression or of herniation of atheromatous intima into the artery wall was not supported by histologic or other morpho-logic evidence and could not be reconciled with the physical incompressibility of solid and liquid plaque material. Precise histologic and morphologic data were therefore needed to de-fine the changes that occur in the plaque and artery wall during balloon angioplasty. Earlier studies were based primarily on angiographic observations before and after dilatation but were not able to define the mechanism since

Supported by NHLBI Grant HL-15062 and NSF Grant CME 7921551.

angiography revealed only the lumen contour and provided no information about the plaque or arterial wall.

Mechanism of Balloon Dilation of Arteries

The mechanism of balloon dilatation was investigated in human iliac, superficial femoral and popliteal arteries obtained at autopsy from freshly amputated limbs. Both normal and diseased arteries were studied. Experimental conditions were designed to approximate those which prevail in the living patient. Arteries were excised, cannulated at both ends, restored to original length, redistended at an intraluminal pressure of 90 - 100 mmHg and maintained at a temperature of 37 °C (3). Angiography was used to locate stenosing plaques and to document the precise position of the balloon, as well as the angiographic changes in lumen contour associated with dilatation. Pressure was maintained throughout the dilatation procedure and each artery was subsequently fixed while distended. Transverse histological sections through the dilated segment were compared with those made at immediately adjacent, nondilated proximal and distal locations and correlated with the angiographic appearances. Although precise quantitation of morphologic changes associated with transluminal angioplasty requires careful control and the study of pressure-fixed arteries (4), the general morphologic changes can be demonstrated in arteries studied in the nondistended state (5).

Normal arteries. Normal arteries demonstrated no significant gross or histologic alterations in the artery wall following balloon inflation to 4 atmospheres, provided the balloon size was not excessive. Endothelial injury or integrity could not be reliably assessed in these preparations. When balloons were considerably larger than the normally distended arterial lumen, disruption of the artery wall occurred. The intima and media tended to rupture earliest and the adventitia was affected only when balloon diameter was sufficiently great. There was little or no cleavage between the intima and media, even in arteries with moderate uniform fibrocellular intimal thickening. This may be due to the similarity in compliance between the intima and media in such vessels.

Arteries with nonstenotic plaques: Balloon dilatation of arteries with nonstenotic fibrocalcific intimal plaques resulted in separation of the intimal plaque from the media and stretching of the artery wall. The uninvolved portion of the artery wall, as well as the media beneath the plaque, was stretched but there was little direct effect on the fibrous plaque itself. It is likely that the plaque is less compliant than the artery wall and, as a result, a shearing force develops at the plaque-media interface causing separation to occur. The separated regions of the plaque protruded into the lumen, revealing a sharp cleavage plane between plaque and media. Such cleavages or dissections could be seen on post-dilatation angiograms in patients undergoing transluminal angioplasty. The media became thinner as it stretched and ruptured if the dilating balloon was sufficiently large, leaving only the adventitia to maintain vessel wall continuity.

Arteries with stenotic plaques: Balloon dilatation of arteries with focal lumen stenoses resulted in marked detachment of the plaque from the underlying media and stretching of the media to enlarge the lumen (Figure 1). There was little or no evidence of plaque compression, molding, extrusion or redistribution (3). Fracture of the intima was in a longitudinal rather than a transverse plane and the plaque inself did not fragment. The plaque remained attached to the artery wall both proximal and distal to the dilated area, as well as its central thickest portion. The persistence of zones of plaque attached may help to account for the clinical finding that dilated arteries tend to remain patent following balloon dilatation despite extensive artery wall disruption and plaque dissection. The favorable clinical results of this procedure would not be predicted on the basis of histologic observations of random sections alone. Multiple serial sections through the dilated area are needed to fully demonstrate the morphologic changes. In instances where an advanced plaque occupied the entire circumference of an artery, the plaque fractured at or near its thinnest point and separation of the remainder of the lesion usually occurred in a plane immediately adjacent to the luminal aspect of the internal elastic lamina. When plaques were extensive and were associated with medial atrophy or degeneration, the dissection plane frequently

occurred at the outer limit of the media leaving only the
adventitia intact.   These are the same planes which are used
to remove lesions when endarterectomy is performed as an open
procedure at operation.   The adventitial layer is nearly
always thickened and more compact in arteries with fibrocalcific plaques and this focal change may contribute to the
capacity of the adventitia to provide sufficient support
to the vessel wall.

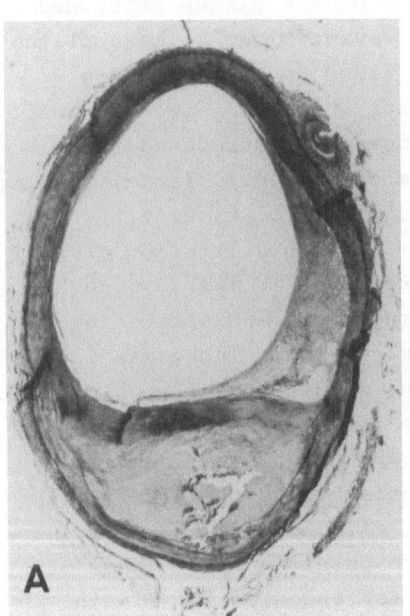 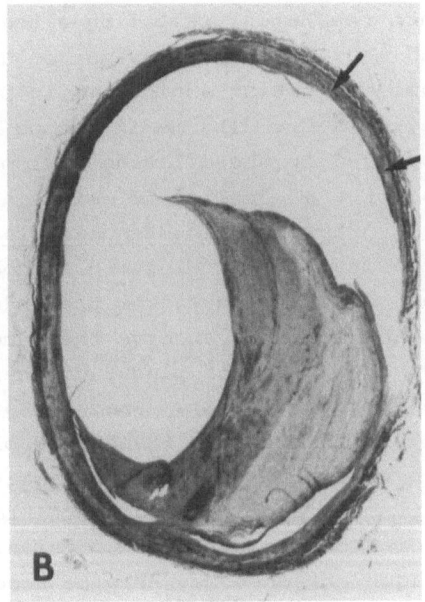

Figure 1.   Transverse sections of human superficial femoral
artery: A) Nondilated segment; b) After balloon dilation:
Note separation of the plaque from the underlying media,
thinning and stretching of the media (arrow) and enlargement
of lumen cross-sectional area.   The plaque protrudes into the
lumen leaving an irregular lumen contour.   The plaque remains
adherent to the media at its thickest point but the plaque
shape and contour are not markedly altered.   (Reproduced with
permission from Vascular Surgery: Principles & Practices by
Samuel E. Wilson, Frank J Veith, Robert W. Hobson and
Russell A. Williams, McGraw Hill, Inc.)

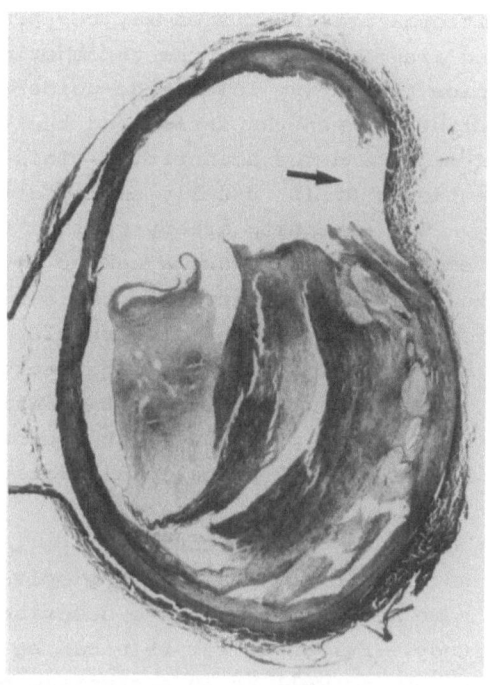

Figure 2. Transverse section of totally occluded superficial femoral artery after balloon dilatation. The media is ruptured (arrow) and the artery wall is stretched and pulled away from the occlusive plaque to create a lumen. Under these circumstances there may be a few or no dissection channels evident. (Reproduced with permission from Vascular Surgery: Principles and Practices by Samuel E. Wilson, Frank J. Veith, Robert W. Hobson and Russell A. Williams, McGraw Hill, Inc.)

Occluded arteries: The lumen area of totally occluded arteries may be completely replaced by complex fibrocalcific lesions or may be partially obstructed by intimal plaque with the remaining lumen occluded by a thrombus. In the presence of a central thrombotic core, dilatation of totally occluded vessels occurs by much the same mechanism as described for a stenotic vessel. The angiographic guide wire travels easily through the soft thrombotic material and remains in the lumen. The dilating balloon catheter follows the course of the guide wire and morphologic changes after balloon dilation are essentially the same as those which occur in a stenotic vessel. Intimal flaps and lumen irregularities associated with plaque separation and intimal dissection are seen, but additional irregularities may be produced by deformation and fragmentation of the thrombotic core. When a plaque occupies the entire lumen, the guide wire frequently travels in a plane between the intima and the atrophic media or between the media and the adventitia. This is the same plane of dissection that is usually employed for operative endarterectomy. The remaining artery wall is therby pulled away from the occlusive plaque and a new or false lumen is created beneath the plaque (Figure 2). As a result, the usual separation plane may not be discernable on angiography. The plaque is therefore effectively "sequestered" away from the new lumen, resulting in a configuration which may resemble that seen in the presence of an eccentric plaque which has not been subjected to balloon dilatation.

Transluminal Angioplasty in Patients

Percutaneous transluminal balloon angioplasty in patients occurs by the same mechanisms as those described in the experimental study. Evidences for this can be found on post-dilation angiograms, as well as in postmortem or post-amputation arteries that have previously been dilated. Angiograms reveal lumen contour irregularities, including intimal flaps corresponding to partial plaque separations and pro-trusion of separated intimal plaque into the lumen. Such lumen irregularities and dissection channels beneath plaques may be seen on 50-60% of post-dilatation angiograms of patients treated by transluminal angioplasty. The initial clinical success rate and subsequent restenosis rate do not, however, appear to be related to the presence, absence, or size of the flaps as seen on angiography (6,7). The presence of intimal flaps may instead indicate that sufficient dilatation has been achieved. According to the Law of La Place (T = Pr), the tangential tension (T) tending to keep the vessel lumen open is closely approximated by the product of the intra-luminal pressure (P) and the vessel radius (r). Thus, wall tension may be increased both by increasing pressure and by increasing radius. The sequence of changes described above suggests that transluminal angioplasty results in an increase in effective lumen diameter due to plaque separation with stretching of the media. Under conditions of marked vessel wall alteration by atherosclerosis, however, the increased level of wall tension resulting from balloon dilation must be sufficiently high to assure persistence of an adequately patent lumen and increased flow. If such a critical increase in diameter is not achieved, immediate clinical failure or restenosis may result. Thus, early restenosis, commonly seen within the first several months after balloon dilatation, may be related to insufficient detachment of plaque corresponding to inadequate stretching of the arterial wall.

Remodeling and Repair

Remodeling and repair processes after arterial disruption by the balloon catheter occur rapidly. Intimal flaps seen on initial post-dilatation angiograms may be entirely resolved as early as three days after the procedure. Subsequent angiography reveals that most dissection planes have resolved by one month. This may occur by reattachment of the intimal flap to the artery wall or by thrombus deposition and organization in the dissection plane. On occasion, residual flaps may persist and protrude into the lumen in association with an unsatisfactory clinical result. Such lesions are usually amenable to repeat dilatation with good long-term results.

Long-term follow-up with repeat angiographic studies of successful dilatation suggest that there is little change in bulk of the plaque and that continued patency appears to depend on persistence of the "overstretched" vessel wall (Figure 3). Vessels that do not have evidence of significant lumen enlargement initially have a higher rate of restenosis, probably due to insufficient disruption and stretching of the artery wall.

Restenosis

Restenosis is a significant problem following balloon dilatation. The one-year patency rate for iliac angioplasty has been estimated to be 77% and for femoral angioplasty, 56% (8). Failure may occur early due to the presence of unfavorable dissection planes or inadequate dilatation as noted above. Following successful dilatation, restenosis occurs as an exponentially decreasing function of time and by five years the patency rate is 63% for iliac angioplasty and 29%

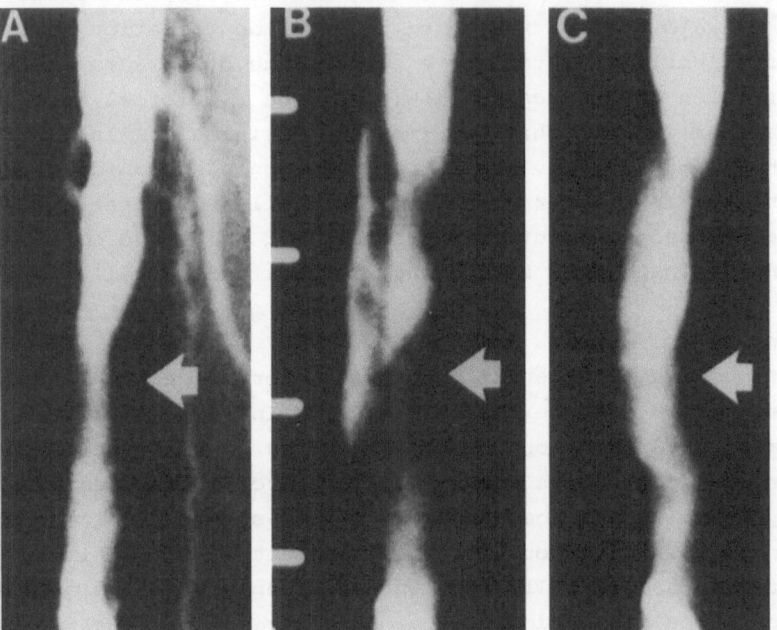

Figure 3.   Superficial femoral artery lesion treated by
balloon dilatation.   (A)   Contour of plaque before dilatation.
Arrow indicates thickest portion of plaque. (B)   Post-
dilatation angiogram reveals plaque disruption with a prominent intimal flap.   The contour of the thickest portion
of the plaque is unchanged (arrow); intimal flaps are located
predominantly on the opposite side.   (C) One year later, the
original plaque contour is still unchanged (arrow) and continued patency corresponds to "overdistension" of the artery
wall opposite the thickest portion of the plaque.   (Reproduced
with permission from Vascular Surgery: Principles and Practices
by Samuel E. Wilson, Frank J. Veith, Robert W. Hobson and
Russell A. Williams, McGraw Hill, Inc.).

for femoral angioplasty (8).   Although it has been suggested

that balloon dilatation may accelerate atherogenesis and

evidence for this has been reported in rabbits (9), morpho-

logic studies of human lesions are thus far inconclusive.

Examination of arteries harvested at autopsy or amputation

as long as 20 months after transluminal angioplasty show

little cellular reaction other than increased penetration

of vasa vasorum at the site of medial disruption.   There is

no evidence of "new plaque" formation or acceleration of

atherosclerosis in previous dilated areas (10).   Some curling

of the thinnest portion of the separated plaque near its

reattachment to the artery wall and blunting of the separated

plaque edges may be seen. Configurational alterations of
lesions caused by the balloon catheter and extension of
dissection planes to adjacent undilated segments of the vessel
may result in an angiographic appearance of "progression" or
"acceleration" of disease without actual changes in the volume
of an intimal plaque. On the basis of current findings, it
is likely that restenosis occurs not by new plaque deposition,
but by retraction or scarification of the disrupted and/or
overstretched artery wall, faulty reattachment of the dissected intima or by thrombus deposition.

CONCLUSION

Transluminal balloon angioplasty is a useful clinical
tool for enlarging the lumen in stenosed or occluded arteries.
Lumen enlargement occurs by: (1) disruption of the plaque
and artery wall, (2) separation of the plaque from the wall
and (3) stretching of the artery wall to enlarge the lumen.
There is little evidence that plaque compression or molding,
herniation or fragmentation of the plaque, or loss of plaque
substance is an important mechanism in achieving lumen enlargement. Thus clinical benefit is achieved not by plaque ameliora-
tion but rather by plaque displacement. Stretching the artery
wall is probably the most important feature of balloon angioplasty and long-term clinical benefit probably depends on
continued "overstretching" of the wall to maintain lumen
enlargement. Restenosis probably results from contraction,
retraction of the scarified media of the overstretched artery
wall or thrombus formation rather than by new plaque deposition.

REFERENCES
1. Dotter CT, Judkins M (1964) Transluminal treatment of
    arteriosclerotic obstruction: Description of a new
    technique and a preliminary report of its application.
    Circulation 30:654.
2. Gruntzig A, Kumpe D (1979) Technique of percutaneous
    transluminal angioplasty with the Gruntzig balloon cathe-
    ter. AJR 132:547
3. Lyon RT, Zarins CK, Lu CT, Yang CF, Glagov S (1981)
    Arterial wall disruption by balloon dilatation: Quanti-
    tative comparison of normal, stenotic and occluded
    vessels. Surg Forum 32:326
4. Lyon RT, Zarins CK, Lu CT, Yang CF, Glagov S (1987)
    Vessel, plaque and lumen morphology following balloon
    angioplasty: A quantitative study in distended post-
    mortem arteries. Arteriosclerosis 7:306-314

5. Castaneda-Zunaga WR, Amplatz KA (1983) The mechanism
    of transluminal angioplasty, In Casteneda-Zunaga WR (ed):
    Transluminal Angioplasty. Thieme-Stratton, New York,
    pp 11-19
6. Turcotte JK, Lu CT, Zarins CK (1981) The role of trans-
    luminal angioplasty in limb salvage and claudication.
    J Surg Res 30:428
7. Rush DS, Gewertz BL, Lu CT, Ball DG, Zarins CK (1983)
    Limb salvage in poor-risk patients using transluminal
    angioplasty. Arch Surg 118:1209
8. Doubilet P, Abrams HL (1984) The cost of underutiliza-
    tion: Percutaneous transluminal angioplasty for peripheral
    vascular disease. N Engl J Med 2:95
9. Faxon DP, Sanborn TA, Weber VJ, Haudenschild C, Gottsman
    SB, McGovern WA, Ryan TJ (1984) Restenosis following
    transluminal angioplasty in experimental atherosclerosis.
    Arteriosclerosis 4:189
10. Zarins CK, Lu CT, Gewertz BL, Lyon RT, Rush DS, Glagov
    S (1982) Arterial disruption and remodeling following
    balloon dilatation. Surgery 92:1086

39

Angioplasty, Laser Probes and Atherectomy

Christian C. Haudenschild, Timothy A. Sanborn, and David P. Faxon

Since the last workshop on the evolution of the
atherosclerotic plaque in 1963, progress in both basic and
clinical research has opened several new and promising ways
of preventing or delaying the development of atherosclerotic lesions. Impressive advances have also been made in
our ability to restore blood flow in vessels where a fully
developed, complicated plaque has already caused a significant narrowing or occlusion of the lumen. At this stage,
two options are available for intervention directly at the
affected vessel segment: a) to bypass the lesion with a
graft (tissue or biomaterials), or b) to penetrate or
disrupt the lesion by catheter, endarteriectomy, angioplasty, lasers, or by means of cutting instruments. While
these techniques have succeeded in immediate re-establish-
ment of channels for blood flow, they have also induced
various degrees of vascular trauma, ranging from endothelial denudation to total arterial wall necrosis. These
injuries can elicit a proliferative response of the vessel
wall which, together with the participation of blood-borne
cells, can lead to restenosis in a shorter time than was
needed for the development of the original obstruction.

In a vascular tissue graft, injury to endothelial
cells and to smooth muscle cells can be minimized by appropriate surgical techniques and vessel relaxation (1), reducing both early, thrombotic, and late proliferative restenosis (2). In balloon angioplasty and other instrumental

recanalizations through the stenosed vessel, massive
vascular trauma cannot be avoided (3); thus, one of the
most effective direct treatments of atherosclerotic vascular
stenosis may initiate the accelerated evolution of a
potentially stenosing lesion. The development of these new
lesions shares many of the pathogenetic mechamisms of
spontaneous atherosclerotic plaques.

It is indeed tempting to consider the response of the
arterial wall to angioplasty as a special case of the development of an atherosclerotic lesion (4). Injury, involvement
of cellular and humoral hemostatic components, inflammatory
cells, growth factors, and migratory, proliferative as well
as synthetic response of the vasular cells, are all present
and are in fact less hypothetical than in the various postulated "response to injury" mechanisms of spontaneous atherogenesis (5). There are, three fundamental differences
between plaque development and the response to angioplasty
which are relevant to the pathophysiology of the mechanically injured vessel, and which are also of practical
significance with respect to treatment after angioplasty
or similar interventions.

First, the nature and the extent of the vascular injury
resulting from angioplasty differ from other known and postulated injuries (6). Denuding or non-denuding, functional
endothelial defects have been suggested as very early events
in the pathogenesis of spontaneous atherosclerosis (6). In
animal models denudation of a large area of endothelium,
probably combined with smooth muscle irritation, can reliably produce intimal thickening resembling in many respects
an atherosclerotic lesion (7), especially when combined
with dietary manipulations (8). After successful angioplasty, a part of the vessel wall is often completely torn,
and the outer circumference is markedly extended (9). De-
endotheliation is complete, exposing basement membrane and
fibrillar collagen, and other extracellular components to
the circulating blood. The smooth muscle cells are subjected to extensive mechanical irritation, partial damage,
or necrosis. Surviving cells react by proliferating. On
the other hand, necrotic cells attract inflammatory cells,
especially monocytes, which can release powerful growth

stimuli. The numbers of necrotic and surviving cells vary; this may explain some of the variability in the extent and location of and location of subsequent reactive hyperplasia.

A second major difference between spontaneous formation of early plaques and the response to angioplasty is that the injury inflicted by the balloon affects a vascular wall which is already abnormal and varies markedly in its composition, physical properties, and reactivity. Bone-hard calcifications, non-distensible collagen, non-compressible lipid accumulations, and fluid-retaining glycosaminoglycans are mixed with stretchable, viable, cellular, and elastic components of the remaining normal vascular wall. In response to the balloon, the atheromatous and sclerotic portions of the original lesion tend to fracture and show little change otherwise, while the viable, elastic, and cellular parts are widely distended and line the new, enlarged lumen(9). These viable parts probably also provide most of the proliferating cells which are a source of the reactive hyperplasia, while the advanced, complicated, necrotic, calcified, plaque, except for fibrocellular caps and as vasa vasorum (10), has few cells which could proliferate. The extent of restenosis may therefore depend on the stimulus received by the reactive, non-sclerotic portions of the vessel, which are usually located at the outer circumference or up- or downstream of the dilated segment. One might ask whether a selective removal of the atheromatous, necrotic inner lesion, if possible at all, is really efficient and desirable without changing the reactivity of the remaining normal smooth muscle cells. Testing of these hypotheses is difficult even in animal models, since most diet/injury-induced vascular narrowings lack extensive necrosis and contain abundant reactive smooth muscle cells which respond by exuberant proliferation and restenose the vessel after angioplasty. In this respect, the animal model is an exaggeration of the problem and can be interpreted as a worst case situation.

While the participation of cellular and humoral components of the clotting system is debated in the formation of the earliest, spontaneous atherosclerotic lesions, thrombosis does play an important role in the complications

of late, ulcerated, calcified lesions, as well as in
experimental intimal denudation. After angioplasty, the
extent of initial thrombosis is probably the most important
factor determining both the initial patency and the late
result. Accumulation of chromium-labeled platelets at the
site of experimental angioplasty is up to a ten-fold increase
compared to the platelets found at the site of a simple
balloon denudation of a normal vessel (11). Slits and
pouches trap platelets and thrombi despite anticoagulant
therapy (Figure 1). If the thrombus is not immediately

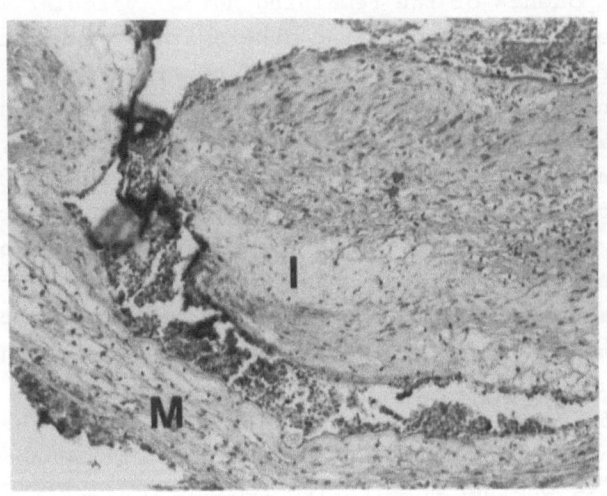

Figure 1. After experimental angioplasty, thrombotic material accumulates on the lumenal surface of the intimal thickening, along the torn intima, as well as in a large space
between intima (I) and media (M). Rabbit iliac artery,
6 weeks after balloon denudation/high cholesterol diet,
3 minutes after balloon angioplasty. Hematoxylin-eosin,
X 220.

obstructive, rapid organization soon leads to a filling of
the available lumenal space. Indeed, restenosis only four
weeks after experimental angioplasty shows the dense, original, torn intimal layers surrounded by a loose, fibrocellular proliferation resembling more an organizing thrombus than an atherosclerotic plaque (Figure 2), but occupy-
iny as much or more of the available lumenal space. It
should be noted that penetration of vasa vasorum into the

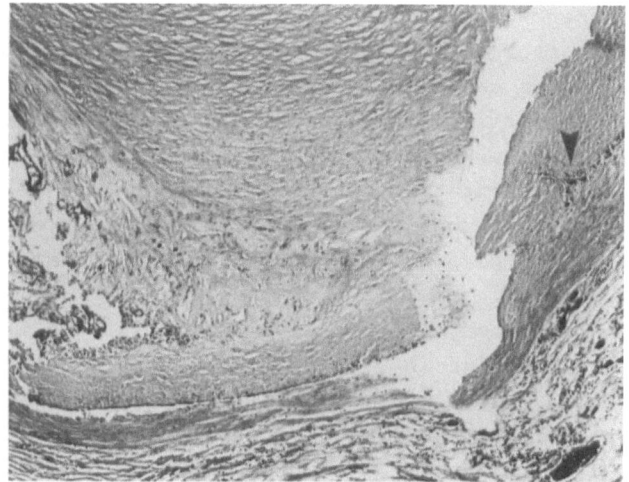

Figure 2. Four weeks after experimental angioplasty in the same rabbit model as in Figure 1. The torn intimal flaps are still visible, and much of the space on both sides of the tear is occupied by foam cells and loose, proliferating tissue resembling an organizing thrombus. van Gieson Elastin. X 30.

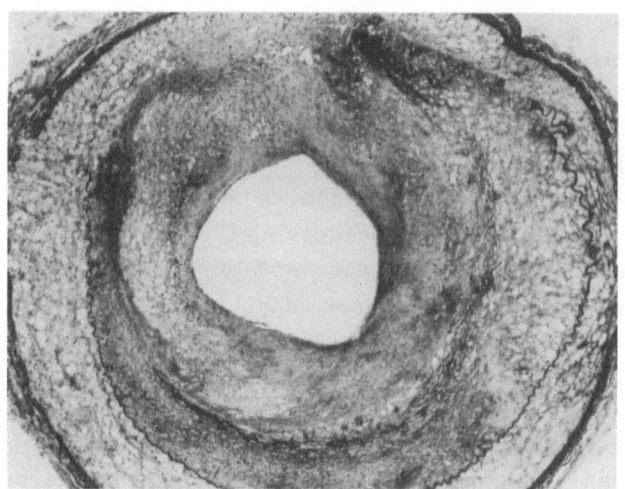

Figure 3. Human coronary artery, 4 hours after angioplasty. Note the tear reaching the adventitia, and the vasa vasorum within the fibrocellular intimal thickening (arrowhead). Hematoxylin-Eosin, X 140.

original atherosclerotic lesion as well as into the healing vessel wall after angioplasty may be an additional source of thrombi which can then undergo cellular organization. While the atherosclerotic rabbit iliac arteries in our diet/injury model are especially rich in vasa vasorum, small blood vessels penetrating into human lesions are less frequent, but must be considered an additional source of hemorrhage into the plaque, both spontaneously and after angioplasty (Figure 3).

Given this recognized role of thrombosis and the known onset of the vascular injury in angioplasty, antithrombotic therapy during, after, and possibly also before the intervention is obviously an effective way of preventing both early and late restenosis. Short term heparin, and aspirin with and without persantine, are currently used empirically in varied combinations for various time periods. A few experimental antiplatelet drugs are under investigation (12). Yet, the overall 30% restenosis rate (13), up to 47% in diabetics (14), indicates that today's post-angioplasty, antithrombotic treatment regimens, are not optimal. Furthermore, it may indicate that even the best regimen may not be insufficient in many cases because thrombosis, though important, is not the only determinant of vascular healing after angioplasty. The re-opening procedures themselves and their direct effects on the diseased vessel wall are continuously being modified.

Many attempts have been made to improve the original angioplasty balloons and procedures with various goals such as better access to the segments affected with a plaque, selective effects on the plaque only, reduction of overall trauma, diminishing of the newly-created thrombogenic surfaces, avoidance of perforation and rupture, and better sealing of the new conduit. We had the opportunity to test two of many recent devices which re-canalize diseased vessels by new mechanisms and therby elicit a different response from the vessel wall. We have used these devices, the Simpson atherectomy instrument and the Trimedyne heated laser probe, in our 6-week diet/injury model of stenosing atherosclerosis in rabbit iliac and carotid arteries, and we have limited preliminary experience with these devices in human use both in peripheral and coronary vessels.

The Simpson atherectomy instrument (15) is a rigid catheter tip with a lateral opening in which a rotating sharp knife can be moved. A balloon on the opposite side of this slit positions the tip tightly to the vessel wall and suction moves a part of the plaque into the slit, where it is cut sharply by the rotating knife. The cuts, in addition to removing plaque material, allow better control of the distention of the remaining wall than the spontaneous tears in response to a conventional balloon. A smooth, cut surface, and the absence of slits and pouches, diminishes initial platelet adhesion. There is a possiblity of directing the sites of the cuts to some extent, and of repeating the procedure under angiographic control within the same session until the lumen is satisfactory. The removed plaque material can be evaluated microscopically (Figure 4). Because of the balloon, which presses the catheter slit against the vessel wall, there is also a certain degree of mechanical dilatation. The procedure requires considerable skill on the part of the operator and anticoagulant therapy. The cuts heal by fibrocellular proliferation, which seems to be self-limiting, without involvement of the entire circumference, resulting in an improved long-term patency.

The Trimedyne heated laser probe is a spheroid metal cap covering the tip of a fiberoptic catheter (16). Unlike other laser devices, in this hot probe the laser energy is converted entirely into heat (400° C) and does not directly affect the vessel wall in the form of light. With this design, the energy can be directed to the sides of the catheter tip as well as forward; the amount of energy can be controlled by continuous or pulsating activation of the laser. Similar to, but entirely the same as direct laser light, the heat probe creates instant heat coagulation of the tissue analogous to an acute burn injury. In addition, there is always some degree of distention, since the tip must touch the vessel wall tightly in order to be effective. The optimal result is an acellular, coagulated region in the lumenal portion of the vessel wall, with a relatively smooth surface without slits, pouches, or cracks. The thrombogeneity

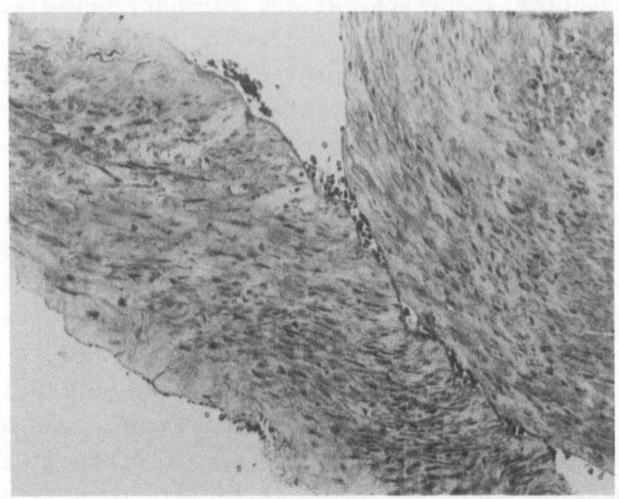

Figure 4. Atherectomy specimens from a stenosing lesion in
a human popliteal artery. Note the fibrocellular nature of
this lesion and the sharp borders obtained by the rotating
knife. Hematoxylin-Eosin, X 360.

of the new surface seems to be slightly less pronounced than
that of non-heated tissue; more important is the band of
coagulated, acellular tissue which establishes a sizable
distance between the platelets and the first viable cells
able to respond to platelet growth factors. The coagulated
tissue layer may also be an obstacle to migration of stimulated wall cells. We assume that these are the major reasons
why, in the best case, intimal proliferation on the top of
the coagulated tissue is minimal after 4 weeks (Figure 5).
Problems in less successful cases include: adhesion of the
heated probe to the tissue, circumferential tears in the
outer wall, plain endarteriectomy with the potential of
embolization of atherosclerotic material, tortuosity of
the vessels, or mismatch between the diameters of the tip
and the lumen. From the viewpoint of plaque evolution and
response of the vascular wall to injury, the heat injury
teaches a surprising, almost trivial lesson: in the absence
of a source of viable cells near the injury, there is no proliferation and thus no late, restenosing intimal thickening!

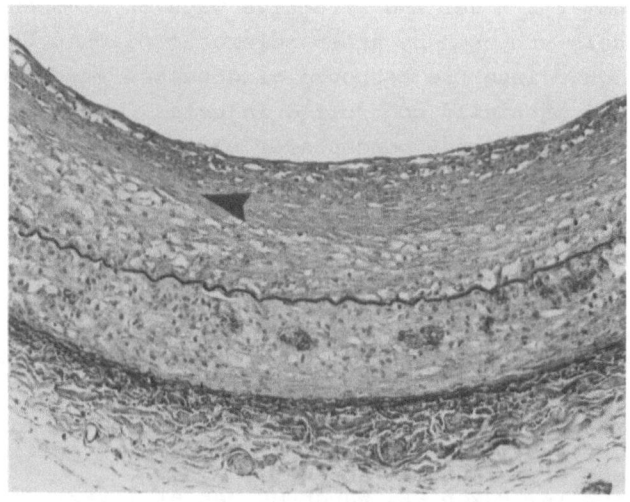

Figure 5. Six-week balloon/cholesterol diet model of rabbit iliac artery lesion, 4 weeks after re-opening of a 50% stenosis with a laser thermal probe. Starting from the lumen (top), the layers represent a thin, probably new, endothelialized foam cell lesion, a dense, largely acellular band (arrowhead), the rest of the intima containing foam cells, the internal elastic lamina (stained black), the media containing prominent vasa vasorum, and the collagenous adventitia (bottom). van Gieson-Elastin, X 140.

One could speculate that some advanced, acellular, extensively teutonic fibrous or calcified, atherosclerotic plaques may become self-limited simply because there are too few cells which can be stimulated to proliferate. Furthermore, the absence of reactive cells in the heat-coagulated tissue band deprives the vessel wall from contractile elements which could narrow the lumen by spasm. An acellular or partly acellular tube created by the heat probe or any other device with a similar effect in partly necrotic plaque tissue may represent a desirable, non-reactive, non-antigenic *in situ* autograft, provided that the resulting conduit is strong enough to prevent eventual excessive aneurysmal dilatation.

In summary, novel and effective ways of re-opening blood vessels stenosed by atherosclerotic plaques have also given insights into the response of diseased vessel walls to known and partially controlled injuries. New and perhaps somewhat unconventional concepts of plaque evolution emerge from the study of the lesions formed after traumatic lesion removal.

REFERENCES

1. LoGerfo FW, Quist WC, Crawshaw HM, Haudenschild CC (1983) Integrity of vein grafts as a function of initial intimal and medial preservation. Circulation 68(pt 2): 117-124
2. LoGerfo FW, Quist WC, Cantelmo NL, Haudenschild CC (1983) Integrity of vein grafts as a function of initial intimal and medial preservation
3. Sanborn TA, Faxon DP, Waugh MD, et al (1982) Transluminal angioplasty in experimental atherosclerosis. Circulation 66:917-922
4. Faxon DP, Sanborn TA, Haudenschild CC (1987) The mechanism of angioplasty and its relationship to restenosis. Amer J Cardiol 60:5B-9B
5. Ross R (1986) The pathogenesis of atherosclerosis - an update.New Engl J Med 314:488-500
6. Reidy MA (1985) A reassessment of endothelial injury and arterial lesion formation. Lab Invest 53:513-520
7. Haudenschild CC, Schwartz SM (1979) Endothelial Regeneration. II. Restitution of endothelial continuity. Lab Invest 41:407-418
8. Faxon DP, Weber VJ, Haudenschild CC, Gottsman SB, McGovern WA, Ryan TJ (1982) Acute effects of transluminal angioplasty in three experimental models of atherosclerosis. Arteriosclerosis 2:125-133
9. Sanborn T, Faxon DP, Haudenschild CC, Gottsman SB, Ryan TJ (1983) The mechanisms of transluminal angioplasty in three experimental models of atherosclerosis. Circulation 68:1136-1140
10. Barger AC, Beeuwkes R III, Lainey LL, Silverman KJ (1984) Hypothesis: Vasa vasorum and neovascularization of human coronary arteries. A possible role in the pathophysiology of atherosclerosis. New Engl J Med 310:175-177.
11. Wilentz JR, Sanborn TA, Haudenschild CC, Valerie CR, Ryan TJ, Faxon DP (1987) Platelet accumulation in experimental angioplasty: Time course and relation to vascular injury. Circulation 75:636-642
12. Sanborn TA, Balleli LM, Faxon DP, Haudenschild CC, Valerie CR, Ryan TJ (1985) Inhibition of 51Cr-labeled platelet accumulation after balloon angioplasty in rabbits: Comparison of heparin, aspirin and CGS 13080, a new thromboxane synthetase inhibitor. J Amer Coll Cardiol 7:934
13. Holmes DR, Vlietstra RE, Smith HC, et al. Restenosis after percutaneous transluminal coronary angioplasty (PTCA): A report from the PTCA Registry of the NHLBI. Amer J Cardiol 53:77C

14. Margolis JR, Krieger R, Glemser E (1984) Coronary angioplsty: Increased restenosis rate in insulin dependent diabetes. Circulation 70(pt 2):175

15. Faxon DP, Simpson J, Thalplyiyal H, et al (1985) *In vivo* evaluation of atherectomy, a new technique to enlarge atherosclerotic vessels. Circulation 72 (Suppl 3):469

16. Sanborn TA, Faxon DP, Haudenschild CC, Ryan TJ (1985) Experimental angioplasty: Circumferential distribution of laser thermal energy with a laser probe. J Amer Coll Cardiol 5:934-938

Evaluation of Lesion Status in Major Arterial Beds

40

Late Changes in Saphenous Vein Aorto-Coronary Bypass Grafts: Clinical, Angiographic, Lipid and Pathological Correlations

Gerald M. Lawrie, George C. Morris, Donald G. Weilbaecher, Jack L. Titus, Joel D. Morrisett, Philip D. Henry, Nan Earle, and Michael E. DeBakey

INTRODUCTION

Coronary bypass surgery has become well established as the most effective form of treatment for relief of angina pectoris and has been shown, in a number of ramdomized studies, to prolong life in certain subsets of patients. Despite the extraordinary success of this operation and its durability in comparison to other forms of operations for atherosclerosis, there is need for enhancement of early and late graft patency and prevention of the late vein graft deterioration which has been observed in a significant portion of patients over a period of 10 to 15 years.

Vein Graft Patency

In our studies (1), graft patency at one month was 92%; at three months 91%; and at six months, 84%. Our studies of pathologic changes showed that early graft occlusion is almost always produced by thrombosis (1). Our angiographic studies showed that the underlying coronary artery usually remains uninvolved in this thrombotic process (2,3).

A variety of perioperative factors may influence early graft occlusion rates. These include the methods used in harvesting and preparing the vein graft, the size of the recipient coronary artery, the presence or absence of severe proximal coronary stenosis, the magnitude of the resting intraoperative vein-graft blood flow, whether significant reactive hyperemic increase in graft flow can be induced and the occurrence of perioperative vein graft and coronary arterial spasm (4-7).

Late occlusion or stenosis of vein grafts are due to a variety of pathological changes in the graft. Late occlusion of the graft also may be due to thrombosis secondary to occlusion from progression of disease in the grafted coronary artery.

The data in Table 1 demonstrates that the prevalence of occlusion and stenosis of vein grafts increases with the passage of time and these procedures are most common in the 7-15 year time interval. Studies of sequential changes in graft patency in a subgroup of 187 of these patients produced results similar to those observed for the entire group. At the first post-operative study at a mean interval of 42.5 $\pm$ 1.8 (SE) months after operation, 80.1% (270/337) of grafts were normal, 3.6% (12/337) were stenotic (more than 20% luminal diameter reduction) and 16.4% (55/337) were occluded. The second post-operative study was at a mean interval of 87.4 $\pm$ 2.2 months from operation and of the 270 grafts patent at the first study, 71.5% (193/270) were normal, 10.0% (27/270) were stenotic, and 18.5% (50/270) were occluded. Of the same group of 337 grafts, 85 grafts underwent a third study, 107.7 $\pm$ 2.3 months after operation. In this subgroup, 58.8% (50/85) of the vein grafts were normal, 5.9% (5/85) of grafts were stenotic and 35.3% (30/85) were occluded.

Statistical analysis showed that the number of vein grafts performed (p < 0.03), the presence of poor preoperative left ventricular function (p < 0.04), the absence of preoperative angina (p < 0.004), vein grafts to right or circumflex coronary arteries (p < 0.05), and higher triglyceride levels (293 $\pm$ 28 vs 228 $\pm$ 13 mg/dl) (p <0.03) were all predictive of graft abnormality but the cholesterol levels were similar: 256 $\pm$ 4.4 mg/dl for normal and 255 $\pm$ 7.6 mg/dl for the abnormal grafts (p < 0.05).

Vein Graft Pathology

Pathological evaluation of vein graft specimens obtained from more than 400 patients either at reoperation or autopsy have documented a variety of pathological changes in the vein grafts.

Table 1: Rates of Patency[a] and Stenosis[b] in 1530 Vein Grafts Up to 179 Months After Operation in 583 Patients

Months After Operation	Catheterization Number	Patent Number	%	Stenosed Number	%
0-11	224	192	85.7	5	2.6
12-23	136	108	79.4	0	0.0
24-35	143	113	79.0	4	2.8
36-47	89	68	76.4	3	3.4
48-59	125	104	83.2	1	0.8
60-71	203	157	77.3	8	3.9
72-83	126	93	73.8	8	6.3
84-95	86	52	60.5	11	12.8
96-107	94	54	57.4	7	7.4
108-119	95	52	54.7	12	12.6
120-131	79	55	69.6	13	16.5
132-143	68	49	72.1	8	11.8
144-155	35	23	65.7	7	20.0
156-167	21	12	57.1	2	9.5
168-179	6	4	66.7	1	16.7
Totals or Mean	1530	1136	74.2	90	5.9

[a] Patency is defined as demonstration of flow through a graft including stenotic grafts.

[b] Stenosis is defined as greater than 20% reduction in luminal diameter

The earliest changes are fibrin depositions on a damaged intima which occurs in a few hours and lasts a number of days. Inflammatory cells are seen in the intima

and media in increased numbers during the first two weeks.
There is patchy necrosis of the intima and media. These
changes are much less severe with newer preservation techniques of the harvested saphenous veins and the postoperative use of aspirin and persantine. These changes are
followed (over the next few days) by a cellular fibromuscular proliferation of the intima. This is a diffuse
process and probably originates from intimal and medial
smooth muscle cells. Acid mucopolysaccharides are a
prominent feature in the cellular intimal proliferation.

In most cases, this cellular intimal proliferation
markedly decreases and ceases after a few weeks to months.
The acid mucopolysaccharide content decreases along with
the intimal cellularity which consist of a mixture of
fibroblasts, fibrous tissue and smooth muscle cells. The
intima usually remains stable for a long time after these
changes. However in some patients complications occur
such as atherosclerosis or dissection. The luminal stenosis
caused by intimal proliferation usually is clinically
insignificant but rarely, cellular intimal proliferation
will continue and the lumen of the graft will become
occluded. This process usually occurs within one year and
often within the first 6 to 9 months. Occasionally
intimal proliferation may be sufficiently asymetrical that
a localized stenosis of clinical significance is produced.

The mechanisms for development of true atherosclerosis
in vein grafts are not well understood. Changes which are
morphologically characteristic of atherosclerosis rarely
develop before 18 months and most take much longer. Most
grafts do have intimal lipid foam cell lesions but
whether this represents the earliest lesion of true atherosclerosis in vein grafts is controversial.

Characteristic changes of atherosclerosis are defined
as the presence of intra- and extra-cellular cholesterol
esters, complex carbohydrates, vascularization and calcification. These changes occur at different times after
operation and to different degrees. Many of the complicated lesions are focal whereas the fibromuscular intimal
proliferation described earlier is diffuse.

A complication which may be the result of or the cause of a lesion resembling atherosclerosis is intimal dissection. This can be localized or extensive, and may lead to acute graft occlusions. Such lesions, which are observed occasionally in native arterial atherosclerosis, are common in vein grafts and have been seen in well over half of the occluded late vein grafts. This lesion is characterized by a plane of intimal dissection in which the false channel is filled with blood and/or the breakdown products of hemorrhage including lipids. The true lumen is markedly narrowed. Often there is an inflammatory response of lymphocytes and plasma cells in the intima and media. Changes characteristic of arterial atherosclerosis are usually absent from the vein wall.

Influence of Plasma Lipids on Vein Grafts

We have been interested for some time in the relation between vein-graft atherosclerosis and serum lipids. In an anatomic study of 99 saphenous-vein grafts recovered at necropsy from 55 patients who survived aortocoronary bypass for 0 to 75 months, we made a comparison between patients with normal and elevated lipid levels in regard to the severity of intimal proliferation in vein grafts and the prevalence of graft atherosclerosis (8). Although intimal proliferation progressed with time in both groups of patients, a greater proportion of severely hyperlipemic patients had high-grade luminal narrowing of vein grafts as the interval after aortocoronary bypass increased. Luminal narrowing did not develop before 12 months in any of the 59 vein grafts from the 27 normolipemic and 5 hyperlipemic patients but did develop in 3 of 26 vein grafts (11.5%) from normolipemic and 11 of 14 vein grafts (78.6%) from hyperlipemic patients 13 to 75 months after surgery. We observed microscopic atherosclerotic changes in saphenour vein grafts in some patients with normal total lipid levels, but we noted that the early onset of atherosclerosis in vein grafts was most likely in those patients with high cholesterol levels in the range of 308-537 mg/dl.

Anatomic and technical factors are the dominant determinants of graft patency. However, in order to

determine the role of lipid levels and other factors on
influence graft patency, we analyzed multiple preoperative
clinical and angiographic variables for 682 patients with
1174 grafts which had been studied angiographically. Mean
interval from operation to recatheterization was 49.3 months
+ 38.8 months. Overall patency was 71.3% (837/1174). Right
coronary graft patency was 70.9% (321/453); left anterior
descending, 74.9% (400/534); and circumflex, 62.0% (116/187).
Overall, 399 patients 58.5%) had all grafts patent, and 565
(82.8%) had one or more grafts patent. Patency of 472
grafts evaluated between 85 and 156 months postoperatively
was 63.1%.

The variables were analyzed by two-way contingency
table analysis to evaluate differences between normal and
abnormal grafts. The number of vessels grafted (p < 0.001)
(increasing number was unfavorable), absence of preoperative angina (p < 0.01), lack of preoperative propranolol
(p < 0.01), and circumflex coronary artery graft (p < 0.01)
were all associated with higher rates of graft occlusion.
Age, sex, smoking, diabetes, or hyperlipidemia were not
predictive of graft failure (p > 0.05). These results
suggest that conventional risk factors including plasma
cholesterol levels had no predictive value as to on the
long-term patency of the grafts of patients included in
this study.

More detailed analysis of the long-term influence of
cholesterol was performed in 322 patients with preoperative
cholesterol data derived from a series of 1447 patients
followed 10-14 years (10). These 322 patients had undergone post-operative graft evaluation at a mean interval
of 65.2 months (1-178 months). Multiple clinical angiographic and laboratory values were similar for these
patients and the remaining 1125 patients. Plasma cholesterol was 249.6 + 53.5 mg/dl in unstudied compared with
256 + 56.9 mg/dl for studied patients (p > 0.12). Patients
were classified angiographically as normal (189 patients)
or abnormal (133 patients). Abnormal patients had one or
more stenotic and/or occluded grafts. Plasma cholesterol
was 251 + 58.8 (SD) mg/dl for normal patients and 264 +
53.8 mg/dl in abnormal patients (p >0.05). A 10-year

Kaplan-Meier analysis was performed for four groups of
patients: cholesterol <200 mg/dl $\geq$200<245, $\geq$245<280, >280
mg/dl (Figure 1). There was no difference in incidence of
graft abnormalities among these four groups (p >0.05). Cox,
two-way table and logistic regression analyses of multiple
variables showed no association between plasma cholesterol
and graft abnormality but triglyceride levels were predictive of graft failure.

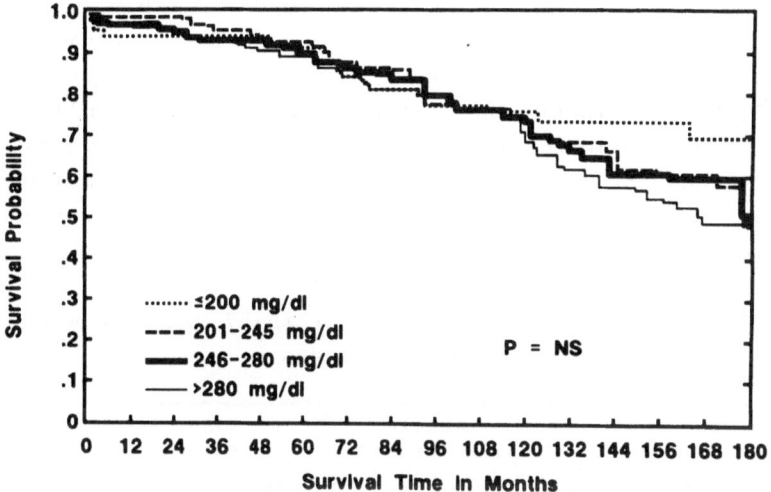

Figure 1.

In order to further investigate these findings and
evaluate the influence of HDL - cholesterol levels, another
study was performed of 1557 patients with vein graft patency data for 2861 grafts up to 15 years after operation
(11). Clinical features and lipid levels of patients with
normal vein grafts were compared to those with occluded and
stenotic vein grafts. Patients with normal grafts had
fewer grafts performed initially: 1.67 compared with 1.96
(p <0.01). Cholesterol and HDL - cholesterol levels of
patients with normal grafts were 241 $\pm$ 54 and 37.4 $\pm$ 12.2
mg/dL compared with 242 $\pm$ 54 and 38.1 $\pm$ 11.7 mg/dL for
patients with occluded grafts (p > 0.05). Triglyceride

levels of patients with normal grafts were 205 ± 129
compared with 219 ± 166 mg/dl for patients with occluded
grafts (p > 0.05). Blood glucose levels were 94 ± 37 and
94 ± 39 mg/dl. Analysis of individual vein grafts showed
similar findings except that triglyceride levels were higher in the occluded group (208 ± 127 vs 224 ± 181 mg/dl
p < 0.06). There were 117 patients with one or more stenosed grafts; their cholesterol level was 266 ± 55 and triglyceride level was 277 ± 33 mg/dl (p <0.01).

In 57 patients with vein graft pathological diagnoses
the plasma cholesterol was 228 ± 61 mg/dl (p > 0.05), and
the triglyceride level was 249 ± 179 mg/dl (p < 0.05). HDL
cholesterol levels were available for 23 of these patients,
and was 36.2 mg/dl in the atherosclerotic group compared
with 37.5 mg/dl in 11 other patients with intimal proliferation. Thus, cholesterol levels were not different for patients without or with vein graft occlusion or atherosclerosis,
whereas the triglyceride level showed borderline elevation in
all groups with vein graft abnormalities (Table 2).

Table 2. Plasma Lipid Levels (mg/dl) in 57 Patients with
          Vein Graft Anatomic Diagnosis

Lipid	Athero-sclerosis	No Athero-sclerosis	P
Total Cholesterol	228 ± 61	241 ± 54	NS
HDL Cholesterol	36.2 ± 11.8	37.4 ± 12.2	NS
Total Triglycerides	249 ± 179	205 ± 129	< 0.05

The results of these studies all consistently suggest
that preoperative levels of total cholesterol and HDL -
cholesterol were not predictive of the presence or absence
of vein graft failure in most patients.

It has been suggested that the level of plasma apoB may
have an effect on vein graft failure (12). Preliminary
analyses of the levels of plasma Lp(a) and apoB levels in
27 of our patients with or without vein graft atherosclerosis diagnosed histologically rather than inferred from

angiographic findings indicate that no significant
difference existed between these two groups in relation to
levels of plasma lipids (Table 3).

Table 3. Plasma Lipid Levels in 27 Patients with an
          Anatomic Diagnosis of Vein Graft Athero-
          sclerosis or Intimal Proliferation

Lipids	Atherosclerosis	Intimal Proliferation	P
Total Cholesterol	174 ± 14.2 mg/dl	184 ± 14.6 mg/dl	NS
HDL Cholesterol	25.4 ± 1.4 mg/dl	27.4 ± 1.6 mg/dl	NS
Apo [a]	153.9 ± 43 µg/ml	126.9 ± 39.9 µg/ml	NS
ApoB	1005.6 ± 82.2 µg/ml	1106.4 ± 75.8 µg/ml	NS
Total Cholesterol	161 ± 25 mg/dl	179 ± 30 mg/dl	NS

These lipid data do not support the conclusions of the
study of Campeau *et al* (12). Like us (9-11), Campeau and
coworkers have found that age, sex, and the prevalence of
hypertension, diabetes, and smoking were similar in patients
with and without progression of atherosclerosis in vein
grafts or native coronary circulation. However, they showed that patients with vein-graft atherosclerosis had elevated levels of total serum cholesterol, low levels of HDL
cholesterol and high levels of apoB (12). Our data do not
indicate a correlation of elevated total cholesterol levels
or reduced HDL cholesterol levels or elevation of plasma
apoB levels with vein-graft atherosclerosis that develops
from 5 to 10 years after operation.

That patients with severe hypercholesterolemia are more
susceptible to saphenous-vein graft atherosclerosis is well
recognized. We were among the first to report a substantial experience with this phenomenon (8). Certainly, most
patients in whom vein-graft atherosclerosis develops in the
first several years after operation have notable elevations
of serum cholesterol, usually over 300 mg/dl. These

patients, however, represent only a very small proportion
of the patients in whom late vein-graft lesions become a
clinical problem. Most patients do not develop vein-graft
lesions until more than five years after operation (Table 1).

Lytle *et al* (13) demonstrated different rates of graft
failure in a study of 502 patients who underwent sequential
graft studies for groups defined by them as either high or
low risk. The low risk group consisted of 212 non-diabetic
patients with plasma cholesterol levels below 300 mg/dl and
triglyceride levels below 180 mg/dl and the high risk group
consisted of diabetic patients with lipid levels above
these values. Interestingly, only 6/502 patients (1.2%)
were found with this combination. They found that 43/502
patients (8.6%) had no diabetes but had cholesterols of
more than 300 mg/dl and triglyceride levels of more than
180 mg/dl. Only in these severely hyperlipidemic patients
could a relationship be demonstrated between lipid levels
and graft failure in their long-term studies. Their finding that patients with severely elevated cholesterol levels
develop more graft lesions is consistent with our own
earlier observations (8).

It is not generally appreciated that most of Campeau
and coworkers' patients (12) were derived from their earliest esperience with coronary bypass surgery in which unfavorable graft patency and graft stenosis rates were reported (14). These data showed that whereas early (less than
one month) graft patency was comparable in both groups,
graft occlusion and stenosis rates were much higher in the
early experience of 300 patients than in the subsequent
experience (Table 4). Of particular note is the fact that
16.5% of grafts had localized narrowing from 6 to 18 months
after operation in the initial experience as contrasted
with only 6% in the subsequent experience. Campeau and
coworkers interpreted these data to indicate a high incidence of technical surgical problems in their initial
experience which were subsequently overcome by technical
refinements (14, 15).

These data are important because they show that injuries
sustained by vein grafts at the time of operation may continue to affect graft function adversely for many years

Table 4. Data from Montreal Heart Institute Studies of Early and Late Angiographic Findings in Two Consecutive Series of Patients[1]

Series	Cumulative graft patency (percent)		
	Within One month	Between 6-18 months	Between 54-88 months
Consecutive series #1	86.3	66.8	57.7
Consecutive series #2	91.9	85.5	83.2
All grafts	86.6	75.9	67.8

Series	Graft narrowing >40% noted between 6 to 18 months after surgery		
	No of patent grafts studied	Grafts with localized narrowing	Grafts with diffuse narrowing
Consecutive series #1	103	No.17 -16.5%*	No.32 -31%
Consecutive series #2	133	No. 8 -6%*	No.17 -12.8%*
All grafts	278	No.30-10.8%	No.58 -20.9%

* p<0.025

[1] From Campeau, L., A generation of Coronary Arteriography, An International Symposium, Cleveland Clinic Foundation, Cleveland, 1979 (pp 133-137).

thereafter. Furthermore, the incidence of late graft problems reported in the most recent study of Campeau *et al* (12) is probably considerably higher than that to be expected with current surgical techniques, and are certainly much higher than documented by us and others (13) both in our overall and sequential studies of graft patency (Table 5).

Another major problem with the study of Campeau *et al* (12) is their failure to analyze the influence of risk factors separately for progression of native coronary disease and graft atherosclerosis; it is important to bear in mind that risk factors may have different effects upon the native circulation and the vein grafts.

Table 5.   Comparison of Results of Sequential Studies of
           Vein Graft Patency

Series	No. Vein Grafts	Normal (%)	Stenosed (%)	Occluded (%)	Interval (mo.)
Montreal Heart Institute[a]	132	37.5 (50/132)	33.0 (43/132)	29.5 (39/132)	120
Baylor College of Medicine[b]	270	71.5 (193/270)	10.0 (27/270)	18.5 (50/270)	108
Cleveland Clinic[c]	645	55 (357/645)	19 (119/645)	26 (169/645)	88

a - Reference 12

b - See text

c - Reference 13

Vein Graft Preparation

Intraoperative endothelial and medial damage to vein
grafts may be substantial and lead to deposition of platelets and fibrin which may initiate further changes. A
number of studies have documented severe damage to the
saphenous veins during harvesting and preparation. Various
techniques have been proposed to minimize this damage but
the results of these studies have been conflicting. In
order to study this subject further we have carried out a
series of experiments evaluating dynamic rather than
structural properties of the saphenous veins.

Our own studies of various methods of intraoperative
preservation of saphenous vein grafts have shown evidence
of serious damage from the use of 0.9 N NaCl solution. This
solution was used routinely in our institution for vein
graft functional integrity, we isolated strips from vein
grafts prepared by different procedures and assessed
venous reactivity to vasoconstrictors or vasodilators that
act on smooth muscle directly or indirectly by release of
endothelium-derived relaxing factor. Preparative procedures evaluated were (6-10 patients/group): I) study of

grafts immediately after vein excision: II) storage in
0.9% saline (22° C) for one hour; III) storage in Plasmalyte
(22° C) for one hour without IIIa) or with pressurization
(400 mm Hg) for lead detection (IIIb); IV) pressurization
and one hour storage in Plasmalyte without (IVa) or with
1μM nitroglycerin (IVb; V) as in IV, either without (Va)
or with 1 μM verapamil (Vb) instead of nitroglycerin. The
results are shown in Table 6. Storage in Plasmalyte compared
to that in saline protected motor and endothelial function
of vein grafts; and storage with nitroglycerin or verapamil
did not prevent the deleterious effects of pressurization.

These results demonstrated that enhanced methods of
vein graft preservation reduce the severity of endothelial
damage. It is conceivable that the intimal proliferative
reaction may be modified and the subsequent development of
stenotic vein graft lesions be reduced. Specimens of
vein grafts obtained 1-5 days after operation have shown
markedly less changes than those seen after preparation
with 0.9 N NaCl.

Table 6.   Results of Studies of Various Methods of Vein Graft
           Preparation

Group	Contraction Phenylephrine (1 uM)	Relaxation, % of Contraction	
		TNG (1uM) EDRF-independent	A23187 (1uM) EDRF-dependent
I Immediate study	2.2±0.4 g (±SE)	91±4%	36±4%
II 0.9% NaCl + 1 hr	1.2±0.2 g *	70±3% *	11±2% *
IIIa Plasmalyte + 1 hr	2.6±0.4 g	88±4%	34±4%
IIIb Plasmalyte + Pressure + 1 hr	1.1±0.9 g * §	69±4% *§	20±3% *§
IVa Plasmalyte + Pressure + 1 hr	1.2±0.8 g *	70±3% *	20±3% *
IVb Plasmalyte + Pressure + NTG + 1 hr	1.3±0.7 g	68±3%*	21±3% *
Va Plasmalyte + Pressure + 1 hr	1.1±0.6 g *	72±2% *	23±3% *
Vb Plasmalyte + Pressure + Verapamil + 1 hr	1.3±0.3 g *	70±4% *	19±4% *

* p < .05 vs. I; § p < .05, b vs. a of the same group.

Lipoprotein Studies of Plasma and Vein Grafts

In our institution we are also carrying out basic
studies of lipoprotein plasma levels and patterns of localization in the walls of vein grafts from patients who have
undergone reoperation. Lp[a] has been of particular interest. Lp [a] is a human lipoprotein whose composition and
structure closely resemble that of human low density lipoproteins (LDL). Both lipoproteins contain apoprotein B
but only Lp [a] contains apoprotein [a]. Previous work
by Morrisett et al (16) and others (17) have demonstrated
that apo [a] is a high molecular weight protein (> 450 kD),
a substantial proportion of which is carbohydrate (> 20%).
In the present study, the involvement of Lp [a] in atherosclerosis has been examined in vein grafts resected from
patients undergoing a second bypass operation.

We have drawn blood after admission from >12 hr fasted
patients and again immediately before surgery. Plasma
lipids were determined by procedures described previously
(18). Plasma apo [a] and apoB were measured using polyclonal antibodies in enzyme linked immunoassays developed
in our laboratories (19). Vein graft tissue resected at
reoperation was immediately placed in a specimen cup (on
ice) containing gauze soaked with saline solution containing the protease inhibitors aprotinin and phenylmethane-
sulfonyl fluroide. Adjacent 5 mm transverse sections were
cut for lipid staining, immunochemical localization, and
electrophoretic quantitation (20). Tissue apo[a] and apoB
were measured with polyclonal antibodies in electroimmuno-
assays described previously (21). The data obtained is
summarized in Table 7.

The mean plasma cholesterol level for 26 patients was
225 mg/dl, 8% below the mean of 245 mg/dl found in a
normal population of comparable age (6). The mean HDL
cholesterol was 32 mg/dl, 24% below the mean of 42 mg/dl
found in a normal population. These values were depressed
about 20% in plasmas obtained from patients in the operating
room immediately before surgery. The plasma levels of
apo[a] and apoB were 183 and 1398 µg/ml, respectively.
These values were more than 50% higher than those of a
normal population of comparable age.

623

Table 7.   Comparison of Plasma and Tissue Levels of Apo Lp [a]
and apoB in Patients Undergoing Coronary Artery Bypass
Reoperation

	Mean	Std. Dev.	N
Patients Age (yrs)	61	8	26
Graft duration (mos)	98	40	25
Total Cholesterol	225	49	26
HDL cholesterol	32	7	25
Plasma apo[a] (ug/ml)	183	200	26
Plasma apoB (ug/ml)	1398	347	26
Plasma apo[a]/apoB	0.124	0.127	26
NSV apo[a] (ng/mg wet wt)	0	0	7
NSV apoB (ng/mg wet wt)	3.5	4.5	7
OVG apo[a] (ng/mg wet wt)	24.0	33.8	28
OVG apoB (ng/mg wet wt)	69.1	47.1	28
OVG apo[a]/apo B	0.314	0.362	28
OVG apo[a]/apoB	2.53	2.85	28
Plasma apo[a]/apoB			

OVG = old vein graft

NSV = new saphenous vein

Apo[a] was not detected in normal saphenous vein samples, and the level of apoB was very low (3.5 ng/ml). In resected old vein graft, the mean tissue level of apo[a] was 24.0 ng/mg, and that of apoB was 69.1 ng/ml. The frequency distribution of tissue apo a differs somewhat from that of plasma apo[a] although both are approximately monotonic functions. Distribution of tissue apoB is bimodal, and not as skewed as that of plasma apoB.

Thus in these studies apo[a] and apoB were virtually absent from normal saphenous vein, but accumulated to significant levels in veins grafted into arterial beds. Apo[a] / apoB is significantly higher in vein graft tissue than in plasma. The greater proportion of apo[a] over apoB retained in the vein graft is of interest because of the high correlation of plasma Lp[a] levels with coronary artery disease.

CONCLUSION

In conclusion, late pathological changes in saphenous
vein grafts have been observed by us at a significant but
much lesser frequency than reported by Campeau et al (11,
13). Our clinical studies indicate a lack of correlation
between graft abnormalities and cholesterol, HDL - cholesterol or apoB levels. Pathological studies in large numbers
of grafts previously diagnosed angiographically as having
atherosclerotic stenosis in fact have developed complications related to the presence of intimal proliferation.
In particular, intramural dissection appears to be an
important mechanism for graft occlusion. Our basic research
on human vein specimens have demonstrated the importance of
improved methods of intraoperative graft preservation. The
implications of the observation that lipid accumulation in
the wall of the vein grafts is present even the absence of
gross atherosclerotic changes requires further investigation.
Of particular interest is the fact that whereas in normal
saphenous vein from the thigh apo[a] is absent, it is
present in large quantities in aorto-coronary vein grafts
removed at reoperation. The manner in which various plasma
lipids interact with the injured saphenous vein requires
further study.

REFERENCES
1. Lawrie GM, Lie JT, Morris GC, Jr, Beazley HL (1976)
   Vein graft patency and intimal proliferation after
   aorto-coronary bypass: Early and long-term angiopathologic correlations. Am J Cardiol 38:856-862
2. Lawrie, GM, Morris, GC, Jr, Chapman DW, Winters, WL,
   Lie JT (1977) Patterns of patency of 596 vein grafts
   up to seven years after aorto-coronary bypass. J
   Thoracic Cardiovasc Surg 73:433-448.
3. Lawrie GM, Morris GC, Jr., Howell JF, Ogura JW
   Spencer WH, Cashion WR, Winters WL, Beazley HL,
   Chapman DW, Peterson PK, Lie JT (1977) Results of
   coronary bypass more than five years after operation
   in 434 patients: Clinical, treadmill exercise and
   angiographic correlations. Am J Cardiol 40: 665-671
4. Roth JA, Cukingnan RA, Brown BG, Gocka E, Carey JS
   (1979) Factors influencing patency of saphenous
   vein grafts. Ann Thoracic Surg 28:176-183
5. Bourassa MG, Lesperance J, Campeau L, Simard P (1972)
   Factors influencing patency of aortocoronary vein
   grafts. Circulation Suppl 45, 46 I 79
6. Mautner RK, Giles TD (1980) Coronary artery spasm:
   A possible cause of graft occlusion in a patient with

fixed obstructive coronary artery disease. Arch
Int Med 140:979-980

7. Baduini G, Marra S, Angelino PF (1981) Sudden occlusion of a saphenous vein bypass graft relieved by
direct injection of nitroglycerine. Catheterization
and Cardiovascular Diagnosis. 7:87-95

8. Lie JT, Lawrie GM, Morris GC, Jr (1977) Aortocoronary
bypass saphenous vein graft atherosclerosis: Anatomic
study of 99 vein grafts from normal and hyperlipoproteinemic patients up to 75 months post-operatively.
Am J Cardiol 40:906-914

9. Lawrie GM, Morris GC Jr, Baron A, Glaeser DH (1985)
Clinical determinants of long-term graft patency:
Analysis of 1174 grafts up to 13 years after operation.
J Cardiovasc Surg 26:21 (abstract)

10. Lawrie GM, Morris GC Jr, Thomas S, Glaeser D (1986)
Influence of cholesterol on late graft patency in 322
patients followed up to 14 years after coronary bypass.
JACC 7:142A (abstract)

11. Lawrie GM, Morris GC Jr, Weilbaecher DW, Titus JL,
DeBakey ME (1986) Long-term influence of lipid levels
on vein bypass graft patency. Circulation 74(2)
(abstract)

12. Campeau L, Enjalbert M, Lesperance M, Bourassa MG,
Kwiterovich PJ, Wacholder S, Sniderman A (1984)
The relation of risk factors to the development of
atherosclerosis in saphenous vein bypass grafts and
the progression of disease in the native circulation.
N Engl J Med 311: 1329-1332

13. Lytle BW, Loop FD, Cosgrove DM, Ratliff NB, Easley K,
Taylor PC (1985) Long-term (5-12 years) serial studies of internal mammary artery and saphenous vein
coronary bypass grafts. J Thorac Cardiovasc Surg
89:248-258

14. Campeau L (1979) Post-operative coronary argiography.
A generation of coronary arteriography, An Interna-
tional Symposium, Cleveland Clinic Foundation,
Cleveland, pp 133-137

15. Campeau L, Enjalbert M, Lesperance J, Vaislic C,
Grondin CM, Bourassa MG (1983) Atherosclerosis and
late closure of aortocoronary saphenous vein grafts:
Sequential angiographic studies at 2 weeks, 1 year,
5 to 7 years, and 10 to 12 years after surgery.
Circulation 68 (supple. 2) 1-7

16. Gaubatz JW,Chari MV, Nava ML, Guyton JR, Morrisett JD
(1987) Isolation and characterization of the two
major apoproteins in human lipoprotein [a]. J Lipid
Res 28:69-79

17. Gaubatz JW, Cushing GL, Morrisett JD (1986) Quantitation, isolation, and characterization of human lipoprotein [a]. Meth Enz 129: 167

18. Habib JB, Bossaller C, Wells S, Williams C, Morrisett
JD, Henry PD (1986) Preservation of endothelium
dependent vascular relaxation in cholesterol fed rabbit by treatment with the calcium blocker PN 200110.
Circ Res 58: 305-309

19. Gaubatz JW, Nava ML, Delavari W, Burdick BJ, Morrisett JD (1986) An enzyme-linked immunoassay for quantitation of apolipoprotein [a].
20. Gaubatz W, Heideman C, Gotto AM, Morriset JD, Dahlen GH (1983) Human plasma lipoprotein [a]: Structural properties. J Biol Chem 258:4582-4589.
21. Cushing GL, Gaubatz JW, Nava ML, Burdick BJ, Bocan TC, Guyton JR, Lawrie GM, Morrisett JD (1986) Localization and quantitation of human apoproteins [a] and B in coronary artery bypass vein grafts resected at reoperation.

41

Atherosclerosis of Saphenous Vein Coronary Artery Bypass Grafts in Relation to Risk Factors

Lucien Campeau, Parise Nadeau, and B. Charles Solymoss

INTRODUCTION

Atherosclerosis of saphenous vein coronary artery bypass grafts is now recognized as a frequent complication (1-7). It is rarely observed during the first postoperative years (1,8,9), but its prevalence increases progressively thereafter. The angiographic diagnosis of these atherosclerotic lesions is based primarily on their late development after the first postoperative year (2,3). The atherosclerotic nature of these lesions has been confirmed on pathology examination by the presence of foam cells and lipid deposits, as well as by classic macroscopic aspects (1,7,10-17).

The following risk factors for coronary artery disease are now universally accepted: family history of premature disease, abnormal lipid plasma levels, smoking, hypertension and diabetes (18-24). Few studies have examined the potential relationship between these factors and late saphenous vein graft atherosclerosis detected either at angiography or on pathology examination.

This report describes our experience based on both postoperative control angiography and pathology studies during the past 15 years. Both studies show a positive relationship between saphenous vein graft atherosclerosis and abnormal plasma lipid levels, but not with the other risk factors.

Methods Common to Both the Angiography and Pathology
Studies

A family history was considered when the father, mother,
brothers or sisters had before age 65 clinical manifestation
of atherosclerosis, identified as coronary, cerebral or
peripheral vascular disease.

Diabetes was recognized in patients receiving active
treatment, or who had fasting serum sugar levels above
120 mg/dL. Hypertension was defined as a systolic pressure
above 150/90, or with lower values in patients receiving
antihypertensive therapy. Smoking included cigarettes,
cigars and pipes.

Serum total cholesterol, triglycerides, HDL-cholesterol
and LDL-cholesterol were determined in our laboratory. Apo B
lipoprotein concentration was assayed at the Royal Victoria
Hospital in Montreal (25) by radial immuno-diffusion (26).
This lipoprotein was determined systematically only in
patients who were included in the prospective angiographic
study. Serum triglycerides and total cholesterol were
measured by enzymatic methods (27,28). HDL-cholesterol was
quantified by dextran sulfate-magnesium precipitation (29).
LDL-cholesterol was calculated as follows: LDL − Total
Cholesterol − (HDL + $\frac{triglycerides}{5}$) whenever the triglyceride
level was below 400 mg/dL.

After surgery, cessation of smoking and an antiathero-
genic diet were recommended. Since the majority were
referred patients and reexamined in our outpatient clinic
at 1 to 3 year intervals only, lipid lowering drugs were
seldom prescribed, and none were receiving these drugs during
the three months preceding the plasma lipid assays. Oral
anticoagulant and platelet-active drugs were rarely given
beyond the first six months after surgery.

Risk factors were assessed before the latest angiographic
examination or reoperation. An average of two to three
measurements was documented in most instances. Values were
expressed as means with $\pm$ 1 standard deviation. Differences
in mean values between groups were tested by t-tests.

Methods and Results of the Angiography Study

It was based on control angiographic examinations obtained 10 to 12 years after bypass surgery in 82 patients selected from a total of 148 subjects who had shown at least one graft still patent at a previous control study carried out near one year following surgery, and who were not reoperated during that interim. Of the initial 148 potential subjects, 66 were not reexamined (45%) for a variety of reasons: age greater than 75, lived too far from center, congestive heart failure or other associated diaease, and finally refusal either by the patient or referring physician. The study group thus consisted of 68 men and 14 women whose mean age at their last angiographic examination was 58 $\pm$ 16. These 82 patients did not differ from those who were not studied with respect to age (58 $\pm$ 16 versus 61 $\pm$ 17), and presence of effort angina 10 to 12 years after surgery (46% versus 41%).

Changes in the walls of patent grafts developing after the first postoperative year were attributed to atherosclerosis (Figure 1). In fact, the atherosclerotic nature of these lesions was confirmed in all 24 grafts of 18 patients who were reoperated. These wall modifications had various angiographic aspects: irregularities, plaques, concentric and eccentric stenosis, spurs, cauliflower-like lesions and focal dilatation (30). Several lesions of various morphology, usually with irregular or sharp borders were commonly present in the same graft. Rarely, single narrowing having smooth contours were undistinguishable from lesions produced by hyperplasia of the intima (Figure 2). Only the late appearance (after the first operative year) favored an atherosclerotic etiology. At 10 to 12 years, these wall alterations reduced the graft lumen by at least 50% in 30 of the 43 patients and diseased grafts (70%), the mean narrowing being 62 $\pm$ 15%. When more than one graft was patent, half were involved by this process.

Late graft closure on the other hand may be caused by either hyperplasia of the intima, atherosclerosis or thrombosis, processes which may act alone or in combination.

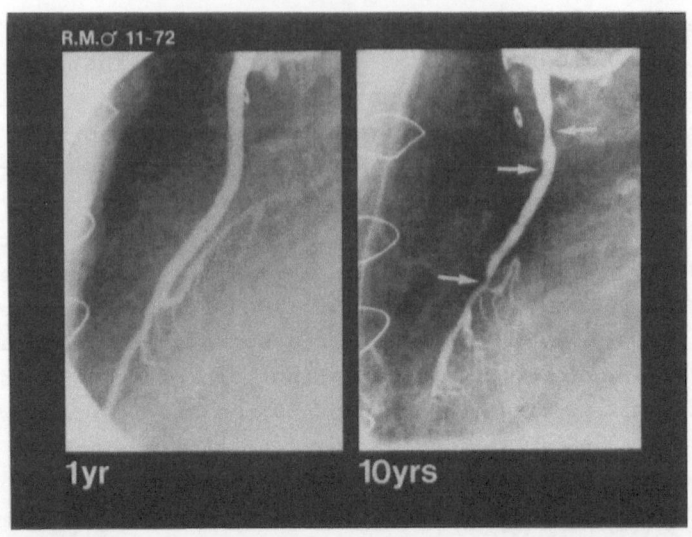

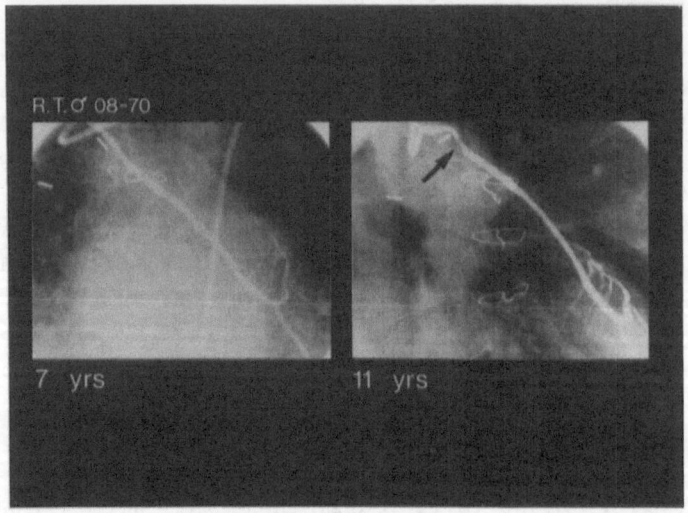

Figure 1. Postoperative cineangiograms of a saphenous vein
coronary bypass graft to the left anterior descending artery.
The appearance is normal one year after implantation. It has
developed several wall irregularities and stenoses at 10 years.
Figure 2. Postoperative cineangiograms of a saphenous vein
coronary bypass graft to the left anterior descending artery.
Normal appearance at 7 years. Development of a single concentric stenosis with smooth contours simulating focal hyperplasia of the intima.

Although atherosclerosis with or without thrombosis frequently causes late occlusion, it was considered as a manifestation
of the disease only in a few instances, namely with late wall
changes had been observed on a previous control angiogram
(Figure 3). Patients were thus divided in three groups:

Group 1: patients having unchanged grafts. No patent
graft showing late wall changes compatible with atherosclerosis, nor total occlusion.

Group 2: patients having at least one patent graft with
wall changes attributed to atherosclerosis, with or without
other closed grafts.

Group 3: patients having at least one totally occluded
graft, without patent atherosclerotic grafts.

As shown in Table 1, no significant differences were
observed with respect to the major risk factors other than
serum lipids. There were significant differences in LDL-
cholesterol, HDL-cholesterol and apo B lipoprotein (Table 2).
Total cholesterol and triglycerides were higher in group 2,
but the differences did not reach statistical significance.

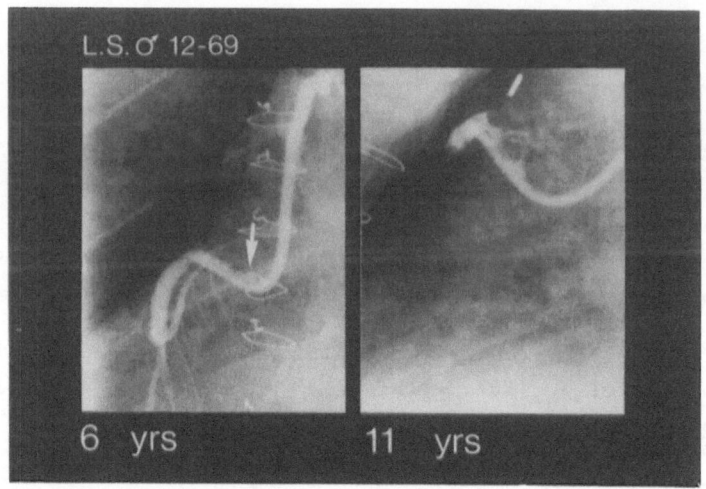

Figure 3. Postoperative cineangiograms of a saphenous vein
coronary bypass graft to the left anterior descending artery.
"Cauliflower like" atheromatous lesion present at 6 years.
Total occlusion observed 11 years after surgery.

Table 1. Prevalence of Risk Factors Other than Serum Lipids in Patients Having Unchanged Grafts (Group 1), with Atherosclerotic Grafts (Group 2), and with Occluded Grafts (Group 3)

	Group 1	Group 2	Group 3
Number of Patients	26	39	17
Age	57 ± 16	59 ± 16	57 ± 12
Sex M/F	21/5	35/4	12/5
Hypertension	3 (11%)	6 (15%)	2 (12%)
Diabetes	1 (4%)	2 (5%)	1 (6%)
Never Smoked	8 (31%)	12 (31%)	2 (12%)
Stopped Smoking	9 (35%)	12 (31%)	6 (35%)
Still Smoking	9 (35%)	15 (39%)	9 (53%)

Table 2. Serum Lipids and Lipoproteins 10-12 Years After Surgery (mg/dL; mean $\pm$ SD)

	Group 1		Group 2		Group 3	
Number of Patients	26		39		17	
Total Cholesterol	244	± 37	280	± 57	270	± 53
Triglycerides	157	± 58	208	± 125	200	± 92
LDL-Cholesterol	163	$\pm 37*$	206	$\pm 52*$	170	± 44
LDL-Apoprotein B	108	$\pm 15**$	162	$\pm 28**$	149	± 19
HDL-Cholesterol	60	$\pm 19*$	47	$\pm 12*$	48	± 13
$\frac{\text{LDL-Cholesterol}}{\text{HDL-Cholesterol}}$	2.9 ± 0.1		4.8 ± 0.2		4.1 ± 0.15	

* p < 0.05
** p < 0.01

Methods and Results of the Pathology Study

Saphenous vein grafts resected at the time of reoperation for coronary bypass surgery are the basis of these observations. In most cases, the entire graft except for the segments adjacent to the anastomoses was available for macroscopic and histologic examinations. Transverse cuts were obtained at 0.5 cm intervals. The diagnosis of atherosclerosis was based on the presence of lipid-laden foam cells in the tunica intima. Of grafts presenting with the above histologic findings, 67% also showed irreversible complicated lesions such as cholesterol clefts, necrosis, and calcifications.

There were 211 grafts removed from 176 patients, of whom 152 were men (82%) and 24 women (14%). Their mean age at the initial intervention was 48.4 ± 7 years.

The interval between operations varied between 1 day and 15 years, with a mean of 7.3 ± 3.5 years. The patient distribution and the prevalence of atherosclerosis during various intervals are detailed in Table 3.

Of the 176 patients, 107 had atherosclerotic grafts (61%). Only 11 patients had more than one graft removed, and all their grafts showed atherosclerosis. The prevalence of atherosclerotic grafts was related to the length of the time interval between the two operations (Table 3).

No significant differences were observed with respect to major coronary risk factors other than serum lipid levels between patients with and those without atherosclerotic grafts (Table 4). Total serum cholesterol, LDL-cholesterol and the LDL-cholesterol/HDL-cholesterol ratio were significantly higher in patients with atherosclerotic grafts (Table 5). Triglycerides and HDL-cholesterol levels however were similar in both groups.

DISCUSSION

Atherosclerosis of Vein Grafts at Pathology

Although atherosclerosis practically never occurs in veins left in their normal location, it develops frequently when placed in the arterial circulation. *In vitro*, canine

Table 3. Proportion of Patients Having Atherosclerotic
          Grafts Related to the Time Interval Between the
          Initial Bypass Surgery and the Reoperation

	Patients Studied	Atherosclerotic Grafts	
		Absent (%)	Present (%)
Time Interval (yr)			
<1	15	15 (100%)	0 (0%)
1 to 3	9	8 (89%)	1 (11%)
4 to 6	27	9 (33%)	18 (67%)
7 to 10	82	23 (28%)	59 (72%)
11 to 15	43	14 (33%)	29 (67%)
All Patients	176	69 (39%)	107 (61%)

Table 4. Graft Atherosclerosis in 176 Reoperated Patients
          Related to Major Risk Factors (other than serum
          lipids)

	Without Atherosclerotic Grafts	With Atherosclerotic Grafts
Number of Patients	71	105
Age at Initial Operation (yrs)	49 $\pm$ 8	48 $\pm$ 7
Sex (M/F)	5.5	7
Family History (%)	63	68
Diabetes (%)	14	12
Hypertension (%)	25	28
Smoking After Grafting (%)	48	59

Table 5. Graft Atherosclerosis in 176 Reoperated Patients
Related to Levels of Serum Lipids and Lipoproteins (mg/dL; mean $\pm$ SD)

	Without Atherosclerotic Grafts		With Atherosclerotic Grafts	
Number of Patients	71		105	
Total Cholesterol	246	$\pm$ 42	267	$\pm$ 49*
Triglycerides	234	$\pm$ 101	250	$\pm$ 125
HDL-Cholesterol	38	$\pm$ 9	39	$\pm$ 10
LDL-Cholesterol	160	$\pm$ 45	187	$\pm$ 59*
$\dfrac{\text{LDL-Cholesterol}}{\text{HDL-Cholesterol}}$	4.3 $\pm$	1.4	5.1 $\pm$	2.2**

 * p < 0.01
** p < 0.05

venous arterial grafts incorporate lipids at accelerated
rates compared with native arteries and veins (31). The propensity for atherosclerosis, particularly in hypercholesterolemic animals is greater in vein grafts as compared to native
coronary arteries (32-35).

Hyperplasia of the intima, which is considered a precursor of an initial stage of atherosclerosis (15,16,36),
develops consistently in aortocoronary bypass grafts (1-7,14,
15). This smooth muscle proliferation and increased hyaline
matrix seems part of a reparative and adaptive process in
response to wall ischemia during vein harvesting and particularly to the subsequent abnormal hydraulic and hemodynamic
conditions of an arterial circulation, for which the vein
structure is not suited. Diffuse thickening of the intima
develops at variable degrees in all aortocoronary bypass vein
grafts during the first postoperative year, but it does not
appear to progress further in subsequent years (37,38).
However, definite evidence of atherosclerosis, as defined by
the World Health Organization (39), is observed mostly in
grafts that have been in place for more than three years.

The first descriptions of graft atherosclerosis were reported
by Brynjolesson, Barboriak et al., and Kern et al. in 1972
(12-14).

Studies using special staining techniques have demonstrated lipid droplets and lipid laden cells as early as
the first operative year. Kern et al. (14) described few
small lipid droplets in a plaque-like intimal thickness of
a graft that had been inserted two months earlier.

Bulkley and Hutchins (15) reported cases of "accelerated"
atherosclerosis where lipid laden macrophages were observed
in one of the four grafts in place for 15 to 30 days that had
circumferencial intimal fibrous plaques. Another graft in
place for 29 months "contained collections of lipid filled
macrophages within the thickened fibrotic intima resembling
early arterial atheromatous plaques". Unni and associates
(16) mention that "special stains reveal only small amounts
of lipid, but none of the 15 grafts in place from one to 19
months showed typical atherosclerotic lesions".

In the pathology study of Lie et al., atherosclerosis
was not observed in 59 grafts in place for less than 13
months. We had not detected this disease in 13 grafts
implanted for less than 24 months, but it was present in 8
of the 19 grafts in place from 2 to 8 years (8). Other
workers have not detected atherosclerosis in grafts in place
for less than 3½ years (9). The proportion of grafts with
atherosclerosis on pathology examination in selected patients
who have died or have been reoperated varies from 17% to 70%,
depending on the time interval after bypass surgery. Klimà
et al. (17) described classic atherosclerotic lesions in 17%
of the 168 grafts removed from 143 patients at reoperation
or after death; three to 84 months after the initial surgery
(mean 48.7 months). Atkinson and associates (6) found
atherosclerotic lesions in 21% of 117 saphenous vein grafts
in place 12 to 168 months prior to death in 56 patients
(mean 62.7 months).

Lie and associates (1) observed "classic atherosclerotic"
lesions in 14 of 40 grafts (35%) at autopsy 13 to 75 months
after implantation. Finally Neitzel and colleagues (7)
reported complex atheromata often associated with thrombosis

in 71% of the 50 grafts removed from 42 patients who underwent revascularization procedure or came to autopsy 6 to 12
years after surgery. In our experience, as detailed in
Table 3, the incidence of graft atherosclerosis was also
related to the time interval after surgery.

Atherosclerosis of Vein Grafts at Angiography

The diagnosis of graft atherosclerosis at angiography
is much less reliable than when based on pathology examination. There are at least three potential sources of error.
Firstly, "normally appearing" grafts, i.e., without late
change after the first postoperative years may have atherosclerosis visible only on histologic study, or produce minor
lesions undetected at angiography. Marshall et al. (11)
reported minimal to severe atherosclerosis in all five grafts
that had a "normal" angiographic appearance before elective
removal 6 to 13 years after the initial grafting in patients
in whom other replaced grafts had shown changes attributed
to atherosclerosis. Another problem is the unknown status
of completely obstructed grafts, which frequently, but not
always have atherosclerosis. Lytle and associates (4) found
atherosclerosis in 9 of 15 grafts (60%) that became completely
occluded at a later angiographic examination performed at a
mean interval of 88 months. In the study of Atkinson et al.
(6) at a mean interval of 63 months after surgery, 10 of the
36 totally occluded grafts had atherosclerotic lesions and
recent thrombus (28%). Loop and colleagues (10) reported
that 80 of the 171 atherosclerotic grafts removed at reoperation at a mean interval of 85 months after surgery were
totally occluded (47%), and thus were not detected at angiography. Thirdly, new narrowings and wall irregularities may
be caused by clots, and less likely by progressive intimal
hyperplasia [as suggested by Guthaner et al. (41)].

In spite of these limitations, we feel that studies
based on angiographic findings remain contributory. The
atherosclerotic nature of late wall changes in patent grafts
has been constantly confirmed on pathology examination.
Palac et al. (2), had confirmation in all 7 grafts that were

examined at pathology. In Marshall and associates study (11), all 11 grafts excised at reoperation and studied at pathology more than 6 years after surgery had classic atherosclerotic lesions which had been grossly under-estimated in 8 on the pre-operative angiograms. Loop et al. (10) had pathology confirmation of atherosclerosis in 91 grafts that had shown wall changes on angiograms performed at a mean interval of 98 months after implantation.

The prevalence of wall changes attributed to athero-sclerosis has been variously reported between 2% and 34% of patent grafts depending on definitions, patient selection, and time interval after bypass surgery. Barner et al. (42) at control reexamination 49 to 105 months (mean 64) reported no new narrowing reducing the lumen by 50% or more in 100 grafts patent at one year. The incidence of less severe lesions is not mentioned. Kouchoukos and associates (43) in control studies at about one year and between 13 to 61 months after the operation (mean 42) reported only two late stenosis in 116 grafts (1.7%). The lack of definition of graft change in their late study except for "stenoses", suggest that only narrowings of 50% or more were considered, a cut-off measure used in their initial study. Seides et al. (44) who studied 22 of 30 consecutive patients with at least one graft patent 3 to 9 months after surgery found minor luminal irregularities in only 2 of the initially 33 patent grafts (6%) at 53 to 84 months after implantation (mean 66).

In a study of 26 unselected patients (from a group of 41 patients who had minimal symptoms and patent grafts at one year) Guthaner et al. (41) found on repeat angiograms near 6 years after operation (65 to 103 months; mean 76) new lesions which they attributed to intimal hyperplasia in 10 of the 39 grafts (26%). We suggest that these changes were caused rather by atherosclerosis as suggested by their late development and appearance.

Palac and associates (2) in repeat angiographic studies performed at 13 ± 5 months and 61 ± 13 months after surgery described progressive narrowing attributed to atherosclerosis in 21 of 61 grafts (34%) and in 15 of these 34 unselected patients (44%).

In our center (45), late changes attributed to athero-sclerosis were observed in 14 of 98 grafts (14%) and 23 of 107 unselected patients (21%) between 5 and 7 years after surgery. Forty-three of 132 grafts (32.5%) in 39 of 82 unselected patients (48%) had developed such late changes by 10 to 12 years (3).

Lytle and colleagues (4) discovered that among a group of 501 patients who had normal grafts at control study near 15 months post-operatively new stenoses or irregularities had developed in 18% of the grafts at 60 to 147 months (mean 88).

Fitzgibbon et al. (5) evaluated within one month, at one year and near five years post-operatively 1179 vein grafts in 353 unselected males having a mean age of 45.5 years at the time of surgery. They found that wall irregularities compatible with atherosclerosis had developed in 33% of the 868 grafts studied between 1 and 5 years.

Atherosclerosis of Vein Grafts and Plasma Lipids

It is reasonable to expect that graft atherosclerosis is related to risk factors for coronary artery disease, family history, cigarette smoking, diabetes, hypertension and hyper-lipidemia. Nevertheless, hyperlipidemia is thus far the only risk factor shown in most studies to be associated with graft atherosclerosis.

Rossiter et al. (46) reported lipid infiltration, abundant foam cells and focal atheroma of both the media and intima in 7 of the 12 grafts from mongel dogs fed on a hyperlipidemic diet (58%), in contrast with absence of atherosclerosis in grafts of animals given a regular canine diet. Vein grafts of both groups showed variable degrees of intimal thickening where atheroma were mostly concentrated. Other workers have also observed atherosclerosis in arterial vein grafts of hypercholesterolemic animals (32-35).

Several authors have found that atherosclerosis of saphenous vein coronary bypass grafts in humans is frequently associated with hyperlipidemia. Lie et al. (1) described evidence of this disease in 11 of the 14 grafts implanted longer than 12 months in hyperlipidemic patients (78%) as compared to only 3 of the 26 grafts from patients whose lipid

levels were normal (11.5%). Among the 14 hyperlipidemic
patients, 4 had type II, 8 had type IV and 1 each had
type III and type V phenotypes. The patients of both groups
were fairly well matched with respect to age, sex, cigarette
smoking and none had clinically documented hypertension or
diabetes.

Barboriak et al. (13) reported two cases where pathology
study carried out 37 and 59 months after surgery had shown
graft atherosclerosis and in whom plasma triglyceride level
was elevated.

Palac et al. (2) compared 15 patients who had angiographic
evidence of graft atherosclerosis with 19 who did not. There
were no significant differences with respect to age, evidence
of hypertension, diabetes or cigarette smoking. Plasma levels
of both triglycerides and total cholesterol were significantly
higher in patients with late graft changes.

Atkinson et al. (6) in a pathology study carried out at
a mean of 62.7 months after surgery in 44 patients who had
accurate documentation of cardiovascular risk factors, found
that patients having atherosclerotic grafts had a significantly higher mean total plasma cholesterol as compared to
those without. Although some degree of fibro-intimal proliferation was found in all atherosclerotic grafts, it did
not reduce the luminal cross-sectional area by more than 25%.
Systemic hypertension was higher in patients with moderate to
severe hyperplasia of the intima (lumen reduction $\geq$ 25%).
Systemic hypertension was more prevalent in patients with
moderate to severe hyperplasia of the intima but not with
atherosclerosis. This discordant relationship is puzzling
since intimal hyperplasia appears to the initial phase of
this degenerative disease. Patients with atherosclerotic grafts
had a higher fasting serum glucose level but the differences
were not statistically significant (163 $\pm$ 38 mg/dL vs 127 $\pm$ 10).
Family history of premature coronary heart disease and smoking
were unrelated to graft atherosclerosis in this study.

Lytle and associates (4) studied the course of vein
grafts that were patent and free of stenosis between 1 and
59 months after surgery (mean 15) and were reexamined between

60 to 147 months (mean 88), they found that 169 of the 645 grafts were occluded (26%) and 119 showed changes compatible with atherosclerosis (19%). A multivariate analysis chose as predictors of occlusion or new stenosis, hypercholesterolemia and hypertriglyceridemia among other variables. The incidence of progression between the two angiographic studies was significantly higher ($p < 0.001$) in the 43 patients having both hypercholesterolemia and hypertriglyceridemia as compared to patients without these plasma lipid abnormalities. Of the six patients who had combined diabetes and elevation of plasma levels of both total cholesterol and triglycerides, 7 of their 9 grafts patent at the early examination showed progression (78%).

Neitzel and associates (7) in a study of 42 patients who underwent a second revascularization or came to autopsy 6 to 12 years after coronary bypass surgery, reported complex atheromata often associated with an acute thrombus in 71% of the grafts. Significantly higher triglyceride and cholesterol levels and lower high density lipoprotein levels were noted in patients undergoing two bypass procedures, in most instances because of graft atherosclerosis. A significantly higher proportion of cigarette smokers and diabetics were also noted in this group. Hypertension did not appear to be a significant risk factor.

In our pathology study, stepwise logistic regression analysis, total cholesterol was chosen as best discriminator for graft atherosclerosis (47). The second choice was the age of the graft. Smoking was the best discriminator for graft thrombosis.

On the other hand, Smith et al. (9), in a pathology study, found no correlation between hyperlipemia and graft atherosclerosis. In an angiographic study, Lawrie and associates (48) reported similar plasma levels of cholesterol in normal grafts and in stenotic or occluded grafts. The interval after surgery however extended from one to 178 months, and no distinctions were made between early and late lesions, nor between partial and total obstruction, so that the study does not concern specifically atherosclerotic changes, which in our view can be identified at angiography only by their late appearance and in grafts that are still patent.

In an earlier angiographic study in patients about six years after surgery, we found no correlation between vein graft atherosclerosis and serum lipid levels (49). The low incidence of these late changes found in only 21% of patients at that relatively short interval after the operation may explain this discrepancy. At 10 to 12 years (3), 48% of the 82 patients had developed graft atherosclerosis, and these were found to have significantly higher plasma lipids (Table 2). New lesions developed in the grafts or the native vessels in 67 patients, but not in the remaining 15 (25). Serum levels of very-low-density lipoproteins (VLDL) and low-density lipoproteins (LDL) were higher, and high-density lipo-protein (HDL) levels were lower in those with new disease than in those without. Univariate analysis showed that plasma total choelsterol and triglyceride levels were significantly higher at the time of surgery and at the 10 to 12 year examination in those with new lesions. Multivariate analysis indicated that among the lipoprotein indexes, levels of HDL cholesterol and plasma LDL apoprotein B best distinguished the two groups. Twelve of the 15 patients without graft athero-sclerosis nor progression of the disease in their nonbypassed coronary arteries had normal plasma lipid and normal plasma LDL apoprotein B levels in contrast with only 5 of the 67 patients with new lesions.

Thus our two studies, based on the one hand on angio-graphic examination, and on the other hand on pathology find-ings, both show positive correlations between vein graft atherosclerosis and serum levels of LDL-cholesterol. Higher serum triglyceride and lower HDL-cholesterol levels are associated with graft atherosclerosis only in the angiography study, a discrepancy that remains unexplained. The higher triglyceride and lower HDL levels in the pathology study may reflect a more advanced disease in these patients who needed reoperation, as opposed to the patients of the angiography study who were unselected.

SUMMARY

Atherosclerosis develops in one-third to half of saphenous vein coronary artery bypass grafts between one and 10 years after surgery. Our findings, based on both control angiographic examination in 82 unselected patients and pathology study of grafts removed at reoperation in 176 subjects, show positive correlations between atherosclerosis of vein grafts and abnormally high serum level of LDL cholesterol. Other risk factors for coronary artery disease have not yet been shown to play a significant role, although few studies have shown an association with cigarette smoking and diabetes.

REFERENCES

1. Lie JT, Lawrie GM, Morris GC Jr (1977) Aortocoronary bypass saphenous vein graft atherosclerosis. Anatomic study of 99 vein grafts from normal and hyperlipoproteinemic patients up to 75 months postoperatively. Am J Cardiol 40:906-914.
2. Palac RT, Meadows WR, Hwang MH, Loeb HS, Pifarre R, Gunnar RM (1982) Risk factors related to progressive narrowing in aortocoronary vein grafts studied 1 and 5 years after surgery. Circulation 66 (Suppl I):I-40-I-44.
3. Campeau L, Enjalberg M, Lesperance J, Vaislic C, Grondin CM, Bourassa MG (1983) Atherosclerosis and late closure of aortocoronary saphenous vein grafts: Sequential angiographic studies at 2 weeks, 1 year, 5 to 7 years, and 10 to 12 years after surgery. Circulation 68 (Suppl II): II-1-II-7.
4. Lytle BW, Loop FD, Cosgrove DM, Ratliff NB, Easley K, Taylor PC (1985) Long-term (5 to 12 years) serial studies of internal mammary artery and saphenous vein coronary bypass grafts. J Thorac Cardiovasc Surg 89: 248-258.
5. Fitzgibbon GM, Leach AJ, Keon WJ, Burton JR, Kafka HP (1986) Coronary bypass fate. Angiographic study of 1,179 vein grafts early, one year, and five years after operation. J Thorac Cardiovasc Surg 91:773-778.
6. Atkinson JB, Forman MB, Vaughn WK, Robinovitz, M, McAllister HA, Virmani R (1985) Morphologic changes in long-term saphenous vein bypass grafts. Chest 88:341-348.
7. Neitzel GF, Barboriak JJ, Pintar K, Qureshi I (1986) Atherosclerosis in aortocoronary bypass grafts. Morphologic study and risk factor analysis 6 to 12 years after surgery. Arteriosclerosis 6:594-600.
8. Solymoss BC, Campeau L, Grondin CM (1979) Morphologic alterations in aortocoronary vein grafts in place for up to eight years. Exc Med Amsterdam Intern Congress Series 491:889.

9.   Smith SH, Geer JC (1981) Morphology of saphenous vein-
     coronary artery bypass grafts 7 months to 8 years post-
     operatively. Circulation 64 (Suppl IV):IV-90 (abstract).
10. Loop FD, Lytle BW, Gill CC, Golding LAR, Cosgrove DM,
     Taylor PC (1983) Trends in selection and results of
     coronary artery reoperations. Ann Thorac Surg 36:
     380-388.
11. Marshall WG Jr, Saffitz J, Kouchoukos NT (1986)
     Management during reoperation of aortocoronary saphenous
     vein grafts with minimal atherosclerosis by angiography.
     Ann Thorac Surg 42:163-167.
12. Brynjolfsson G (1972) Pathologic changes in venous
     coronary bypasses. Proc Inst Med Chic 29:79-80 (abstract).
13. Barboriak JJ, Batayias GE, Pintar K, Tieu TM, Van Horn DL,
     Korns ME (1972) Late lesions in aorta-coronary artery
     vein grafts. J Thorac Cardiovasc Surg 64:596-601.
14. Kern WH, Dermer GB, Lindensmith GG (1972) The intimal
     proliferation in aortic-coronary saphenous vein grafts.
     Am Heart J 84:771-777.
15. Bulkley BH, Hutchins GM (1977) Accelerated "atherosclero-
     sis". A morphologic study of 97 saphenous vein coronary
     artery bypass grafts. Circulation 55:163-169.
16. Unni KK, Kottke BA, Titus JL, Frye RL, Wallace RB, Brown
     AL (1974) Pathologic changes in aortocoronary saphenous
     vein grafts. Am J Cardiol 34:526-532.
17. Klima T, Beard EF, Milan JD, Reul CJ Jr, Cooley DA (1979)
     Atherosclerosis of aortocoronary artery saphenous vein
     bypass grafts. Cardiovascular Diseases, Bulletin of
     the Texas Heart Institute 6:318-323.
18. Doyle JT (1972) Cigarette smoking and coronary athero-
     sclerosis. In: Likoff W, Segal BL, Insull W (eds)
     Atherosclerosis and Coronary Heart Disease. New York:
     Grune and Stratton, p. 35.
19. Epstein FH (1967) Hyperglycermia, a risk factor in
     coronary heart disease. Circulation 36:609.
20. Freis ED (1969) Hypertension and atherosclerosis.
     Am J Med 46:735.
21. Epstein FH (1969) Hereditary aspects of coronary heart
     disease. Am J Med 46:735.
22. Kannel WB, Castelli WP, Gordon T, McNamara PM (1971)
     Serum cholesterol, lipoproteins, and the risk of
     coronary heart disease. The Framingham Study. Ann
     Intern Med 74:1.
23. Gordon T, Castelli WP. Hjortland MC et al. (1977) High
     density lipoprotein as a protective factor against
     coronary heart disease. The Framingham Study. Am J
     Med 62:707.
24. Roberts WC, Ferrans VJ, Levy RI, Fredrickson DS (1973)
     Cardiovascular pathology in hyperlipoproteinemia.
     Anatomic observations in 42 necropsy patients with
     normal or abnormal serum lipoprotein patterns. Am J
     Cardiol 31:557.
25. Campeau L, Enjalbert M, Lesperance J, Bourassa MG,
     Kwiterovich P, Wacholer S, Sniderman A (1984) The
     relation of factors to the development of atherosclerosis
     in saphenous vein bypass grafts and the progression of
     disease in the native circulation. N Engl J Med 311:
     1329-1332.

26. Sniderman A, Teng B, Jerry M (1975) Determination of B protein of low density lipoprotein directly in plasma. J Lipid Res 16:465-467.
27. Siedel J, Schlumberger H, Klose S, Ziegenhorn J, Wahlefeld AW (1981) Improved reagent for the enzymatic determination of serum cholesterol. J Clin Chem Clin Biochem 19:838.
28. Sampson EJ, Demers LM, Krein AF (1975) Faster enzymatic procedure for serum triglycerides. Clin Chem 21:1983-1985.
29. Warnick GR, Benderson J, Albers JJ, Baillie EE, Sexton B, Schaefer EJ, Carlson D, Hill M, Brewer HB, Wiebe DA, Hazlehurst J, Cooper GR (1982) Dextran Sulfate-Mg^{2+} precipitation for quantitation of high-density-lipoprotein cholesterol. Clin Chem 28:1379-1388.
30. Enjalbert M, Campeau L, Lesperance J, Grondin CM, Bourassa MG (1984) Angiographic features of saphenous vein aortocoronary bypass graft atherosclerosis. J Am Coll Cardiol 3:529 (abstract).
31. Larson RM, Hagen PO, Fuchs JCA (1974) Lipid bio-synthesis in arteries, veins and venous grafts. Circulation 50 (Suppl 3):529 (abstract).
32. Sako Y (1961) Susceptibility of autologous vein grafts to atheromatous degeneration. Surg Forum 12:247-249.
33. Friedman M (1963) Spontaneous atherosclerosis and exerpimental thrombo-atherosclerosis Arch Pathol 76:571-577.
34. Scott HW Jr, Morgan CV, Bolasny BL, Lanier VC, Younger RK, Butts W (1970) Experimental atherosclerosis in auto-genous venous grafts. Arch Surg 101:677-682.
35. King P, Boyle JP (1972) Autogenous vein grafting in atheromatous rabbits. Cardiovasc Res 6:627-633.
36. Ross R, Giomset JA (1973) Atherosclerosis and the arterial smooth muscle cell. Proliferation of smooth muscle cell is a key event in the genesis of the lesions of atherosclerosis. Science 180:1332.
37. Lawrie GM, Lie JT, Morris GC Jr, Beazley HL (1976) Vein graft patency and intimal proliferation after aortocoronary bypass: Early and long-term angiopathologic correlations. Am J Cardiol 38:856-862.
38. Lesperance J, Bourassa MG, Saltiel J, Campeau L, Grondin CM (1973) Angiographic changes in aortocoronary vein grafts. Lack of progression beyond the first year. Circulation 48:633-643.
39. World Health Organization (1958) Classification of atherosclerotic lesions: Report of a study group. Technical Report Series. Publication 143. Geneva: World Health Organization, pp. 3-20.
40. Batayias GE, Barboriak JJ, Korns ME, Pintar K (1977) The spectrum of pathologic changes in aortocoronary saphenous vein grafts. Circulation 56 (suppl II):II-18-II-25.
41. Gunthaner DF, Robert EW, Alderman EL, Wexler L (1979) Long-term serial angiographic studies after coronary artery bypass surgery. Circulation 60:250-258.
42. Barner HB, Swartz MT, Mudd JG, Tyras DH (1982) Late patency of the internal mammary artery as a coronary bypass conduit. Ann Thorac Surg 34:408-412.

43. Kouchoukos NT, Karp RB, Oberman A, Russell RO Jr, Alison HW, Holt JH (1978) Long-term patency of saphenous veins for coronary bypass grafting. Cardiovascular Surgery, 1977 Supp. to Circulation 58 (Suppl I):I-96-I-99.

44. Seides SF, Borer JS, Kent KM, Rosing DR, McIntosh CL, Epstein SE (1978) Long-term anatomic fate of coronary-artery bypass grafts and functional status of patients five years after operation. N Engl J Med 298:1213-1217.

45. Campeau L, Lesperance J, Corbara F, Hermann J, Grondin CM, Bourassa MG (1978) Aortocoronary saphenous vein bypass graft changes 5 to 7 years after surgery. Cardiovascular Surgery, 1977. Supp. to Circulation 58 (Suppl I):I-170-I-175.

46. Rossiter SJ, Brody WR, Kosek JC, Lipton MJ, Angell WW (1974) Internal mammary artery versus autogenous vein for coronary bypass graft. Circulation 50:1236-1243.

47. Solymoss BC, Nadeau P, Campeau L (1987) Factors related to atherosclerosis of saphenous vein coronary bypass grafts. J Am Coll Cardiol 9:85A.

48. Lawrie GM, Morris GC Jr, Thomas S, Glaeser D (1986) Influence of cholesterol on late graft patency in 322 patients followed up to 14 years after coronary bypass. J Am Coll Cardiol 7:142A.

49. Grondin CM, Campeau L, Lesperance J, Solymoss BC, Vouhe P, Castonguay YR, Meere C, Bourassa MG (1979) Atherosclerotic changes in coronary vein grafts six years after operation. J Thorac Cardiovasc Surg 77:25-31.

42

Femoral Lesion Change in Relation to Measured Risk Factors in the Stockholm-Uppsala Trial

Anders G. Olsson, Uno Erikson, Gunnar Helmius, Anders Hemmingsson, Ingar Holme, and Gunnar Ruhn

INTRODUCTION

Our access to highly efficient drugs against hyperlipoproteinemia (1,2) and to a high resolution femoral
angiography technique (3) prompted us to study the effect
of pronounced serum-lipid lowering on the development of
femoral atherosclerosis in hyperlipoproteinemia.

Efforts were made to adopt computer assisted image
processing (3) but as stated elsewhere reproducibility was
not sufficient with this early method due mainly to biological facts: crossing contrast filled arterial branches,
inhomogeneous contrast mixing, variable vessel diameter
between examinations, local spasm, etc. (4,5). For a
computer assisted image analysis to be successful, therefore, every effort must be made to eliminate biological
variability. One example is to syncronize the x-ray exposure
to the cardiac cycle. Also powerful enough computers must
be used allowing algorithms for crossing branches, etc.

In this report we will give the results of one
year's treatment with serum-lipid lowering by drugs on
femoral atherosclerosis development compared to dietary
treatment.

Dr. Olsson's current address is Department of Internal
Medicine, University Hospital, S-581 85 Linköping, Sweden

MATERIALS AND METHODS

Subjects

Sixty-three male patients (mean age at entry 53 years, range - 35 to 65) with fasting serum cholesterol above 9.5 mmol/L and/or triglycerides above 3.5 mmol/L were allocated into the study. All except two were asymptomatic with regard to symptoms of coronary and peripheral artery disease. Two subjects had intermittent claudication in addition to hyperlipoproteinemia. The distribution on types IIA, IIB and IV hyperlipoproteinemia (6) was 21, 18 and 24, respectively.

Design of Study

Patients were admitted to medical ward for one week at 0, 6 and 18 months, respectively, for femoral arteriography. At the first visit patients were given moderate advice regarding their living habits. At six months patients were randomly allocated to treatment group (n = 31) or control group (n = 32). Patients in the treatment group received a combination of nicotinic acid in successively increasing dosage to 1 g four times daily and fenofibrate 0.2 g twice daily. Patients in the control group received two placebo tablets twice daily identical with the fenofibrate tablets. The study, thus, had a single blind design. Serum lipo-protein concentrations were followed every second month during the course of the study.

Arteriography

Femoral arteriography was performed as described elsewhere (5). When the study was finished visual estimation was performed on all angiograms.

Three radiologists made independent scoring of athero-sclerosis on four segments of the femoral artery (upper and lower segments of superior and inferior parts, respectively): 0 = no atherosclerosis, 1 = single plaque < 50% of diameter, 2 = more than one of one, 3 = single plaque of > 50% of diameter, 4 = more than one of three and 5 = complete occlusion. Consensus evaluation was required between the radiologists.

Change of atheroma size was estimated in pairs of femoral arteriograms and in random order with regard to group. For each segment regression, progression and no change were given the values -1, +1 and 0, respectively. The sum of segment changes was divided by the number of segments scored. Change of atherosclerosis score (0-5) merited to -2 or +2 as this always indicated a big change in atheroma size.

The results will be given both on a segment basis (all segments calculated) and on patient basis (sum of scores divided by number of segments judged for each patient). As atherosclerosis as imaged on the arteriogram is a focal process involving different segments of the artery to different extents in our experience, it was felt that using only the individual as basis for observation on atheroma size and change would cause information loss.

Serum Lipoproteins

Serum lipoprotein determination was performed as described previously (7). Lipid extraction was performed using a two-phase system (Folch extraction). Cholesterol (8) and triglyceride (9) concentrations were determined on each lipoprotein fraction. The mean variation of double estimation of HDL triglycerides, the tiniest triglyceride fraction, was less than 10%.

RESULTS

Exclusions

Sixteen patients were excluded from the study, the reason being (treatment/control groups): no visible atherosclerosis (8/6), unwillingness to continue one year's treatment (1/1). One patient developed allergic symptoms to the contrast medium at the first arteriography and could therefore not be investigated. No significant differences between treatment and control groups were seen after six months on regimen with regard to age, smoking, systolic and diastolic blood pressure and serum lipoprotein concentrations.

Serum Lipoproteins

The serum lipoprotein concentration after six months of regimen and after twelve months of drug/placebo in patients completing one year of drug treatment is given in Figure 1.

After twelve months on drugs significantly lower serum lipoprotein levels were seen in the treatment group when compared to the control group in all lipoprotein lipids except LDL triglycerides and HDL cholesterol.

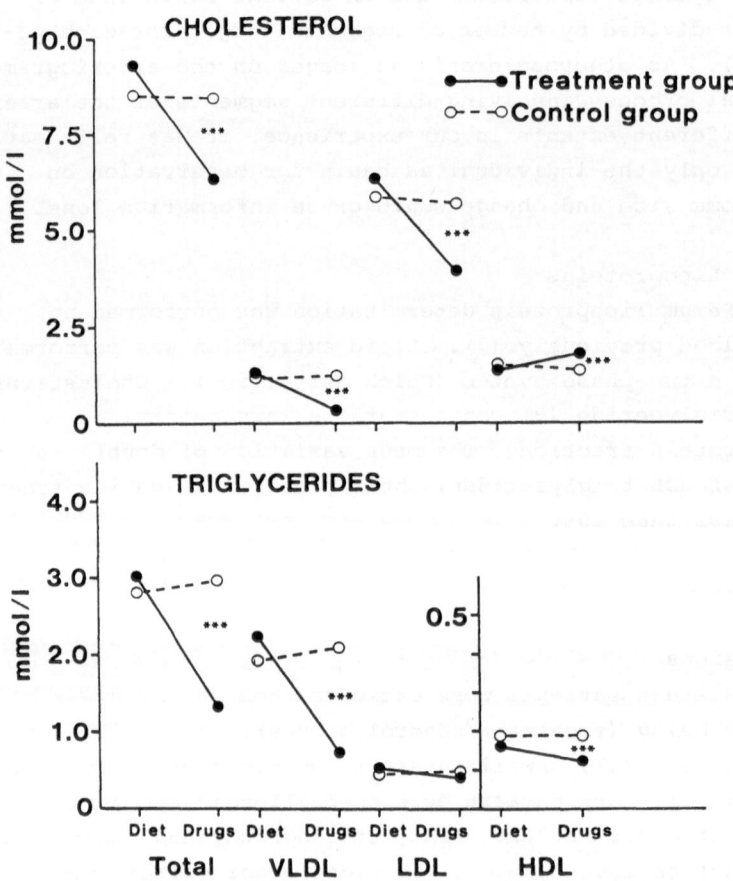

Figure 1. Mean total serum and lipoprotein cholesterol and triglyceride concentrations after six months diet (Diet) and twelve months additional drug or placebo treatment (Drugs). *** Indicates significant difference at the p < 0.001 between treatment and control groups, respectively (Wilcoxon).

Atherosclerosis at Baseline

Before drugs, 14 of the 63 patients were free from
visual atherosclerosis [i.e., 80% of hyperlipidemic middle-
aged asymptomatic men (n = 61) have the disease in that
location]. The distribution of atherosclerosis score
between treatment and control groups is given in Figure 2.
Many of the patients had only minor changes (score 1).
There was no significant difference in the atherosclerosis
distribution between control and treatment groups.

**STOCKHOLM-UPPSALA REGRESSION STUDY
VISIBLE ATHEROSCLEROSIS AT BASELINE**

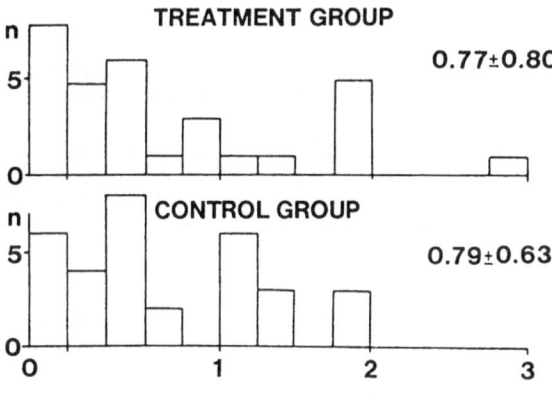

Figure 2. Distribution of atherosclerosis score with visual
estimation in treatment and control groups.

Before drugs, 193 femoral arterial segments were studied in
the 47 patients with visual atherosclerosis present.
Atherosclerosis was found in 110 segments (i.e., 57%).

The localization of the atheromatosis changes varied
between the segments studied. Table 1 shows the involvement
of the four femoral segments in all 63 patients. The more
distal the segment, the more atherosclerosis was seen.

Table 1. Atherosclerotic Involvement of Different Parts of
          the Femoral Artery in 63 Hyperlipidemic Patients

	US	LS	UI	LI
%	43	55	56	82

S = superior part
I = inferior part
U = upper segment of part
L = lower segment of part

Atherosclerosis Change

Changes in femoral atheroma were seen in 11 of the 47
patients with visual atherosclerosis. The distribution of
the subjects with regard to change on treatment and control
groups is given in Table 2.

Table 2. Number of Subjects with Regression and Progression
          in Treatment and Control Groups, Respectively

Group	Regression	Progression	All
Treatment	2	1	3
Control	1	7	8
All	3	8	11

With Fisher's exact test, Mann-Whitney test and
Student's T-test p values for one-sided tests were p = 0.15,
p = 0.15 and p = 0.09, respectively. Thus the effects on
atheroma development on atherosclerosis change was not
statistically significant in this small group of patients.

Of the 110 segments with atherosclerosis, changes were
seen in 24. The distribution of the segment changes in
treatment and control groups is given in Table III. According to x^2 the distribution was highly unlikely to be caused
by chance (p < 0.001). Treatment and control groups differed

mainly with regard to the number of segments progressing, which was largely prevented by treatment.

Table 3. Number of Segments with Regression and Progression in Treatment and Control Groups, Respectively

Group	Regression	Progression	All
Treatment	4	2	6
Control	2	16	18
All	6	18	24

x^2 $p < 0.001$

During the observation time of one year, four segments demonstrated new atheroma, all changing score from 0 to 1. Three of them belonged to the control group without lipid-lowering drug treatment; one to the treatment group. Of the four segments showing new atheroma, two were in patients who were initially completely free from visual atherosclerosis.

Subgroup Analysis

Subgroup analysis was performed on subjects, not segments.

The mean concentrations of VLDL and HDL triglycerides decreased significantly more in those whose atheroma regressed (n = 3) and HDL cholesterol increased significantly more than those whose atheroma progressed (n = 8) (Table 4).

Correlation analysis showed that significant correlations existed between regression and decrease in HDL triglycerides (r = -0.78) (Figure 3) and decrease in total cholesterol (r = -0.58). Correlation of borderline significance were seen between regression and decrease in LDL cholesterol (r = -0.49) and in HDL cholesterol (r = 0.48).

Multiple regression analysis demonstrated that 94% of the variability in femoral atheroma (R^2 = 0.94) could be explained by the multiple changes in HDL triglycerides (p < 0.01), total triglycerides (p < 0.001) and VLDL triglycerides (p < 0.001).

Table 4. Mean Serum Lipoprotein Changes in Patients
Showing Regression, Progression or no
Atherosclerosis change, mmol/L

Lipoprotein		Regression n=3	p^1	Progression n=8	No change n=36
VLDL	triglyceride	-1.78	<0.05	-0.21	-0.75
LDL	cholesterol	-1.48	n.s.	-0.41	-1.53
HDL	cholesterol	0.40	<0.02	0.01	0.11
HDL	triglyceride	-0.05	<0.03	-0.01	0.00
Total	cholesterol	-2.44	n.s.	-0.60	-1.72
Total	triglyceride	-1.40	n.s.	-0.35	-0.76

[1] Calculated according to Wilcoxon

DISCUSSION

Using patients as an observation unit, no significant
effect of serum-lipid lowering was found on femoral atheroma
development for one year when compared to placebo treated
controls. This was a small number of asymptomatic men with
hyperlipidemia and changes in atheroma size was seen in only
one-fourth of the patients. Due to the small number, the
type 2 error of probability is high.

However, using arterial segments as basis for the
observation, a highly significant difference in progression/
regression distribution was found between the treatment group
and the control group. Although the arterial wall in all
four femoral segments is exposed to the same concentration
of lipoproteins and toxic smoking products and essentially
the same blood pressure, atherosclerosis is a focal disease

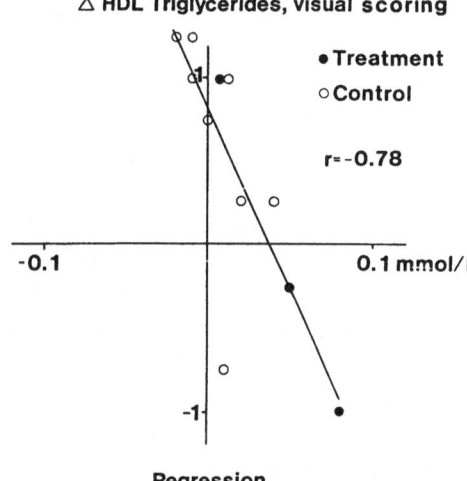

Regression

Figure 3. Relation between change in HDL triglycerides and change in atherosclerosis score after one year's treatment.

in which local factors must play an important role. In this paper we also demonstrate that different segments of the femoral artery display different tendency to atheroma. We have, therefore, found it justified to give results also on a segment basis, well aware of the statistical implications this may have as discussed elsewhere in this volume (10).

Subgroup analysis based on patient observation showed interesting relations between atheroma change and effects on serum lipoproteins. The decrease in the HDL triglyceride concentration was highly significantly related to regression but also the triglyceride content of other lipoprotein fractions was of importance in multiple regression analysis. These findings are in agreement with results of Barndt et al. (11). They reported in an uncontrolled study that patients with regression after treatment for a period similar to that of the present study had significant decrease of their serum triglyceride concentrations. An explanation for the unexpectedly high correlation between plaque change and

the triglyceride content of lipoproteins, especially HDL
triglycerides, cannot be given. It is of interest that HDL
triglyceride has been reported to be a significant independent risk factor for ischemic vascular disease and this
lipoprotein lipid may be an index of the accumulation of
atherogenic lipoproteins and of impaired reverse cholesterol
transport (12).

Our data indicata that atheroma, which change after one
year's observation show strong relations to the changes in
triglyceride content of lipoproteins. We would like to
put forward the following hypothesis: Estimation of femoral
atheroma change after only one year's treatment of a mixed
hyperlipidemic population with "early" changes introduces a
selection of plaques which are particularly sensitive to
volume changes. Regression studies with longer duration are
needed to establish whether there exist different subpopulations of femoral atheroma with regard to mobility proneness
and alterations in the atheroma environment.

REFERENCES

1. Olsson AG, Walldius G, Wahlberg G (1986) Pharmacolo-
    gical control of hyperlipidaemia: Nicotinic acid and
    its analogues – mechanisms of action, effects and
    clinical usage. In: Fears R (ed) Pharmacological
    Control of Hyperlipidaemia. J Prous Science Publishers,
    pp. 217-230.
2. Rössner S, Olsson AG (1980) Effects of combined pro-
    cetofene-nicotinic acid therapy in treatment of hyper-
    triglyceridaemia. Atherosclerosis 35:413-417.
3. Ruhn G, Erikson U, Helmius G, Hemmingsson A (1982)
    Computerized quantitation of atherosclerosis in an
    experimental model. Acta Radiol (Diagn) 23:621-625.
4. Olsson AG, Erikson U, Helmius G, Hemmingsson A,
    Ruhn G (1984) Regression of femoral atherosclerosis
    in humans: Methodological and clinical problems
    associated with studies on femoral atherosclerosis
    development as assessed by angiograms. In: Manilow MR,
    Blaton VH (eds) Regression of Atherosclerotic Lesions:
    Experimental Studies and Observations in Humans.
    New York: Plenum Press, pp. 311-328.
5. Erikson U, Helmius G, Hemmingsson A, Olsson AG, Ruhn G
    Arteriography of patients included in a regression
    study. Workshop on the Evolution of the Human Athero-
    sclerotic Plaque. Rockville, Maryland, September 1986.
6. Beaumont JL, Carlson LA, Cooper GR, Fejfar Z,
    Fredrickson DS, Strasser T (1970) Classification of
    hyperlipidaemias and hyperlipoproteinaemias. Bull
    WHO 43:891.

7. Carlson K (1973) Lipoprotein fractionation. J Clin Path 26 Suppl (Ass Clin Path) 5:32-37.

8. Zlatkis A, Zak B, Boyle AJ (1953) A new method for the direct determination of serum cholesterol. J Lab Clin Med 41:486-492.

9. Fletcher MJ (1968) A colorimetric method for estimating serum triglycerides. Clin Chim Acta 22:393-397.

10. Kelsey S Problems and strategies for statistical analysis of angiographic data: Issue of changes in individual lesion versus individual patients. Workshop on the Evolution of the Human Atherosclerotic Plaque. Rockville, Maryland, September 1986.

11. Barndt R, Blankenhorn DH, Crawford DW, Brooks SH (1977) Regression and progression of early femoral athero-sclerosis in treated hyperlipoproteinemia patients. Annals of Internal Medicine 86:139-146.

12. Little JA, Kakis G, Feather T, Breckenridge CW (1985) Plasma high density lipoprotein triglyceride (HDL-TG) as a risk factor for ischemic vascular disease in a prospective study. Proceedings of Poster Communications, 7th International Symposium on Atherosclerosis, Melbourne October 1969.

43

Arteriography of Patients Included in a Regression Study

Uno Erikson, Gunnar Helmius, Anders Hemmingsson, Anders G. Olsson, and
Gunnar Ruhn

For a long time femoral arteriography has been used to
visualize atherosclerosis. The criteria were very rough from
the beginning, since the technique was used for preoperative
evaluation and in the operative cases most of the lesions
were total or subtotal occlusion of the arteries.

A more patho-chemical approach to the disease has
emphasized the need for a more precise early diagnosis. We
have long been interested in optimizing angiographic techniques and in 1961 pharmaco-angiography was introduced (1,2).
This included intraarterial injection of bradykinin, acethyl-
choline and histamine in order to dilate the arteries and
increase the contrast filling of peripheral arteries (3,4).

Measurement of the blood flow in the leg by means of
venous occlusion pletysmography showed that increased information of arterial anatomy (i.e., contrast filling of the
arteries) was obtained by using the previously mentioned vasoactive drugs.

We also studied the influence of the contrast agents,
and developed the principle of dimeric contrast agents. One
of these dimeric contrast agents, which is now widely used,
is Hexabrix (5).

An important step in improving the angiographic technique was the development of an x-ray tube with a small focal
spot (0.1 x 0.1 mm) enabling high resolution magnified angiography. This was the basis for our study of regression of

atherosclerosis. The angiograms were more informative with this technique and it was thus possible to evaluate very small early changes. By these means, visual judgement could be used for comparison of angiograms with more accuracy and could be combined with defined measurements of intraarterial diameters (6).

A regression study was started in 1978 in which we tried to combine the ocular analyses with a more objective computerized one, encouraged by the results of Crawford and colleagues (7). In this investigation of 31 treated and 32 untreated men, with a mean age of 53 years (range 36 to 65 years) repeated arteriograms were performed at 6 months intervals (Project Lipanthyl®, Lab. Fournier, Dijon, France). All patients had fasting serum cholesterol above 9.5 mmol/L and/ or triglycerides above 3.5 mmol/L. Altogether 210 examinations were performed and the maximum observation time was 3 years. No complications occurred from the procedure, including the arterial puncture, but one patient had a slight allergic urticaria, possibly caused by the contrast agent. The reaction subsided very soon.

This report is preliminary regarding the result of treatment with Lipanthyl. We found a significant positive effect in the treatment group with a high frequency of regression and a low frequency of progression.

Subjective ocular analysis can be critized since repeated consensus viewing only gives an identical result in about 70% (6). But a comparison between two similar pictures is much safer even when using an ocular method. The ocular analysis was made with the images randomized in the series for one patient and without knowledge of treatment group.

In viewing the material, we find it important to emphasize some technical aspects and a need for definition of the disease. In comparison to the analysis of the arterial lumen at arteriography, NMI, CT and PET may show a more complete picture of the disease in the future.

In our study we also applied a computerized method which was a modification of the method introduced by Crawford and his group (7). We cut out a film from the angiogram

661

(125 x 125 mm) and by means of a rotating drum scanner
(Optronix), this image was digitized. From the scans, estimates of the amount of atherosclerosis was obtained.

A model study encouraged us but we very often found it
difficult to analyze the angiograms because of biological
reasons, crossing branches, etc. (8,9). We were very often
computerizing a short and normal segment. Pronounced lesions
only   a short distance from the normal segment could, however, sometimes not be computerized because of the crossing
branches.

A further study showed the importance of using the ECG
triggered exposure technique (10). This increased the correlation coefficient in double estimations from 0.75 to 0.94.

My conclusion up to now is that a skilled eye is
surprisingly accurate in evaluating atherosclerotic lesions.
There is, however, a need for a large field scanner and image
analyzing equipment in order to have more reliable and
objective results. We have just received equipment of that
type (Imtec, Epsilon) and it will be used in an on-going
study. From the pilot study, started in 1978 and ended in
1985, we may conclude that a serum lipid lowering treating
agent causes a regression or decreased progression of the
atherosclerotic lesions in the femoral artery.

REFERENCES
1. Erikson U, et al. (1962) Föredrag Upsala Allm.
    Läkarförening 21/1: Cirkulationsstudier på
    amputationsstumpar.
2. Erikson U, et al. (1962) Föredrag Medicinska Riksstämman:
    Angiografisk bild och genomblödning i amputationsstumpen
    hos lår- och underbensamputerade patienter.
3. Erikson U (1965) Circulation in traumatic amputation
    stumps. An angiographical and physiological investiga-
    tion. Acta Ragiologica, Suppl:238.
4. Erikson U (1965) Peripheral arteriography during brady-
    kinin induced vasodilation. Acta Radiologica Diagnosis
    3:193.
5. Erikson U, Hemmingsson A (1981) Experiences with
    ioxaglate (Hexabrix) in cardioangiography and peripheral
    angiography. Acta Radiol Diagnosis 22:673.
6. Erikson U, Ericsson M, Persson R (1979) On the relation
    between peripheral atherosclerosis and serum lipoproteins.
    Upsala J Med Sci 84:95.

7. Crawford DW, Brooks SH, Selzer RH, Barndt R, Beckenbach
    ES, Blankenhorm DH (1977) Computer densitometry for
    angiographic assessment of arterial cholesterol content
    and gross pathology in human atherosclerosis. J Lab
    Clin Med 80:378.
8. Olsson AG, Carlsson LA, Erikson U, Helmius G,
    Hemmingsson A, Ruhn G (1982) Effets de l'abaissement
    des lipides par le fenofibrate et par l'acide nicotinique
    sur l'atherosclerose apprecies a l'ordinateur dans des
    cas d'hyperlipidemia asymptomatique. Etude en cours.
    3e Colloque International 13-14 Mars, Dijon. Regression
    de la plaque atheromateuse. Gazetts Medicale de
    France, p. 107.
9. Ruhn G, Erikson U, Helmius G, Hemmingsson A (1982)
    Computerized quantitation of atherosclerosis in an
    experimental model. Arteriography and microdensitometry.
    Acta Radiologica Diagnosis 23:621.
10. Nilsson S, Berglund I, Bylund H, Erikson U, Helmius G,
    Hemmingsson A, Holme I, Stenport G, Walldius G
    Quantitation of atherosclerosis in femoral angiography
    with ECG-gated exposures. (In preparation)

44

Ultrasound Lesions of the Carotid Artery and Risk Factors in Men

William Insull, Jr., M. Gene Bond, Sharon Wilmoth, Jean Fishel, and Jay Herson

Non-invasive ultrasonographic evaluation of carotid artery atherosclerosis provides a method for prospectively determining lesion growth characteristics and of correlating rate of disease change with risk factor dose and duration. Although epidemiological studies have reported variable patterns of association between clinical carotid artery disease and risk factors, the most consistent relationship has been with hypertension (1). B-mode ultrasound evaluation presents a powerful tool and the unique opportunity to prospectively monitor lesion growth and to relate these changes to risk factors. Recent refinements in ultrasound instrumentation, standardized protocols for lesion measurement, and validation by comparing *in vivo* measurements of disease extent and severity with pathology measurements, enable measurement of human carotid arteries with high accuracy and precision (2,3).

This study was based on the concepts that atherosclerotic lesions show progressive growth over time, and that after medical intervention, lesion growth can show regression, stabilization, retardation or no effect.

The purposes of this study were fourfold

1. To examine the feasibility of measuring plaque growth in human carotid arteries using serial B-mode ultrasonography in high risk subjects with asymptomatic lesions.

2. To evaluate and compare arterial size characteristics with clinical observations of subjects.

3. To identify risk factors for the growth of carotid artery plaques in men.

4. To provide basic information for the design of B mode ultrasound studies aimed at evaluating efficacy of treatment on carotid arteries with lesions.

The design of the study was to measure, using B mode ultrasound, artery wall thickness (intima, media and adventitia) at a single carotid artery site in thirty-six middle-aged men during a sixteen month period. The growth of each site was estimated by comparing four serial measurements performed at intervals of four to seven months. No treatments for atherosclerosis were administered during this observation. Twenty-eight men had complete observations for growth measurement. Twenty-seven men had complete measurements of risk factors. Twenty-six men were used for evaluation of risk factors, omitting one individual whose baseline measurement of thickness appeared unrealistic.

METHODS

Ultrasonographic interpretation of carotid artery lesions was performed with a 10 MgHz B-mode ultrasound instrument (Horizons Research Laboratories) by a single examiner (MGB) using a standard protocol. The same instrument was used throughout the study. Critical elements of the procedure were that the interpreter was blinded to each subject's identity at time of examination. Subjects were requested to refrain from consuming coffee and tobacco products before the examination and were resting in a reclining position at least ten minutes before the examination started. Blood pressure in the reclining position was demonstrated to be stable by measurements before and after each study. One interpreter performed all measurements and was assisted by two experienced sonographers who did the scanning procedure. Multiple angles of view were routinely obtained on longitudinal images of each artery. The instrument gain was set for optimum lesion detection based on experience based on *in vitro* experiments and on validity (models) experiments in animals. In each subject measurements were performed at the site of a single lesion which was readily located on subsequent scans from constant

anatomical references, (recognizable features in the ultrasound images, i.e. (flow divider). Uniform sonographic
criteria based on *in vitro*) studies of human plaques and
in vivo studies of animal models were used to identify the
tissue interfaces necessary for measurement of wall thickness. Using these techniques of variance of replicate
measurements, (mean ± standard deviation) was determined
for total wall thickness, measured on both near and far walls
at each examination, as 0.19 ± 0.18 mm and for lumen diameter
as 0.37 ± 0.36 mm. Measurements performed at intervals of
four to seven months over the period of sixteen months demonstrated at each plaque site progressive and statistically
significant increases in wall thicknesses (Figure 1). This
increase in wall thickness was significant by analysis of

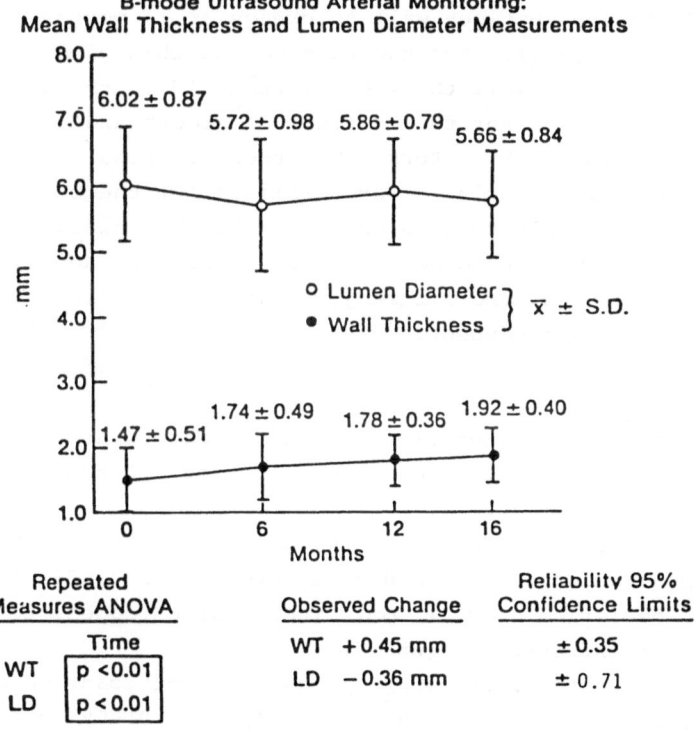

Figure 1. B mode ultrasound monitoring of carotid artery
plaques over 16 months. Measurements of carotid wall thickness and lumen diameter, respectively WT and LD, performed
at a single site in each of 28 subjects. The evaluation of
change by analysis of variance, and confidence limits of
replicate measurements is summarized.

variance. By the sixteenth month the increase exceeded the
95 percent confidence limits for replicate measurements.
The decrease in lumen diameter was significant by analysis
of variance, but failed to exceed the 95 percent confidence
limits for replicate measurements.

Impingements of plaques into the carotid artery lumen
averaged 15%, with a range of about 5 to 30%. No clinically
significant carotid stenoses were observed in the study
subjects.

Fasting plasma lipids were measured by modified LRC
procedures performed under quality control surveillance of
the CDC Lipid Standardization Program (4).

Three measures of growth of the individual plaques were
available: 1) Slope of wall thickness over time; 2) ratio
of wall thickness at 16 months to wall thickness at baseline;
3) the difference between wall thickness at 16 months and
at baseline ($T_{16}-T_0$). For the purposes of this paper, the
difference between wall thickness between 16 months and
baseline was chosen for the analysis of growth and its
association with risk factors. Thirteen potential risk
factors, listed in Table 1, were examined for their relationship with the 16-month difference in wall thickness.

The study was approved by the Institutional Review Boards
for Human Research, and all subjects were volunteers who
signed an informed consent.

RESULTS
The subject characteristics and the cardiovascular
disease risk factors in the men at the start of the study
are summarized in Table 1.

The distribution of 16-months growth of wall thickness
for 26 men ranged from 0 to 0.8 mm, average of 0.438 mm,
standard deviation of 0.219 mm. These values appear to have
a normal distribution (Figure 2).

The 16-month growth ($T_{16}-T_0$) had a significant negative
correlation with baseline thickness, T_0 ($r = 0.609$; $p = 0.001$).
Thus, the arteries with thicker walls had less growth than
those with thinner walls.

Analyses of the correlation between 16-month growth and
risk factors showed a significant correlation only for the
baseline systolic blood pressure, ($r = -0.636$, $p < 0.0001$).

Table 1. Subject Characteristics, Risk Factors, in
          Men at Baseline

Characteristics	Mean + SD	Range
Age	55 ± 6	39 - 60
Quetelet Index (Wt/Ht^2)	2.55 ± .26	2.0 - 3.0
Systolic BP mmHg	130 ± 10	116 - 160
Diastolic BP mmHg	81 ± 8	68 - 100
Total Plasma Cholesterol mg/dl	276 ± 46	213 - 395
Total LDL Plasma Cholesterol mg/dl	185 ± 51	79 - 295
Total HDL Plasma Cholesterol mg/dl	47 ± 15	28 - 87
Plasma LDL/HDL	4.16 ± 1.43	1.6 - 7.3
Plasma Cholesteryl Ester Fatty Acids		
Palmitic %	11 ± 7	918 - 12.4
Oleic %	19 ± 2	13 - 23
Linoleic %	55 ± 4	48 - 64
Arachidonic %	9 ± 2	5 - 15
Carotid Wall Intial Thickness mm	1.4 ± .5	.90 - 2.5

Figure 2. Frequency distribution of 16-month growth in carotid
artery wall thickness of 26 men.

    Thus, it appears that men with lower baseline systolic for
blood pressure have higher 16-month growth than men with high
baseline pressures. Additional analysis has shown statistically significant positive correlation between baseline

systolic pressure and baseline wall thickness (r = 0.506, p = 0.008). Thus, men with low baseline systolic blood pressure tend to have small baseline wall thickness, and these are the men predicted to have larger 16-month growth than those with higher baseline wall thickness.

Analyses for the association of the 16-month growth with plasma lipids as single independent variables showed marginal significance only for the 16-month growth with the ratio of LDL cholesterol to HDL cholesterol at base-line, r= -.372 and p = 0.0614. There were no significant associations of the 16-month growth with the other risk factors.

DISCUSSION

This study has demonstrated that significant growth of carotid wall thickness at the site of ultrasound-diagnosed atherosclerotic plaques can be measured over a 16-month period.

Analysis of factors influential for this growth has demonstrated that greater growth was observed in arteries which at baseline had thinner walls and lower systolic blood pressure. Analyses for the association of 16-month growth with other single risk factors showed only the ratio of plasma LDL cholesterol to HDL cholesterol to have marginal significance. All other potential risk factors were not significant.

An analysis of interaction between the baseline wall thickness and systolic blood pressure revealed that the nega-tive relationship between baseline wall thickness and 16-month growth might not apply to men with systolic blood pressure greater than 145 mmHg. Only 2 of the 26 men in the study had systolic blood pressure greater than 145 mmHg.

The negative correlation of growth with the initial wall thickness indicates that there may be an upper limit to the potential amount of wall thickness.

The identification and evaluation of carotid plaque risk factors by short-term observation demonstrates that the technique of serial high-resolution ultrasonography can be used to increase knowledge and understanding of the pathogenesis of carotid plaque in man. The prominent role

of pre-existing alterations of the vessel wall, greater
thickness, is emphasized. The importance of systolic blood
pressure and the relatively weak effect diastolic blood
pressure are noted. The potential effect of plasma lipids,
particularly the roles of LDL and HDL cholesterol, as
expressed in their ratio, is revealed.

To extend these concepts, further studies are needed,
using more subjects with a greater range of risk factor values
and for a longer period of observation.

In conclusion, this pilot study accomplished its purposes. Measurement of growth of asymptomatic plaques in
the human carotid artery using serial B mode ultrasonography
over a reasonable time period is feasible. The size characteristics of lesions can be evaluated and compared with
clinical characteristics. Risk factors for plaque growth
can be identified. The basic characteristics of studies of
growth and risk factors were identified and can be used to
design future studies of plaque growth and to guide the
design of studies to evaluate treatment of plaques.

REFERENCES

1. Epstein FH (1986) Risk factors for peripheral and
    cerebral atherosclerosis: Similarities and differences
    with coronary atherosclerosis. Monograph, Atherosclerosis
    14:1-5
2. Pignoli P, Tremoli E, Poli A, Oreste P, and Paoletti R
    (1986) Internal plus medial thickness of the arterial
    wall: A direct measurement with ultrasound imaging.
    Circ 74:1399-1406
3. Hennerici M, Rautenberg W, Trockel U, Kladetzky RG
    (1986) Spontaneous progression and regression of small
    carotid atheroma. Lancet i:1415-1419
4. National Heart and Lung Insitute (1974) Manual of Labora-
    tory Operations, Vol 1, Lipid and Lipoprotein Analysis.
    Bethesda, MD: National Institutes of Health, (Lipid
    Research Clinics Program) (DHEW publication no. NIH
    75-628

45

Clinical Trials in Atherosclerosis: Summary and Overview

Stanley P. Azen and David H. Blankenhorn

INTRODUCTION

There are two general strategies to test the efficacy
of drugs or dietary regimens which retard or reverse the
progression of atherosclerosis in man. The first is to
study effects on atherosclerosis-related morbidity or mortality. This strategy assumes that therapy effects will be
powerful enough to emerge despite the presence of advanced
complicated lesions, the known anatomic substrate for atherosclerosis morbidity and mortality. The second strategy is
to measure the rate of atherosclerotic lesion change. In
this case, it is assumed that therapy effects will be more
pronounced on early stage lesions, but that long-range
benefits will accrue if growth of these can be reversed or
retarded.

Clinical trials which have utilized the first strategy
include: (a) the World Health Organization trial of clofibrate on the incidence of ischemic heart disease in
15,475 males aged 20 to 59 years (1); (b) the Coronary
Drug Project which studied the effects of five drug regimens
and a placebo in 8,341 men aged 30 to 64 years who had
recovered from one or more episodes of myocardial infarction
(2); (c) the Multiple Risk Factor Intervention Trial which
tested the effect of a multifactor intervention program
on mortality from coronary heart disease in 12,866 high-risk
men aged 35 to 57 years (3); (d) the Lipid Research Clinics
Primary Prevention Trial which studied the effects of

Table 1. Summary of Published Clinical Trials

Principal Investigator	Random- ized	Entry Criterion	Total Number	Angiogram Vessels	Angio- Interval (years)	Therapy Under Test	Endpoint Measurement
Arntzenius	No	Angina	52	Coronary	2	Diet with linoleic acid	Computerized angiograms (Utrectht)
Brown	Yes	Coronary bypass	127	Coronary	1	ASA + dipyridamole	Computerized angiograms (Washington)
Cohn	Yes	Coronary angiogram positive	40	Coronary	1	Clofibrate	Visual reading of angiograms
Duffield	Yes	Type II, III	24	Femoral	19 mo	Cholesty- ramine, Clo- fibrate	Panel, Computerized angiograms
Frick	Yes	Angina	78	Coronary	5	Surgery	Visual reading of angiograms
Kuo	No	Type II, IV, mixed	40	Coronary	4	Colestipol	Panel reading of angiograms
Nash	No	Coronary angiogram positive	42	Coronary	2	Colestipol, Clofibrate	Panel reading of angiograms
NHLBI	Yes	Type II	116	Coronary	5	Cholesty- ramine	Computerized angiograms (Washington)
Nikkila	No	Chol > 278 2-3 vessel athero.	48	Coronary	5	Clofibrate, nicotinic acid, or both	Visual reading of angiograms

cholestyramine and placebo on 3806 men aged 35 to 59 who
were free of clinical evidence of coronary heart disease on
entry (4); and (e) a study of Gemfibrozil in 4080 dyslipidemic
Finnish men which is now in progress. Clinical trials utilizing this strategy can also test therapy designed to reduce
morbidity or mortality from associated conditions such as
cardiac arrythmia which increase the hazard resulting from
coronary atherosclerosis. A recent trial of this sort was
the Beta-Blocker Heart Attack Trial which tested the efficacy
of long-term therapy with propranolol in survivors of an
acute myocardial infarction (5).

There are 23 trials that are either in progress or have
recently been completed which utilize the second strategy
of assessing drug effects in atherosclerosis by lesion change
(Tables 1 and 2). The rationale for these trials is based
in part on evidence obtained in animal models that significant reduction in atherosclerotic lesions can occur within
six months to a year after the atherogenic stimulus is
withdrawn (6-8). Additional evidence from angiographic
reports of lesion regression in man supports these trials (9).

This paper reports on the status of clinical trials in
atherosclerosis. In Section II a summary of the completed
trials is given. Section III reviews the status of on-going
clinical trials. Section IV comments on design issues for
future clinical trials.

Published Trials

The following summarizes the design and results of the
trials which have been published. Table 1 presents an
overview of these trials.

1. The Arntzenius Study (10)

Arntzenius and co-workers studied the effect of
lowering cholesterol on coronary artery atherosclerosis.
This trial differs from all other trials in that lipid levels
were lowered solely by dietary measures. Thirty-nine patients
under 60 years of age with stable angina pectoris in whom
coronary angiography had demonstrated severe narrowing of the
diameter (>50%) of one or more major coronary arteries were
studied. Patients were excluded if they had undergone coronary bypass surgery, or if they had disease of the left main

Table 2. Summary of Clinical Trials in Progress

Principal Investigator	Random-ized	Entry Criterion	Total Number	Angiogram Vessels	Angio-Interval (years)	Therapy Under Test	Endpoint Measurement
Alderman	Yes	Coronary bypass	240	Coronary	3	Risk factor intervention	Computerized angiograms (Stanford)
Blankenhorn	Yes	Coronary bypass	160	Femoral coronary carotid	2	Colestipol, niacin	Computerized angiograms, panel, ultra-sound (JPL/USC)
Blankenhorn	Yes	Coronary artery disease	210	Coronary	4	Mevinolin	Computerized angiograms (JPL/USC)
Brown	Yes	95th perc. β-apo. HLP	100	Coronary	2	Colestipol, niacin	Computerized angiograms (Washington)
Buckwald	Yes	Myocardial infarct	800	Coronary pelvic	3,5	Ileal bypass	Panel reading of angiograms morbidity, mortality
Carlson, Erikson, Olsson	Yes	Hyperchol-esteremia, femoral athero.	240	Femoral	1,2,3	Probucol, cholestrya-mine	Computerized angiograms (Uppsala)
Cheseboro	Yes	Coronary angioplasty	600	Dilated coronary segment	6 mo-1 yr	ASA + dipyridamole	Computerized angiogram (Washington)

Table 2 (continued)

Gerstenoblith	Yes	Coronary bypass	150	Coronary	1	Nifedipine	Panel reading of angiograms
Havel	Yes	Type II	70	Coronary, femoral	4	Colestipol, niacin	Computerized angiograms (UCSF and JPL/USC)
Kane	Yes	Type II	90	Coronary, femoral	2	Colestipol, niacin	Computerized angiograms (Washington)
Lichtlen —	Yes	Mild CAD	420	Coronary	3	Nifedipine	Computerized angiograms (Rotterdam)
Mc Callister	Yes	Coronary angioplasty lesions 50%	280	Coronary	1	Diltiazem	Computerized angiograms (Washington)
Olsson, Erikson	Yes	Type II, III, IV	40	Right femoral	0.5	Niacin, phenofibrate	Computerized angiograms (Uppsala)
Waters	Yes	Coronary angio with mild diffuse disease	400	Coronary	3	Nicardipine	Computerized angiograms (Rotterdam)

coronary artery, coexisting valvular or nonischemic myocardial disease, or insulin-requiring diabetes. Intervention consisted of a vegetarian diet in which the ratio of polyunsaturated to saturated fatty acids was at least 2, and the dietary cholesterol was less than 100 mg per day. Coronary arteriography was performed pre-and post-treatment at 24 months. Films were assessed virually by two experienced observers who estimated the percentage of obstruction in each lesion in increments of 5 percentage points. The severity of coronary obstruction was scored by calculating the mean of the percentages of obstruction in each patient. In addition, computer-assisted analysis was carried out. The severity of coronary obstruction was expressed relatively as the percentage of reduction of a vessel's diameter, and absolutely as the minimal diameter at the site of obstruction. Both types of assessment indicated progression of disease in 21 (54%) of 39 patients but no lesion growth in 18 (46%). Coronary lesion growth was correlated with total/HDL cholesterol ($r = 0.5$, $P < 0.001$), but not with blood pressure, smoking status, alcohol intake, weight, or usual drug therapy ($e.g.$, beta-blockers, diuretics, digitalis, etc.) Disease progression was significant in patients who had values of total/HDL cholesterol that were higher than the median throughout the trial period. No coronary lesion growth was observed in patients who had lower values for total/HDL cholesterol throughout the trial or who initially had higher values that were significantly lowered by dietary intervention.

   2.   The Brown Study (11)

      Brown and co-workers studied the effect of platelet inhibiting drugs on thrombus formation in the arterial circulation. One hundred twenty-seven coronary bypass patients were studied in a randomized, double-blind, risk-stratified, placebo-controlled prospective trial evaluating the effect on graft patency of 325 mg tid aspirin (ASA) plus 75 mg tid dipyridamole (DP) or ASA alone. The follow-up period was one year. A logistic regression model was used to determine the effects of 28 different measured variables on graft patency and to adjust for these effects in determining the relationship between antiplatelet therapy and graft occlusion. The results of the study showed that no patient-specific variable contributed significantly to the prediction of occlusion in either the placebo or the treated group. Six graft-specific variables (arterial diameter, severity of stenosis, graft flow, reactive hyperemia, presence or absence of collaterals, and graft type) did contribute to the prediction model. Relative to the placebo, the relative risk of graft occlusion with ASA was 0.47 (p = .04); with ASA + DP, it was 0.50 (p = 0.4). The authors concluded that early postoperative ASA appears to be a simple, inexpensive, and effective form of therapy. It is not clear whether the addition of DP to the regimen improves the results.

3. The Cohn Study (12)

Cohn and co-workers studied 65 patients who already had had selective coronary angiography and, in all but two patients, coronary artery surgery. Patients were paired by age and randomized to one of two treatments: clofibrate or placebo. Forty patients completed the study, 16 in the clofibrate group and 24 from the placebo group. Coronary angiography was performed preoperatively and after one year. Two observers visually determined change in coronary artery pattern. Progression, as defined when greater obstruction or total occlusion of a main artery or one of its branches could be clearly delineated, was observed in 15 out of 24 patients (63%) of the placebo group, and in 11 out of 16 (69%) of the clofibrate group. Ninteen out of 64 (30%) coronary arteries in the clofibrate group showed progressive narrowing, and 24 out of 96 (25%) arteries manifested progressive narrowing in the placebo group. No regression of coronary artery disease was seen. The authors concluded that clofibrate did not significantly influence the rate of progression of coronary artery disease in a one-year period.

4. The Duffield Study (13)

Duffield and co-workers studied men and women presenting with a history of hyperlipidemia and with stable intermittent claudification for at least six months. Twenty-four patients were randomly assigned to usual care and treatment groups, the latter receiving dietary advice and cholestyramine, nicotinic acid, or clofibrate depending

on their lipoprotein phenotype. Arteriography was performed
when the study began and after an average period of 19 months.
Angiograms were assessed both visually and by computerized
analysis. For the latter, disease progression or regression was based on an index of edge irregularity. Visual
assessment demonstrated that significantly fewer arterial
segments showed detectable progression of atherosclerosis in
the treatment group (p < 0.06), and that the mean increase
in plaque area in the treatment group was one third of that
in the usual - care group. Computerized analysis indicated
that the mean increase in edge irregularity index in the
treatment group was only 40% of that in the usual care group
(p < 0.05). Twice as many arterial segments showed improvement in the treatment group. Finally, regardless of the
treatment group, changes in edge irregularity index were
directly related to plasma LDL cholesterol concentration.
However, concern was expressed by Blankenhorn *et al* (14)
that statistical analyses were performed assuming independence of segments.

5. The Frick Study (15)

Frick and co-workers studied 100 males under 65 years
of age, with angina pectoris despite medical treatment
with nitrates and beta-blocking agents, a positive exercise
test, significant (>50%) coronary artery stenosis in at
least two arteries, and suitable coronary anatomy for grafting. Subjects were randomly assigned for medical therapy
or bypass surgery. The medical patients were reexamined
after 5 years and the surgical patients 3 weeks, 1 year and
5 years after operation. Coronary lesions were scored on
the basis of reduction in luminal diameter as: 0-49%, 50-
74%, 75-90%, subtotal obstruction, and complete occlusion.
Progression of the disease was considered to have occurred
if the degree of narrowing increased by at least 1 grade, or
if a new lesion had developed. Sixty-seven percent (67%)
of the medical patients and 68% of the surgical patients had
progression. The frequency of new lesions in initially
normal segments after 5 years was 6.7% versus 4.1% in
ungrafted normal segments in the surgical group (p < 0.05).
The frequency of progression in abnormal arteries was 24.1%
in the medical group versus 22.6% in the ungrafted arteries

of the surgical group. The rate of progression of obstructed sugments proximal to the fraft over 5 years was 43% versus 27% of the corresponding segments in the medical group (p <0.01).

6. The Kuo Study (16)

Kuo and co-workers studied eighteen male and 12 female atherosclerotic patients, aged 38-65 years with Type II hyperlipoproteinemia. Patients were randomized into drug (colestipol) and placebo groups. All subjects were placed on a low cholesterol, low saturated fat and limited simple-carbohydrate diet. Coronary brachiocephalic and peripheral arteriograms were performed in 12, three and four patients, respectively before and 3-4 years after institution of the treatment. Each coronary arteriogram and angiogram was reviewed by three observers at the same time to reach a consensus. Long-term colestipol and diet treatment reduced the xanthoma size and stabilized serially angiographically visualized atherosclerotic lesions in 21 of 25 patients who showed a satisfactory hypolipemic response (average drop in total cholesterol = -108.4 mg/dl, in LDL cholesterol = -98.8 mg/dl).

7. The Nash Otudy (17)

Nash and co-workers studied 42 (out of 61) subjects, each of whom demonstrated significant (>50%) narrowing of a non-grafted coronary artery and a baseline cholesterol level >250 mg%. Patients were excluded if they exhibited major diverticular, thyroid, liver, renal or malignant disease. Treatment consisted of colestipol hydrochloride therapy and a cereal based, low-fat, low-cholesterol diet. Twenty-five patients who had sustained at least 15% reduction of serum cholesterol levels after one month of therapy were placed in the colestipol hydrochloride treatment group and con-tinued this therapy for two years. Seventeen patients who demonstrated less than a 15% reduction were switched to avicel placebo. Coronary arteriograms were performed on all patients pre- and post-treatment. Progression, regression, and stability was visually determined separately on ungrafted major coronary vessels. Progression steps were considered as interval changes of 0 to 25%, 25 to 50%, 50 to 75%, 75 to 90%, 90 to 99%, and 99 to 100% obstruction in luminal diameter. A minimum of two steps of progression

were required to classify the patient. Three of the drug-
treated patients showed progression, while 8 of the 17
placebo treated patients demonstrated progression (p = 0.11).

8. The NHLBI Coronary Intervention Study (4)

Patients with Type II hyperlipoproteinemia and
coronary artery disease were randomly assigned to a low-
cholesterol, low fat diet and drug (cholestyramine) or to
the same diet and placebo. Coronary lesions were assessed
by coronary angiography at entry into study and after five
years of therapy. Results are given for 116 out of 143
patients. (Sample size calculations indicated a desired
study sample of 250 patients). Baseline and follow-up
angiograms were reviewed visually by three separate panels,
each consisting of three angiographers. Segments were
classified for the presence and extent of a lesion. Segments
were also classified as normal or as exhibiting one or
multiple lesions. Panels recorded the change, if any, in
luminal diameter for each lesion on the two sets of films.
A confirmed change required at least two or three of the
panels to agree that a change occurred. Once a definition
of lesion change was established the following definitions
were used: Definite progression--at least one lesion with
progression and no lesion with regression; probable pro-
gression--at least one lesion with probable progression and
no lesion with regression or definite progression; probable
regression--at least one lesion with probable regression and
no lesions with definite regression or any progression;
definite regression--at least one lesion with definite
regression and no progression; mixed response--regression and
progression; no change. When only definite progression was
considered, 35% of the placebo-treated patients versus 25% of
the drug-treated patients exhibited definite progression.
When the analysis was performed with adjustment for baseline
inequalities of risk factors, effect of treatment was more
pronounced. Of lesions causing 50% or greater stenosis at
baseline, 33% of placebo-treated with 12% of cholestyramine-
treated patients manifested lesion progression (< 0.05).
Similar analyses with other endpoints all favored the
cholestyramine-treated group.

9. The Nikkila Study (18)

Nikkila and co-workers studied 41 patients with
coronary artery disease of two or three vessels and with

serum triglyceride concentration exceeding 177 mg/100 ml.
Patients considered for surgical treatment and those with
clinical diabetes, poor left ventribular function, cardiac
failure, or uncontrolled hypertension were excluded. These
patients were treated with diet and lipid-lowering drugs
(clofibrate or nicotinic acid, or both). A non-randomized
control group was formed from 20 patients with coronary
disease participating in another prospective study carried
out at the same time at the same hospital. Patients in this
group had angina pectoris, a positive exercise test, stenoses
of more than 50% in at least two coronary arteries, and
hyperlipidemia. They received medical treatment for coronary
artery disease but no treatment to reduce lipid concentrations. Coronary arteriography was done before entry to the
study and after two and seven years. Seven coronary arteries were analyzed for each patient. Obstruction was estimated as the proportional reduction in the luminal diameter.
The progression of coronary lesions at repeat angiography
was assessed visually as the total increase in proportional
luminal narrowing. Progression was said to be present if
the luminal narrowing at a lesion had increased by a minimum
of 20% or if a subtotal obstruction had advanced to total
occlusion. In addition, the number of major arterial segments
showing progression was counted and related to the number of
segments at risk for progression. By all criteria coronary
lesions progressed significantly less in the treated patients
than in the non-randomized controls. The angiographic
state remained completely unchanged in 32% of the patients
compared with 8% of the controls. Of the arterial segments
at risk, 16.5% progressed in the patients compared with 38%
in the controls ($p < 0.001$), and the coronary obstruction
increased less in patients than in controls ($p < 0.05$).
Survival was 89% in seven years in the patients compared
with 65% in five years in the controls ($p < 0.01$).

Trials in Progress
     There are fourteen angiographic clinical trials which
are currently in progress (see Table 2 for a summary). In
all current studies, selective arterial angiography is used
to measure lesion change and, although there is good reason

to believe that angiography will eventually be augmented
or replaced by less invasive, more flexible procedures,
the nature of angiography largely determines the characteristics of these studies. Thus, all current studies tend to
restrict the number of measurements which can be made per
subject and also the number of subjects included in the
trial. Consequently, the therapies selected have generally
been chosen with the expectation that they will produce a
major alteration in atheroclerosis growth rates.

Of the trials listed in Table 2, the major criterion
for entry is either an elevation of blood lipid levels or
manifest atherosclerosis. Thus, the primary entry criteria
are: coronary bypass (3), hyperlipidemia (3), coronary
artery disease (2), and angioplasty (2). Other entry
criteria include the upper 5th percentile of the distribution of β-apolipoprotein (1), myocardial infarction (1), and
hypercholesteremia and femoral atherosclerosis (1). Projected sample sizes range from 40 to 800. All fourteen
trials are randomized.

In most of the trials (10), only one vascular bed is
under evaluation of that correlation of atherosclerosis
change across vessels will not be possible. The primary
site for the evaluation of treatment effect are the coronary
vessels (18), while two trials are evaluating the femoral
arteries. Of the remaining four trials, two are evaluating
both the coronary and femoral vessels, and one study is
evaluating the coronary and pelvic vessels. The only trial
which evaluates three vessel sites (coronary, femoral, and
carotid) is the Cholesterol Lowering Atherosclerosis Study
(CLAS) of the University of Southern California.

Most trials are attempting to produce a major change
in lipid levels through use of vigorous drug therapy (7)
or partial ileal bypass (1). The lipid lowering drugs are:
niacin and colestid (4), niacin and phenofibrate (1),
mevinolin (1), and probucol (1). Four trials are testing
the effect of calcium blockers: (nifedipine (2), nicardipine
(1), and diltiazem (1). One trial is studying the effect
of platelet inhibiting drugs on thrombus formation in the
arterial circulation. Finally, one trial is examining the
efficacy of risk factor intervention.

The distribution of the angiographic interval for the first follow-up angiogram is: one year (5), two years (3), 3 years (4), and 4 years (2). Two trials call for more than one follow-up angiogram (the Buckwald study and the Carlson, Erikson, and Olsson study).

The majority (11) of the trials employ computerized angiographic measurements of lesions. In the remaining trials(2), a panel of human readers is used to interpret films. It is noteworthy that the CLAS study plans to utilize three modes of evaluation: computer, panel, and ultrasound.

Planning for Future Trials

From the published and to-be-published studies, insight will not only be gained into the question of the efficacy of drugs or dietary regimens in retarding or reversing the progression of atherosclerosis in man, but valuable information will also be gained for the planning of future trials. First and foremost information will be able to be obtained for the omnipresent question of the adequacy of sample size. For that reason, it is important that methods of measurement and variance estimates are reported along with estimates of change in lesion growth. Ideally, variance estimates for factors influencing total variability should be published, *e.g.*, measurement variance, within-subject variance, variability over time, and between-subject variance.

Second, information may be obtained as to the appropriateness of the experimental design. Most studies utilize one post-treatment measurement of the endpoint. If lesions grow in a linear fashion, then it would be possible to detect progression, stability, or regression. If, on the other hand, lesions do not regress or progress linearly, but rather grow in episodes, the pre-post design may be inappropriate, since changes in lesion growth may be missed. Unfortunately, data from animal studies are cross-sectional in nature and do not provide this needed information. A model for testing treatment effects with multiple angiograms (proposed by Holme (19) could possibly provide information regarding whether lesion change--either regression or progression--occurs in episodes, as well as provide a method for testing small treatment effects.

Third, as measurement methodology becomes more advanced, non-invasive imaging techniques (e.g., ultrasound, magnetic resonance, isotopic imaging) may become available for evaluating lesion growth. This would permit more follow-up determinations to be made which would reduce sample size needs for agents which produce large changes, and would also allow for testing of less drastic therapies. This would be of particular importance in testing effects of diet. In addition, the non-invasive aspect of the techniques may improve the recruitment process.

Possibly the largest potential benefit from advances in imaging methodology will be to allow physiologic processes operative within the vessel wall and atheroma to be measured. Current procedures which measure luminal intrusion provides only an overall estimate of the process. Studies of this type could be complimented by the introduction of intermediate steps such as infiltration of LDL or adherence of platelets with release of platelet-derived growth factor.

REFERENCES

1. Oliver MF, Heady JA, Morris JN (1978) A cooperative trial in the primary prevention of ischemic heart disease using clofibrate. Br Heart J 40:1069
2. The Coronary Drug Project Research Group (1975) Clofibrate and niacin in coronary heart disease. J Amer Med Assoc 231:360
3. Multiple Rick Factor Intervention Trial Research Group (1982) Multiple risk factor intervention trial. Risk factor changes and mortality results. J Amer Med Assoc 248:1465
4. The Lipid Research Clinics Coronary Primary Prevention Trial Results: I. Reduction in Incidence of Coronary Heart Disease. J Amer Med Assoc 251:351-354
5. Beta-Blocker Heart Attack Research Group (1984) Beta-Blocker Heart Attack Trial: Design, Methods, and Baseline Results.
6. Fritz KE, Augustyn JM, Jarmolych J, Daoud AS, Lee KT (1976) Regression of advanced atherosclerosis in swine. Arch Pathol Lab Med 100:380-385
7. Adams CWM, Morgan RS (1977) Regression of atheroma in the rabbit. Atherosclerosis 28:399-404
8. Vesselinovitch D, Wissler RW, Hughes R, Borensztajn J (1976) Reversal of advanced atherosclerosis in rhesus monkeys. Part 1. Light-microscopic studies. Atherosclerosis 23:155-176
9. Manilow MR (1984) Atherosclerosis: Progression, regression, and resolution. Am Heart J 108:1523-1537

10. Arntzenius AC, Kromhout D, Barth JD *et al* (1985)
    Diet, lipoproteins and the progression of coronary
    atherosclerosis: The Leiden Intervention trial.
    New Engl J Med 312:805-811

11. Brown BG, Cukingnan RA, DeRouen T *et al* (1985) Improved
    graft patency in patients treated with platelet-
    inhibiting therapy after coronary bypass surgery.
    Circulation 72:138-146

12. Cohn K, Sakai FJ, Langston MF (1975) Effect of
    clofibrate on progression of coronary disease: A
    prospective angiographic study in man. Amer Heart
    J 89:591-598

13. Duffield RGM, Miller NE, Brunt JNH, Lewis B, Jamieson
    CW, Colchester ACF (1983)   Treatment of hyperlipidaemia
    retards progression of symptomatic femoral atherosclero-
    sis: A randomized controlled trial.   The Lancet 2(8351):
    639-642

14. Blankenhorn DH, Azen SP, Neissim SA (1983) Letter to
    Editor: Treatment of hyperlipidaemia and progression
    of atherosclerosis.   The Lancet 2(8360):1193

15. Frick MH, Valle M, Pekka-Tapani H (1983) Progression
    of coronary artery disease in randomized medical and
    surgical patients over a 5-year angiographic follow-
    up.   Amer J Cardiol 52:681-685

16. Kuo PT, Hayase K, Kostis JB, Moreyra AE (1979) Use of
    combined diet and colestipol in long-term (7-7 1/2
    years) Treatment of patients with Type II Hyperlipo-
    proteinemia.   Circulation 59:199-211

17. Nash DT, Gensini G, Esente P (1982) Effect of lipid-
    lowering therapy on the progression of coronary
    atherosclerosis assessed by scheduled repetitive
    coronary arteriography.   International Journal of
    Cardiology 2:43-55

18. Nikkila EA, Viikkinkoski P, Valle M, Frick MH (1984)
    Prevention of progression of coronary atherosclerosis
    by treatment of hyperlipidaemia: a seven year prospec-
    tive angiographic study.   Br Med J 289:220-223

19. Holme I (1986) Power computations for multipoint
    measurement studies of atheroma development in femoral
    arteries.   In: Fidge NH and Nestel PJ (Eds).
    Atherosclerosis VII. Amsterdam, Elsevier, pgs 95-97

Current and Prospective Methods for Detecting Plaque Change

46
Ultrasonic Evaluation of Arterial Wall Dynamics

Ward A. Riley, Jr.

INTRODUCTION

In discussions of current and prospective approaches
to detecting, non-invasively, changes in arterial wall and
plaque characteristics, attention is often focused on the
acquisition of anatomical or structural information. This
approach, in a general sense, provides static information
about the size, location and, indirectly, the composition
of arterial wall features which could be useful in conducting studies of progression or regression. In this paper,
I wish to focus on a second approach which involves the
gathering of physiological or functional information pertain-
ing to the arterial wall. This approach provides dynamic
information about the wall and quantitates the stress/
strain behavior or the stiffness of the wall at specific
sites.

The stiffness of arterial walls is determined by a
rather large number of factors (1). These include the

Acknowledgement: I would like to acknowledge the encouragement and assistance of numerous investigators conducting
research programs over the last decade within the Cerebrovascular Research Center at the Bowman Gray School of
Medicine in Winston-Salem, North Carolina and the SCOR-
Arteriosclerosis at the Louisiana State University Medical
Center in New Orleans. I would like to express special
appreciation to Dr. James F. Toole, Dr. Ralph W. Barnes,
and Dr. Gerald S. Berenson.

elastin and collagen content, the elastin-collagen ratio,
the number of smooth muscle cells present, and the various
activation mechanisms. The measurements arising from this
approach are thus gross measures of the collective effect
of these various determinants.

OBJECTIVE

The overall objective of this approach is two-fold and
can be stated as follows: to reliably measure arterial wall
motion at specific predilective sites: (A) prior to plaque
development in order to identify dynamic wall characteristics which might predispose to disease, and (B) During
plaque progression or regression to characterize the mechanical properties of existing plaques. In this paper, I
wish to focus on objective (A) and emphasize the current
and potential application of ultrasonic methods in improving
our ability to assess risk for cardiovascular disease at a
relatively early period of life.

METHODS

Reports of non-invasive ultrasonic measurements of
arterial wall motion at a specific site have begun to
accumulate since the late 1960's with work being reported
from several countries and for several arterial sites: the
carotid, the aorta and the femoral (2-8). The results I
will discuss here were obtained on the common carotid
artery. This site was selected because of its relatively
simple and symmetric geometry (nearly cylindrical), its
convenient anatomical location (close to the skin surface
and accessible to ultrasonic energy) and its proximity to
the carotid bulb (a site predisposed to disease development).
However, the techniques can be applied to other arterial
beds which are accessible to ultrasound.

Examples of the high quality of data which can be
obtained with these methods are shown in Figure 1A and 1B.
These graphs show several cycles of the carotid artery lumen
diameter change pulse wave in both the right and left
carotid arteries of a young boy and girl. The artery diameters stretch about 0.8 mm between diastole and systole,
and very similar pulse wave contours are detected

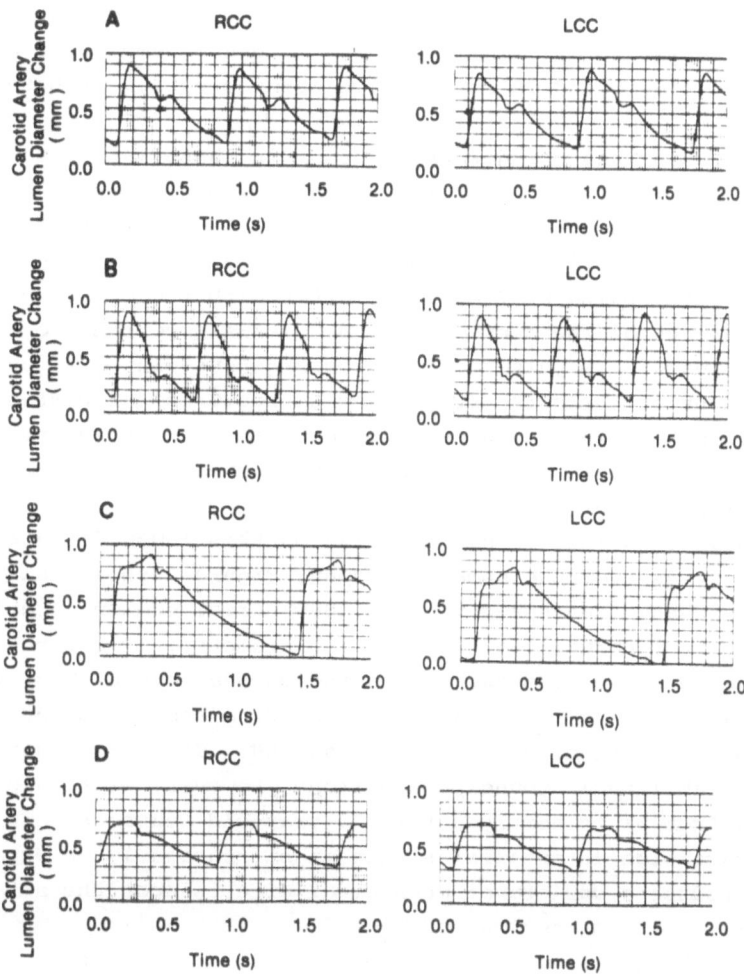

Figure 1 A–D. Detailed comparison of the strip chart
recordings of the lumen diameter changes occurring in the
right (RCC) and left (LCC) common carotid arteries in:
(A) a 10-year-old male subject; (B) a 14-year-old female
subject; (C) a 19-year-old female subject; and (D) a 25-
year-old female subject. Subject (C) was a highly trained
runner. Small diameter variations near the base of the
dicrotic notch approximately 10 μm in amplitude (B) are
frequently observed on both sides. (Reprinted from Preventive
Medicine 13:173, 1984 by permission of Academic Press).

independently on both sides. With these methods, dicrotic
notch details as small as 10-20 micrometers in amplitude can
be reliably detected in consecutive cardiac cycles in both
carotids.

The principal changes which occur in these waveforms
with age are: a significant reduction in lumen diameter
change during the cardiac cycle, shown in Figure 1D to be
only 0.4 mm in a 25-year-old woman, and a significant modification of the pulse wave contour, often with the complete
disappearance of the dicrotic notch. It is important to recognize that these pulse wave contours depend, in part, on
reflections of the pulse from arterial features far distant
from the site being measured, and thus can contain information about arterial characteristics both proximal and distal
to the measurement site.

To give an idea of how the size of this lumen diameter
change varies over the human lifespan, Figure 2 shows this
diameter change, measured in over 1000 normal common carotid
arteries, but normalized to diastolic diameter. The percent
increase in lumen diameter during the cardiac cycle is plotted
versus age showing mean values varying from about 14% for
young children to only 2% or 3% by age 60. There is significant variability in young people alone, however, with values
ranging from 6% to nearly 20% in 20-year-old subjects. This
large variation in arterial strain might reasonably be expected to produce a variety of mechanical effects upon the arterial wall over long periods of time.

Several quantities are commonly used to define the
elasticity of arteries (9,10). Three of the most common are:
arterial distensibility, arterial compliance, and pressure-
strain elastic modulus. Arterial distensibility (AD) is
defined as the fractional volume increase occurring within
the artery during the cardiac cycle divided by the arterial
pulse pressure. For a simple model of an artery consisting
of a thin-walled cylindrical tube, having systolic and diastolic lumen diameters equal to Ds and Dd, respectively, and
systolic and diastolic blood pressures equal to Ps and Pd,
respectively, the arterial distensibility is defined as:

$$AD = (Ds^2 - Dd^2) / [Dd^2 (Ps - Pd)]$$

Arterial distensibility is independent of the length of the arterial segment.

Arterial compliance (AC) is defined as the absolute volume increase occurring within the artery during the cardiac cycle divided by the arterial pulse pressure. Thus, the arterial compliance per unit length for our simple arterial model would be:

$$AC = \eta \ (Ds^2 - Dd^2) \ / \ [4 \ (Ps - Pd)]$$

Longitudinal extension of the artery is assumed to be negligible.

The pressure-strain elastic modulus, Ep, is defined as the arterial pulse pressure divided by the circumferential arterial strain (CAS) imposed on the artery during the cardiac cycle. This definition becomes:

$$Ep = (Ps - Pd) \ / \ CAS$$

where the circumferential arterial strain is:

$$CAS = [(Ds - Dd) \ / \ Dd)]$$

or, in fact, the fractional increase in arterial diameter during the cardiac cycle. As an artery becomes stiffer, the distensibility and compliance decrease, whereas the elastic-modulus increases.

The four parameters required to determine these measures of elasticity are thus Ds, Dd, Ps and Pd. The first two, arterial lumen diameters, can be measured directly with noninvasive ultrasonic methods (2-8). The values of Ps and Pd must be measured indirectly, normally in an adjacent artery. The values of Ep for the common carotid artery are reported in this paper with values of Ps and Pd being determined in the left brachial artery using an oscillometric technique (11). The values of AD and AC could also be calculated, however, from the same data. Any artery accessible to ultrasonic evaluation could be studied in a similar manner.

RESULTS AND DISCUSSION

In Figure 3, the elastic modulus, denoted by E(p), is plotted as a function of age showing the path along with carotid artery stiffness changes over the human life span

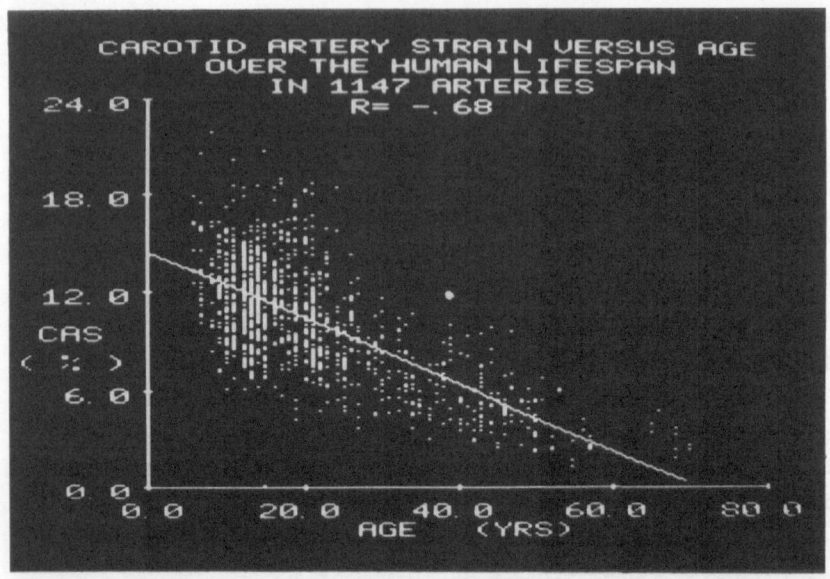

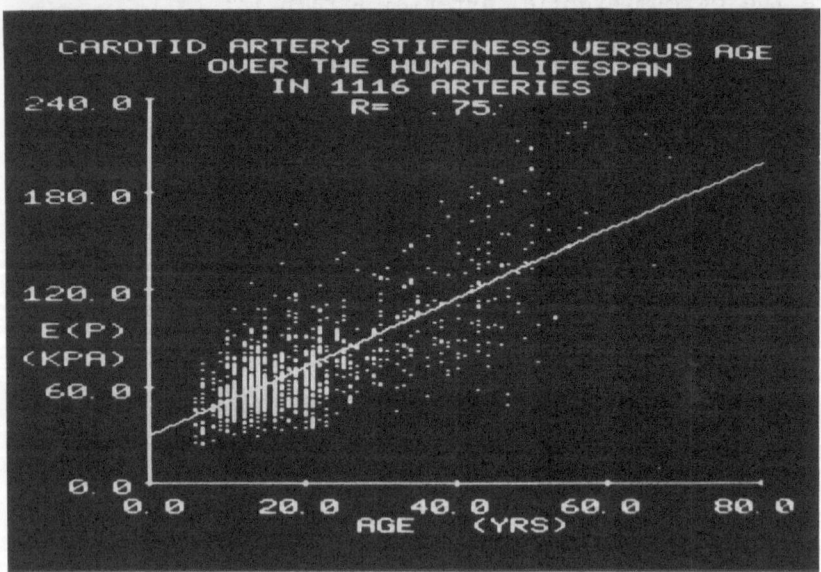

Figure 2. Variation of the carotid artery strain (CAS) with age over the human lifespan in 1147 arteries. The CAS in this figure is equivalent to the fractional lumen diameter change occurring during the cardiac cycle expressed as a percentage of the diastolic diameter.
Figure 3. Variation of the carotid artery stiffness (as measured by the pressure-strain elastic modulus), E(p), with age over the human lifespan in 1116 arteries.

in individuals without significant carotid bifurcation lesions, tripling from about 40 kPa at age 10 to about 120 kPa by age 40. The variability is great, however, and for young people around 20 years of age, varies from a low value of about 30 kPa to over 120 kPa. To determine how much of this variability is due to measurement error, and how much is related to true differences in the stiffness of arteries, reliability studies were conducted.

Table 1 provides a comparison of the reliability of measurements of diastolic blood pressure, a common risk factor, and E(p) made on participants in the Bogalusa Heart Study with a two-week interval between measurements (12). The final column shows that, in both cases, the variability within the population is more than three times that which can be attributed to measurement variability alone within individuals. The two parameters are thus essentially equivalent in terms of reliability of measurement.

Table 1. Comparison of the Reliability of Measurements of Diastolic Blood Pressure and E(P)

Bogalusa Heart Study

	Mean	Standard Deviations		
		Inter-Individual	Intra-Individual	Inter/Intra
DBP (mmHg)	62.5	11.8	3.6	3.3
E(p)	61.0	17.7	5.2	3.4

One could next ask, since this variability in
arterial stiffness is real, might it possess a significant
genetic component? One way of approaching this question is
to compare the correlation of E(p) in sibling-pairs and non-
sibling pairs after matching for age and gender. Results
of such a comparison in teenagers in Figure 4 shows insignificant correlation of 0.72 in sibling pairs. Thus a strong
genetic component is suggested by these results.

Another genetic-related question arises of great
importance to the topic of this meeting: can young people
with elevated carotid artery stiffness be linked to clinical
disease based on genetic background? A way of approaching
this question is to compare the relative frequency of parental myocardial infarction of offspring having low E(p)
values to those having high E(p) values. Results of such
a comparison involving the lower and upper tertiles of E(p)
in Figure 5 showed a more than five-fold higher frequency
of parental MI in young people with stiffer arteries,
suggesting a possible genetic link of E(p) with CVD (12).

In addition to parental MI, a number of other CVD risk
factors have shown significant associations with E(p):
including age, gender (male arteries stiffer than females),
race (blacks stiffer than whites), and a combination of
elevated total serum cholesterol and systolic blood pressure
(12). In fact, on the average, a black male, with elevated
TSC and SBP at age 13 has an artery which is 25% stiffer
than a white female with low TSC and SBP. This is equivalent, in terms of the average increase with age, of a seven
year difference in effective arterial age.

Much attention has also been paid recently to aerobic
exercise as a possible contributor to cardiovascular health,
particularly in persons over 40 years of age, and ultrasonic
methods now permit possible associations with arterial wall
function to be studied. In one such study conducted at Wake
Forest University in 1984, we found that chronic exercisers
who had run at least 25 miles a week for at least two years
had significantly more elastic carotid arteries compared to
sedentary individuals, independent of gender, as shown in
Figure 6. In addition, as shown in Figure 1C, the diameter
change waveform in chronic exercisers is characteristically

CORRELATION OF E(p) in
NON-SIBLINGS AND SIBLINGS
MATCHED FOR AGE AND GENDER
AGE: 10 - 19 YEARS

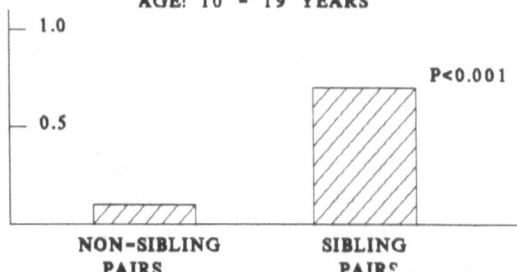

ASSOCIATION OF E(P) WITH
PARENTAL HISTORY OF DISEASE
BOGALUSA HEART STUDY

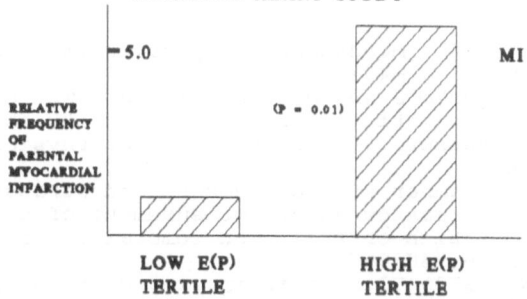

ASSOCIATION OF E(P) WITH
AEROBIC EXERCISE IN BOTH SEXES
(25 MILES PER WEEK FOR 2 YEARS)
AGE: 40-49 YEARS

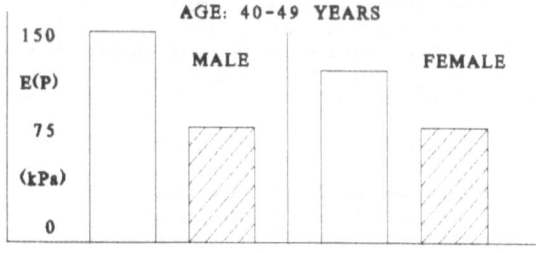

Figure 4.(upper) Comparison of the correlation in arterial
stiffness, E(p), among siblings and non-siblings, matched
by age and gender.
Figure 5.(center) Comparison of relative frequency of
parental myocardial infarction with carotid artery stiffness
in a subpopulation participating in the Bogalusa Heart Study.
Figure 6.(lower) Comparison of arterial stiffness in sedentary individuals and chronic exercisers of both genders.

different from sedentary individuals. These results demonstrate the potential value of research in this area to help
define exercise prescriptions to meet a variety of health-
related objectives.

Over the next several years, studies on populations
from five communities are being planned as: (A) a component
of the Bogalusa Heart Study in Louisiana, where 200, 10-17-
year-olds will be studied; and as (B) a component of the
Atherosclerosis Risk In Communities study in Maryland,
Minnesota, Mississippi and North Carolina, where 16,000
45-64-year-olds will be studied. These data will provide
an important resource for assessing risk for CVD and better
understanding of the atherosclerotic disease process.

REFERENCES

1. Dobrin PB (1978) Mechanical properties of arteries.
   Physiol Rev 58:397-459
2. Arndt JO, Klauske J and Mersch F (1968) The diameter
   of the intact carotid artery in man and its change
   with pulse pressure. Pflugers Arch Ges Physiol
   300:230-240
3. Mozersky DJ, Sumner DS, Hokanson DE and Strandness
   DE Jr (1972) Transcutaneous measurement of the
   elastic properties of the human femoral artery.
   Circulation 46:948-955
4. Buschman W (1973) Ultrasonic imaging of arterial wall
   echoes. Ultrasound Med Biol 1:33-43
5. Lunt MJ, Rueben JR, du Boulay EPGH (1978) Preliminary
   report on some ultrasonic methods for detecting carotid
   artery disease. J Med Eng Technol 2:289:297
6. Riley WA, Barnes RW, Schey HM (1984) An approach to
   the noninvasive periodic assessment of arterial
   elasticity in the young. Prev Med 13:169-184
7. Imura T (1985) Non-invasive measurement of the elastic
   properties of the abdominal aorta and the analysis of
   aging change. Hokkaido Tgaku Zasshi 60:653-661
8. Reneman RS, van Merode T, Hick P et al. (1986) Age-
   related changes in carotid wall properties in men.
   Ultrasound in Med & Biol 12:465-471
9. Guyton AC (1981) Textbook of Medical Physiology, 6th
   edition, W.B. Saunders, Philadelphia
10. McDonald DA (1974) Blood Flow in Arteries. Williams
    and Wilkins, Baltimore
11. Borow KM, Newburger JW (1982) Noninvasive estimation
    of central aortic pressure using the oscillometric
    method for analyzing systemic artery pulsatile blood
    flow. Amer Heart J 103:879-886
12. Riley WA, Freedman DS, Higgs NA et al. (1986) Decreas-
    ed arterial elasticity associated with cardiovascular
    risk factors in the young. Arteriosclerosis 6:378-386

47

Role of Doppler Ultrasound in Monitoring Atherosclerotic Disease Progression

D.E. Strandness, Jr.

INTRODUCTION

The atherosclerotic plaque produces problems by two possible mechanisms: 1) a reduction in blood flow, and 2) release of materials either attached to the surface or from the contents of the plaque itself. For vascular beds such as the lower extremity, the visceral arteries and the renal circulation, the sequelae of the lesion depends primarily upon the extent of narrowing and its effect on blood flow to the organ. This occurs when the plaque has reached sufficient size to reduce both the perfusion pressure and flow beyond the lesion. This degree of narrowing is commonly referred to as a "critical stenosis".

While there is no doubt that emboli originating from the plaque can also produce problems in these vascular beds, the clinical consequences are appreciated only when the total amount of the embolic material is sufficient to obstruct vital end arteries which are essential in maintaining tissue nutrition. An example in the limbs is referred to as the blue toe syndrome where the digital arteries may become occluded and lead to rest pain and ulceration. It is also known that microemboli to the kidney and gut can occur but a clinical event such as hematuria, or intestinal infarction is a very uncommon event.

In the case of the brain, the situation is different because of the critical nature of neural tissue and its sensitivity to even small areas of ischemia. The most

common and easily recognized manifestation of intermittent
cerebral ischemia is amaurosis fugax where the embolic
fragments may be observed in the retinal circulation. It
is also known that an acute reduction in carotid blood flow
can also lead to cerebral infarction as a second mechanism
for the production of transient ischemic attacks and
strokes.

Atherosclerosis and Clinical Practice

It is now accepted that the lesion responsible for most
clinical events is the complicated plaque. The earlier
lesions with an intact fibrous cap are rarely the cause of
events. At what stage and for what reason(s), the fibrous
plaque degenerates to form the dangerous lesion is unknown.
Thus, at the present time, it is reasonable to assume that
a patient presenting with symptoms or signs of atherosclerosis will have the far advanced lesion as the underlying
cause.

The scenario which is repeated daily throughout the
world is as follows:

1. The presenting complaints - if these are compatible
with a tentative diagnosis of atherosclerosis, the patient
will undergo arteriography - to define the location and
extent of the involvement.

2. The therapy to be employed depends upon several
factors. Regardless of the therapeutic approach, the
follow-up consists of assessing the extent to which the
symptoms and signs have been relieved.

3. Repeat arteriography to assess the results of
therapy is rarely done unless the clinical sequelae demand
it. Thus, an asymptomatic patient is rarely studied again.
This produces an interesting and frustrating situation for
the physician. Disease progression is rarely recognized
or documented leaving the feeling - which is obviously
incorrect - that atherosclerosis is a relatively static
process or at best progresses very slowly. This has led to
the common concept that atherosclerosis requires years to
develop and further years to progress after it is discovered.
While this may be true, it has never been proven.

The Role of Noninvasive Testing

None of the indirect (non-imaging) noninvasive tests are suitable for documenting disease progression. This is due to the fact that they become positive only for high grades of disease. There is no gradation with reference to the degrees of involvement. They are either positive or negative. Thus, of all the testing modalities available only the direct imaging and Doppler techniques hold any promise in monitoring disease progression.

While it seems intuitively obvious that an imaging approach would provide the best, most certain method of monitoring changes over time, this is not necessarily the case. Unfortunately, the atherosclerotic plaque is irregular, non-axisymmetric and unpredictable in the pathway it takes to reach an advanced stage. In addition, as noted above, it is not a uniform structure that easily lends itself to standard imaging approaches. This process is further compounded by the fact that calcium is a regular almost constant constituent of the advanced plaque. This poses a potentially serious problem for ultrasound since the presence of calcium can seriously affect our ability to visualize all components and dimensions of the lesion. The acoustical shadowing which may result is always a potential problem that can limit the use of ultrasonic imaging.

While there have been improvements in ultrasonic image processing, they are not yet to the point where "image alone" analysis is sufficiently accurate to permit reliable monitoring of changes over time. This is also true for angiography which is the most commonly used diagnostic test. Because of the risks of angiography, it is unlikely that this method will ever be used to assess the change in atherosclerotic lesions over time.

Our approach to this problem has been different. While the nature of the plaque with its constituents and covering are critical determinants of outcome, there is little evidence that we can reliably monitor these over time by any current imaging method.

On the other hand, the fact that any change in the dimensions of plaque has to result in a change in the velocity in the narrowest portion of the lesion is important.

If we can selectively sample from the point of the highest velocity in the vicinity of a plaque, this must represent its narrowest portion. In addition, any further change in the dimensions of the stenosis will have to produce a corresponding change in velocity.

On the basis of these hypotheses, we have utilized changes in velocity in the narrowest portion of a vessel as the most sensitive and objective measures we currently have for progression of the disease (1,2). Our only experience to the moment is with the carotid artery.

Carotid Bifurcation Atherosclerosis

While stroke remains the third most common cause of death in this country, the role of the carotid bifurcation with atherosclerosis is in considerable dispute, particularly with regard to management. As noted above, these lesions may produce problems by either release of emboli from areas of ulceration or when the internal carotid artery becomes totally occluded secondary to acute thrombosis.

The risk of carotid atheroma to the patient depends upon several factors which are as follows:

1. the lesions responsible for symptoms are the complicated plaques. These are the fully developed, advanced lesions;

2. in the patients with TIA's and strokes secondary to emboli, it is likely that the risk tends to diminish with the passage of time presumably because the lesion has the capability to heal;

3. the risk for an ischemic event is on the order of 4%/year when the patient's carotid disease is discovered incidentally by the presence of a bruit;

4. the natural history is unknown.

The Asymptomatic Patient with a Carotid Bruit (3)

When the patient is found to have a carotid bruit, several questions are always raised: 1) is it secondary to a high grade stenosis?; 2) what is its potential for causing trouble?; 3) should we be aggressive in working it up in terms of the location and severity of the lesion?; and 4) how should it be managed?

To investigate the relationship between disease progression and clinical events, we carried out two prospective
trials examining patients with disease documented by Duplex
scanning. The two populations included the asymptomatic
patient with a cervical bruit and the carotid artery on
the side contralateral to endarterectomy. All patients
underwent the studies in our laboratory which has a standard
approach and protocol for studying this problem.

All patients were classified into one of the following
categories based upon the detected velocity changes in the
narrowed region of the plaque: 1) normal; 2) 1-15%
diameter reduction; 3) 16-49% stenosis; 4) 50-79%;
5) 80-89%; and 6) total occlusion. We have been involved
in several prospective validation trials to evaluate the
accuracy of the velocity changes as predictors of the degree
of stenosis. The sensitivity of Duplex scanning exceeds 95%.
Its specificity is currently in the range of 90% (1). It
must be noted that when false positive studies occur, the
error is in predicting minimal disease and not high grade
lesions. The criteria used for each category of disease
has been published so will not be dealt with further.

The Contralateral Carotid Artery and the Asymptomatic
Patient (4)

There are often differences in the extent of involvement
when two sides are the site of atherosclerosis. In addition,
the potential of these lesions for causing problems may also
be different. A useful patient population to study are those
patients who have undergone endarterectomy on one side only.
To examine this issue, we serially studied 134 such patients
with duplex scanning extending up to 48 months. There were
nine deaths, none of which were stroke related. By life
table analysis, the mean annual rate of progression for all
categories of disease was 12.6% and 7.6% for progression to
a greater than 50% reduction in diameter. Symptoms occurred
in 13 patients for an overall incidence of 10% giving a mean
annual rate estimated at 5%. These were all TIA's - there
were no strokes. There was a strong relationship between
the development of symptoms and the presence of a greater
than 80% stenosis either at the initial examination or
secondary to disease progression.

In a parallel study, we investigated the natural history of carotid atheroma in 167 asymptomatic patients with cervical bruits followed up to 36 months. During follow-up there were 10 patients who became symptomatic (six with TIA's, four with strokes). In eight patients, the development of symptoms was associated with progression of the disease. The mean annual rate of progression to a greater than 50% of stenosis was 8%. For the entire study group, the mean annual rate for symptoms was 4%.

It was significant that for outcome, there was a significant relationship between degree of stenosis and endpoints. The presence of or progression to greater than 80% stenosis, was highly correlated with the development of TIA's, strokes and total occlusion of the internal carotid artery (p = 0.00001) (Figure 1). The major risk factors associated with progression were diabetes mellitus, age (< 65 years) and cigarette smoking.

DISCUSSION

These ultrasonic studies utilized velocity changes recorded from a stenosis as the best marker for disease progression. However, this approach provides no insight concerning the pathologic changes responsible for the evolution of the lesion. Nonetheless, the changes in velocity appeared to be a more accurate marker for the degree of stenosis and its change over time than ultrasonic imaging of the plaque.

The accuracy of using velocity indices to document the degree of stenosis has been covered in previous studies (1). While there has been uncertainty for the classification between normal and the minimal disease categories, this approach is very accurate for higher grades of stenosis and total occlusion.

The surprises in these studies can be summarized as follows:

1. carotid artery disease progression occurs at a rate which exceeds that expected on clinical grounds alone. For example, a progression rate of 8%/year from less than to a greater than 50% stenosis is rather phenomenal;

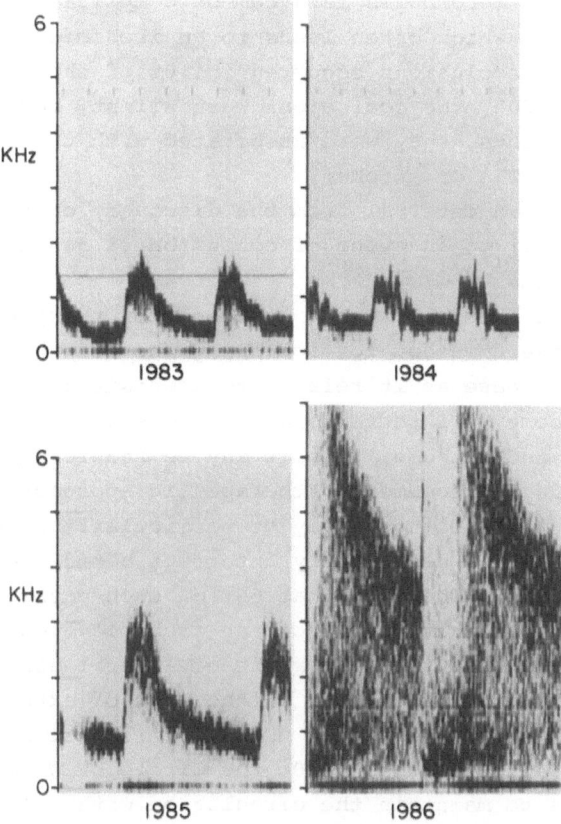

Figure 1. These Doppler spectra were recorded from the
right internal carotid artery of a 65-year-old woman who had
undergone a carotid endarterectomy on the left side in 1983.
In 1983 both the arteriogram and the velocity data were
nearly normal. By 1985, there was an apparent increase in
the peak systolic velocity which represented a real change.
However, when restudied in 1986, the result was very dramatic
with both the peak systolic and end diastolic velocities
compatible with a greater than 80% stenosis. This was confirmed by repeat arteriography followed by endarterectomy.

2. in some patients, the progression may occur very
rapidly. For example, in one of our patients with a minimal
lesion (1-15%), progression to an asymptomatic total occlusion occurred within a 12-month period;

3. there appears to be a relationship between the
degree of stenosis and outcome. The very tight lesions (> 80%)
were the most likely to lead to TIA's, strokes and total
occlusions. This should not be surprising since it is now

well known that thrombosis is a common complication in atherosclerosis which often leads to an ischemic event;

4. total occlusions occurred in 10% of the asymptomatic patients. In 60%, the occlusions were silent, but in the remaining patients, they were associated with the development of either TIA or stroke;

5. the mean interval from the discovery of the tight stenosis (> 80%) to an event of occlusion is quite short, being 4.9 months.

What does this all mean? At least for the present it appears we have a method for following the step-wise progression of disease as it relates to stenosis diameter and clinical outcome. If there is a relationship between degree of narrowing and outcome, then it may be feasible to utilize these criteria to recommend a therapeutic approach. For example, the tight stenosis may be particularly susceptible to thrombosis which may acutely interrupt blood flow and lead to ischemia. The fact that 60% of such patients may sustain this complication without an ischemic event further supports the important role for the collateral circulation in maintaining nutrient flow even in the fact of extensive extracranial arterial disease. However, it must not be forgotten that in the remaining 40% the Circle of Willis may be inadequate to maintain the circulation with resulting TIA's and strokes. Unfortunately, we have no methods at the moment which can be used to reliably assess the status of the Circle of Willis.

REFERENCES

1. Langlois YE, Roederer GO, Chan ATW, et al. (1983) The concordance between pulsed Doppler/Spectrum analysis and angiography. Ultrasound in Med and Biol 9:51-63.
2. Roederer GO, Langlois YE, Jager A, et al. (1984) A simple spectral parameter for accurate classification of severe carotid disease. Bruit 6:174-178.
3. Roederer GO, Langlois YE, Jager KA, et al. (1984) The natural history of carotid arterial disease in asymptomatic patients with cervical bruits. Stroke 15:605-613.
4. Roederer GO, Langlois YE, Lusiane L, et al. (1984) Natural history of carotid artery disease on the side contralateral to endarterectomy. J Vasc Surg 1:62-72.

48
Ultrasonic Evaluation of Arterial Intima and Media Thickness: Development and Validation of Methodology

Paolo Pignoli

Atherosclerosis results in arterial wall thickening. The evaluation of lesion geometry and the monitoring of changes thus entail measuring wall thickness (1,2). This can be accomplished in two ways (Figure 1). The direct approach involves measuring arterial wall tunicas from pathology specimens. Plaque thickness can also be evaluated indirectly, e.g., contrast angiography, from measurements of the residual lumen, by comparing the diameter at the site of the lesion with than presumed to be the normal diameter. This indirect approach allows calculation of lesion extent into the lumen. However, this method has several known limitations and drawbacks.

Arterial dilation during atherosclerosis progression (3) or secondary to aging may complicate what has previously been considered a straightforward inverse relationship between

Supported in part by CNR grant 85.01493.57.115. Special thanks to M.G. Bond, Department of Anatomy, J.F. Toole, Department of Neurology, and Dr. W. McKinney and Dr. W. Riley, Center for Medical Ultrasound and Department of Neurology, Bowman Gray School of Medicine, Winston-Salem, North Carolina; Dr. R. Paoletti, Institute of Pharmacological Sciences, and Dr. T. Longo, Department of Surgery, University of Milan; Dr. V. Villa, Merate Hospital; Professor A. Satori, Emeritus Chief of Surgery and Principal Investigator, Merate Atherosclerosis Prevention Project, Merate Hospital; the Carle Family and the Carle and Montanari Spa; and finally, to my wife, Antonella.

direct   indirect

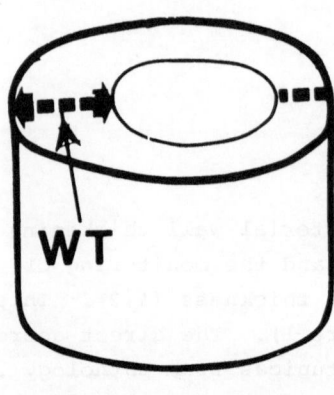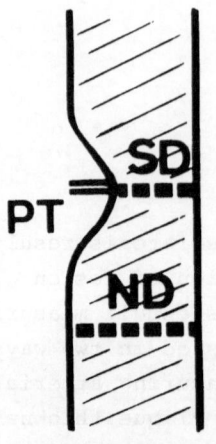

PT = ND-SD

Figure 1. The direct measurement of arterial wall thickness (WT) on the left versus the indirect evaluation of plaque thickness (PT) on the right. This is calculated from measurement of normal diameter (ND) and stenotic diameter (SD).

wall thickness and residual lumen. Percent lumen stenosis may therefore, not be a valid index of the extent or severity of an atherosclerotic lesion. Vessel tapering and the complex geometry which characterized arterial bifurcations may also produce significant errors in stenosis calculations (4). There are some other disadvantages which are important but do not involve measurement problems. Diffuse arterial wall thickening can occur without localized stenosis (5). Four different arterial conditions are possible (Figure 2): normal wall, diffuse wall thickening, a combimation of diffuse wall thickening and localized stenosis and localized stenosis alone. At present the relationship between diffuse wall thickening and localized plaque is not known. This relationship along with the effect of risk factors and aging on

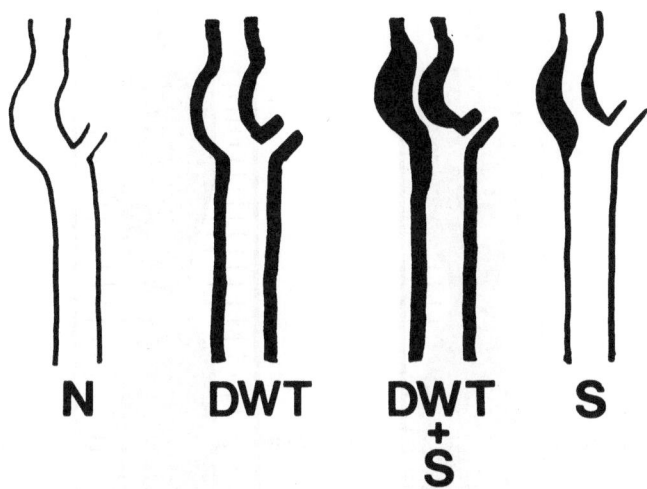

Figure 2. Four different conditions of the artery wall
(common carotid artery with bifurcation): normal (N), diffuse
wall thickening (DWT), diffuse wall thickening with stenosis
(DWT+S) and stenosis along (S).

diffuse wall thickening require further definition in prospective investigations. The clinical significance of diffuse
wall thickening is unknown, but it appears to effect arterial
wall dynamics and left ventricular afterload (6).

The concept of a normal artery as shown by angiography (Figure 3) may be adequate for understanding the
biology of atherosclerosis. The artery wall may be diseased
and thickened exactly where the lumen is indicated as normal
because it is large when compared to a stenotic site. However
the concept of normal diameter based on lumen characteristics
alone may be very different from that of normal artery wall.
This may be defined by taking into account other locations of
the same artery, the same location at a different time, other

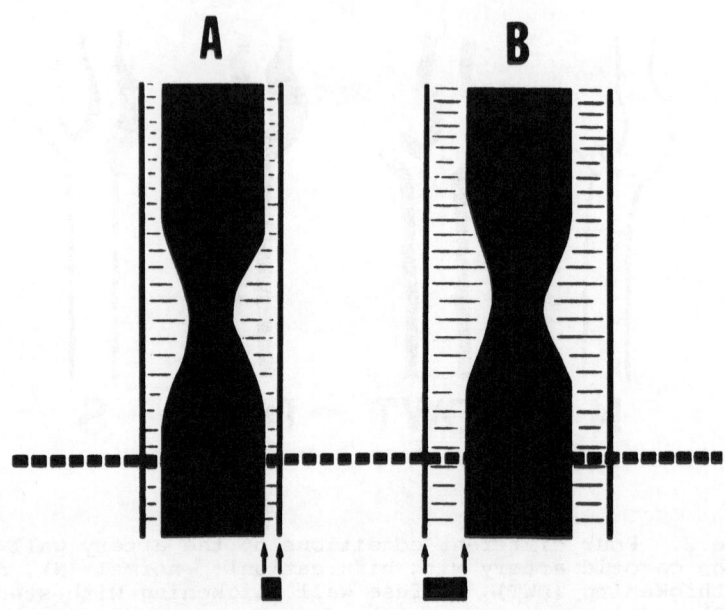

Figure 3. Two different conditions of an artery generating the same angiographic appearance. In B, at the level of the dotted line, the wall is thicker than in A.

locations of other arteries in the same subject, different subjects of the same age, etc., and compare these.

Any method of evaluating arterial wall thickness directly *in vivo* could be potentially very useful. At the American Heart Association meeting in Silver Springs queries arose (7) about the feasibility of evaluating and measuring wall thickness with ultrasound B mode imaging; some previous investigations having suggested that this might be practicable.

Methodology Development

The intimal and medial acoustic impedence has been shown to be relatively constant with reflection coefficients being similar to those reported for muscle (8). Stepwise acoustic impedence changes at the luminal interface was reported by

Murakami and Beretsky (8,9) and Barber (10) using an ultrasonic microprobe. These studies evaluated the directivity
of interfaces and focal areas of homogenous tissue within
the artery wall, and found high amplitude angle dependent
echoes at the water/fibromuscular cap, at the adventitia/
media interface and within the adventitia. The media/plaque
transition did not generate such type of direction sensitive
echoes. These findings, in part explain the influence of
incident beam position on echo amplitude and B-mode image
quality of the arterial wall.

Several studies have evaluated the acoustical properties
of normal and diseased arterial walls (11-15). The range of
ultrasound velocities (1492-1558 m/sec) found by Greanleaf
may be the source of a 4% error in wall thickness measurement
using B-mode imaging (11). Calcium and cholesterol arterial
wall content have also been found to be determinant factors
influencing acoustic properties (12-14). Grossly calcified
lesions may diffract ultrasound and completely attenuate
its propagation (12). The correlation between high amplitude
echoes with acoustic shadows for calcified lesions has been
reported by Wolverson (16) who showed that low level echoes
were generated by fibrous connective tissues whereas high
amplitude echoes without shadowing were observed in sudanophilic stained areas.

Others (17,18) have reported the presence of an intimal
echogenic line along the surface of the carotid artery wall
in vivo. The anatomic nature of this line, however, has not
been determined. Bond et al. (19), validating a real time
B-mode instrument *in vitro* and measuring cross sections of
human common carotid arteries, found a correlation coefficient
of 0.30 between the gross pathology and the ultrasound wall
thickness values. This "unexplained variability" was considered to be due to the limited resolution of the ultrasound
unit (5 MHz), and to the relatively small size of the
arteries as well as to other artifactual and interpretative
errors. Better correlation between gross pathology and
ultrasound wall thickness values has been reported (20) with
a precise description of the interpretative criteria which

allow wall thickness measurement to be carried out on the
artery wall B-mode image.

B-Mode Imaging Instrumentation. Concepts Relevant for Application to Arterial Thickness Measurements

Echoes are generated at interfaces where the density
and elasticity of the medium changes. In the current biomedical application of B-mode imaging, the main source of
information is represented by shapes defined by echoes
originating from high amplitude angle dependent specular
reflections (21). These echoes are generated by interfaces
with a radius greater than ultrasound wavelength, and are
determined by relatively macroscopic structures, such as the
tunica intima and media. Smaller structures, i.e., cells and
macromoles, generate very low amplitude echoes (22).

The time necessary for an echo to reflect back to the
transducer is measurable and allows the determination of
interface depth. Axial resolution is "the minimum spacing
of two reflectors along the axis of the ultrasound beam at
which two reflectors can be resolved and remain resolved
for all the greater spacings using either the barely
resolvable or clearly resolvable criterion" (23). Axial
resolution depends essentially on transducer frequency and
bandwidth which determine pulse length. This acoustic and
electric parameter is influended by receiver gain and by
impedence mismatch at a specific interface (24). Commercially available broadband transducers allow generation of
very short pulses, i.e., 0.3-0.4 mm, for a mid-frequency
range of 5-8 MHz (Figure 4). When a second pulse is reflected
at a deeper interface, if very closely spaced, it may occur
within the tail of the first pulse. The second pulse may be
detected as separate one if the distance between the two
interfaces is equal to or larger than the axial resolution
(Figure 4).

Precision is a concept quite different from resolution
(24). Axial precision defines the minimum distance along
the ultrasound beam depth axis that can be detected. For
example, in the upper panel of Figure 4, the minimum

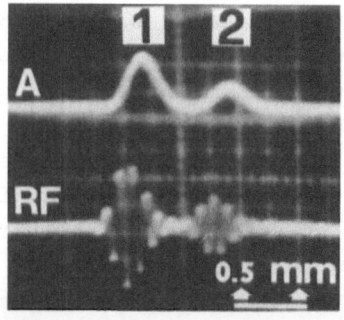

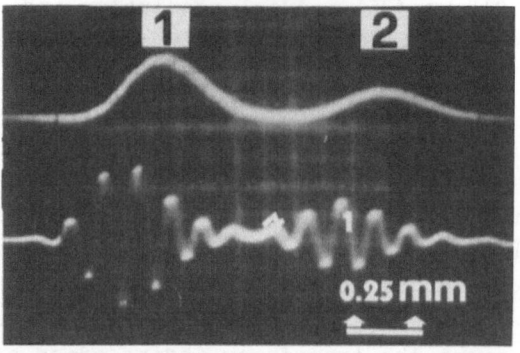

Figure 4. Amplitude mode (A) and radiofrequency (RF) oscilloscope presentation of signals representing two echoes (1,2)
generated by two specular interfaces located at different
depths along the ultrasound beam. The different time base
scale of the two panels is shown.

detectable distance is larger than that of the lower panel,
because of different magnification obtained. Precision depends
essentially on object magnification, the light spot spread
function, and ultrasound speed in the tissue (24,25). Obviously precise measurements can only be performed on interfaces
which spaced equal to or exceed the axial resolution. In our
laboratory, A-mode and B-mode precisions have been found to
be 0.018 and 0.090 mm respectively when measuring a sharp

object (a polythene pipe in water) with a 0.5 microsec/div
calibrated Tektronix Oscilliscope and a 24" standard B/W
monitor (where a 2.0 mm real distance is magnified to
21.5 mm). The reading error was found to be ± 2.0 mm in
21.5 mm equal to ± 4.6%. A more sophisticated system using
both digital and optical processing for magnification, pseudo-
color for display and computerized morphometry for measurement is now available and allows measurement of combined
intima plus media thickness with a reading resolution (precision) or ± 0.015 mm (26). Axial resolution and axial
precision depend also on lateral resolution and beam thickness (27).

Validity
    An artery is geometrically similar to a polythene pipe.
In a longitudinal B-scan image, four interfaces are present
which define the wall boundary (Figure 5). Cross sectional or
transverse B-scan images do not allow visualization of the
lateral walls and have less imaging potential (Figure 6).
The distance between the transducer facing edges of two lines
corresponds to wall thickness. The thickness of a single
echogenic line, i.e., an interface, has no relationship to
wall thickness by itself, and depends only on pulse length
which varies depending on time gain settings (24).
    In a similar way two lines are expected to border the
artery wall. If a pressure perfused common carotid artery
is scanned in a tank of saline at room temperature a typical
and reproducible B-mode image is obtained (Figure 7). The
superficial and deep walls can be seen as echogenic complexes
separated by the anechoic lumen. The far wall shows two
parallel echogenic lines separated by an hypoechoic space
(20,28).
    This double line pattern was found in all the common
carotid arteries evaluated *in vitro* and in all the relatively
normal aorta specimens studied (28). When the artery wall
was the site of an atherosclerotic plaque the double line
pattern was present and typical in 56% of the specimens,
present but complex in 24% and absent in 20%. When

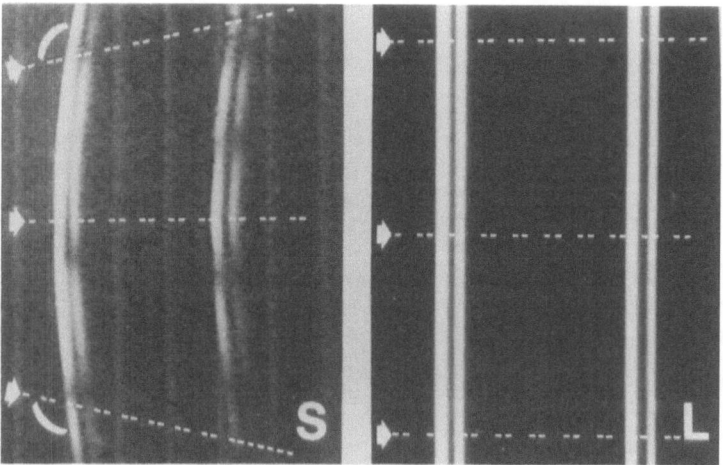

Figure 5. B-mode image of longitudinal scan of a polythene pipe in a water bath. In the left panel (S) the distortion introduced by a mechanical sector scanner (Biosound) is apparent as compared with the image of the same object generated with a linear array (L).

calcification and fibrosis are present, strong echoes, in some cases with shadowing occur, in the usually anechoic interline space, and the outer line may be undetectable. The same B-mode image with the double line pattern was obtained in blood as well as in saline during *in vitro* experiments using a wide range of gain settings. This indicates that only an unnecessarily high gain setting can fill the interline space. Otherwise this space shows a remarkably constant thickness.

Experiments were performed (28) to identify the anatomic structures generating the two echogenic lines in the double line pattern. The amplitude of these echoes was found to be closely dependent on the incident beam angle, with high values for orthogonal incidence (Figure 8). This means

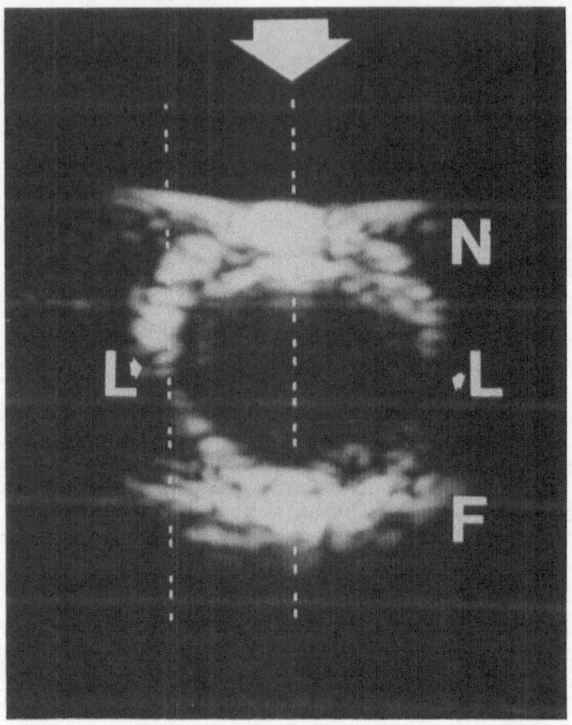

Figure 6. B-mode image of the cross sectional scan of a polythene pipe. Note the absence of the lateral (L) walls even at high gain settings which worsen the lateral resolution at the near (N) and far (F) walls.

macroscopic structures with a relatively large radius (8,21) like the arterial tunicas are responsible for the interfaces generating those angle-dependent echoes rather than very small interfaces like cells or macromolecular fibers. Dissection experiments (28) performed on the intima showed that the inner line is generated by the lumen-intimal transition, while removal of the adventitia was followed by the

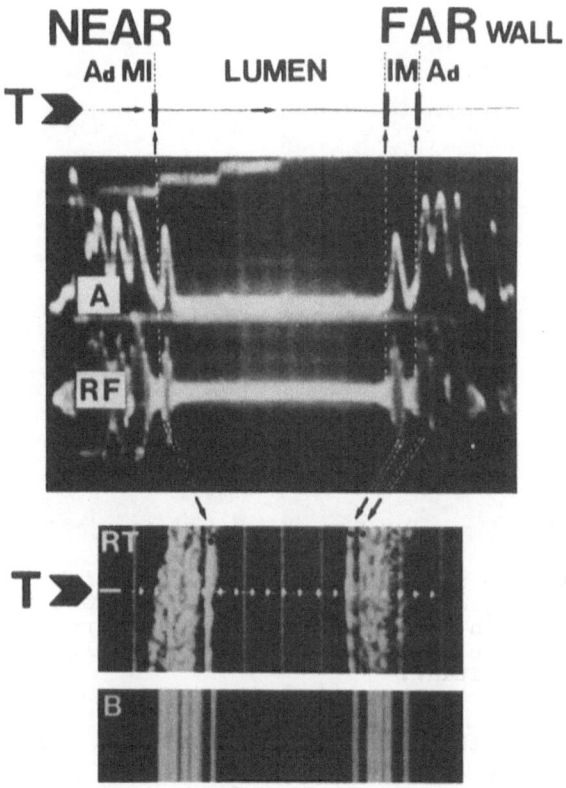

Figure 7.   Top panel: A-mode (A) and radiofrequency (RF) oscilloscope presentation of the echoes generated by inter- faces present in a normal pressure perfused common carotid artery in a water bath.   Lower panel: B-mode presentation of the echoes present in the single ultrasound beam line shown in the top panel.   The position of this beam is defined by the T line in the middle panel, representing the B-mode real time (RT) image resulting from the scanning of the beam.   IM = intima plus media, Ad = adventitia, T = transducer.

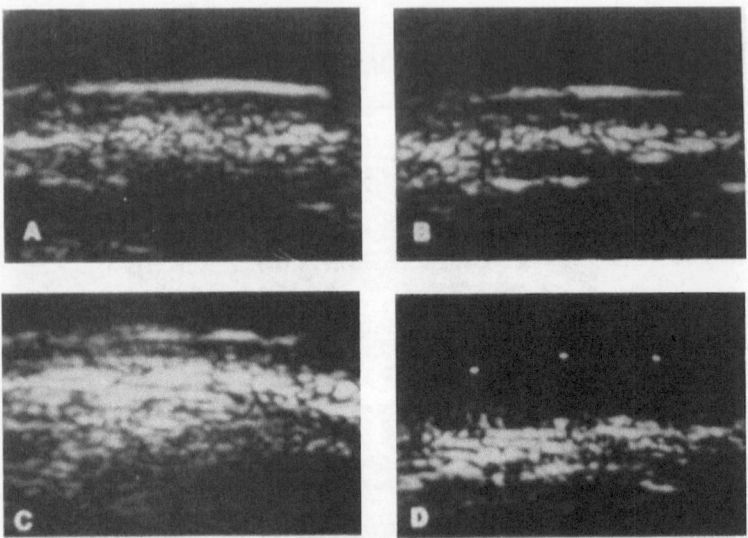

Figure 8. B-mode image of the artery wall with different
incident beam angles. From A to D the incident angle becomes
less orthogonal in relation to the intima surface. The inner
line is more angle dependent that the outer line (corresponding to the adventitia).

disappearance of the outer line. This outer line is therefore generated by the innermost layer of the adventitia.
In order to corroborate these qualitative findings, the
distance between the transducer facing edges of the two
echogenic lines was measured and compared in each sample
with measurements of the thickness of each tunica and combinations of tunicas determined from gross pathology and/or
histology (Figure 9). The best correlation was found with
the intima plus media combination. The other tunicas and
their combinations showed lower correlations with ultrasound
measurements. These data (28) again support the hypothesis
that at the far wall (Figure 7) the distance between the
two echogenic lines is equivalent to the intima plus media
thickness.

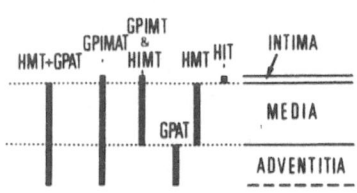 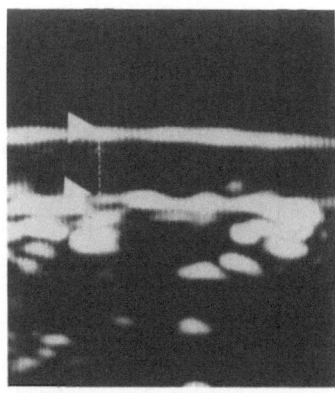

Figure 9. The right panel represents the typical B-mode
image of the arterial wall. Dotted line between white
triangles = B-mode imaging intima plus media thickness.
On the left a schematic representation of the histology (H)
or gross pathology (GP) measured intima (I), media (M),
adventitia (A) thickness (T) and their combinations.

At the level of the near arterial wall (Figure 7) the
interfaces sequence encountered by the incident ultrasound
pulse is very different when compared to that of the far
wall. Instead of the lumen-intima-media-adventitia interfaces sequence, these are present in inverse order within
the near wall. Echoes generated by the innermost fibers
of the adventitia extend into the media (deeper in relation
to pulse propagation) (Figure 7). The adventitia/media
interface cannot be defined in any way within the near
wall. The acoustically silent media and lumen allow the
identification of the echoes generated by the media/intima

or intima/lumen interfaces. The transducer facing edge of the echogenic line, resulting from these echoes in B-mode presentation, indicates the location of this interface. The thickness of this line depends only on pulse-length and impedance mismatch of the interface (M-I or I-L). The convexity of the near wall determines the divergence of the reflected ultrasound beam and therefore is responsible for the low amplitude of echoes present at this location as compared to those occurring in the far wall.

It is neither easy or frequent to obtain a double line arterial pattern both within the near and far walls simultaneously. A scanning plane which is orthogonal to both near and far walls is required to generate such an image and this is difficult, because of pulsating arterial movements. Both the evaluation of residual lumen and methods for arterial diameter monitoring to measure compliance (which are based on tracking of B-mode, A-mode or rf signals during the cardiac cycle) depend on accurate detection of rapidly moving intima/lumen interfaces. (This interface does not frequently generate an echo which may disappear for some time during a cardiac cycle.) The ultrasound measurements of lumen and wall thickness should be validated *in vitro* under conditions simulating *in vivo* movement before they can be validly applied *in vivo* for research and diagnosis (29,30).

The *in vitro* accuracy of the method was tested by comparing ultrasound data with gross pathology gold standard values (28). Typical double line images showed better accuracy than complex images frequently found in atherosclerotic arteries. The method described here is therefore more accurate in evaluating normal and less diseased arterial walls. [For more severe lesions the accuracy of B-mode ultrasound for wall thickness measurement is reported to be low (31-36)].

Is the method feasible *in vivo*? To evaluate the effect of superficial tissues (skin, adipose tissue, muscles and fasciae) on the transmission of ultrasound and on the generation of the double line pattern, *in situ* experiments were performed on pressure perfused carotid arteries in cadavers.

The *in situ* B-mode intima plus media thickness measurements
performed on unexposed arteries were very close to those
obtained in the same but exposed arteries after removal of
the superficial tissues and to the *in vitro* measurements
which showed a 10% reduction owing to pressure fixation (28).
Finally, B-mode intima plus media thickness was measured in
ten young normal subjects at the lower and upper thirds of
the common carotid artery in two orthogonal planes (anteroposterior and lateral). These values did not differ from
those obtained *in vitro* with B-mode imaging, gross pathology
or histology in common carotid arteries dissected from
cadavers of subjects of the same age (28).

Reliability

In order to detect and monitor changes in arterial wall
lesions the reliability of the method must be defined so as
to differentiate a true change in the objects' geometry and
size from an error, or variability, in the measuring
technique.

All measurement apparatus tends to produce systematic
and random errors (37). In the following discussion we
shall ignore the possible occurrence of phenomena which may
induce unexpected changes in the geometry and size of the
lesions even in short term variability studies covering only
few days or hours (38). These phenomena tentatively are:
thrombus formation, local active or passive vasomotion, and
changes in mean and differential pressures and distal
vascular impedance (39).

Systematic errors of B-mode images are intrinsic to
the apparatus (27). These include errors in calibration and
registration of the x and y coordinates, errors arising from
image distortion due to beam divergence in sector scanners
(Figure 5) vis-a-vis a linear scanner, errors due to differences in lateral resolution at varying depths dependent on
the shape of the ultrasonic beam and gain settings, and other
errors (39). Investigators must be aware of these systematic
errors which need to be investigated in appropriate validation
and quality control experiments. However, until they become

really stable in time they should not influence the repeatibility of the measuring apparatus, provided that some precautions are taken, e.g., locating the object under investigation in the same position within the B-mode image during different examinations, and using instrument controls at fixed settings derived from calibration procedures performed on phantoms.

The most significant random errors encountered in evaluating the geometry of the arterial wall and measuring its size are basically caused by the almost complete lack of any objective and quantitative knowledge about the coordinates of the two-dimensional B-mode scanning plane in relation to the three-dimensional geometry of the artery. It is obvious that if an arterial lesion is eccentric rather than concentric the two-dimensional B-mode image of the arterial wall may differ considerably, depending on the angle of the scanning plane (Figure 10). Such differences may well explain much of lesion regression and progression detected by ultrasound (40). At the present time this is a very critical issue in the use of B-mode imaging *in vivo* for clinical and research applications.

Consecutive serial parallel transverse scanning planes have been used to generate a three-dimensional reconstruction of the artery (41). However, this technologically relatively simple approach may have limited potential for *in vivo* application because transverse scanning of the artery does not allow artery's lateral walls to be imaged (Figure 6). Even the near and far walls show degrading effects due to the limited lateral resolution of even the better instruments. In order to generate an image of the arterial wall and lumen with the best available resolution, multiple parallel and non-parallel longitudinal scanning planes are required. The location of these in relation to a three-dimensional coordinate system that is fixed to the patient's artery during each examination, is determined on-line by a non-mechanical probe position sensing device. An automatic or manually operated edge tracking system may be used depending on the complexity and purpose of the system. A working prototype

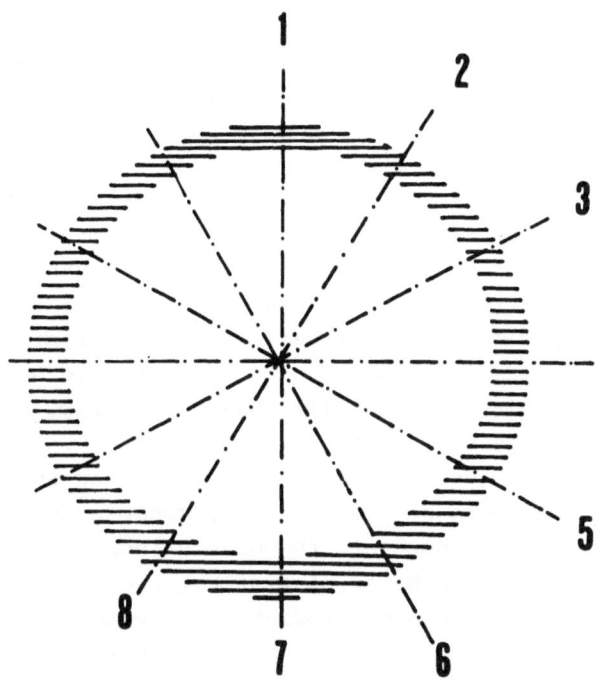

Figure 10. Effect on wall thickness measurement of different radial planes scanning an eccentrically developed thickening of the arterial wall.

has been developed in this laboratory and is now under test.

Even so, until the problem of repeatibility is solved through the equipment described, which should be ready for clinical application within the next two years or earlier, the method of arterial intimal plus medial thickness measurements with B-mode imaging should be used with an

acceptable methodological background to explore its biological and clinical potential. It may be used in single-
examination protocols, in which the variability effect is
less significant than in monitoring studies involving at
least two examinations. The effect of variability in
measurements may be decreased (but not eliminated) by
comparing the mean B-mode imaging intima plus media thickness (BMIMT) values of two groups of subjects rather than
those obtained at two different examinations in a single
subject at a specific artery location. The statistical
averaging process allows intrasubject variance to be
reduced (37). This approach will obviously allow the overall mean difference between the two groups of subjects to be
detected. Some subjects in each group will show underestimated BMIMT and others an overestimate, because of measurement
error (variability). However, the mean values measured blind
should be reliable enough for statistical averaging. If this
approach is followed in a monitoring study with two examinations the mean change will be significant whereas individual
intragroup changes may be the result of variability in
measurement and hence of no statistical value. The number
of subjects in each group will depend on the design of the
study and the required statistical power (42).

Measurement variability should be larger in subjects
with thicker arterial walls than that found in a group
with thinner intima plus media. This factor should be taken
into account in the study design in order to determine the
size of the population and control group.

With B-mode imaging the thickness of the far arterial
wall can be measured in different radial and longitudinal
planes (Figure 11) in the following arteries: common carotid
artery, carotid bifurcation, proximal internal and external
carotid arteries; abdominal aorta and common and external;
and common and superficial femoral arteries and popliteal
artery (Figures 12-14). *In vitro* the coronary arteries show
a typical double line pattern when scanned with a high
frequency/high resolution system. Some arteries can be
imaged in a larger number of planes than others. This may

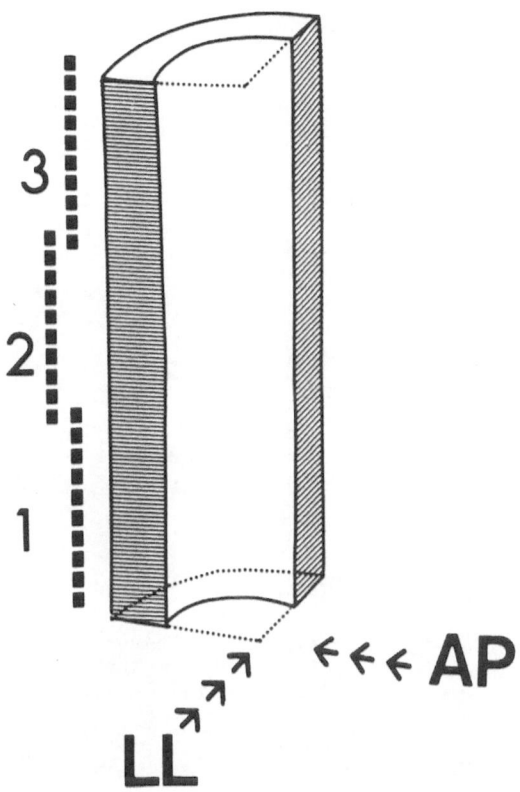

Figure 11. Schematic representation of two anteroposterior
(AP) and laterolateral (LL) radial scanning planes and
three (1,2,3) different longitudinal positions of these
planes.

be an advantage or a disadvantage depending on the questions
the study aims at answering.

The B-mode image may be transferred to a digital memory
where it may be submitted to image processing and/or quantitative evaluation (computerized morphometry). Image processing or B-mode arterial wall images is being extensively
used and is under development in this laboratory in order to
define the most suitable algorithms for extracting the most

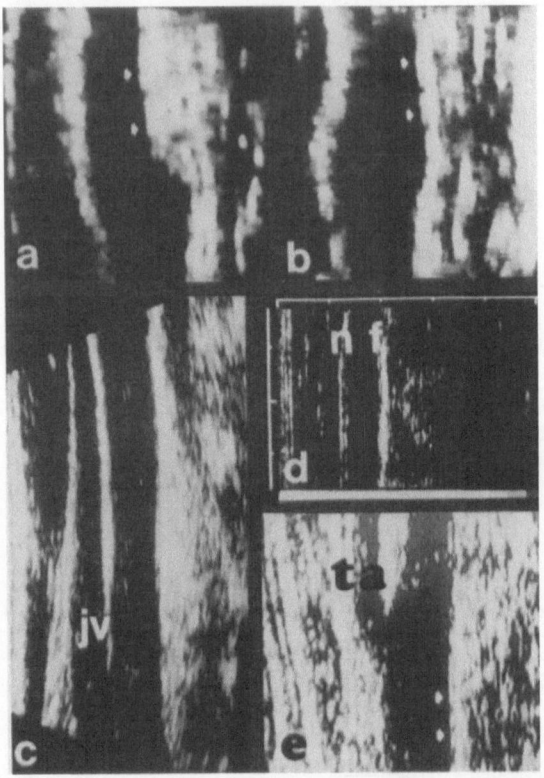

Figure 12. B-mode images of different arteries showing the
double line pattern (DLP) at the level of the far (F) wall.
In D panel the DLP is present also in the near (N) wall.
A) External carotid artery. B) Internal carotid artery.
C) Common carotid artery with jugular vein (JV). D) Superficial femoral artery. E) Popliteal artery with the
anterior tibialis artery (ta). All images obtained with
a 5 MHz Aloka SSD-210 linear array except the C) panel
obtained with a 7.5 MHz Aloka sector scanner.

information possible from the image (i.e., tissue characterization, edge enhancement, etc.) and automatic tracking of
the artery wall and lumen.

Using computerized morphometry the maximal, minimal and
mean thickness of the arterial wall can easily be measured
as can indirect parameters. The area between the two lines
of the B-mode image of the arterial wall can be digitalized,
after its contour has been defined by an operator-driven
cursor.

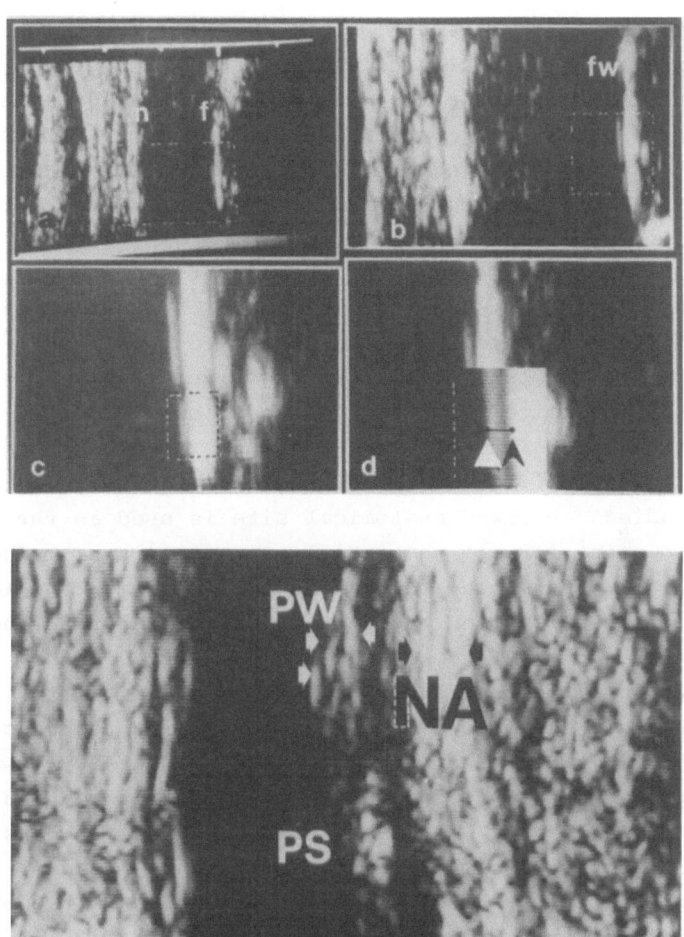

Figure 13. B-mode images of abdominal aorta near (N) and
far (F) walls at different magnifications. Images obtained
with a 5 MHz Aloka linear scanner.
Figure 14. B-mode image of the common femoral artery at
the level of a dacron prosthesis anastomosis. PW = prosthesis
wall, NA = native artery, PS = cross section of a prolene
suture line.

A critical issue regarding the reliability of these measurements is the degree of accuracy by which we can determine the location of the scanning planes along the longitudinal axis of the artery (e.g., the lower or upper third of the common carotid or superficial femoral arteries) (Figure 11). Lateral resolution of the most highly focused transducers is in the order of 0.6-1.5 mm at the focal distance with significant deterioration at other depths. An electronic device has been devised in our laboratory which allows different radial scanning planes to be accurately located along the longitudinal axis of the artery in relation to a fixed anatomical site such as the flow divider of a bifurcation or collateral branch. A more simple approach is however feasible if only a short segment of artery is required to be studied. A fixed anatomical site is used as the reference point for all the radial scanning planes. The upper margin of the clavicle can be followed with the lower border of the ultrasound probe as an anatomical reference to evaluate the lower 2-4 cm of the common carotid artery depending on probe configuration. This may be, at the present time, the only acceptable method of performing reproducible measurements in different radial planes without 3D reconstruction. The flow divider of the carotid bifurcation is present in only a few planes and cannot therefore be used as a reference point for multiple radial scanning planes. This anatomical reference site is hardly ever found in two orthogonal radial planes.

Preliminary *In vivo* Measurement Protocol

In this laboratory the following scanning protocol has been developed and used in measuring arterial wall thickness with B-mode imaging *in vivo* with an acceptable methodological approach (pending the clinical availability of a 3D reconstruction system).

1. The subjects are placed in a supine position, with the head slightly extended but without any pillow in order to increase the head-trunk angle. The head is slightly rotated with the nose at $60°$ towards the contralateral side.

2. Scanning is performed in the anteroposterior and lateral planes of the lower common carotid artery with the lower margin of the probe on the upper border of the clavicle (shoulder relaxed with arms along the thorax). A single image is obtained in each plane by optimizing beam incidence with subtle movements.

3. A goniometer is used to measure 90° between the two radial planes.

4. Only the far wall is imaged for evaluation.

5. A frozen digital image is obtained at peak diastole with a small parts 5 MHz linear array instrument. This instrument has been previously positively tested and validated *in vitro* on pathologic specimens.

6. The frozen B-mode image is projected onto the graphic tablet (HiPad-Houston Instruments) interfaced with an Apple 2e computer. An operator-driven cursor then allows the arterial wall borders to be digitalized.

7. The computer calculates the area of the defined contour and its mean thickness. Other parameters are available but have not been used in the following study.

Correlation Between Age and B-Mode Intima Plus Media Thickness

Using the protocol previously described, a preliminary *in vivo* study was performed in order to evaluate the correlation between age and B-mode intima plus media thickness (BMIMT). The population studied comprises 148 unselected consecutive patients of ages ranging between 18 and 85 years, presenting in the outpatient clinic of a general surgical department for ailments not primarily related to vascular disease. Some of the subjects displayed clear signs and symptoms of symptomatic atherosclerotic disease of the coronary, cerebral or lower limb arteries. In its present form this study does not allow conclusions to be drawn about the relationship between arterial wall thickness and other risk factors other than age and indeed this was not the aim of the study. As can be seen in Figure 15, there was a significant correlation between age and intimal plus media thickness (43) as would be expected from the available

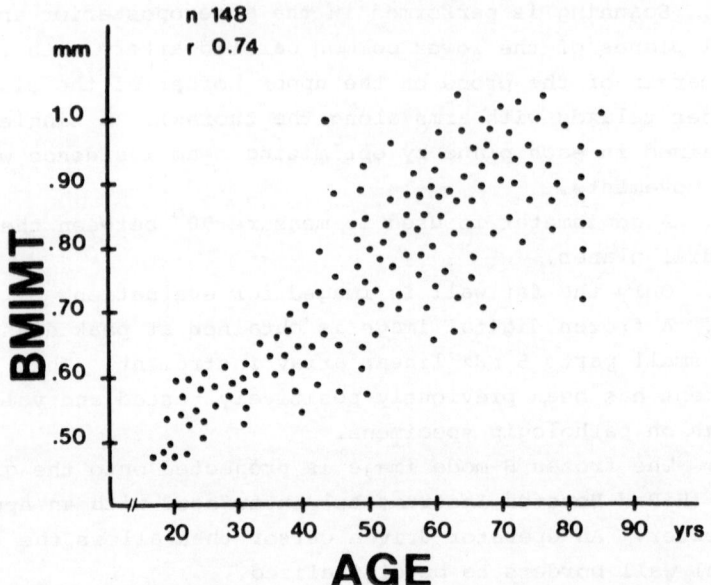

Figure 15. Correlation between age and B-mode imaging intima plus media thickness (BMIMT).

pathologic data (44,45). Widespread distribution occurs indicating a different propensity for wall thickening among subjects of the same age, and possibly the presence of "thickening factors" in different amounts. At the present time we do not know whether these are the same as those proposed and accepted for the development of localized atherosclerotic plaques or subsequent clinical ischemic events.

CONCLUSION

The method described has considerable potential for the detection and measurement of early changes in arterial intima plus media thickness which are likely to lead to more advanced and often localized atherosclerotic lesions.

This method does not exclude the application of more conventional approaches involving residual lumen evaluation with B-mode imaging, or flow disturbances detected with Doppler ultrasound. Disturbed flow may not only be an effect of an arterial lesion, but may be involved with its pathogenesis (45). More advanced Doppler technology (46) may play a significant role in the detection and quantification of local hemodynamic "risk factors" which may complete the subject risk profile in addition to the more widely accepted traditional risk factors (47).

In the near future, B-mode and Doppler imaging will find support from emerging ultrasound technology (FM imaging, RF tissue characterization, Time delay spectrometry) (48-50) to investigate atherosclerosis, and integration of this method with nuclear magnetic imaging is also expected to occur (51). At the present time, however, NMR appears to be an expensive and time consuming technique with limited potential for widespread screening application in asymptomatic subjects.

REFERENCES

1. Wissler RW (1984) Principles of pathogenesis of atherosclerosis. In: Braunwald E (ed) Heart Disease: A Textbook of Cardiovascular Medicine. Philadelphia: Saunders, p. 1183.
2. Pignoli P (1986) Ultrasound evaluation of atherosclerosis. Methodological problems and technological developments. Eur Surg Res 18:238-253.
3. Bond MG, Adams MR, Bullock BC (1981) Complicating factors in evaluating coronary artery atherosclerosis. Artery 9:21-29.
4. Forster FK, Chikos PM, Frazier JS (1985) Geometric modeling of the carotid bifurcation in humans: Implications in ultrasonic Doppler and radiologic investigations. J Clin Ultrasound 13:385-390.
5. Ferrans VJ (1980) Vascular structure. In: Patel DJ, Vaishnav RN (eds) Basic Hemodynamics and Its Role in Disease Processes. Baltimore: University Park Press, pp. 105-154.
6. McDonald DA (1974) The elastic properties of the arterial wall. In: McDonald DA (ed) Flow in Arteries. Baltimore: The Williams & Wilkins Company, pp. 238-282.

7. Insull W Jr (1983) Universal reference standards for measuring atherosclerotic lesions. The quest for the "gold standard". In: Bond MG, Insull W Jr, Glagov S, Chandler AB, Cornhill JF (eds) Clinical Diagnosis of Atherosclerosis. Quantitative Methods of Evaluation. New York: Springer Verlag, pp. 551-559.

8. Murkami R (1973) Analytical and experimental determination of acoustic reflecting characteristics of normal aortic walls. Thesis submitted in partial fulfillment of the requirements for the degree of Master of Science in Electrical Engineering, University of Washington, Seattle, Washington.

9. Beretsky I (1977) Detection and characterization of atherosclerosis in human arterial wall by Radiographic technique. An *in vitro* study. In: White D, Brown R (eds) Ultrasound in Medicine. New York: Plenum Press, V3B, p. 1597.

10. Barber FE (1977) Scattering from arterial tissue by ultrasonic microprobe. In White D, Brown R (eds) Ultrasound in Medicine. New York: Plenum Press, V3B, p. 1979.

11. Greanleaf JF, Duck FA, Samayoa WF, Johnson SA (1974) Ultrasonic data acquisition and processing system for atherosclerotic tissue characterization. In: 1974 Ultrasonics Symposium Proceedings, IEEE cat 74CH0896-1SU.

12. Hartley DJ, Strandness DE (1969) The effects of atherosclerosis on the transmission of ultrasound. J Surg Res 9:575.

13. Rooney JA, Gammel PM, Hestenes JD, Chin HP, Blankenhorn DH (1981) The use of ultrasonic spectroscopy to characterize calcified lesions. IEEE Trans Sonics Ultrasonics SU 28:219.

14. Rooney JA, Gammel PM, Hestenes JD, Chin HP, Blankenhorn DH (1982) Velocity and attenuation of sound in arterial tissue. J Acoust Soc Am 71:462.

15. Geleskie JV, Shung KK (1982) Further studies on acoustic impedance of major bovine blood vessel walls. J Acoust Soc Am 71:467.

16. Wolverson M, Bashiti H, Sunderam M, Heiberg E, Grider R (1980) Ultrasonic tissue characterization of atheromatous plaques using a high resolution real time scanner. Presented at the 25th Scientific Session, American Institute of Ultrasound in Medicine, New Orleans, September 15-19.

17. Zwiebel WJ (1982) High resolution B-mode and Duplex carotid sonography. In: Zwiebel WJ (ed) Introduction to Vascular Ultrasonography. New York: Grune & Stratton, p. 103.

18. James EM, Earnest IV, Forbes DF, Houser OW, Folger WN (1982) High resolution dynamic ultrasound imaging of the carotid bifurcation: A prospective evaluation. Radiology 144:853.

19. Bond MG, Riley WA, Barnes RW, Kaduck JM, Ball MR (1982) Validation studies of a non invasive real time B scan imaging system. In: Berson AS, Budinger TF, Ringquist I, Mock MB, Watson JT, Powel RS (eds) Non invasive Techniques for Assessment of Atherosclerosis in Peripheral, Carotid and Coronary Arteries. New York: Raven Press, p. 197.

20. Pignoli P (1984) Ultrasound B mode imaging for arterial wall thickness measurement. Atherosclerosis Rev 12:177.
21. Kosoff FG, Garrett WJ, Carpenten DA (1976) Principles and classification of soft tissues by grey scale echography. Ultrasound Med and Biol 2:89.
22. Wells PTN (1977) Scattering by biologic materials. In: Wells PTN (ed) Biomedical Ultrasonics. London: Academic Press
23. Carson OL, Zagzebsky JA (1980) Pulse Echo Ultrasound Imaging Systems: Performance Tests and Criteria. Published for the American Association of Physicists in Medicine. New York: American Institute of Physics, p. 5.
24. Wells PTN (1977) Dynamic range, swept gain and resolution. In: Wells PTN (ed) Biomedical Ultrasonics. London: Academic Press, p. 147.
25. McDicken WN (1981) Using A-scan instruments. In: McDicken WN (ed) Diagnostic Ultrasonics. Principles and Use of Instruments. New York: John Wiley and Sons, p. 113.
26. Pignoli P, Villa V, Paoletti R, Tremoli E (1983) Ultrasound B mode and A mode quantitative evaluation: Accuracy level for polythene pipe wall thickness measurements. Abstracts of the International Cardiovascular Congress IV, Scottsdale, Arizona, February 14-16, p. 39.
27. McDicken WN (1981) Performance of real-time scan instruments. In: McDicken WN (ed) Ultrasonics. Principles and Use of Instruments. New York: John Wiley and Sons, p. 209.
28. Pignoli P, Tremoli E, Poli A, Oreste PL, Paoletti R (1986) Intimal plus medial thickness of the arterial wall: A direct measurement with ultrasound imaging. Circulation 74:1399-1406.
29. Blankenhorn DH, Rooney JA, Curry PJ (1983) Non invasive assessment of atherosclerosis. Prog Cardiovas Dis 26:295.
30. Riley WA, Freedman DS, Higgs NA, Barnes RW, Zinkgraf SA, Berenson GS (1986) Decreased arterial elasticity associated with cardiovascular disease risk factors in the young. Bogalusa Heart Study. Arteriosclerosis 6:378.
31. Comerota AJ, Cranely JJ, Cook SE (1981) Real time B mode carotid imaging in diagnosis of cerebrovascular disease. Surgery 89:719.
32. Zwiebel WJ, Austin CW, Sackett JF, Strother CM (1983) Correlation of high resolution, B mode and continuous wave Doppler sonography with arteriography in the diagnosis of carotid stenosis. Radiology 149:523.
33. Hobson RW, Berry SM, Katocs AS, O'Donnel J, Jamil Z, Savitsky JP (1980) Comparison of pulsed Doppler and real time B mode echo arteriography for non invasive imaging of the extracranial carotid arteries. Surgery 87:286.
34. Evans TC, Taezner JC (1979) Ultrasound imaging of atherosclerosis in carotid arteries. Applied Radiology March-April;106.
35. Cooperberg PL, Robertson WD, Fry P, Sweeney V (1979) High resolution real time ultrasound of the carotid bifurcation. J Clin Ultrasound 7:13.

36. Leopold GR, Bernstein EF (1982) Ultrasonic imaging for occlusive carotid disease. In: Bernstein EF (ed) Non Invasive Diagnostic Techniques in Vascular Disease. St. Louis: The CV Mosby Company, p. 265.

37. Barford NC (1967) Experimental Measurements: Precision, Error and Truth. London: Addison-Wesley Publishing Company

38. Brown BG, Bolson EL, Dodge HT (1984) Dynamic mechanisms in human coronary atherosclerosis. Circulation 70:917-922.

39. O'Rourke MF (1982) Arterial Function in Health and Disease. Edinburgh: Churchill Livingstone

40. Hennerici M, Rautenberg W, Trockel U, Kladetzky (1985) Spontaneous progression and regression of small carotid atheroma. The Lancet, June 22:1415-1419.

41. Blankenhorn DH, Chin HP, Strikwerda S. Bamberger J, Hestenes JD (1983) Work in Progress: Common carotid artery contours reconstructed in three dimensions from parallel ultrasonic images. Radiology 148:533.

42. Brooks SH, Blankenhorn DH, Chin HP, Sanmarco ME, Hanashiro PK, Selzer RH, Selvester RH (1980) Design of human atherosclerosis studies by serial angiography. J Chron Dis 33:347-357.

43. Toli A, Tremoli E, Colombo A, Satari N, Pignoli P, and Paoleti R (1988) Ultrasonographic measurement of the common carotid artery wall thickness in hypercholesterolemic patients: A new model for the quantitation and follow-up of preclinical atherosclerosis in living human subjects. Atherosclerosis 70:253-261.

44. Muratori G, Rossatti B (1951) Modificazioni dimensionali e strutturali delle arterie anonima, succlavia e carotide comune con l'eta'. Boll Soc Biol Sper 27:540-545.

45. Zarins CK, Giddens DP, Bharadvaj BK, Sottiurai VS, Mabon RF, Glagov S (1983) Carotid bifurcation atherosclerosis. Quantitative correlation of plaque localization with flow velocity profiles and wall shear stress. Circ Res 53:502-514.

46. Powis RL (1986) Angiodynography. A new real time look at the vascular system. Applied Radiol Jan-Feb:33.

47. Solberg LA, Strong JP (1983) Risk factors and atherosclerotic lesions. A review of autopsy studies. Arteriosclerosis 3:187-198.

48. Ferrari LA, Jones JP, Gonzalez V, Beherens M (1982) Acoustical imaging using the phase of echo waveform. In: Acoustical Imaging. New York: Plenum Press, pp. 635-641.

49. Landini L, Sarnelli R, Picano E, Salvadore M (1986) Evaluation of frequency dependence of backscatter coefficient in normal and atherosclerotic aortic walls. Ultrasound in Med and Biol 12:397-401.

50. Heyser Rc, LeCroissette (1974) A new ultrasonic imaging system using time delay spectroscopy. Ultrasound Med Biol 1:119-131.

51. Kaufman L, Crooks LE, Sheldon PE, Rowan W, Miller T (1982) Evaluation of NMR imaging for detection and quantification of obstruction in vessels. Invest Radiol 17:554-560.

49

Multicenter Validation Study of Real Time (B Mode) Ultrasound, Arteriography, and Pathology: I. Methods and Materials

Mauricio Calderon-Ortiz, Matthew D. Rifkin, Daniel H. O'Leary, James F. Toole, M. Gene Bond, Fred A. Bryan, Jr., Tarle Holen, Michael L. McCartney, Robert A. Kane, J.M. McWhorter, Eric Schenk, Alfred Kurtz, and Marta W. Goodison

ABSTRACT

This study was designed to determine whether B-mode ultrasound imaging is accurate for identifying and quantifying localized atherosclerosis using angiography and pathological findings for validation and correlation assessments. Twelve hundred sixty-nine (1269) patients were enrolled and 1099 (87%) carotid and 170 (13%) iliofemoral arteries were studied. Eleven percent were designated by random selection to assess repeatability/variability. The remainder were used for evaluation of sensitivity/specificity.

At the site of minimum residual lumen, lesion width, length and tissue characteristics, as well as normal dimensions at other standard locations were quantified. Three hundred seventy (370) specimens from carotid endarterectomies were used for validation of B-scan and arteriography. No previous study has reported comparative pathology measurements of carotid atherosclerotic lesion location and extent in combination with B-scan imaging and angiography.

Acknowledgments: The names of the many people who helped with this study are listed in the Appendix.

INTRODUCTION

In 1972, the Task Force on Atherosclerosis of the National
Heart, Lung and Blood Institute (NHLBI) of NIH emphasized the
need for developing noninvasive techniques for detection and
quantification of atherosclerosis by stating; "B-mode ultrasound imaging is potentially a powerful clinical and research
tool for determining the extent and severity of atherosclerosis in arteries that can be imaged. We hope it will prove to
be useful for tracking lesion progression or regression."
Solicitations for noninvasive instrument research and development were first made in 1975. In 1980, the NHLBI's Division
of Heart and Vascular Diseases solicited proposals for assessment of noninvasive real time B-scan ultrasound imaging vis-
a-vis arteriography and pathology. In May 1981, five clinical
centers, one animal center and a data coordinating center
(DCC) were awarded contracts for a multicenter randomized
program (1).

OBJECTIVES

The primary goal was to determine the relative value of
B-mode ultrasound imaging for detecting and quantifying
atherosclerotic lesions in human beings and in animal models.

The objectives of the clinical and animal centers were
to collect sufficient data, under standardized conditions,
to determine the sensitivity, specificity, repeatability and
variability of B-mode imaging relative to arteriography and
pathology gathered from the interrogated arterial segments.
Determination of the role of adjunctive noninvasive functional
evaluation was identified as a secondary goal.

A detailed description of this program including its
Manual of Operations, is on file with the National Technical
Information Services (NTIS) at 5258 Port Royal Road,
Springfield, VA 22161.

A blinded, randomized, multicenter standardized program
was designed to measure the worth of ultrasonic B-scan
imaging for both diagnostic evaluation and longitudinal
follow up.

Hypotheses

The hypotheses to be tested were:

1. B-scan imaging is accurate in diagnosing the presence or absence of atherosclerosis within 15 mm of the carotid bifurcation when compared to angiography and/or anatomic pathology.

2. B-scan imaging can define the extent of atherosclerotic lesions and severity by measurement of minimum residual lumen diameter, lesion width and length.

3. The accuracy and predictive value of B-scan imaging is equivalent to that of arteriography and descriptive pathology in the areas investigated.

4. Prior knowledge of the clinical history and functional studies improves the accuracy and predictive value of B-scan imaging by influencing its performance and interpretation.

Pilot Study

Each clinical center was assigned 32 cases, of which eight were randomized for repeatability/variability (R/V) data (2,3). The balance provided data for sensitivity/specificity (S/S) analysis (3,4). All S/S cases underwent functional testing and B-scan imaging. Reasons for termination from the study were identified and categorized. The remaining cases formed the basis for the revision of forms, modification and standardization of B-scan and angiographic procedures, definition of measurable variables, and revision of technique for procurement and handling of endarterectomy specimens for pathology analysis. Additional standardized training of the program's staff, and the establishment of a quality control program were also implemented.

R/V cases were randomly assigned to operators and readers of angiograms and B-scans, and a sample of these angiograms or B-scans were obtained and classified at random as A or B; seven independent interpretations were then performed: 5 readings within the originating center (scan A read by two different interpreters and scan B read 3 times by the same two operators in alternate fashion), and at a second randomly selected center (2 readings by different interpreters.)

Single angiographic studies of the R/V cases were interpreted
in similar fashion, three times at the originating center
and twice at a second center. Thirty-nine (39) of the 160
carotid cases, in the pilot study, were assigned to R/V.
Because of attrition due to refusals to have tests, the
final number was 34.

However statistical analysis determined that a lesser
number of interpretations was adequate and that the second
B-scan was not necessary.

Main Study

1. Any patient scheduled for B-scan functional testing
and angiographic evaluation of the carotid or iliofemoral
arteries was eligible for enrollment. Physician and informed
patient consent were always obtained.

2. Enrollment occurred the date of the first procedure
(angiogram or B-scan) or on the completion of the History
and Physical (H & P) form. (In most cases, the H & P was
taken at the same time as the B-scan/functional; therefore
on the diagrammatic figures, only angiography or B-scan are
considered as first or second procedures.)

3. The two kinds of randomizations were:

a. R/V or S/S cases. R/V studies provided an
intramodality evaluation of the within-reader repeatability
and the between-reader variation. S/S studies provided an
intermodality comparison of the various techniques for detection and quantification of lesions.

b. Either "Yes-prior-knowledge" (YPK), or "no-prior-
knowledge (NPK) of the information obtained on the history,
physical examination and functional testing with Doppler,
phonoangiography, ophthalmoplethysmography or dynamic studies
of the lower extremities. This was true only for those carotid
and lower extremity cases randomized for S/S studies. All
cases randomized for R/V studies were carotid cases and NPK.

4. For those cases in which carotid endarterectomy was
performed on S/S or R/V carotid patients specimens were
handled in standardized fashion (vide infra).

5. Angiograms, B-scans, and surgery were to be performed
within 14 days of each other to minimize the change of having
a "significant clinical event" or lesion change which might

destroy comparability. When this limit was exceeded, individual case reviews were made to determine whether there had been any intervening event.

6. When the same staff member both performed and read either B-scan image or angiography at least 14 days elapsed between performance and reading.

7. One additional reading was done by another reader at a randomly selected referral center in all R/V cases.

8. The areas of interrogation for this program were as follows:

a. Carotid: from 15 mm proximal to the carotid bifurcation, to 6 mm distal to the bifurcation along the internal carotid artery. The CCA/ICA axis was the segment on which the readings concentrated primarily, unless the reader noted the external carotid artery as the site of an isolated lesion.

b. Lower extremity: The distal external iliac (if visualized) common femoral, superficial femoral, and popliteal arterial segments. Each was measured at three different levels: proximal, mid, and distal segments.

9. Operators knew that they were performing an R/V case, but the reader did not.

10. All completed cases had a dataset of completed forms: randomization envelope/control sheet, history and physical examination, functional, B-scan performance and measurement, and angiography performance and measurement. Any angiography or B-scan procedural difficulty or adverse effects, and surgery complications and pathology measurements and were forwarded to the DCC. If the case terminated, the appropriate form was completed as well.

11. The following were reasons for termination:

a. Died before either angiography or B-scan (incomplete study).

b. Patient refused either angiography or protocol B-scan.

c. Physician refused either scheduled angiography or protocol B-scan; e.g., procedure cancelled.

d. Angiography or B-scan incomplete, due to unforeseen complications; e.g., allergy to contrast agent, equipment failure, etc.

    e. Significant clinical event intervened between the B-scan and angiography procedures.

    f. Angiography or B-scan below standard and unacceptable for measurement, unless acceptable pathology data were included for overall intertechnique comparison.

    g. Time intervals between angiography B-scan and endarterectomy were exceeded.

Quality Control

Quality control of the B-scan Imaging Assessment Program took four forms:

Training: During the Pilot Study, the interim period, and especially at the beginning of the Main Study, multiple training meetings were held for the different members of the clinical staff, (Data Coordinators, B-scan Operators, B-Scan Readers, Angiographers, Angiography Readers, Surgeons, and Pathologists). During these meetings, methods and procedures were reviewed in detail and any discrepancies in operational routines were discussed. Special instructional workshops were held for sonographers which contributed to the development of a final protocol. Criteria for identification of reference points reviewed from non-optimal angles, for establishing interfaces at the base of lesions and for describing various tissue characteristics from B-mode images were standardized as much as possible.

B-Scan Phantoms. The second form of quality control was assessment of the continued quality of the B-scan images being recorded in the various Clinical Centers. The importance of having a quantitative basis for comparison among the various B-scan instruments was recognized early in the program. At the initiation of the pilot study, identical phantoms (devices with bubble structures and wire arrays of known sizes and spatial relationships, suspended in a medium that mimics the ultrasonic character of tissue when insonated) were distributed to each center. Data from each instrument were submitted to the DCC. At this stage these data were qualitatively evaluated to insure that adequate images of the phantom structures could be obtained with each Center's instruments. The operators and readers were instructed to employ the phantoms to monitor ongoing equipment performance.

This was achieved by obtaining a phantom image as an initial portion of each case's B-scan evaluation during the data acquisition phase.

In addition, a second phantom device was circulated among the Clinical Centers. Detailed measurements of all structures in this device were performed at each Clinical Center. Hard copies of B-scan images from this phantom were sent to the DCC for quantitative evaluation of instrument resolution by comparison with the actual dimensions of the phantom elements. Axial resolution of 0.5 mm at the focal point of the ultrasound beam was generally maintained, as required by the protocol.

Angiographic "Dimensional Markers". The third form of quality control provided for the elimination of magnification discrepancies associated with angiographic technique, in order to permit valid comparative measurements. Dimensional markers of known sizes were always included in the field of view of each film. A magnification factor was found and employed prior to analysis to convert the measurements from the films to true anatomic dimensions. Some centers used steel ball-bearing markers of 5 mm diameter while others used dimes. Readers were required to submit diagrams and operating instructions describing their measurement methods and their technique for compensating for parallax image deformation.

Standardization of Data Records and Reports. The fourth form of quality control dealt with the collective reporting and recording of data. Once completed, each of the data collection instruments was reviewed at the originating Clinical Center by the Data Coordinator.

Data sets were reviewed for a second time after receipt by the DCC. Notifications of "outliers", exceeding expected ranges predefined during the Pilot Phase experience, were returned to the Originating Center for review and verification. Case studies which contained significant variations between B-scan and angiography measurements were also flagged and returned to the individual Clinical Center for review. The probable cause for disparity was identified and recorded.

Following visual edit at the DCC, all data forms were keyed directly to machine readable form at the CRT data

terminal. All data were 100% verified by rekeying at data
entry. In the event of disparity between the initial and
the rekeyed data, the CRT terminal was programmed to lock up
until the discrepancy was identified and resolved.

Definitions. Precise definitions of terms used for
measurement of the carotid bifurcation were developed during
the pilot study. Standard lumen (SL): lumen diameter measured 15 mm below the carotid flow divider. This point was
chosen because it is often disease-free and can be used to
compare measurements from minimally diseased arteries. Lesion
width (LW): the total thickness of the plaque combined for
both walls (near and far) and measured at the point of minimal residual lumen. Minimal residual lumen (MRL): the smallest lumen diameter present in the internal or common carotid
artery. Normal arteries: vessels with no lesion visible on
the angiograms or ultrasound examination. For normal arteries, lesion width was recorded as zero and minimal residual
lumen was not measured. Occluded artery: no measurable
residual lumen (MRL=0). Lesion width for an occluded artery
was the measured diameter of the artery. The degree of lumen
stenosis was derived from the residual lumen and lesion width
by the formula:

$$\% \text{ Stenosis} = \left(1 - \frac{MRL}{MRL + LW}\right) \times 100$$

MATERIALS AND PROCEDURES - MAIN STUDY

Population Enrolled

The target population was patients with signs and/or
symptoms indicative of carotid and/or lower extremity arterial occlusive disease who were scheduled for noninvasive
functional studies, B-scan imaging and either standard or
digital subtraction angiography. The goal was 1250-1500
patients during the 18 month enrollment based on the Pilot
Study experience.

Twelve hundred sixty-nine (1269) cases were entered,
of whom 1099 were carotid and 170 were common femoral arteries. Nine hundred eighty-two of the carotid cases were
randomized into the S/S subset but 82 terminated. Of 117 in
the R/V subset, 9 were terminated leaving 108. Of 170
lower femoral cases enrolled, 37 were terminated leaving 133
cases.

Data gathered by history and physical examination provided uniform information on demographics, risk factors, signs and symptoms, and medication history. Of the population enrolled, 60.2% (764) were male and 39.8% (505) were female. Their mean age was 65 years (range 9-89 years). Eighty-seven percent (87%) of the total population was 50 years or older. Racial distribution was 95% white, 4.7% black and 0.3% other.

The prevalence of associated risk factor was: hypertension - 61.2%, cardiac disease - 52.8%, diabetes mellitus - 28.0%, current smoking - 41.6%, previous smoking - 33.9%. The prevalence of stroke previous to enrollment was 27.8%, and that of transient ischemic attacks was 51.6%. Of those patients enrolled for carotid studies 62.4% had cervical bruits.

Noninvasive Functional Tests

Oculoplethysmography, periorbital Doppler flow analysis, phonoangiography, and spectral analysis of Continuous Wave and/or Pulsed Doppler flow were used to obtain measurements in the carotid cases. Segmental Doppler pressures and pulse volume recordings at rest and after exercise were also obtained for the lower extremities. Functional tests varied from Center to Center and were so recorded.

Arteriography Methods

At least two views of the carotid bifurcation were routinely obtained at arteriography. Circular markers of known dimensions were placed on the skin adjacent to each · vessel to permit precise correction for X-ray magnification. At the discretion of the examiner, patients were examined by either conventional arterial injection and filming or by arterial or venous injection and digital subtraction filming.

B-Scan Method

Ultrasound imaging was performed with 7.5 or 10-MHz transducers having axial resolutions of at least 0.5 mm. For each image the depth from the skin to the far arterial wall was recorded together with the arterial lumen diameter

and lesion width at standard locations (common carotid
artery 15 mm below the bifurcation, and the common femoral
artery at the groin crease in the lower extremity). For the
carotid an additional lumen diameter and lesion width was
obtained 6 mm distal to the bifurcation at peak systole. The
lumen diameter was defined at standard locations which 1)
could be reliably reproduced by different operators and
2) where disease was least and most likely to be found. For
angiographic measurement only the vascular lumen diameters
could be obtained for comparative measurements at these
standard sites.

It was determined that lengthy recording of B-scan data
was not useful for determination of lesion parameters.
Therefore, operators were encouraged to concentrate on visualization of the structures in the area of observed disease.
As a routine, operators traversed all arterial segments and
then determined the best angles for visualizations of the
area in which lesions were seen using the probe angle which
provided the best images. In most cases transverse, arterio-
oblique, lateral and postior-oblique planes were visualized.

Because gain affects apparent wall thickness, variation
in settings was done periodically to determine the optimum
and this was noted on the voice channel in order to allow
the interpreter to decide at what point the apparent change
in wall thickness was related to the gain setting.

For the lower extremity studies the external iliac artery,
the common femoral, the superficial femoral, and the popliteal artery in each leg were examined by both arteriography
and real-time B-mode. The profunda femoris artery was not
studied after the pilot phase, since the vessel was infrequently seen by B-scan. During the pilot phase it was only
visualized in 31 of 90 cases or 34%, and all of these were
interpreted as "normal".

The location of the minimum residual lumen associated
with a lesion was then located. For each modality the
following measurements were obtained (Figure 1): <u>Minimum
Residual Lumen (MRL)</u>- the transverse lumen diameter at the
point of maximum lumen encroachment by the atherosclerotic
lesion, <u>Lesion Length</u> - the sum of the distance measured
from the maximum disease point (MRL) to the proximal and

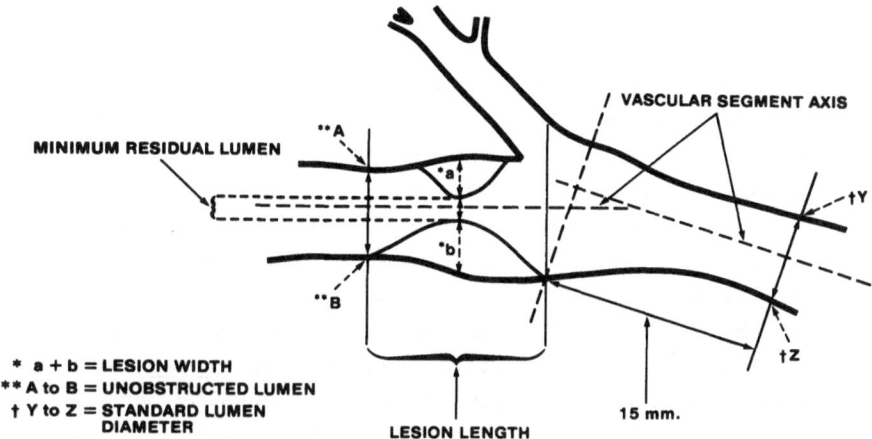

Figure 1. Schematic representation of the measurements obtained from B-scan ultrasound and angiography. All measurements were made with calipers to the nearest 0.5 mm.

distal lesion margins, <u>Lesion Width (LW)</u> - the combined width of anterior and posterior arterial wall lesions at the level of MRL, and <u>Unobstructed Lumen Diameter</u> - measured in the segment of normal caliber at the nearest lesion margin from the MRL point. <u>Reference Distance (RD)</u>- the distance from the flow divider to the specific site in the common or internal carotid artery that contained the minimum residual lumen. The location of the lesion (near wall, far wall, both, or circumferential involvement) was recorded. Arterial wall movement such as radial wall motion proximal and distal to the lesion, and longitudinal plaque motion were recorded for B-scan images.

Lesion surface characteristics were classified in the B-scan studies as smooth or irregular and/or pocketed. For the angiographic studies lesion surface was classified as smooth, irregular, or ulcerative.

The intramural ultrasonographic character of each atherosclerotic lesion was evaluated for sonic reflectivity

(minimal, moderate, high) and attenuation (minimal, high).
For angiographic studies plaque characteristics were
evaluated for presence or absence of calcification and/or
intramural filling defects.

Videocassette recorders with frame freeze capability
were used by the readers for the analysis of Videotapes of
B-scan images. A phantom was used whenever possible to
standardize calibration. In some centers internal calibration methods were used instead of the phantom.

When the arterial site containing the minimal residual
lumen was identified, the reader proceeded to <u>freeze</u> the
most representative frame with its image, manually performed
the measurements from the CRT image, multiplied the screen
measurements by the conversion factor previously obtained
and recorded the absolute dimensions of each parameter under
study.

At the end of the B-scan or angiographic measurement the
reader classified the quality of the images obtained (standard or above, below standard, or unacceptable), and described
any difficulties encountered in making the required measurements.

Measurement data were reported only if the side was
not occluded and a lesion was present. If a reader judged
the ultrasound or angiogram to be below standard or unacceptable, the study was excluded from analysis. Analysis was
limited to measurements made on diseased but patent arteries
with the lesion having its minimum lumen within 15 mm of the
flow divider.

Ultrasound and angiography readers were unaware of the
patient's history, physical findings and functional studies.
For each modality, the reader was required to choose the
frame or film which they determined best demonstrated the
MRL. Measurements were made from the ultrasound image to
the nearest 0.5 mm and characteristics of lesions at the MRL
were described. One of the two readers was randomly assigned
to reread each frame for a total of three readings. In order
to prevent carry over knowledge, a minimum of 14 days was
interposed between rereadings.

No standardization of the angiographic technique was
attempted. Sixty-nine percent of the carotid patients

underwent selective common carotid injections of contrast
media with magnification views of the carotid bifurcation.
The remaining 31% underwent digital subtraction angiograms
after intravenous injection of contrast media.

For angiographic measurements, the reader was supplied
with hard copy films from the biplane angiographic studies,
and utilizing the dimensional marker included in the field
of view of each film, proceeded to calculate the conversion
factor for correction of magnification and measure actual
dimensions.

Surgery

Because this study was not designed to evaluate the
endarterectomy procedure, no attempt was made to standardize
operative technique or anesthesia. Whenever possible,
plaques were removed intact with minimal surgical artifacts.
In some instances a single longitudinal slit was made
through the endarterectomy specimen, which was otherwise
removed intact.

Pathology

Four hundred seventy-eight carotid endarterectomies
were performed. In 88 the specimen was either fragmented or
the MRL was found in the external carotid artery. An
additional 20 specimens corresponded to cases with incomplete
data sets and were excluded. Of the remaining 370, 37 were
from R/V cases, while 333 were from S/S cases. After further
exclusions (B-scan or angio unacceptable quality), the remaining 289 specimens were analyzed.

Endarterectomy specimens were photographed, x-rayed in
the fresh state and immersion fixed in 10% neutral buffered
formalin for not less than 72 hours. Specimens that had a
single surgically induced longitudinal slit were identified
as split but were measured. In a subset, specimens were
again photographed and x-rayed after fixation and again
after decalcification to assess shrinkage artifact. Each
photograph and x-ray contained dimensional markers of
known size within the field of view so that calibration
factors for subsequent quantification could be determined.

A first coronal cut of the specimen was made at or slightly below the estimated position of the bifurcation in the common carotid artery. The location of the flow divider was then noted by looking upward through the lumen. Cross sectional tissue slices were then made at 3 mm intervals along the course of each specimen, with a cutting angle perpendicular to the longitudinal axis of the artery.

To compensate for artifactual collapse of the lumen, and in view of the fact that a common finding in the specimens evaluated was the presence of collapsed and distorted lumens, both among and within specimens, geometric lumen reconstruction was performed. The length of the lumen perimeter was measured and the diameter of the circle with that circumference was arithmetically calculated. This method assumes that lumen shape in pressurized atherosclerotic vessels *in vivo* most closely resembles a circle or an ellipse in which the minor-major diameter ratio approaches 1. From cross sections of the site of the minimum residual lumen, the lumen diameter and wall thicknesses were measured from four different angles. These angles duplicated the B-scan lateral, anterolateral, anterior, and posterolateral views and the angiographic anteroposterior, posterolateral, lateral, and anterolateral projections. Details are provided in a separate paper (5).

Tissue characteristics were evaluated as being present or absent including: mural/thrombus recent, mural/thrombus old, intramural hemorrhage recent, intramural hemorrhage old, fibrosis, necrosis, lumen surface smooth, lumen surface irregular, and ulceration. A detailed description of methods and findings will be published in a companion paper (4).

Statistical Analysis

The basic unit of observation for the carotid cases was patent side upon which carotid artery measurements were made. For lower extremity cases each one of three (iliofemoral, superficial femoral, and popliteal), or four (when external iliac artery was imaged), segments studies per side was an independent study unit.

Statistical Techniques. Measurement data were analyzed using analysis of variance, variance component analysis and Wilcoxon rank tests. The S/S data were summarized using mean, standard error, range, correlations and absolute differences. The R/V data were summarized using the following measures of inter- and intra-reader variability: variance, mean absolute difference and correlations. The statistical significance of sources of variation such as operator, arteries within patient, and center were also assessed.

Statistical Measures. Classificatory type of data (presence of ulcerations or disease, classification of artery based on stenosis, etc.) were analyzed using methods applicable to data presented in the form of multiple contingency tables (log linear models, logistic regression). The data were summarized using simple contingency tables, kappa statistics, sensitivity, specificity, positive and negative predictive values.

Follow Up Phase

A second phase of this multicentric study is still in progress. From 12/01/84 through 9/30/86, additional second and third real-time B-scan imaging procedures are being performed in those patients who are carotid cases and have remained eligible (at least one non-operated vessel that is not occluded continued patient and physician cooperation with the study, etc.). Analysis of the ability of B-scan imaging to detect progression/regression of atherosclerotic lesions and definition of the natural history of cervical carotid atherosclerosis as documented by B-scan imaging in this group of patients are the objectives of this phase.

REFERENCES
1. National Heart, Lung, and Blood Institute, NIH (1980) Request for proposal RFP NHLBI 80-10. Assessment of ultrasonic B-scan imaging for detection and quantification of atherosclerotic lesions in human carotid and iliofemoral arteries of animals.
2. O'Leary DH, Bryan, FA, Goodison MW, Goldberg BB, Gramiak R, Ball M, Bond MG, Dunn RA, Rifkin M, Toole JF, Wheeler HG, Gustafson NF, Eckholm S, and Raines J (1989) Multicenter Validation Study of Real-Time (B Mode) Ultrasound, Arteriography and Pathology II.

Repeatability/Variability Assessment, this volume
Chapter 52

3. O'Leary DH, Bryan FA, Goodison MW, Rifkin M, Gramiak R,
   Ball M, Bond MG, Dunn RA, Goldberg BB, Toole JF,
   Wheeler HG, Gustafson NF, Eckholm S, and Raines J (1987)
   Measurement of variability of carotid atherosclerosis:
   Real-Time (B mode) Ultrasonography and arteriography.
   Stroke 18:1011-1017

4. Ricotta JJ, Bryan FA, Bond MG, Kurtz A, O'Leary DH,
   Raines JK, Berson AS, Clouse ME, Calderon-Ortiz M, Toole
   JF, DeWeese JA, Smullens SN, and Gustafson NF (1989)
   Multicenter validation of real-time (B mode) ultrasound,
   arteriography and pathology III. Sensitivity and
   specificity Assessment, this volume, Chapter 53

5. Ricotta JJ, Bryan FA, Bond, MG, Kurtz A, O'Leary DH,
   Raines JK, Berson AS, Clouse ME, Calderon-Ortiz M,
   Toole JF, DeWeese JA, Smullens SN,and Gustafson NF (1987)
   Multicenter validation study of real-time (B mode
   ultrasound, arteriography and pathologic examination.
   J Vascular Surgery 6:512-520

6. Schenk E, Bond M, Artez T, Angelo J, Choi H, Rynalski T
   and Bryan F (Unpublished data) Pathologic evaluation of
   endarterectomy specimens: How good is the gold standard?

APPENDIX

Dr. Calderon-Ortiz and colleagues wish to thank the following people who assisted with this study.

Bowman Gray School of Medicine: Jean Angelo, M.D., M. Gene Bond, Ph.D., Marshall Ball, M.D., Gary Harpold, M.D., Catherine Nunn, R.N., R.V.T., Janice Frye-Pierson, R.N., CNRN, Kelley Williamson, William M. McKinney, M.D., J.M. McWhorter, M.D.

Jefferson University Hospital: Barry B. Goldberg, M.D., Hong Choi, M.D., Huynh T. Doan, M.D., Carlos Gonzalez, M.D., Alfred Kurtz, M.D., Esmond M. Mapp, M.D., Matthew D. Rifkin, M.D., Stanton N. Smullens, M.D., Robert M. Steiner, M.D., Debra Ahrensfield, Shanlee Pollack, Gerardo Rodriguez

Miami Heart Institute: Jeff Raines, Ph.D., F.A.C.C., Marta W. Goodison, M.P.A., Mauricio Calderon Ortiz, M.D., Maria Correa, RN, R.V.T., Jerry Stolzenberg, M.D., Alan Drexler, M.D., Marc Epstein, M.D., Jerome Benson, M.D., Thomas Rynalski, M.D., Debra St. Louis

New England Deaconess: Daniel H. O'Leary, M.D., Hugh G. Wheeler, Ph.D., Melvin E. Clouse, M.D., H. Thomas Aretz, M.D., Robert A Kane, M.D., Miguel Alday, M.D., Jeffrey Potter, B.S., Deborah Pinel, R.D.M.S., Barbara Zaias, M.D., Gary Gibbons, M.D., Tessa Hedley-White, M.D., Kenneth Stokes, M.D., David Mikulis, M.D., Sally Edwards, B.A., Jill Hoffman, B.S., Nancy Vindetti, B.S., Terry Hanlon, B.S., Roger Pezzuti, M.D.

University of Rochester: Raymond A. Gramiak, M.D., Eric Schenk, M.D., Harle Holen, M.D., Sven Eckholm, M.D., Mary LaRose, R.N., Data Coordinator, Marsha W. Senges, M.S., Data Coordinator, Sandra A. Roe, R.T., R.D.M.S.

Animal Center: M. Gene Bond, Ph.D., Janet K. Sawyer, M.S.C., Marshall Ball, M.D.

Data Coordinating Center: Fred A. Bryan, Jr., Ph.D., A. Vijaya Rao, Ph.D., Judith A. Katzin, Nancy F. Gustafson, M.S., Barbara J.G. York, M.S., David L. Myers, Ph.D., Debra M. Fleishmann, Ph.D., Michael L. McCartney, Sc.D.

NHLBI: Alan S. Berson, Ph.D., Rosalie Dunn, Ph.D.

Data Review Board: Colin Schwartz, M.D., Marian Fisher, Ph.D., James Halsey, M.D., Gerardo Heiss, M.D., Ph.D., Robert Hobson, M.D., Sheldon Schaffer, Ph.D., Marvin C. Ziskin, M.D.

A detailed description of this program including its Manual of Operations, is on file with the National Technical Information Services (NTIS) at 5258 Port Royal Road, Springfield, VA 22161.

50

Multicenter Validation Study of Real Time (B Mode) Ultrasound, Arteriography, and Pathology: II. Repeatability/Variability Assessment

Daniel H. O'Leary, Fred A. Bryan, Marta W. Goodison, Barry B. Goldberg, Raymond Gramiak, Marshall Ball, M. Gene Bond, Rosalie A. Dunn, Matthew Rifkin, James F. Toole, Hugh G. Wheeler, Nancy F. Gustafson, Sven Eckholm, and Jeff Raines

INTRODUCTION

In 1981 the National Heart, Lung, and Blood Institute awarded contracts to five clinical centers to establish the capabilities of high-resolution B mode ultrasound imaging for detecting and quantitating atherosclerotic lesions in the carotid and iliofemoral arteries of human subjects. This chapter details the repeatability/variability (R/V) component of the carotid artery studies and permits intramodality evaluation between and within-reader variation. The within-technique repeatability procedures described here were limited to evaluation of carotid arteries using B mode ultrasound and angiography.

MATERIALS AND METHODS

Details of the methods for patient selection and examination techniques for this study are given in the preceeding paper.

Data Analysis

The primary objective of the statistical analysis was to determine the within- and between-reader variability in B mode ultrasound imaging and angiography assessment of lesion parameters. Secondary assessments addressed other sources of variation such as differences between arteries of a patient, differences among patients within a clinical setting (center), differences among clinical settings, and in the case of B mode imaging, differences among sonographers.

Three measures of variability were used to assess the measurement data: the variance (the average squared deviation of measurements of an artery from its mean) and the 95% confidence interval; the absolute difference (the mean of the absolute differences between pairs of measurements), and the correlation coefficient (Pearson correlation coefficient between pairs of measurements).

The kappa statistic and its 95% confidence interval were used to summarize the categorical data (1). This statistic is a standardized measure of agreement between the classifications of the same artery in excess of chance, and as such, can also be interpreted as the correlation between the classifications of the same artery. Thus, the within-reader kappa statistic is the correlation among repeated independent classifications of any artery by the same reader and measures the agreement in excess of chance. The between-reader kappa statistic is the correlation between independent classification of any artery by multiple readers and also measures the agreement among single readings of any artery by different readers, in excess of chance.

Following Landis and Koch (2) the following labels are used to indicate the relative strength of agreement associated with range of kappa indicated in parentheses: poor (0-0.2); fair (0.21-0.40); moderate (0.41-0.60); substantial (0.61-0.80); and almost perfect (0.81-1.0). Although these labels are somewhat arbitrary, they do provide useful benchmarks.

The data were analyzed using analysis of variance techniques (3). The components of the variation in measurements were estimated using variance components model. Within-reader variability in this chapter describes the variability among independent measurements of an artery by a reader. Between-reader variability describes the variability among independent (single) readings in the same artery by multiple readers.

RESULTS

1099 patients were enrolled in the carotid portion of the ultrasound B mode ultrasound assessment program; 117 of these were randomly assigned to the reliability/variability

study. Nine percent of angiograms and 16% of B mode images
were considered below standard or unacceptable and were
excluded from analysis. Selected arterial studies were done
in 74% of these cases and digital venous studies in 26%.
These results are combined for the purposes of this report.
The maximum number of observations available for analysis was
6 per patient, 3 each for the right and left carotid artery.

   The unit of analysis was one side of a patient (artery).
A patient's side was excluded from analysis if only one reading
was available on that side or if all the reported readings
on a side did not address the same arterial segment. The
internal carotid artery and common carotid artery were considered as the same arterial segment for this purpose.

   Furthermore, sides classified as normal or occluded on
any of the readings were excluded from the analysis of variability of residual lumen, lesion width, stenosis and reference
distance. The number of observations in the analysis varied
little among various measurements. For the analysis of
residual lumen, there were 297 observations on 80 patients
with angiographic data and 283 observations on 74 patients
with B mode data.

Categorical Data
   The within and between reader agreement for lesion
detection for both B mode and angiography was substantial,
with the exception of between-reader agreement for the external
carotid artery which was only fair for B mode and moderate
for angiography (Table 1).

   For both B mode and angiography the within-reader agreement was substantial for the 0-49% and 75% occluded categories
but was moderate in the 50-74% category (Table 2). For angiography, the between-reader agreement was also substantial in
the 0-49% and 75-100% categories, and moderate in the 50-
74% category. For B mode, however, the between-reader agreement was substantial in the 75% occluded category, moderate
in the 0-49% category, and only fair in the 50-74% category.
For both within and between reader comparisons, the overall
agreement was substantial for angiography and moderate for
B mode ultrasound.

Table 1. Within- and Between-Reader Agreement on Detection of Lesions: Kappa Statistics

Segment	N*	Within-Reader Agreement (95% Confidence Interval)	N*	Between-Reader Agreement (95% Confidence Interval)
B Mode				
CCA	170	0.69 (0.58-0.80)	166	0.58 (0.46-0.71)
ICA	165	0.73 (0.62-0.83)	164	0.65 (0.53-0.77)
ECA	145	0.64 (0.49-0.79)		0.34 (0.15-0.52)
Angiography				
CCA	177	0.74 (0.64-0.83)	187	0.59 (0.48-0.71)
ICA	173	0.82 (0.72-0.92)	182	0.66 (0.54-0.79)
ECA	172	0.60 (0.47-0.73)	181	0.58 (0.45-0.70)

* Number of arteries

Reprinted from O'Leary, D.H. et al, Stroke 18; 1011-1017, 1987 by permission of the American Heart Association, Inc.

Table 2. Within- and Between-Reader Agreement for Stenosis Categories: Kappa Statistics

Stenosis Category	N*	Within-Reader Agreement (95% Confidence Interval)	N*	Within-Reader Agreement (95% Confidence Interval)
			B Mode	
0-49%	99/98	0.67 (0.55 - 0.78)	106/99	0.53 (0.40 - 0.66)
50-74%	42/39	0.43 (0.27 - 0.59)	34/40	0.34 (0.17 - 0.51)
75% Occluded	27/31	0.62 (0.52 - 0.82)	26/27	0.66 (0.51 - 0.82)
All Categories Combined	168	0.59 (0.48 - 0.70)	166	0.50 (0.38 - 0.62)
			Angiography	
0-49%	114/118	0.82 (0.73 - 0.91)	126/125	0.76 (0.66 - 0.86)
50-75%	21/33	0.53 (0.34 - 0.72)	23/19	0.46 (0.26 - 0.66)
75%	40/34	0.83 (0.73 - 0.93)	35/40	0.78 (0.67 - 0.90)
All Categories Combined	175	0.76 (0.67 - 0.85)	184	0.71 (0.61 - 0.81)

* Number of arteries, First Reading/Second Reading;
The N appropriate for this statistic is that for all categories combined.

Reprinted from O'Leary, D.H. et al., Stroke 18; 1011-1017, 1987 by permission of the American Heart Association, Inc.

Table 3 presents the within and between reader agreement on the presence of ulcerations. For the analysis, a lesion was classified as ulcerated if pocketing or irregularity was reported. While within-reader kappa statistics for the diagnosis of ulceration were substantial for both B mode (0.64) and angiography (0.67), the between-reader agreement was poor for B mode (0.11) and fair to moderate for angiography (0.41).

Measurement Data

The within-reader and between-reader measures of variability are given in Tables 4 and 5 respectively. The within-reader variances for B mode measurements of residual lumen, lesion width, reference distance and standard lumen are larger than the within-reader variances for the corresponding angiographic measurements (p less than .05 for each measurement); the absolute differences also show the same ordering. The within-reader correlations for B mode measurements of residual lumen, reference distance and standard lumen are smaller than the correlations for the corresponding angiographic measurements (p less than .05 for each measurement). The within-reader correlation for B mode measurement of lesion width is larger than the corresponding angiographic measurement.

Table 3. Between- and Within-Reader Agreement on Presence of Ulceration: Kappa Statistics

	N*	Within-Reader Agreement (95% Confidence Interval)	N*	Within-Reader Agreement (95% Confidence Interval)
B Mode	88	0.64 (0.45 - 0.82)		0.11 (0 - 0.33)
Angiography	107	0.67 (0.53 - 0.81)		0.41 (0.22 - 0.59)

* Number of arteries

Reprinted from O'Leary, D.H. *et al*, Stroke 18; 1011-1017, 1987 by permission of the American Heart Association, Inc.

Table 4. Within-Reader Variability

Measurement	Mean Absolute Difference ± SE	Variance (95% Confidence Interval)	Correlation (95% Confidence Interval)
	B Mode		
Residual Lumen (mm)	0.89 (0.10)	0.78 (0.60 - 1.09)	0.76 (0.65 - 0.84)
Lesion Width (mm)	0.81 (0.10)	0.71 (0.54 - 0.99)	0.74 (0.63 - 0.82)
Stenosis (%)	9.9 (1.0)	102 (77 - 141)	0.77 (0.66 - 0.84)
Reference Distance (mm)	2.49 (0.33)	7.5 (5.7 - 10.6)	0.76 (0.66 - 0.84)
Standard Lumen (mm)	0.64 (0.07	0.44 (0.33 - 0.60)	0.72 (0.60 - 0.81)
	Angiography		
Residual Lumen (mm)	0.35 (0.05)	0.17 (0.13 - 0.24)	0.94 (0.91 - 0.96)
Lesion Width (mm)	0.61 (0.07)	0.37 (0.28 - 0.52)	0.72 (0.60 - 0.81)
Stenosis (%)	8.1 (0.9)	0.70 (53 - 106)	0.85 (0.78 - 0.90)
Reference Distance (mm)	1.34 (0.22)	3.05 (2.33 - 4.22)	0.87 (0.80 - 0.91)
Standard Lumen (mm)	0.48 (0.05)	0.20 (0.16 - 0.28)	0.89 (0.84 - 0.93)

Adapted from O'Leary, D.H. *et al*, Stroke 18; 1011-1017, 1987 by permission of the American Heart Association, Inc.

The between-reader variance in B mode measurements of all parameters except reference distance were larger than the variance in the corresponding angiographic measurements (p less than .05 for each); the same ordering is reflected in the mean absolute differences of the two modalities. The between-reader correlations for B mode measurements of residual lumen, stenosis, and standard lumen are smaller than the correlations for the corresponding angiography measurements (p less than .05 for each measurement).

Table 5. Between-Reader Variability

Measurement	Mean Absolute Difference ± SE	Variance (95% Confidence Interval)	Correlation (95% Confidence) Interval)
		B Mode	
Residual Lumen (mm)	1.2 (0.11)	1.0 (0.79 - 1.32)	0.61 (0.45 - 0.73)
Lesion Width (mm)	1.3 (0.12)	1.48 (1.15 - 1.99)	0.56 (0.39 - 0.69)
Stenosis (%)	13.7 (1.3)	149 (117 - 197)	0.62 (0.47 - 0.74)
Reference Distance (mm)	3.3 (0.40)	10.10 (7.94 - 13.42)	0.65 (0.50 - 0.76)
Standard Lumen (mm)	1.0 (0.08)	0.78 (0.61 - 1.04)	0.48 (0.30 - 0.63)
		Angiography	
Residual Lumen (mm)	0.6 (0.08	0.42 (0.33 - 0.56)	0.85 (0.78 - 0.90)
Lesion Width (mm)	0.8 (0.07)	0.54 (0.43 - 0.70)	0.64 (0.50 - 0.75
Stenosis (%)	9.1 (0.09)	82 (66 - 106)	0.85 (0.78 - 0.90)
Reference Distance (mm)	3.8 0.39)	10.01 (7.82 - 13.40)	0.56 (0.40 _ 0.68)
Standard Lumen (mm)	0.5 (0.05)	0.29 (0.23 - 0.38)	0.83 (0.76 - 0.88)

Adapted from O'Leary, D.H. *et al*, Stroke 18;1011-1017,
1987 by permission of the American Heart Association, Inc.

Sources of Variation in Measurements

The B scan data were also analyzed with a model which
partitioned the total variance in measurements into the
following components: Clinical center, operator, patient
side (artery), reader and error (Table 6a). The angiographic
model for the same analysis included all components of the
B mode model except the operator (Table 6b). These components of variance are additive and when summarized express
the total measurement variance.

Table 6a. Variance Components for B-Mode Measurements (as Percent of Total Variance)

Source	Min. Res. Lumen	Lesion Width	Stenosis	Ref. Distance	Standard Lumen
Center	4	9	7	12	21
Operator	5	0	3	0	0
Patient	12	0	0	39	33
Artery	48	50	56	19	0
Reader	7	22	11	8	20
Error	25	20	23	22	26
Total Variance	3.2	3.6	433	33.5	1.7
Mean	3.7	4.1	52	1.8	7.4
Coefficient of Variation (C.V.%)	29	21	24	178	12
N	283	283	289	278	291

Table 6b. Variance Components of Angiographic Measurements (as Percentage of Total Variance

Center	13	5	7	6	8
Patient	22	0	0	32	64
Artery	51	59	79	22	12
Reader	9	11	2	28	5
Error	6	25	12	12	11
Total Variance	2.8	1.5	564	25.3	1.8
Mean	3.0	2.4	45.7	3.4	6.7
Coefficient of Variation (C.V.%)	21	30	20	93	8
N	297	295	302	298	303

The center component of variance reflects the possible effects due to differences in type of patients referred to the centers, clinical environment, etc. Although this component is statistically significant (p less than .05 for each measurement) for all B mode and angiographic measurements, the range in total variances 5 to 13% for angiographic measurements and 4 to 21% for B mode measurements, are relatively similar.

The effect due to possible differences in the extent and severity of disease among different centers is reflected in the patient component of variance. The artery component reflects the differences in the extent of disease between the two sides of a patient. The sum of these two components reflects the major portion of the disease component of variance. For angiography, the sum accounts for 75% of the total variance for residual lumen, 58% for stenosis, 54% for reference distance and 76% for standard lumen. For B mode the sum of the patient and artery components accounts for 50-60% of the total variance for lesion related measurements and 33% of the variance of standard lumen measurements. Thus, the disease related components appear to account for a larger portion of variation in the angiographic measurement than for B mode.

The effect attributable to technical skill of sonographers is reflected in the operator component and is statistically significant (p less than .05) only for residual lumen (5%) and stenosis (3%). The reader component for B mode measurements accounted for 20% of the total variance of standard lumen, 22% for lesions width and less than 12% for the total variance of each of the measurements except reference distance, for which it was responsible for 28%.

The error component reflects random variations in a manner similar to within-reader variance discussed above, and accounted for 20-26% of the total variance of B mode measurements but 12% or less for angiographic measurements with the exception of lesion width, for which it accounted for 25%.

Tables 6a and b also give the mean, total variance, number of arteries (N), and coeffieient of variation (CV) for all B mode and angiography measurements. The mean B mode measurements were larger than the corresponding mean angiography measurements for all measurements except the reference distance. When these means were calculated only for arteries with measurements by both methods (comparing Table 6a and b), the mean difference between the B mode and angiography measurements were: 0.7 mm for residual lumen, 1.7 mm for lesion width, 6.3% for stenosis, 1.6 mm for reference distance and 0.7 mm for standard lumen.

The coefficient of variation (CV) for lesion-related measurements are in the range of 20-30% for both methods, but are larger for ultrasound than for angiography with the exception of lesion width. Thus, the angiographic measurements were more reproducible for all categories except lesion width. For both B mode and angiography, the most precise and least precise measurements were the standard lumen (B mode 12% and angiography 8%) and the reference distance (B mode 178% and angiography 93%), respectively. The coefficients of variation for percent stenosis were 24% for B mode and 20% for angiography.

DISCUSSION

Because B mode ultrasound is used as a noninvasive method to diagnose carotid artery atherosclerosis, the accuracy of the ultrasound measurement must be known. Previous studies attempting to quantitate this have used angiography as the standard for comparison, but our findings suggest that measurement using the angiograms cannot necessarily be relied upon. Although we have found that angiographic measurements were more reliable than B mode measurements for all parameters except lesion width, the variations within each modality were in fact, similar for most components.

Both angiography and B mode showed substantial within-reader agreement in measurements of lesion parameters, in categorization of arteries according to stenosis, in diagnosis of lesions within arterial segments, and in the diagnosis of ulceration. Between-reader differences in the measurements by both methods were statistically significant for lesion width and standard lumen diameter. The B mode measurements were on average larger than the corresponding angiography measurements and also varied significantly depending on the artery being measured.

These results are consistent with other reports
addressing the issues of observer variability in angiographic
interpretation. In the largest such study of carotid angiography yet reported, Chikos *et al*, found a similar degree of
within and between-reader variability in estimates of percent
stenosis (4). Their 64 cases were drawn from a larger set
of 100 consecutive patients, 36 angiograms then being put
aside because of their relatively poorer technical quality,
with each case viewed twice by three readers. All studies
were selective arterial injections. The single best view
from each projection was preselected, and each reader was
given this set of films. All measurements were made with
calipers. Their within-reader correlation coeffieicnt for
percentage of stenosis was .94 compared to our value of .85.
Their average within-reader variability in estimating percentage of stenosis was .92% and their absolute difference
in percentage of stenosis was 7.2%. Our corresponding figures are .85 and 9.1%. These differences are not great when
one considers t hat our study is a multicenter study without
preselection criteria for inclusion, and with full latitude
for the reader to select the specific film to be read.

Slot,*et al* utilized the kappa statistic to analyze
between-reader agreement among 11 observers in the interpretation of 21 single-plane translumbar arteriograms (5).
The kappa value ranged from 0.51 for the left superficial
femoral artery to 0.07 for the right profunda bifurcation.
They concluded that except for recognition of occlusion, so
little agreement was found between observers as to raise
serious doubt about the utility of angiography for clinical
decision making. In a study of coronary angiography, Zir
et al found a marked degree of between-observer variability
in quantifying the percentage of coronary artery stenosis,
and noted that observer agreement decreased with an increasing
percentage of positive findings (6). They suggested that
observer agreement would increase if the percentage of normal
vessels were higher, or if only a single vessel were studied.
They also focused on the difficulty of identifying normal
segments for determining percentage of arterial stenosis in
disease vessels.

Angiographic and B mode images still differ greatly in quality, primarily due to the physical principles upon which X-ray and acoustic transmissions and deflection are based. Fundamentally, X-rays form sharper images because they scatter less than do sound waves. Theoretical resolution is also greater for X-rays because of smaller wave lengths. Other considerations are the properties of biologic tissues which affect the transit of X-rays and sound. For arterial imaging, angiography produces images by using contrast material to alter transmission properties of the blood within the vessel. With this method, the properties of the vessel wall are not altered, and thus atherosclerotic lesions and the underlying artery wall are not distinguished from the surrounding tissue. B mode imaging can differentiate surfaces of lesions and vessel walls by acoustic reflections that occur at the lumen-intima, media-adventitial, and adventitial-periadventitial interfaces.

These differing capabilities offer some clues regarding differences between angiography and B mode measurements for lumen diameter and lesion width, both of which are greater for B mode. For angiographic images, lesion width must be calculated by comparing lumen diameter at the lesion with the diameter at an assumed normal location. Because the base of the atherosclerotic plaque is not seen, this calculation reveals only that part of the lesion which encroaches into the lumen and whether the normal segment chosen is, in fact, normal is an assumption. For B mode images, lesion width is measured directly from the lesion/lumen interface and the lesion-adventitial interface, the sum of lesion and arterial wall dimensions. Explanation of why lumen diameter is observed to be greater by B mode than angiography is more difficult. One hypothesis is that some arterial interfaces are delineated with less clarity using B mode, particularly the weak reflection from the intima-blood interface. However a stronger signal is usually reflected from the media-adventitial interface, and this interface may be incorrectly construed as defining lumen boundaries.

The method of measurement is another factor which limits resolution as are also the physical characteristics of X-ray

or acoustic radiation. For both angiography and B mode, the
readers used calipers or a scale, and were asked to make
measurements within 0.5 mm. In neither case was this resolution attained in practice because observers tended to round
their measurements to the closest 0.5 mm.

Also, there is a loss in image quality when comparing
videotapes with real-time B-mode images. Furthermore, ultrasound readers were at a relative disadvantage because measurements were made by viewing a videotape and then freezing one
frame. Considering the thousands of frames to choose from,
it is unlikely that repeat readings were made from the same
frame. On the other hand, angiography readers were presented
with very few images, and the likelihood of choosing the same
one for repeat readings was high.

Ultrasound readings were done without knowledge of
Doppler, or other ancillary information. The following
chapter by Ricotta et al. details the sensitivity/specific-
ity results and shows that interpretation of B mode images
is improved by prior knowledge of the results of these
functional studies. During protocol development we attempted
to develop means by which to identify the precise location
of a lesion within an arterial segment for comparison of
modalities and for future identification of specific arterial
sites. For the carotid artery, flow divider provided the
best anatomic reference landmark. However, our data regarding
locating the most significant lesion with respect to this
reference by B mode and arteriography are among the poorest
in reproducibility. Both B mode and angiographic measurements yielded the poorest coefficients of variation for reference distance i.e. the distance from the reference point to
the site being measured (Table 6). The explanation for this
variability may lie in single plane views, and depending on
the angle, external and internal carotid arteries may overlap for varying distances. The best view of the flow divider
is often different from that angle which best defines a lesion
or the minimum residual lumen. For angiography or B mode,
the single plane of view selected by the sonographer/inter-
preter is that which displayed the minimum residual lumen
and often that view does not display the reference flow divider
clearly. Zir and his colleagues had similar difficulty

identifying reference locations and suggest that this was
a major source of error (6). One may speculate that the
differences in distances from the reference point to the
site being measured, combined with variability in the angle
interrogation between B mode and arteriography probably
explains a majority of the differences in measurement
between the two techniques.

The reproducibility of identifying ulceration was much
poorer than that for dimensional data because criteria for
designating smooth, irregular, or pocketed surfaces were not
developed precisely. This is consistent with reports of
other investigators (7,8). Until better ways are found for
establishing these criteria, the difficulty will persist.

High resolution B mode ultrasonography has been
suggested as a potential method for monitoring anatomic
changes in atherosclerotic lesions over time. From our data,
we calculate that to be confident of disease change (p .05
level and a power of 85%), using the clinical methods described
here, the minimum change in lumen diameter required for angiography is $\pm$ 2.7 mm and for ultrasound is $\pm$ 3.2 mm. Large
scale epidemiological assessments will involve many sonographers and readers. Because of this, assessments of plaque
change involving multiple sonographers and readers should
probably use the operator, reader and error components of the
variance for angiographic assessments. Because angiography
measurements are generally more precise than B mode measurements, the sample sizes needed for detecting changes in the
mean are larger for B mode than angiography. For example,
the sample sizes needed for detecting relative changes (with
a probability of .90 and error (alpha) of .05) of the same
magnitude by angiography will be about 15% smaller than that
required for B scan. With a sample of 500 patients, one can
detect a 4.3% change in the mean angiography residual lumen
or a 5.9% change in B mode residual lumen.

In clinical practice the same reader and sonographer
are more likely to be involved in longitudinal follow-up of
individual patients. Assuming no change in personnel, procedures or instrumentation between evaluations, it may be
more realistic to use within-reader variabilities to determine changes one can detect by measurements alone. One

can detect smaller changes by angiography than B mode.
For example, one can detect a 9% (0.6 mm) change in standard
lumen with a probability of .90 and an alpha error of .05
by angiography and a 17% (1.3 mm) change in standard lumen
by B mode.

This study was carried out in five different clinical
centers. Because entry criterion was for the patient to be
scheduled for carotid angiography, no data were excluded
unless a reader considered the quality of a study to be
unacceptable. Therefore, these results have a wider applicability than single-centered studies done under more controlled circumstances. The safety and repeatability of B
mode commends its wide use as a diagnostic screening procedure and our results suggest that B mode is an acceptabl-
supplement for angiography and a reliable substitute in
appropriate circumstances.

REFERENCES
1. Fleiss J (1981) Statistical methods for rates and
    proportions, 2nd Ed, New York, John Wiley & Sons,
    Inc
2. Landis JR, Koch GG (1977) The measurement of observer
    agreement for categorical data. Biometrics 33:159-174
3. Rao CR (1965) Linear statistical inference and its
    applications. New York, John Wiley & Sons, Inc
4. Chikos PM, Fisher LD, Hirsch JH, et al (1983) Observer
    variability in evaluating extracranial carotid artery
    stenosis. Stroke 14:885-892
5. Slot HB, Strijbosch L, Greep JM (1981) Interobserver
    variability in coronary angiography. Circulation
    53:627-632
6. Zir LM, Miller SW, Dinsmore RE, et al (1976) Inter-
    observer variability in coronary angiography.
    Circulation 53:627-632
7. Zwiebel WJ, Austin CW, Sackerr JF et al (1983) Correla-
    tion of high-resolution, B-mode and continuous-wave
    Doppler sonography with arteriography in the diagnosis
    of carotid stenosis. Radiology 149:523-532
8. Eikelboom BC, Riles TR, Montzer R et al (1983) Inaccuracy
    of angiography in the diagnosis of carotid ulceration.
    Stroke 14:882-885

Addendum

    After this manuscript was completed, aspects of this
study were reported by O'Leary et al in Stroke 18;1011-1017,
1987.

51

Multicenter Validation Study of Real Time (B Mode) Ultrasound, Arteriography, and Pathology: III. Sensitivity and Specificity Assessment

John J. Ricotta, Fred A. Bryan, M. Gene Bond, Alfred Kurtz, Daniel H. O'Leary, Jeffery K. Raines, Alan S. Berson, Melvin E. Clouse, Mauricio Calderon-Ortiz, James F. Toole, James A. DeWeese, Stanton N. Smullens, and Nancy F. Gustafson

INTRODUCTION

One of the most promising technologies for the study of atherosclerosis is high-resolution, realtime ultrasound. Developed in large part over the last decade, this methodology has been successful in imaging a variety of body organs including blood vessels. It is non-invasive and associated with minimal risk and radiation. If ultrasound images are an accurate representation of arterial anatomy they could provide an excellent method of identifying and following changes of atherosclerotic disease. To test this methodology, the National Heart, Lung and Blood Institute sponsored a multi-center validation study of realtime ultrasound in the carotid and ileofemoral arteries in human subjects. This report summarizes the comparisons made among ultrasound, angiography, and pathology in evaluation of atherosclerosis of the carotid bifurcation.

MATERIALS AND METHODS

The design of the overall study, which included 1269 patients, is reported separately (1). Of this larger group, a cohort of 892 patients were selected to study the sensitivity and specificity of realtime ultrasound with respect to angiography and examination of pathologic specimens in the extracranial carotid arteries. Eighty-two (82) patients were withdrawn from this cohort for failure to meet all inclusion criteria leaving 900 patients for analyses.

In all cases, interpretation of data were performed
by ultrasound or arteriography readers who were randomly
assigned cases and who were not aware of the clinical data
or measurements made from the other techniques. In one
exception to this rule, one half of the ultrasound images
were interpreted with the knowledge of other non-invasive
information such as doppler spectral frequency data.

Data Analysis

The data were analyzed to determine agreement between
the interpretations of B-scan and angiography by comparing
lesion length and width; MRL; standard lumen; and degree of
diameter stenosis. The statistical summary measures used
in these comparisons included the difference (B-scan minus
angiography), absolute difference and correlation coefficients
as well as linear regression of B-scan measurements with
angiographic measurements; and measures of association
between angiographic and B-scan classification of arteries
based on stenosis, including the Kappa statistic, specifically
value,and sensitivity.

The data were analyzed using analysis of variance for
measured anatomic dimensions; standard lumen, MRL, LW, and
contingency tables for classification of degree of diameter
stenosis, $e.g.$, mild, moderate, severe. Statistical significance of important parameters was determined after correct-
ing for effects of design factors such as clinical center
and access to functional studies data.

RESULTS

Angiography - Ultrasound Comparisons

Angiograms acceptable for interpretation were performed
in 99% of cases and 93% were described as "high quality".
High quality ultrasound examinations were encountered 87% of
the time, 12% of examinations were acceptable and only 1%
could not be interpreted. Total time for performance and
interpretation of the ultrasound examination was approximately
one-half that required with angiography (51 minutes vs 105
minutes). Angiography and ultrasound adequately demonstrated
the common carotid artery in over 99% of cases and the internal carotid in 98.8% and 97.6% respectively. Complications

occurred in 5 of 900 angiogram procedures and 6 of 900 ultrasound examinations (0.7%). There was no permanent morbidity from either examination in this study.

Standard lumen (SL) was chosen to represent a relatively uniform, disease free area of the common carotid artery. A priori it was felt that SL measurements would show the closest correlation between angiography and ultrasound. Measurements of SL in Table I show that these were consistently smaller when measured angiographically. This was true for both intravenous and intraarterial angiography. The difference in the mean (Ultrasound-Angiography) of SL measurement was significant for both the intraarterial and intravenous groups (p<0.0001). Correlation coefficients for SL between ultrasound and angiography varied between centers but were generally poor (r=0.28 - 0.43) suggesting a rather weak predictive ability of ultrasound for this measurement.

A similar trend was seen with measurements of minimal residual lumen (MRL) and lesion width (LW), both parameters being larger when measured by ultrasound (Table 2). Again, the difference in mean measurement values was highly statistically significant (p<0.0001). There was some center variation in the correlation between MRL and LW, with the differences being largest in measurements of lesion width (Table 3). In no instance however, did the correlation coefficient indicate that ultrasound measurements were strongly predictive of those made angiographically.

It was postulated that some of this poor correlation could be due to difficulty of ultrasound in quantitating severe disease, as has been suggested by other authors (3,4). In Table 4 the absolute difference between ultrasound and angiographic measurements is presented for LW and MRL, stratified on the basis of % angiographic stenosis. Contrary to prior assertions, no effect of severity of stenosis was seen on this correlation.

A more qualitative comparison of ultrasound and angiography is presented in Table 5.

In this case, the percent diameter stenosis determined by ultrasound is compared to the angiographic stenosis as a standard. Correlations are best in the normal and occluded categories. Ultrasound is able to detect angiographically

Table 1. Comparisons of Standard Lumen Diameter (mm) by Arterial Angiography, IV-Digital Subtraction Angiography, and B-Scan

Lumen Measures	Arterial Angiography	B-Scan	IV Angiography	B-Scan
Mean ± SD	6.9 ± 1.3	7.3 ± 1.2	6.2 ± 1.4	7.9 ± 1.3
Range	1.5 - 13.1	2.0 - 11.0	1.9 - 15.1	4.2 - 12.0
Observations	1169	1169	478	478
Significance*	p<0.0001		p<0.0001	

* Significance of the difference: B-Scan - Angiography

Table 2. Measurements Correlations

	Lesion Width (mm)		Minimum Residual Lumen (mm)	
	Ultrasound	Angiography	Ultrasound	Angiography
Arteriography				
Mean ± Std. Dev.	4.2 ± 1.9	2.5 ± 1.3	3.5 ± 2.0	3.1 ± 1.8
Range	0.5 – 11.8	0.1 – 7.4	0.1 – 10.5	0.3 – 11.4
Observation	667		673	
Significance*	p<0.0001		p<0.0001	
Digital Subtraction Angiography				
Mean ± Std. Dev.	4.4 ± 1.8	2.7 ± 1.4	3.5 ± 1.6	2.6 ± 1.5
Range	1.0 – 11.0	0.1 – 8.2	0.1 – 8.2	0.2 – 7.4
Observations	291		292	
Significance	p<0.0001		p<0.0001	

* Significance of the difference: B-Scan – Angiography

Table 3. Center Differences Between B-Scan and Angiographic Measurements

		Lesion Width				Minimal Residual Lumen		
Center	N**	Mean Difference (mm)	Mean Abs. Difference (mm)	Corr. Coef.* (r Value)	N**	Mean Difference (mm)	Mean Abs. Difference (mm)	Corr. Coef.* (r Value)
A	228	2.1	2.3	0.34	232	0.3	1.3	0.55
B	157	1.3	1.6	0.35	158	0.7	1.5	0.43
C	226	2.0	2.3	0.17	227	0.8	1.6	0.37
D	152	2.0	2.2	0.28	154	-0.1	1.3	0.46
E	195	1.1	1.8	0.27	194	0.9	1.7	0.40
All	958	1.8	2.1	0.28	965	0.5	1.5	0.46

* B-Scan versus Angio

** Number of observations

Table 4. Comparisons of Degree of Diameter Stenosis

Degree of Stenosis on Angiogram	Lesion Width (mm) Means ± S.D.					Minimum Residual Lumen (mm) Means ± S.D.				
	N*	Ultrasound	Angiogram	Difference**	Absolute Difference	N*	Ultrasound	Angiogram	Difference**	Absolute Difference
<50%	502	3.7 ± 1.8	1.7 ± 0.8	2.1	2.2	501	4.2 ± 1.9	4.2 ± 1.4	-0.04	1.4
50%-74%	299	4.7 ± 1.7	3.2 ± 1.0	1.6	2.0	299	3.1 ± 1.6	2.1 ± 0.4	1.0	1.4
75%-99%	157	5.2 ± 1.6	4.1 ± 1.2	1.2	1.9	157	2.5 ± 1.6	0.9 ± 0.4	1.6	1.7

* Number of observations

** B-Scan minus Angio

Table 5. Percent Diameter Stenosis. Angiography/Ultrasound

	ULTRASOUND						
	Normal	<50	50 – 74	75 – 99	Occl.	Total	Kappa
Normal	174	123	36	8	4	345	0.38
<50	115	268	181	52	6	622	0.18
50-74	22	89	130	80	11	322	0.13
75-99	13	17	75	65	13	183	0.22
Occl.	6	11	12	28	39	96	0.46
Totals	330	508	434	233	73	1,578	

detectable disease (without regard to its severity) with a sensitivity of 88% (1077/1233) and overall accuracy of 79.3% (1251/1578). It is interesting to note that disease was demonstrated by ultrasound in 171 cases (50%) in which the angiogram was interpreted as normal. In the majority of these cases (123), the disease was in the "mild" (50% stenosis) category. Sensitivity of ultrasound varied between 77%-97% between centers while differences in overall accuracy for identification of disease was more uniform (77-83%).

Ability to correctly identify angiographic stenosis >50% diameter was 453/611, or a sensitivity of 74.1%. The specificity of ultrasound in this category was 70.3% (680/967) and overall accuracy was 71.8% (1133/1578). Of the 279 patients with severe (>75% or occluded) angiographic disease, ultrasound identified 232 (83.2%) as having stenosis >50%. While only 41% (39/96) of angiographically occluded arteries were identified as occluded by ultrasound, 86% (63/73) of arteries felt to be occluded by ultrasound had angiographically significant disease (>50% stenosis).

The addition of functional studies to high resolution ultrasound improved its sensitivity for detecting severe stenosis and occlusion and improved the correlation between ultrasound and angiography for MRL and % stenosis (Table 6).

Correlation of plaque characteristics, specifically ulceration, between ultrasound and angiography was poor. Lesions noted as irregular or ulcerated by angiography were compared to those noted to be irregular or pocketed by ultrasound (Table 7). While the sensitivity of ultrasound to angiographically detectable ulcerations was 72%, sonographic findings of irregularity or pocketing were frequent and specificity was only 32%.

Comparisons with Pathology

Results of LW, MRL and % stenosis obtained by both angiography and ultrasound were compared to data derived from the study of specimens retrieved at the time of carotid endarterectomy. Comparisons could be made in 196 cases for LW, 201 for MRL and 216 for percent diameter stenosis. Data are presented in Table 8 showing results for each center as well as overall comparisons for all the data. The thickness of

Table 6. Effect of Functional Studies on B-Scan – Angiography Correlations*

	Without Functional Studies	With Functional Studies	p Value
Sensitivity >50% Stenosis	51%	64%	<0.05
Specificity >50% Stenosis	86%	86%	NS
Sensitivity Occlusion	26%	58%	<0.05
Specificity Occlusion	97%	97%	NS
Mean Absolute Change MRL (B-Scan – Angio)	1.56 mm	1.34 mm	0.05
r Value	0.38	0.54	--
Mean Absolute Change % Stenosis (B-Scan – Angio)	0.20	0.17	0.05
r Value	0.36	0.53	--

* Sensitivity and specificity for detecting an abnormal artery or ulceration were not effected by functional studies.

Table 7. Detection of Ulceration

Comparison of Ultrasound – Angiography

		Angiography		
		Ulcer	No Ulcer	Total
Ultrasound	Ulcer	273	392	665
	No Ulcer	107	188	295
	Total	380	580	960

Table 8. Comparison of LW, MRL, and Percent Stenosis Measured by Angiography, B-Scan, and Pathology

Center	Lesion Width (Mean ± S.D.)			Minimum Residual Lumen (Mean ± S.D.)			Percentage of Stenosis (Mean ± S.D.)		
	Angiography	B-Scan	Pathology	Angiography	B-Scan	Pathology	Angiography	B-Scan	Pathology
A	3.2 ± 1.2 ***1/	5.6 ± 1.4 ***2/	6.7 ± 1.5 N = 39	1.3 ± 1.1	2.1 ± 1.1	1.7 ± 1.6 N = 44	71 ± 20 ***	73 ± 14 ***	81 ± 17 N = 42
B	2.7 ± 1.7 ***	3.5 ± 1.5 **	5.0 ± 1.6 N = 23	2.1 ± 1.7	2.9 ± 1.2 ***	1.6 ± 1.2 N = 21	56 ± 27 **	54 ± 21 ***	77 ± 16 N = 24
C	3.5 ± 1.1 ***	5.3 ± 2.5	5.9 ± 1.7 N = 44	1.6 ± 1.1 **	3.0 ± 1.9 **	2.0 ± 1.4 N = 47	68 ± 19 *	63 ± 24 **	74 ± 16 N = 49
D	3.1 ± 0.6 ***	5.0 ± 2.0	5.5 ± 1.8 N = 27	1.4 ± 0.9	1.5 ± 1.3	1.7 ± 1.3 N = 34	71 ± 13	76 ± 22 *	77 ± 15 N = 34
E	3.7 ± 1.1 ***	3.8 ± 2.4 ***	5.3 ± 1.9 N = 63	2.0 ± 1.1	3.6 ± 1.8 ***	1.8 ± 1.2 N = 55	63 ± 19 ***	47 ± 28 ***	72 ± 17 N = 67
Total	3.3 ± 1.2	4.6 ± 2.3	5.7 ± 1.8 N = 196	1.7 ± 1.2	2.7 ± 1.7	1.8 ± 1.3 N = 201	66 ± 20	61 ± 26	76 ± 16 N = 216

1/ Significance for test of equality of angiography and pathology measurements (paired sample t-test)

2/ Significance for test of equality of B-scan and pathology measurements (paired sample t-test)

Asterisks indicate levels of significance of differences in measurements:

* p<.05

** p<.01

*** p<.001

the endarterectomy specimen was uniformly greater than estimated by either angiography or ultrasound although in 2 centers (C & D) differences between ultrasound and pathology were not significant. Differences in measurement of LW between angiography and pathology were uniformly significant (p<0.001).

Measurements of MRL by angiography more closely approximated specimen measurements than did those made by ultrasound. In only one center did angiographic measurement of MRL, differ significantly from pathology while this was true in 3 centers with ultrasound measurements. In all centers both angiography and ultrasound "underestimated" % stenosis when pathology was used as a standard.

Using absolute differences, it was found that LW by ultrasound was within 1 mm of pathology measurements in 34% of cases and within 2 mm in 61%. For angiography 20% of LW measurements were within 1 mm of pathology and 47% showed <2mm difference in LW when compared to the endartectomy specimen. Absolute differences in MRL were smaller for both ultrasound and angiography when compared to pathology data (data not shown). MRL by angiography agreed with pathology within 1 mm in 64% of cases and within 2 mm in 91%. For ultrasound - pathology 40% of cases corresponded within 1 mm and 68% within 2 mm.

DISCUSSION

The technology of high resolution ultrasound imaging has developed steadily over the last decade (5-7) spurred at least in part by programs sponsored by the National Institutes of Health. Techniques for imaging the arterial wall and lumen have been developed and studies by Hobson (3), Camerota (4,8), Zwiebel (9), and others (10-13) have demonstrated the clinical ability of this technology in the characterization of atherosclerosis at the carotid bifurcation. Their results have supported high resolution ultrasound as a potential non-invasive methodology for the identification, quantification and longitudinal study of human atherosclerotic plaque. If ultrasound fulfilled these expectations, it would provide a unique heretofore unavailable technology for research on the mechanisms and development of atherosclerosis.

In an effort to validate the efficacy of ultrasound technology, the National Heart, Lung and Blood Institute sponsored a multi-centered trial which would study ultrasound in animal models and in the human carotid and ileofemoral arterial system. The trial involved five clinical centers, one animal center and a data coordinating center. Its purpose was to compare ultrasound description of atherosclerotic plaque with those available by angiography and examination of specimens by pathologists. The study was divided into segments involving evaluation of non-human primates, investigation of measurement repeatability and variability in both primate and human arterial systems, and comparison of angiography, pathology and ultrasound as descriptors of clinical atherosclerosis in the carotid and ileofemoral arterial systems in man. Details of the methodology of these trials and organizations of the multicenter groups are published elsewhere (1).

The data reported here included comparisons between angiography, ultrasound and pathology in a group of 900 patients with carotid atherosclerosis. Our aim was to test the capabilities of ultrasound in the clinical setting in which it is most often employed. Therefore, we studied patients with suspected carotid atherosclerosis, usually symptomatic, who had been selected by their physician for angiography. While standard examination techniques were developed, they were purposely made similar to those used in clinical practice. It was for this reason that intravenous digital angiography, which had become widely used clinically during the trial, was deemed an acceptable angiographic technique.

There were several implications of the aforementioned study design. Many patients with advanced atherosclerosis were evaluated and evaluation was performed by a number of individuals in five different centers. Pathology specimens were removed by a number of surgeons using differing techniques and even when intact, were studied by necessity in a nonpressure fixed state. Because of variation in time and personnel, it was often difficult to absolutely identify lesion location and insure correct spatial orientation, which compounded some measurement comparisons. It is apparent

that data from this study can not be compared to work done
in the non-human primate model. The latter provides insight
into the limits of current ultrasound technology under optimal controlled experimental conditions, while data presented
here gives a more accurate estimate of the reliability of
such measurements performed under optimal clinical conditions.
As a large scale multi-center blended comparison of ultrasound
with the standard diagnostic technique, angiography, and examination of removed endarterectomy specimens, this study stands
as a unique effort.

A number of conclusions can be drawn about ultrasound as
a technology for assessing carotid atherosclerosis. It is a
practical technique which requires one half the time of angiography, and can identify the common and internal carotid
artery in virtually all cases. Morbidity associated with
ultrasound examination is minimal, suggesting that it is well
suited to evaluation and longitudinal followup of large populations at risk for atherosclerosis. The ability to identify
angiographically apparent atherosclerotic disease is good
with a sensitivity of 88% and accuracy of 79%. In addition,
our data suggest that ultrasound may be more sensitive than
angiography in detecting minor degrees of atherosclerosis,
since 50% of normal angiograms were found to have disease
on ultrasound examination.

Quantitative comparisons between ultrasound, angiography
and pathology were disappointing. Lesion width, minimal
residual lumen and standard lumen were all larger when measured sonographically than by angiographic techniques.
Furthermore, the predictive ability of ultrasound with respect to angiographic findings was modest. There was evidence to suggest that the addition of functional studies,
specifically doppler frequency analysis, improved correlations of MRL, % stenosis and diagnosis of occlusion. Both
diagnostic techniques underestimated lesion width and over-
estimated MRL when compared to data obtained by endarterectomy specimens, although ultrasound more closely approximated LW and angiographic data correlated better for MRL.
While O'Donnell (12), Reilly (13), and others (3) have
suggested that ultrasound can reliably detect ulceration in
atherosclerotic plaques, in our experience, ability to

consistently identify ulceration was poor with both techniques. While some differences were apparent among centers, trends were similar throughout the trial.

A variety of reasons may explain these differences. Error is associated with each measurement technique, and our analysis of measurement error with these techniques is reported elsewhere (14-16). Shadowing by calcified plaque remains a significant problem with sonography, and boundary definition can be difficult with both techniques although this is less true with angiography. The majority of atherosclerotic lesions are eccentric and variation in orientation at the time of interrogation can compound measurement differences. While every attempt was made to standardize measurement angle by all three techniques, variability in the topography of the carotid bifurcation made this impossible to ascertain. Artifactual distortion of the pathologic specimens, especially luminal collapse, further compounded measurements of what was to be the "gold standard" (16).

It is apparent from these studies that comparisons between ultrasound and angiography in patients with clinically suspected atherosclerosis must at present remain qualitative rather than quantitative. Data presented elsewhere (14,15) suggest that differences in lesion dimension of approximately 3 mm must be observed before a change can be predicted with confidence in this patient population, although this decreases to <1.5 mm if a single individual is involved in repetitive followup. These data have particular significance when planning longitudinal study of patient populations at risk for progression of atherosclerosis.

With these caveats however, the general clinical utility of high resolution ultrasound has been confirmed. It is apparent that this utility can be increased by combining ultrasound with other studies such as doppler frequency analysis. While a negative ultrasound cannot completely exclude angiographic disease, a positive examination is a significant finding and should prompt further clinical investigation. Similarly, although we were unable to confidently predict angiographic occlusion by ultrasound examination, the presence of an occlusion on ultrasound was almost always associated with significant angiographic disease.

At present, we suggest that sonography is most useful clinically as a screening test to evaluate patients with suspected atherosclerosis and determine the extent of further evaluation.

One of the most encouraging findings of this study was confirmation of ultrasound's ability to define lesion width. Because angiography focuses on lumen size and contour, most clinical interest has been centered on % lumen stenosis. It is apparent that this focus excludes the majority of the atherosclerotic process itself. High resolution sonography provided a reasonable approximation of lesion measurements made on endarterectomy specimens. While characterization of the constituents of atheroma by ultrasound was not a primary focus of this study, it is currently a topic of considerable investigative interest and effort. It is likely that sonographic techniques will make their greatest impact in this area in the future.

REFERENCES

1. Calderon-Ortiz M, Rifkin MD, O'Leary DH *et al* (1989) Multicenter validation study of real time (B-mode) ultrasound: Arteriography and Pathology. I Materials and Methods, this volume, Chapter 51
2. DeWeese JA, May AG, Lipchick ED, Rob CG (1970) Anatomic and hemodynamic correlations in carotid artery stenosis. Stroke 1:149-157
3. Hobson RW II, Berry SM, Katocs AS, O'Donnell JA, Jamil Z, Savitsky JP (1980) Comparison of pulsed Doppler and real time B-mode echo arteriography for noninvasive imaging of the extracranial carotid arteries. Surgery 87:286-293
4. Comerota AJ, Cranley JJ, Cook SE (1981) Realtime B-mode carotid imaging in diagnosis of cerebrovascular disease. Surgery 89:718-729
5. Mozersky DJ, Hokanson DE, Sumner DS, *et al* (1972) Ultrasonic visualization of the arterial lumen. Surgery 72:253-259
6. Barnes RW, Bone GE, Reinertson J, *et al* (1976) Noninvasive ultrasonic carotid angiography: prospective validation by contrast arteriography. Surgery 80:328-335
7. Green PS, Taenzer JC, Ramsey SD, Holzemer JF, Suarez JR, Marich KW (1977) A realtime ultrasonic imaging system for carotid arteriography. Ultrasound Med Biol 3:129-142
8. Comerota AJ, Cranley JJ, Katz ML *et al* (1984) Realtime B-mode carotid imaging. J Vasc Surg 1:84-95
9. Zwiebel WJ, Auston CW, Sackett JF, Strother CM (1983) Correlation of high resolution, B-mode and continuous wave Doppler sonography with arteriography in the diagnosis of carotid stenosis. Radiology 149:523-532

10. James EM, Earnest F IV, Forbes GS, Reese DF, Houser DW,
    Folger WN (1982) High resolution dynamic ultrasound
    imaging of the carotid bifurcation: A prospective
    evaluation. Radiology 144:853-858
11. Jacobs NM, Grant ES, Schellinger D, Byrd MC, Richardson
    JD, Cohan SL (1985) Duplex carotid sonography: criteria
    for stenosis, accuracy, and pitfalls. Radiology
    154:385-381
12. O'Donnell TF Jr, Erdoes L, Mackey WC, *et al* (1985)
    Correlation of B-mode ultrasound imaging and arterio-
    graphy with pathologic findings at carotid endarterec-
    tomy. Arch Surg 120:443-449
13. Reilly LM, Lusby RJ, Hughes L, Ferrell LD, Stoney RJ,
    Ehrenfeld WK (1983) Carotid plaque histology using
    realtime ultrasonography. Am J Surg 146:188-193
14. O'Leary DH, Bryan FA, Goodison MW, Goldberg BB,
    Gramiak R, Ball M, Bond MG, Dunn RA, Rifkin M, Toole JF,
    Wheeler HG, Gustafson NF, Eckholm S, and Raines J (1989)
    Multicenter Validation Study of Real-Time (B-Mode)
    Ultrasound, Arteriography and Pathology II. Repeatability/
    Variability Assessment, this volume, Chapter 52
15. O'Leary DH, Bryan FA, Goodison MW, Rifkin M, Gramiak R,
    Ball M, Bond MG, Dunn RA, Goldberg BB, Toole JF,
    Wheeler HG, Gustafson NF, Eckholm S, and Raines J (1987)
    Measurement Variability of Carotid Atherosclerosis:
    Real-Time (B-Mode) Ultrasonography and Arteriography.
    Stroke 18:1011-1017
16. Schenk EA, Bond MG, Aretz TH, Angelo JN, Choi HY,
    Rynalski T, Gustafson NF, Berson AS, Ricotta JJ, Goodison
    MW, Bryan FA, Goldberg BB, Toole JF, and O'Leary DH
    (1988) Multicenter Validation Study of Real-Time
    Ultrasonography, Arteriography, and Pathology: Pathologic
    Evaluation of Carotid Endarterectomy Specimens.
    Stroke 19:289-296

52
Multicenter Validation Study of Real Time (B Mode) Ultrasound, Arteriography, and Pathology: IV. Comparison of B Mode Ultrasonic Imaging with Arteriography in Lower Extremity Arteries

S.N. Smullens, J.K. Raines, D.H. O'Leary, M. Ball, J.J. Ricotta, N.F. Gustafson, M.G. Bond, A. Berson, R.A. Kane, B.B. Goldberg, M. Calderon-Ortiz, B.J.G. York, C. Nunn, and J.A. DeWeese

INTRODUCTION

In 1980, the National Heart, Lung and Blood Institute (NHLBI) issued a proposal for the assessment of ultrasonic B-scan imaging for detection and quantification of athero-sclerotic lesions in human carotid and iliofemoral arteries (1). [In response to this, contracts were issued in 1981 to five clinical centers, one animal center, and a data coordinating center (2). The project consisted of several phases extending over three years.] Although the original NHLBI contract was to be equally dividen between the carotid and iliofemoral systems, the six-month pilot phase demon-strated that the major emphasis would be in the carotid system. Several reasons for this were present.

Firstly, clinical interest was highest in the carotid system, since stroke is the third leading cause of death in the United States. In addition, many studies have emphasized that the pathophysiology of symptomatic carotid disease relates both to embolization as well as flow reduction through the carotid system (3). Further work has suggested that specific anatomic reatures such as ulceration or the presence of hemorrhage may also have a high correlation with the pre-sence of symptoms (4,5). In the lower extremities, however, flow reduction through high grade stenosis or occlusion is the single most important consideration in the development

Supported by USPHS NHLBI contracts 12904, 12912-17

of symptoms. Whereas prevention and, therefore, early
detection of disease is a major consideration in the
carotid system, this is not a factor in the lower extremities, since treatment begins only after limb threatening
symptoms develop. An important additional reason for the
carotid emphasis was that pathologic data would be lacking
in the lower extremity cases, since bypass, rather than
endarterectomy, is the usual treatment modality. As a
consequence of this, no atherosclerotic plaques would be
available for review of comparison following the operative
procedure.

Because of these limitation, only three of the five
clinical centers participated in this study. These were the
Thomas Jefferson University Hospital, the New England
Deaconess Hospital, and the Miami Heart Institute. Of the
total 1269 patients enrolled in the overall study, 170
patients comprised the total lower extremity real time
B-mode population (2).

Design and Study Hypothesis

Because of the size constraints, only a sensitivity/
specificity (S/S) study was undertaken, as compared to both
S/S and R/V (repeatibility/variability) studies in the carotid
portion (6,7). Because of the lack of pathologic material,
arteriography, rather than pathology as in the carotid study,
became the diagnostic standard. Various study hypothesis
were tested and analyzed:

1. That real time B-mode ultrasound can visualize the
   lower extremity arteries comparable to arteriography.
2. That real time B-mode can identify diseased versus
   normal arteries.
3. That B-scan can identify categories of diseased
   arteries.
4. That B-scan real time imaging can quantitate the
   atherosclerotic disease found in these vessels.
5. That there is clinical utility in the use of real
   time B-scan ultrasound in lower extremity atherosclerosis.

MATERIALS AND METHODS

Patients were included for study if they had symptomatic atherosclerosis of the lower extremities and were to
undergo arteriography. All B-scan real time examinations
were performed within two weeks of the primary arteriogram. In contrast to the carotid study, all patients
(after the pilot phase) had conventional arteriography and
no digital arterial or venous studies were used for the
main study in the lower extremities. The technique of
arteriography was standardized between the centers and
is briefly described in an accompanying paper in this
volume (Chapter 51). In addition, a circular marker of
known dimensions was placed on the arteriograms to allow
accurate measurement compensation for magnification. The
technique of B-scan examination was also standardized, as
described elsewhere in this series (Chapter 52). Typically, the external iliac artery, the common femoral, the
superficial femoral, and the popliteal artery in each leg
were studied by both arteriography and real time B-mode.
The profunda femoris artery was not studied after the pilot
phase, since the vessel was infrequently seen by B-scan.
During the pilot phase it was only visualized in 31 of 90
cases, or 34%, and all of these were interpreted as "normal".

The data collected for both B-mode imaging and arteriography were evaluated for categories of disease in each of
the segments and characterized as either being: not
applicable (N/A), not visualized, normal, having non-
intrusive arterial disease (NIAD), stenotic, occluded or
aneurysmal. Venous or prosthetic bypass grafts, when
present, were also categorized. Quantitative measurements
were made to the nearest 0.5 mm when stenotic, occlusive, or
aneurysmal lesions were identified. Infrequent aneurysms
were seen and no significant data were collected regarding
these lesions. Bypass grafts were also infrequently seen.
Since no grafts were identified both in B-mode and arteriography, comparisons between these techniques for this aspect
of the study were not possible. Quantitative measurements
were carried out for lesion length (LL), minimal residual

lumen (MRL), lesion width (LW) at the point of the MRL, and unobstructed lumen (UL) obtained in each segment. The degree of luminal stenosis was derived from LW and MRL using the formula:

$$\% \text{ Stenosis} = 1 - \left(\frac{MRL}{MRL + LW} \right) \times 100$$

An additional measurement, standard lumen (SL), was measured over the common femoral artery at the groin crease (Figure 1). This was selected to allow a fixed point for comparison of arteriography to B-scan.

B-mode studies were performed by an experienced examiner assigned by the Data Coordinating Center. All instruments were high resolution scanners, and calibrations maintained by use of ultrasonic phantom. A 10 MHz probe was used when possible, and a 7.5 MHz substituted for deeper vessels. Interpretation and measurement of both arteriogram and real time scans were done by randomly assigned readers who were blinded to the results of the opposite study. Measurements were made with calipers to the nearest 0.5 mm directly from the x-ray or tape. Data evaluation was carried out for sensitivity, specificity, positive predictive value, negative predictive value, accuracy, and prevalence. Verification of data quality was accomplished by reviewing a 20% random sample of the complete data set.

RESULTS

1. Visualization of the Iliofemoral Arteries. The ability of B-mode to visualize the different arteries varied. The external iliac artery was visualized by B-mode 45% of the time, the common femoral 98%, the superficial femoral 97%, and the popliteal 90%.

2. Ability to Identify Normal Versus Diseased Arteries. The overall study showed a sensitivity of 89%, a specificity of 42%, a positive predictive value of 83%, a negative predictive value of 54%, and an overall accuracy of 78%. The prevalence was high overall at 76% (Table 1).

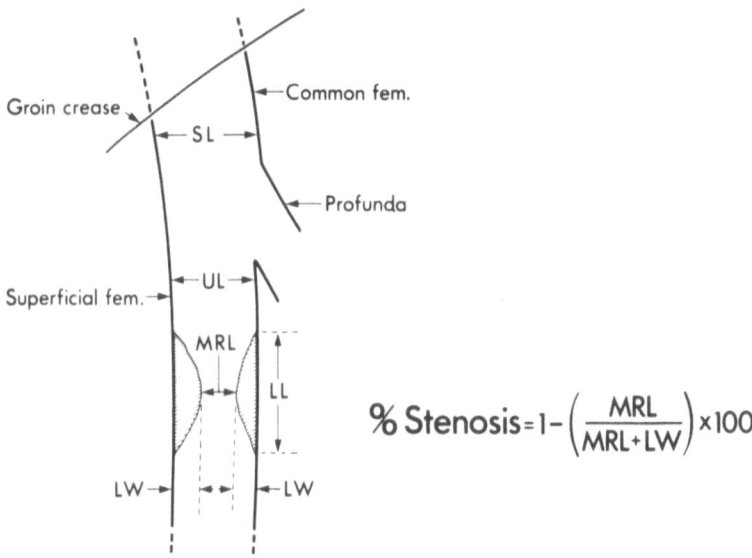

$$\% \text{ Stenosis} = 1 - \left(\frac{MRL}{MRL + LW}\right) \times 100$$

Figure 1.

A breakdown by segments showed similar findings. However, the best results were obtained in the superficiel femoral artery, where the sensitivity was 93%, the negative predictive value was 28%, the accuracy was 91%, with a high overall prevalence of 93%. The improvement in sensitivity and positive predictive value for this section reflects this high prevalence.

    3. <u>Ability to Detect Categories of Disease</u>. This was poor in all levels, including normal vessels, NIAD, stenotic, occluded and aneurysmal. The worst results were found in the stenotic lesions. The best overall results were found in occluded vessels where an accuracy of 62% was identified (Table 2).

    4. <u>Ability to Quantitate Degree of Atherosclerosis</u>. The correlation was poorest with SL with a correlation coefficient (r) of 0.26. This was a disappointment since

Table 1. Presence of Disease in Lower Extremity Arteries

	Arteriography	
ULTRASOUND	Normal	Diseased
Normal	75	63
Diseased	102	502

Sensitivity	89%
Specificity	42%
Positive Predictive Value	83%
Negative Predictive Value	54%
Accuracy	78%
Prevalence	76%

Table 2. Matrix of Disease Categories Ultrasound/Arterio-
graphy

	Arteriography					
ULTRASOUND	NL	NIAD	Sten	Occl	Aneur	Totals
NL	75	49	12	12	0	148
NIAD	72	104	103	25	3	307
Sten	22	49	32	20	1	124
Occl	7	34	27	94	0	162
Aneur	1	2	0	0	0	3
TOTAL	177	238	174	151	4	744
Correctly Identified	42%	44%	18%	62%	0%	Kappa 0.2

it was thought this parameter would yield consistent
results. In a subgroup of 38 cases in which both the
right and left leg standard lumens were measured, only
a small difference between arteriography and B-scan
occurred (0.3 mm) but correlation remained poor (Table 3).
MRL had a correlation of 0.46, percent stenosis r = 0.35,
and LL r = 0.37. The best results were found in UL with
a correlation coefficient of 0.62, and in LW with a
correlation coefficient of 0.71 (Table 4).

Measurements by real time tended to be larger than
those by arteriography in all categories except LL and SL.
However, when comparisons were made in the measurements of
disease by Center, the reason for the difference in LL was
apparent. In Center A, there was a large discrepancy in
LL by arteriography as compared to real time, whereas, in
both Centers B and C, the larger measurement by B-mode prevailed (Table 5). In a separate evaluation in which LL in
both the right and left side in identical cases was evaluated,
here again, B-mode measurements were larger than arteriography (Table 3).

DISCUSSION

Although a large literature has developed in evaluating
the carotid artery by real time B-mode ultrasound imaging,
a paucity of work has been done in the lower extremities.
This disproportion was apparent in our study, in which 1099
patients were enrolled in the carotid S/S study, 117 randomly
assigned to the carotid RV study, and 170 patients comprising
the total lower extremity population.

Interesting differences were noted in the visualization
of the various arterial segments. In a paper published by
Hobson in 1981, 88% of the common femoral arteries were
visualized, as compared to 98% in our study (8). In his
report, the superficial femoral artery was visualized 100%
of the time when it was patent, and 70% when it was occluded.
An overall 97% visualization was achieved by real time in
our study, with no difference noted between patency or
occlusion. The popliteal artery, a deeper vessel than the

Table 3.   Standard Lumen by Sides in Similar Cases (mm)

	Left		Right	
	Arteriogram	B-Mode	Arteriogram	B-Mode
Mean	6.95	7.06	6.98	7.27
Standard deviation	1.64	2.30	1.69	1.91
Number of observations	38	38	38	38
Mean difference		0.09		0.30
Correlation coefficient		0.41		0.25

superficial or common femoral artery, was visualized 90%
in our study. The external iliac was the poorest visualized
and was seen in only 46% of cases. The difference in
visualization of the various segments is felt mainly due to
the depth of the vessels, a problem similar to that of
real time imaging of the coronary arteries, where depth is
a major factor (9).

Real time ultrasound did well in detecting presence of
disease, with an overall sensitivity of 89%, a specificity
of 42%, a positive predictive value of 83%, a negative predictive value of 54%, and an accuracy of 78%. The overall
prevalence disease was high at 76%. This prevalence reflects
the population studied, all of whom had symptomatic lower
extremity atherosclerosis. The best results were in the
superficial femoral artery, where the prevalence of
disease was quite high at 93%, and where 77% of the vessels
were either classified as stenotic or occluded.

Although real time ultrasound did detect the presence
of disease, it did poorly in categorizing the extent of
disease. Although most reports show that real time ultrasonic imaging does best in minimal or mid-range disease, our
studies suggest that obstructed vessels are more accurately

Table 4.   Quantitative Measurement of Disease (mm)

STANDARD LUMEN (SL)

	Arteriogram	B-mode
Mean	7.14	6.94
Standard deviation	2.03	2.15
Number of observations	101	101
Mean difference		0.20
Correlation coefficient		0.26

MINIMAL RESIDUAL LUMEN (MRL)

	Arteriogram	B-mode
Mean	2.47	3.00
Standard deviation	1.37	1.1
Number of observations	27	27
Mean difference		0.53
Correlation coefficient		0.46

LESION LENGTH (LL)

	Arteriogram	B-mode
Mean	14.61	12.33
Standard deviation	18.11	6.16
Number of observations	27	2⁷
Mean difference		2.28
Correlation coefficient		0.37

UNOBSTRUCTED LUMEN (UL)

	Arteriogram	B-mode
Mean	4.68	6.43
Standard deviation	1.98	1.98
Number of observations	27	27
Mean difference		1.75
Correlation coefficient		0.62

% STENOSIS

	Arteriogram	B-mode
Mean	49.9%	55.0%
Standard deviation	17.2%	12.2%
Number of observations	25	25
Mean difference		5.17%
Correlation coefficient		0.35

LESION WIDTH (LW)

	Arteriogram	B-mode
Mean	2.32	3.85
Standard deviation	1.35	1.64
Number of observations	26	26
Mean difference		1.53
Correlation coefficient		0.71

Table 5.   Differences* in Measurement of Disease
           by Center (mm)

Parameter	Center		
	A	B	C
MRL	-0.22	-0.82	-0.48
LW	-1.12	-2.10	-1.10
% stenosis	-5.6%	-8.1%	0.8%
LL	13.01	-4.16	-1.51
UL	-0.79	-2.59	-1.69

*   Refers to difference in mm in means between
    arteriogram and B-mode measurements. Negative
    value reflects a larger measurement by B-mode.

identified (10-14). The reason for this is difficult to
determine, but the relatively superficial nature of the
thigh vessels and the high prevalence of disease, particularly in the severe categories, probably was the major
determining factor in the accuracy of this portion of
protocol.

    Quantitative measurements were, unfortunately, few
due to the large number of occlusions found. In addition,
the design of the study where long segments of lower extremity vessels were evaluated in a blinded-fashion, did not
allow frequent comparisons to be made, since many times
analogous lesions were not studied by both real time and
arteriography. In general, the real time B-scan measurements were larger than arteriography, except in LL. In
two of the three Center, however, LL was also larger by
real time. The one Center, Center A, showed a large
difference in which the arteriography study showed much
larger measurements than real time. The reason for this
consistent trend may be due to differences between the two
measurement modalities, in which the vessel wall, as well
as plaque thickness, is detected by real time imaging, but
only the lumen by arteriography (15,16). Difficulties in
detecting the plaque to lumen interface with real time, as

compared to detecting the lumen with arteriography, are repetitive problems. Pathologic evaluations in the carotid portion of the study suggest that lesion width is more accurately defined by real time B-mode, but that MRL is more closely correlated with arteriography (17). The better correlation with LW and UL may, in part, relate to the relatively small area involved in these measurements as compared to LL. This latter is a more difficult parameter to define, since it is a longitudinal rather than a transverse measurement. Poor correlation with percent stenosis may arise since there are two measurement variables, MRL and LW, which are used to determine this parameter, and each introduces its own inherent variability. Poor correlation with SL was a disappointment. Although the measurement means were quite close (a difference of 0.2 mm), the correlation remained poor. This may be due to difficulties in anatomically detecting the femoral artery at the groin crease because of variability in thickness of the subcutaneous tissue, the variability in the bifurcation of the femoral, and difficulty in correlating the image seen by B-mode as compared to arteriography.

CONCLUSIONS

1. Real time B-mode ultrasound visualizes the external iliac artery in less than one-half of the vessels studied, but visualizes the common femoral, the superficial femoral, and the popliteal arteries in over 90% of the cases. Although not part of the main study, B-mode ultrasound visualized the profunda femoris artery in about one-third of the cases during the pilot phase.

2. A diseased lower extremity artery can be separated from a non-diseased artery, with a sensitivity of 89%, a specificity of 42%, a positive predictive value of 83%, a negative predictive value of 54%, and with an overall accuracy of 78%. Real time B-mode ultrasound performed particularly well in the superficial femoral artery where the highest prevalence of disease occurs.

3. Real time B-mode ultrasound however, does not accurately separate categories of disease as compared to arteriography. However, it does best at detecting obstructed arteries, particularly in the superficial femoral artery.

4. Quantitative measurements do not correlate well with arteriography, except in regards to UL and LW. Real time B-mode tends to measure not only a larger LW but also a larger MRL and UL, as compared to arteriography.

5. Finally, clinical utility of real time B-mode in the lower extremities is limited by the clinical need for functional as well as purely anatomic information. However, B-mode can accurately detect the presence of disease in symptomatic subjects below the inguinal ligament. In addition, quantitative information is obtainable, appears to be reproducible, and can be used safely and inexpensively to track *in vitro* atherosclerotic disease of the lower extremities.

REFERENCES

1. National Heart, Lung, and Blood Institute, NIH (April 1980) Assessment of Ultrasonic B-scan Imaging for Detection and Quantification of Atherosclerotic Lesions in Human Carotid and Iliofemoral Arteries and in Arteries of Animals: Request for Proposal RFP NHLBI 8-10.
2. Calderon-Ortiz M, Rifkin M, O'Leary D, Toole J, et al. (1989) Multicenter validation study of real time (B-mode) ultrasound, arteriography and pathology: I. Methods and materials, in this volume, Chapter 51.
3. Moore WS, Hall AD (1970) Importance of emboli from the carotid bifurcation in pathogenesis in cerebral ischemia attacks. Arch Surg 101:708-716.
4. Imparato AM, Riles TS, Gorstein F (1979) The carotid bifurcation plaque: Pathologic findings associated with cerebral ischemia. Stroke 10:238-245.
5. Reilly LM, Lusby RJ, Hughes L, et al. (1983) Carotid plaque histology using real-time ultrasonography: Clinical and therapeutic implications. Am J Surg 146:188-193.
6. O'Leary D, Rao A, Raines J, Goldberg B, Gramiak R, Ball M, et al. (1989) Multicenter validation study of real time (B-mode) ultrasound: II. Repeatability/variability assessment, in this volume, Chapter 52.

7. Ricotta J, Bond MG, Bryan F, McKinney W, Kurtz A, O'Leary D, et al. (1989) Multicenter validation study of real time (B-mode) ultrasound: III. Sensitivity/sensitivity assessment, in this volume, Chapter 53.

8. Hobson RW, Berry SM, Katocs AS, et al. (1981) Real time B-mode ultrasonography of the femoral arteries: Comparison to contrast arteriography. Am Surg 47:262-267.

9. Blankenhorn DH, Curry PJ (1982) The accuracy of arteriography and ultrasound imaging for atherosclerotic measurement: A review. Arch Pathol Lab Med 106:483-489.

10. Comerota AJ, Cranley JJ, Cook SE (1981) Real time B-mode carotid imaging in diagnosis of cerebrovascular disease. Surgery 89:718-729.

11. Comerota AJ, Cranley JJ, Katz ML (1984) Real time B-mode imaging: A three year multicenter experience. J Vasc Surg 1:84-95.

12. James EM, Ernest F, Forbes GS, et al. (1982) High resolution dynamic real time imaging of the carotid bifurcation: A prospective evaluation. Radiol 144:853-858.

13. Cooperberg PL, Robertson WD, Fry P, Sweeney V (1979) High resolution real time ultrasound of the carotid bifurcation. J Clin Ultrasound 7:13-17.

14. Anderson DC, Loewson R, Yock D, et al. (1983) B-mode real time carotid ultrasonic imaging: Correlation with angiography. Arch Neurol 40:484-488.

15. Wolverson MK, Heiber E, Sundaram M, Tantansirvionese S, Shield JB (1983) Carotid atherosclerosis: High resolution real time sonography correlated with angiography. Am J Radiol 140:355-361.

16. Zwiebel WJ, Austin CW, Sackett JF, Strother CM (1983) Correlation of high resolution B-mode and continuous-wave Doppler sonography with arteriography in the diagnosis of carotid stenosis. 149:523-532.

17. Schenk EA, Bond MG, Aretz TH, Angelo JN, Choi HY, Rynalski T, Gustafson NF, Berson AS, Ricotta JJ, Goodison MW, Bryan FA, Goldberg BB, Toole JF, O'Leary DH (1988) Multicenter validation study of real-time ultrasonography, arteriography, and pathology: Pathologic evaluation of carotid endartectomy specimen. Stroke 19:289-296.

53

Multicenter Validation Study of Real Time (B Mode) Ultrasound, Arteriography, and Pathology: V. Pathologic Evaluation of Endarteroctomy Specimens and of Perfusion Fixed Carotid Arteries

Eric A. Schenk, John Ricotta, M. Gene Bond, Thomas Aretz, Jean Angelo, Hong Y. Choi, Thomas Rinalski, Nancy Gustafson, Alan Berson, Fred A. Bryan, Barry Goldberg, James F. Toole, and Daniel H. O'Leary

During the implementation of an NIH sponsored contract program titled "Assessment of Ultrasonic B-Scan Imaging for Detection and Quantification of Atherosclerotic Lesions in Human Carotid Arteries", 289 endarterectomy specimens became available for pathologic examination at five participating centers (Miami Heart Institute, Bowman Gray School of Medicine, New England Deaconess Medical Center, Jefferson Medical College, and University of Rochester Medical Center). These specimens were fixed in 10% neutral buffered formalin, decalcified, and cross-sectioned at 3 mm intervals. An overlay template was used to measure lumen diameters and near and far wall thickness in four planes.

Quality control measures used in the pathologic evaluation included the identification of outlier cases where angiography and pathology measurements of the smallest lumen diameter (minimum residual lumen - MRL) differed by more than 1 mm. Table 1 summarizes such cases by center and shows that a difference in MRL greater than 1 mm was found in 101 of the 289 cases (35%). A difference greater than 2 mm was found in 26 of the 289 cases (9%). Each of the outlier cases at one center (Rochester) was remeasured and reviewed for the purpose of identifying problems which might have contributed to a lack of accuracy and/or precision in the pathology measurements.

Supported by NHLBI Contracts: N01-HV 12904, 12912-12917.

Table 1. Angiography Minimun Residual Lumen Compared to Pathology Minimum Residual Lumen

Difference	Center and Number of Cases					
	1	2	3	4	5	All
< 1 mm	33(66%)	23(62%)	43(64%)	28(63%)	61(67%)	188(65%)
1-2 mm	13(26%)	10(27%)	20(30%)	11(25%)	21(23%)	75(26%)
> 2 mm	4(8%)	4(11%)	4(6%)	5(11%)	9(10%)	26(9%)
n	50	37	67	44	91	289

Four potential and real problems were identified:

1. <u>Artifacts produced by fixation and decalcification</u>.
At two centers (Bowman Gray and Rochester) the diameters at
3 mm intervals, length, perimeter, and area were measured
by computerized planimetry in 40 whole specimens in the
fresh state, after fixation in formalin, and after decalcification. The data expressed as percent change in dimensions
after fixation and decalcification are presented in Table 2.

Table 2.   Effect of Formalin Fixation and Decalcification of
Specimen Size

| | Percentage of Change | | | |
	Outer Diam*	Length	Perimeter	Total Area
Fresh vs Formalin Fixed				
Mean	-0.14	-1.2	-1.0	2.0
(SD)	(2.9)	(5.5)	(5.0)	(5.1)
Formalin Fixed vs Decalcified				
Mean	-3.0	-4.5	-5.0	-9.0
(SD)	(3.0)	(2.4)	(1.9)	(5.0)

* Outer diameter measured at 3 mm intervals on each specimen

Formalin fixation resulted in no significant changes. Decalcification, however, did produce a 5% average shrinkage in
diameter and length and a 10% shrinkage in area. All specimens were x-rayed and the amount of calcification was reported
semiquantitatively on a scale of 0 to +4. No correlation was
found between the amount of calcium present (and removed by
the decalcifying solution) and the degree of shrinkage (data
not shown).

2. <u>The nature of endarterectomy specimens</u>. Many specimens were received in a fragmented state and of no use for
determining either the site or size of the minimum residual
lumen. Even intact specimens were frequently split longitudinally during surgical removal. Surgical techniques varied

from center to center: in one only 7% of the specimens were intact, in another 90% were removed intact.

Measurement of lumen size in split specimens was possible only by using a computer-based reconstruction process whereby the lumen perimeter was measured and made equal to the circumference of a circle (Figure 1). Even in intact specimens, eccentrically located lumina often showed artifactual infolding of a thin wall along one side (Figure 2). Again, computer-based circularization had to be used to allow measurement of lumen diameters.

3. <u>Non-round lumina in intact specimens</u>. "D"-shaped, ovoid, irregularly shaped and slit-like lumina were present in over one-half of all intact specimens (Figures 3 and 4). The view that all non-round lumina are artifacts due to loss of perfusion pressure was held by some of the pathologists but rejected by others. This problem was dealt with by allowing each pathologist to decide which lumina were artifactually non-round and then to use computer-based reconstruction and circularization.

4. <u>Matching of planes of interrogation used by angiography and by pathology</u>. Measurement of lumen diameters were made along four planes which were fixed by orienting the specimen so that the external carotid artery was always medial (right or left) to the internal carotid artery. Since this orientation does not correspond to the anatomic position of these vessels, which, furthermore is variable from patient to patient, it was not possible to select the measurements along any given plane as representative of those obtained from either the AP or lateral angiographic views. The solution decided on was to use whatever pathology plane had the smallest lumen (and thickest wall). This approach allowed the evaluation of how often angiography can find the smallest lumen rather than how accurately angiography can measure lumen diameter.

Autopsy Studies

To resolve the problem of non-round lumina and effect of loss of perfusion pressure, carotid arteries were obtained

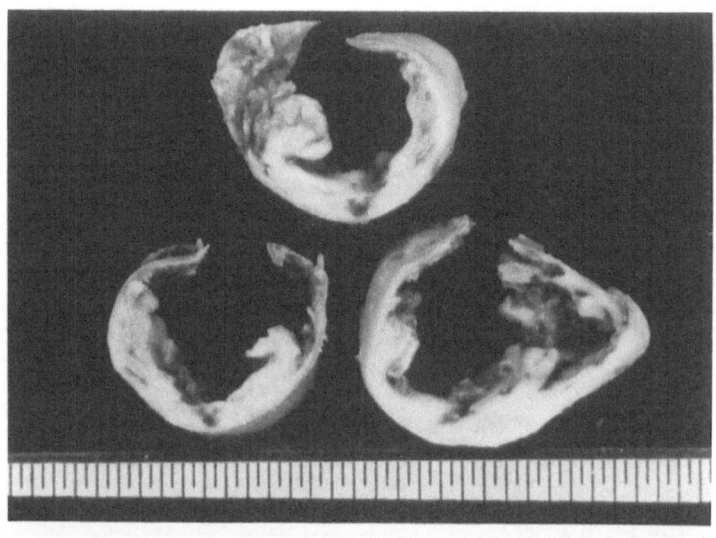

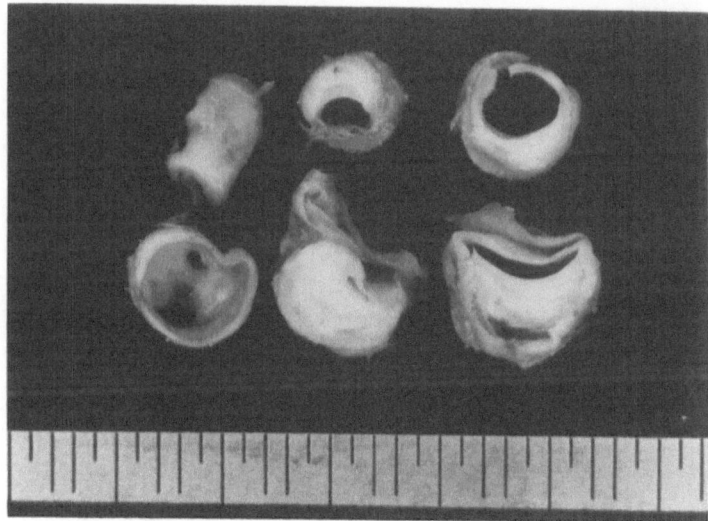

Figure 1.   Endarterectomy specimen split during surgical removal, requires reconstruction and circularization to allow measurement of lumen diameter.
Figure 2.   Artifactual infolding of a thin wall along one margin of an eccentric lumen is seen in two of the cross-sectional slices.   Reconstruction and circularization utilizing perimeter measurement made equal to the circumference of a circle is required.

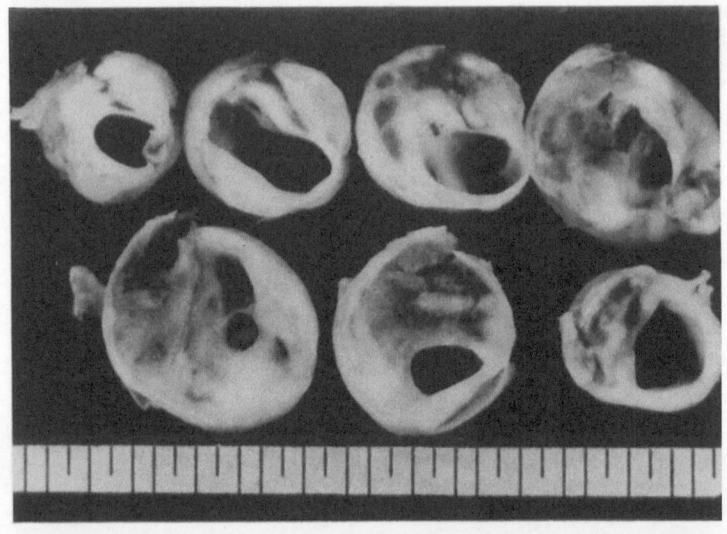

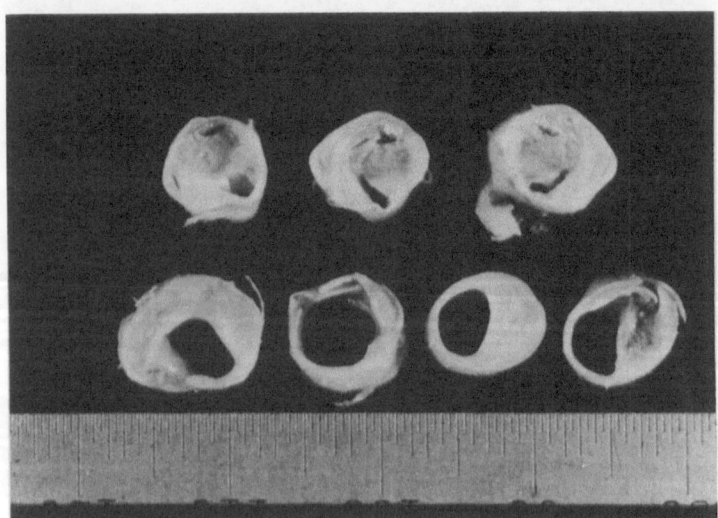

Figure 3. Ovoid and "D"-shaped lumina are present in a
number of the cross-sectional slices in this specimen.
Figure 4. In addition to ovoid and "D"-shaped lumina,
irregular shaped slit-like lumina are seen in two of the
cross-sectional slices.

from 30 unselected autopsy cases. Patients ranged in age
from 22 to 92 and included 19 females and 11 males. The
entire common carotid artery and internal carotid artery to
near the base of the skull was removed bilaterally and perfusion fixed with warm 10% neutral buffered formalin at
150 mmHg pressure for six hours. The arteries were then
serially sectioned at 3 mm intervals. The cross-sections
were x-rayed for calcium content and localization and used
to obtain measurements of external vessel diameter, lumen
diameter, and wall thickness.

Data from these measurements in the common carotid
artery 6 mm below the bifurcation, at the level of the
bifurcation, and in the internal carotid artery at 6 mm
and at 18 mm above the bifurcation are shown in Figures 5
and 6. Measurements recorded are for the smallest lumen
diameter and largest wall thickness found at these locations.
Wall thickness (i.e., plaque size) is represented by the
difference between outside and lumen diameter (illustrated
by the length of the line joining these two points). The
common carotid arteries at -6 mm and at the bifurcation,
and the internal carotid arteries at +6 mm when free of any
recognizeable plaques had a total wall thickness (near and
far wall) of 1 mm. The internal carotid artery at +18 when
free of plaque had a total wall thickness of 0.5 mm.

In the carotid artery 6 mm below the bifurcation, 19 of
57 (33%) vessels had a normal wall, 26 (46%) showed a wall
thickness of 1.5 to 2.5 mm (slight plaque) and 12 (12%)
vessels had a wall thickness of 3 mm or more (moderate to
marked plaque). At the bifurcation 12 of 57 (21%) vessels
were free of plaque, 25 (44%) had slight, and 20 (35%) had
moderate to marked plaque. In the internal carotid artery
6 mm above the bifurcation 30 of 51 (56%) vessels were
normal, 15 (28%) had slight and 6 (49%) had moderate to
marked plaque formation. In the internal carotid artery
18 mm above the bifurcation 14 of 55 (25%) vessels were
normal, 34 (62%) had slight and 7 (13%) had moderate to
marked plaque. Three of the 58 vessels showed luminal
occlusion; in one case the entire artery was occluded, in
another the occlusion extended from the bifurcation to

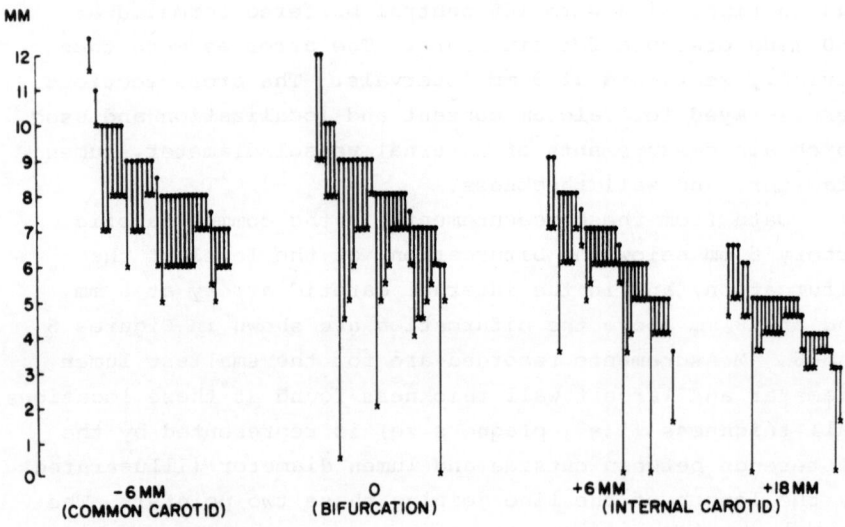

RIGHT CAROTID

• OUTSIDE DIAMETER
× LUMEN DIAMETER
n = 30

MM

-6 MM
(COMMON CAROTID)

0
(BIFURCATION)

+6 MM
(INTERNAL CAROTID)

+18 MM

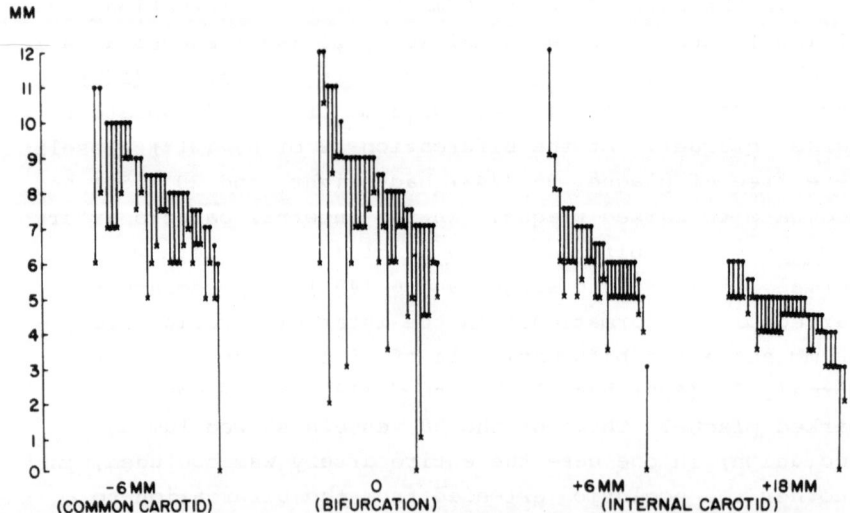

LEFT CAROTID

• OUTSIDE DIAMETER
× LUMEN DIAMETER
n = 28

MM

-6 MM
(COMMON CAROTID)

0
(BIFURCATION)

+6 MM
(INTERNAL CAROTID)

+18 MM

Figures 5 and 6. Measurements of outside diameter and lumen diameter at four levels in right and left carotid arteries obtained at autopsy and perfusion fixed at 150 mmHg. The length of the lines reflect the wall thickness and the amount of atherosclerotic plaque. Of note is the marked variability in vessel size at any given level among these cases, independent of the amount of plaque.

+18 mm, and in the third case the occlusion involved the
internal carotid from +6 to +18 mm. Ovoid, "D"-shaped,
irregularly shaped, and slit-like lumina were found in 11 of
the 58 (19%) perfusion fixed arteries (Figure 7). A further
observation was the marked variability in vessel size at
any given level, which was unreleated to the extent of
plaque formation. For example, in the common carotid artery
at 6 mm below the bifurcation, the outside diameter of
vessels without evidence of plaque ranged from 12.5 mm to
7 mm. Corresponding luminal diameters for these were 11.5 mm
and 6 mm. These differences in vessel size were also not
related to the presence of plaques at any other level and
thus represent individual variability unrelated to disease.

SUMMARY

Examination of endarterectomy specimens is still the
gold standard to be used in evaluating the accuracy of
various diagnostic procedures. However, this standard is
not without problems which both those who examine and measure
the specimens as well as those who use data thus derived,
must be aware of.

1. Fixation with formalin does not cause significant
   distortion; decalcification does result in shrinkage
   of about 15% in linear dimensions.
2. In many institutions intact specimens are rare and
   reconstruction and circularization are necessary to
   obtain measurement of lumen diameters (and of
   percent stenosis).
3. Reconstruction and circularization are also necessary
   when there is artifactual infolding or distortion
   of a thin plaque wall.
4. Non-round, "D"-shaped, ovoid, and slit-like lumina
   are not uncommon, and very likely represent the
   in vivo state rather than artifactual collapse due
   to loss of perfusion pressure since similarly
   shaped lumina can be demonstrated in perfusion
   fixed and pressurized vessels obtained at autopsy.
   These non-round lumina are almost always found in

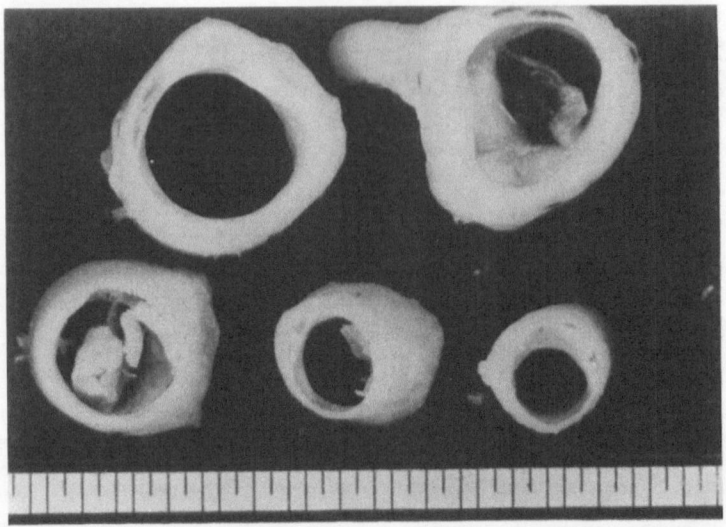

Figure 7. Autopsy specimen of carotid artery which has been pressure perfusion fixed shows "D"-shaped and slit-shaped lumina.

   association with intramural hemorrhage and/or
   mural thrombosis, events which are exceedingly
   common in the complicated plaques found in
   endarterectomy specimens (1,2).

5. The problem of determining matching planes of
   interrogation remains unresolved. It will be
   necessary to devise some strategy for accomplishing
   this in studies which utilize specimens for determining the usefulness of various diagnostic procedures
   in characterizing plaque composition and plaque
   ulceration.

6. Anatomic variations which have been described
   include both the position of the external carotid
   artery relative to the internal carotid artery at
   the bifurcation (3) and differences in the size
   of these vessels. Whereas, wall thickness remains
   constant in the absence of disease, vessel and
   lumen diameter may vary by as much as 100%.

REFERENCES

1. Lusby RJ, Ferrell LD, Ehrenfeld WK, Stoney RJ, Wylie EJ (1982) Carotid plaque hemorrhage. Arch Surg 117:1479-1488.
2. Ricotta JJ, Schenk EA, Ekholm SE, Green RM, DeWeese JA (1986) Angiographic and pathologic correlates in carotid artery disease. Surgery 99:294-292.
3. Prendes JL, McKinney WM, Buonanno FS, Jones AM (1980) Anatomic variations of the carotid bifurcations affecting Doppler scan interpretation. J Clin Ultrasound 8:147-150.

REFERENCES

1. ...
2. ...
3. ...

54

Lessons Learned, Unresolved Problems and Future Opportunities. U.S. Multicenter Assessment of B Mode Ultrasound Imaging

James F. Toole, M. Gene Bond, and Daniel O'Leary

By contracting for a study to validate B-mode ultra-sound imaging using arteriography and pathology as standards, the Devices and Technology Branch of the NHLBI led the way with the first attempt to formally and quantitatively assess this new diagnostic modality. One has only to observe the technical and scientific exhibits at the World Congress of Cardiology, the American Heart Association, Society for Vascular Surgery, the American Academy of Neurology and the American Neurological Association, to realize that non-invasive assessment of the carotid arteries using ultrasound has achieved acceptance which may exceed our understanding of its role in detecting and preventing progression of atherosclerosis, and in managing patients with carotid lesions. Unlike previous technologies which were customarily evaluated within medical centers before general distribution, Doppler and B-mode ultrasound instruments were marketed before their place in the health care delivery system had been defined, perhaps with the thought that the utility of these examinations was self-evident. This has led to the establishment of noninvasive laboratories, at times under the direction of individuals with heterogeneous experience and training, to perform and interpret the tests, and to recommend patient management. Currently, some well-intentioned groups sponsor screening programs to identify asymptomatic

Supported by NHLBI contract N01-HV-12916, N01-HV-12904

individuals with carotid artery lesions without the requisite
understanding of what should be done if lesions are found.
In many cases, the relationship between imaging results,
physical findings, and patient prognosis requires further
study and evaluation. This has presented clinicians with
unresolved questions regarding patient management which are
paramount questions for future clinical research. Intervention trials designed to ascertain these relationships
are of extraordinary importance. To its further credit, the
NIH has implemented two phases of this needed work, the
Atherosclerosis in Communities (ARIC) study and the Asymptomatic Carotid Atherosclerosis Study (ACAS). One aspect of
ARIC, an observational community-based cohort study, is to
determine the natural history of ultrasonographically
measured atherosclerosis. The ACAS study by contrast, is
a randomized controlled trial of surgical vs medical treatment for asymptomatic individuals with carotid stenosis
determined by Doppler ultrasound, Ophthalmoplethysmography
and arteriography.

Organization of Multi-Institutional Cooperative Studies
     It is obvious but sometimes forgotten that goals and
timetables must be set down in a form agreed to by all
participants. Active committees must be established at once
to ensure that tasks are accomplished efficiently. Committee
interaction will soon identify those who will be enthusiastic
and productive workers. Emphasis must be placed on producing
a standardized written protocol and a detailed procedure
manual. Only such a document, supported by training and
monitoring, assures that all centers carry out functions
uniformly. Many investigators have only minimal experience
with such a venture involving scientists from diverse
disciplines and geographic locations. Adhering to the study's
goals can be difficult during a 5-year study in which sub-
goals and new ideas continue to be generated. Frequent
communication and finely tuned administrative skills are
needed to meet the group's objectives and to prevent undue
frustration along the way. In theory, it is desirable that
each center have a representative on each committee; but

functional units of four of five individuals should be
fostered for greater efficacy. Moreover, committees must
have frequent meetings to report on progress to the Steering
Committee which in turn reports to higher authorities. The
time commitment for such meetings and for the liaison
required is often not recognized nor is it compensated.

The Steering Committee must insure that those individuals assigned to a specific task understand the goals and
objectives and that they are properly instructed and compe-
tent to carry out their tasks. This can only be achieved
by continuing interactions at all levels among institutions.
Resources must be designated as part of the contract for
this process of education and ongoing quality control.

In a multicenter study, data quality can be diluted by
one substandard institution or observer, as well as introduce
bias. In order to avoid this, there must be continuing
audits and in-course corrections rather than waiting until
the termination of the study for analyses when it is too
late to consider modification and improvements. One aspect
of this is continuing training of personnel and then recertification throughout the project.

Enthusiasm can be maintained and augmented by a news-
letter or frequent conference calls, but no matter what the
mechanism, a network for continuous communications is a vital
ingredient for a successful multi-institutional, multidisciplinary study. An important method for increasing team
spirit is the publication of analyses of work in progress,
rather than waiting until the end of the study will all the
changes in interest and perhaps investigators that occur
during a 5-year project.

The dedicated efforts of many individuals who contributed
enormous amounts of time and effort must be rewarded at all
academic levels. Not being listed as an author may stunt
academic advancement. The problems related to proper
recognition have often been sidestepped by substituting a
term such as the "Cooperating Group" which insures equity
at the price of anonymity and suggests that the group cannot
agree on ranking of authors. In such cases, all suffer
equally. A common but perhaps unjust system is to list the

most prolix writer first. However, the writing task is
sometimes far less time consuming or difficult than the
tasks of others less facile with the pen, who devoted
extensively of their academic efforts to the project. Yet,
the latter are usually given a lesser position in the author-
ship ranking. We used a random selection process to order
the collaborating institutions and through its internal
mechanisms, the institution chose who would be listed as
author. This gives recognition to internal realities in
which certain individuals will have contributed much effort
behind the scene and therefore deserve more recognition than
would appear to the outside observer. This system worked
well and we recommend it for others.

The development of manuscripts acceptable to all participants is an arduous one requiring great amounts of conference time. Funds should be earmarked specifically in the
contracting mechanism for preparation of graphics and writing
should be initiated early after beginning the project.
Materials should be constructed in draft form at the beginning,
so that the data can be accumulated in a proper fashion for
later publication.

Unresolved Problems

An important aspect of studies such as ours is that
technology often improves during the course of its evaluation;
yet instruments chosen at the beginning must be used to the
end so that the methods can be kept constant. In our case,
this is particularly evident with the introduction of duplex
scanning which can be used to increase specificity, particularly in patients with high grade stenosis which are sometimes
misdiagnosed as occlusion.

Our longitudinal data set from the cohort of B-scan and
arteriogram patients accumulated from five geographically
separated locations with follow-up for at least two years,
will soon be available for analysis. Among areas to be
investigated are such intriguing questions as the degree to
which plaques progress or regress over time and whether
plaques located in different positions on the arterial wall
have varying propensities for change, $i.e.$, does a near wall

plaque in the internal carotid artery change at the same rate as one on the far wall in the common carotid artery. In patients who have apparent plaque regression defined by percent lumen diameter stenosis, is the change due to a reduction in lesion size or increase in lumen diameter because of arterial dilatation? When plaques change, is this related to changes in blood lipids, blood pressure, cessation of tobacco consumption or modification of other risk factors identified at the time of the first examination? It seems reasonable to believe that patients who have lesions brought to their attention will modify their habits by ceasing or decreasing tobacco use, increasing physical exercise, changing dietary habits and exposing themselves to medical care and pharmacologic intervention. Do these individuals reduce their rate of progression of atherosclerosis? Partial answers may be in our data set. The pathophysiologic processes believed to result in clinical expression of extracranial carotid artery atherosclerosis are at least twofold. The first is mechanical resulting in hemodynamic change, and lesion severity is expressed as "percent lumen diameter stenosis." The second, considerably less quantitated and much debated, is plaque degeneration with intramural hemorrhage, necrosis and/or ulceration, which may result in subsequent thrombosis and embolization. Our study was not designed to clarify these mechanisms but some cogent observations can be made. B-mode ultrasound examinations can, with few exceptions, approximate percent lumen diameter stenosis with an accuracy sufficient for clinical use; however, no single method evaluated in this study, *i.e.*, ultrasound, angiography, or pathology, is by itself the flawless standard that most clinical and basic scientific investigators seek, because each method supplements the other and provides unique information on different features of the atherosclerotic process.

For the clinician interested primarily in degree of stenosis, it is inconsequential that a lesion causes wall thickening without intruding upon the lumen. Yet, it is precisely in this determination that B-mode imaging is superior to angiography. However, in some cases of plaque

mineralization, lumen-intimal interfaces and sometimes
arterial walls cannot be imaged because of high reflectivity
thus diminishing the clinical utility of B-mode scanning.
Furthermore, recently developed thrombi or acute plaque
hemorrhage cannot be differentiated with consistency by
B-mode imaging. For all these reasons, Doppler ultrasound
is an important adjuvant for B-mode in the clinical setting.
The need to differentiate lesions causing stenosis exceeding
70% from occlusion is self-evident. B-mode ultrasound by
itself, and an some instances, pathology evaluation of
endarterectomy specimens, are unable to separate severe
stenosis from occlusion. Doppler ultrasound may be a useful
adjunct in this regard, despite its dependence upon lumen
configuration and severity of plaque mineralization which
may obscure flow imaging.

Our data demonstrate that we can quantitate atherosclerotic involvement in terms of lumen diameter, plaque
thickness, and tissue characteristics which has caused
great interest in studies for monitoring changes in atherosclerosis over time. To some degree, discrepancies can be
explained by the different methodologies for measuring
plaque using B-mode ultrasound, angiograms and pathologic
specimens. For example, radiologists measured the minimum
residual lumen diameter from x-rays and compared this with
a second diameter from an assumed but not necessarily
"normal" distal segment of artery. Furthermore, the part
of the plaque which is seen as encroaching on the lumen
may not represent actual lesion thickness. In contrast,
sonographers measured plaque thickness more accurately.
Therefore, criteria for establishing the denominator of the
stenosis equation were not identical for radiologic and
ultrasound measurement, so that one should not expect too
close agreement between the two methods. A further level
of complexity is added when attempting to compare measurements of lumen diameters and plaque thickness from
endarterectomy specimens with those made *in vivo*. Surgical
removal of specimens resulted in collapsed or at least
decreased lumen diameter, the extent of which could not be
estimated accurately in our samples. This combined with

fixation and decalcification shrinkage contributed to
some lack of correlation between the two. Shrinkage would
result in greater stenosis scores from pathology specimens,
as was found.

Although the specimens demonstrated the circumferential
nature of lesions, the thickness of plaques varied with the
angle of interrogation and on the location along the length
of the specimen at which measurements were made. In many
cases, we were unable to assure ourselves that the angles
of interrogation, or the specific sites from which measurements were made by the three modalities were the same. The
assumption that lesions *per se*, or plaque thickness are
randomly distributed along the length and circumference
of the extracranial carotid arteries remain to be documented.
Until this information, as well as the variability of lesion
distribution within the extracranial carotid arteries
becomes available, statistical analyses that are dependent
on assumptions of random distribution must be interpreted
with care. Another explanation for the differences observed
both among and within methods concerns standard procedures
within and among Centers and investigators. The reproducibility of data is dependent on using standard methods and
criteria for evaluation. Our study documented that arteriography is more reproducible for measuring arterial diameters
as was expected. This method has been standardized for many
years. The fact that ultrasound gave less reliable measurements may be due in part to the different ways the two are
measured. Whereas radiologists had a single "frame" to
evaluate twice, sonographers had to reselect the frame they
measured from hundreds of possibilities, and secondly, the
arteries for establishing specific arterial wall interfaces
to be measured, as well as instrument settings which best
demonstrated them. This indicates that greater emphasis on
standardization of methods is needed before the potential
of B-mode ultrasound can be fully realized.

Future Opportunities

Our study has demonstrated the utility of B-mode ultrasound methods for clinical diagnosis. It has also helped

to define the requirements for future studies, such as the NHLBI's Atherosclerosis Risk in Communities Program, one aspect of which is aimed at determining the incidence, prevalence and natural history of extracranial carotid atherosclerosis using standardized protocols which are currently being established as an outgrowth of data garnered by the U.S. Multicenter Assessment of B-mode Ultrasound Imaging.

B-mode ultrasound imaging, when used in a research setting for evaluating asymptomatic extracranial carotid artery atherosclerosis, has been demonstrated to be a valid and reliable method for detecting and for monitoring arterial change over time and, as such, will provide investigators with a unique and important tool with which to define who has, and who does not have atherosclerosis, and secondly, to investigate "risk" factors which may be important for onset of atherosclerosis and for plaque progression or regression.

55
Computer Image Processing Methods to Quantify Atherosclerosis Change: Problems and Prospects

Robert H. Selzer

INTRODUCTION

Clinical studies of atherosclerosis that require quantitative estimates of lesion change from images have moved strongly in the direction of automated techniques in the last five years. Angiogram analysis is the most widely used approach with more than 10 research groups reporting development of computer methods to assess coronary lesion change from cineangiograms (1-10) and at least two groups reporting methods for femoral angiogram analysis (11,12). Computer-aided lesion assessment from B-mode ultrasound has also been developed and used clinically in the U.S. Multicenter Ultrasound Assessment Program (13). Other imaging methods such as magnetic resonance imaging (14) and nuclear imaging (15) have the potential to be used in clinical studies of lesion change but are still under development and have not been tested.

The purposes of this paper are (1) to illustrate some possibly overlooked methodological problems associated with the relatively mature field of automated cineangiographic analysis (2) to describe potential problems in automating lesion measurement from ultrasound images and (3) to discuss the prospects for solving these problems with image processing methods.

Measurement of Lesion Change from Coronary Angiography

Existing automated methods to measure coronary lesion change from cineangiograms involve tracking the vessel image and computing changes in lumen geometry either from the detected vessel edges or on the film density within the lumen shadow. The accuracy and precision of such measurements, which is a major concern in clinical trials since the required number of subjects and trial duration increase rapidly as the measurement variability increases (16), has not been completely determined. In phantom studies, diameter accuracies of two to three percent have been reported but there is serious question as to whether these numbers can be applied to clinical angiograms. In studies of repeat angiograms taken over varying periods of time, Reiber (17) reports stenosis measurement precision (standard deviation of the difference of measurement pairs) from 6.5 to 8.3 percent. Comparable results for repeat angiograms were reported by Kirkeeidi (18).

In these studies, as well as in most other studies to date, lesions within a vessel segment were assessed from a single cine frame, usually selected in mid- or end-diastole. Spears and Sandor (19) suggest that measurement precision can be improved by assessing multiple sequential frames for each segment and then averaging the results. What is not clear is whether the best strategy is to average measurements from similar frames or to average measurements from frames showing the vessel in different orientations. To obtain data on which to develop a frame selection strategy, a study was initiated to estimate the variability of the existing lesion measurements within the cardiac cycle and from cycle to cycle. This study involves application of the computer measurements to every frame in at least two cardiac cycles for a representative number of subjects. This work is not complete, but as discussed below, a number of cyclic and random changes in the angiograms have been observed that strongly influence measurement variability.

Computer Coronary Measurements

The JPL/USC approach to coronary lesion measurement, which is based on detection of the lumen boundaries in cine-angiograms, has been described in detail elsewhere (20) and

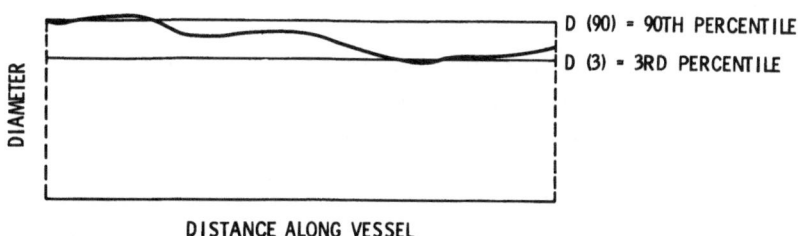

$$\text{STENOSIS} = \left[1 - \frac{D(3)}{D(90)}\right] \times 100$$

Figure 1. Definition of stenosis measurement from computed diameter values. D90 represents the "normal" vessel width and LD3 represents the minimum vessel width.

will not be repeated here. Briefly, arterial edges are selected as the points of maximum film density gradient computed along straight-line paths perpendicular to the vessel midline. A series of vessel diameters are computed from the detected edge points and as shown in Figure 1, stenosis is computed from a reference diameter called D90 which represents the 90 percentile value of the computed diameters and a minimum diameter called D3 which is assigned the 3rd percentile value.

Factors That Influence Measurement Variability

Factors that may cause changes in the computer-detected lumen geometry between two or more frames from the same angiogram include the following.

1. Vessel pulsation
2. Changes in vessel orientation
3. Changes in vessel position between the x-ray tube and the image intensifier
4. Overlapping shadows
5. Wash-in and wash-out of the x-ray contrast medium
6. Transient mixing artifacts
7. Photon noise in the image

Cyclic Factors

To illustrate cyclic changes in the lumen measurement that may occur, consider the plot in Figure 2 showing the D90, D3, average diameter, and computed stenosis (computed as [1-D3/D90] * 100) of an LAD segment for 92 consecutive cine frames covering more than 2 cardiac cycles. In this figure, the light lines show the individual diameter and stenosis measurements while the darker lines indicate a 5 point smoothing of the individual values. Cyclic diameter changes of approximately 10 percent are indicated in all

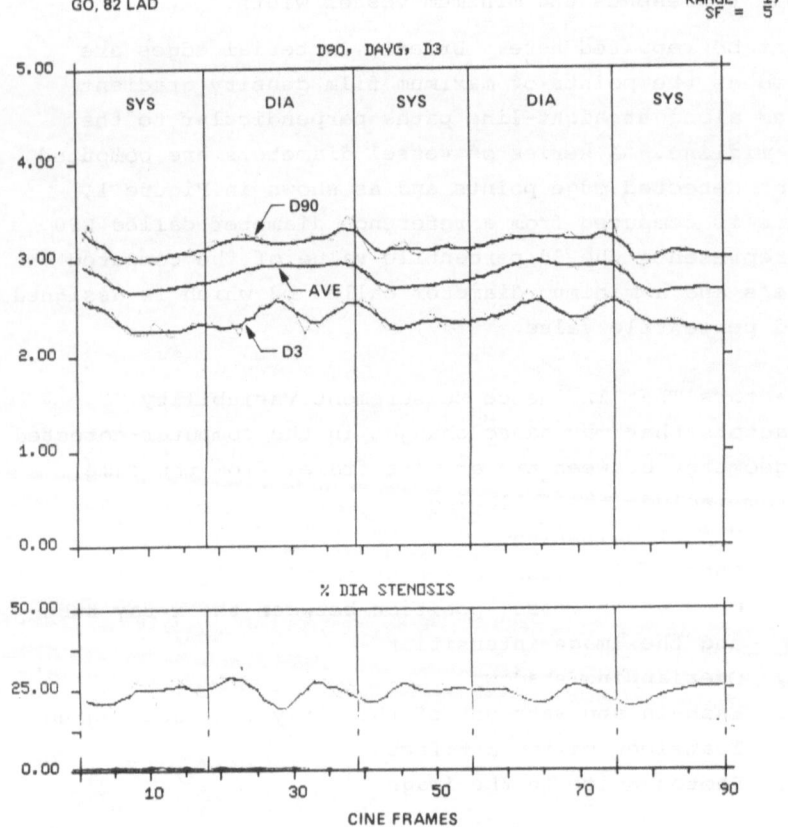

Figure 2. Plot of D3, average diameter, D90 and stenosis for 90 sequential frames for LAD segment. Light curves represent unfiltered values and dark curves represent five point average values.

measurements. In addition, evidence of a non-symmetric lesion may be indicated by the change in D3 during mid-diastole which is not present in D90.

The cyclic changes shown in Figure 2 probably result from a combination of factors including vessel pulsation, changes in lesion orientation, changes in radiographic magnification or geometric distortion in the image intensifier, optical system or video digitizer camera. The individual contributions were not measured although in this and other examples discussed below, the effects of image intensifier distortion were minimized by exluding vessels whose recorded images appeared outside an area on each frame corresponding to the central 20 percent area of the image intensifier.

Correction of geometric distortion in the image intensifier is fairly straight-foreward and is commonly applied. The other sources of geometric variability are more difficult to measure and correct. Clearly, cyclic variation in measurements can be avoided by selection of single matched end-diastolic frames but care must be exercised in the interpretation of absolute diameter measured under these circumstances. In addition, matched end-diastolic frames cannot always be found and in these cases, information about the variation of the measurements with cardiac phase becomes important. An argument can also be made that end-diastole may not be the best part of the cardiac cycle for measurement. Consider the relatively rapid change in measured stenosis at end-diastole for the case shown in Figure 3.

Transient Mixing Artifacts

Incomplete x-ray contrast mixing occurs which is not obvious from visual inspection of the film but causes substantial errors in lesion measurement. This type of artifact, which is more common in bypass grafts, may make it necessary to possess several sequential frames and to derive a composite boundary that represents the maximum lumen of the processed frames (20).

Effects of X-Ray Contrast Wash-In and Wash-Out and Effects of Vessel Dilation

Errors from wash-in and wash-out of x-ray contrast generally take the form of a low-frequency increase or decrease

of apparent arterial dimensions. Vessel dilation will of
course cause a similar change in the measurements. In most
cases, framed sequences in which wash-in or wash-out occurs

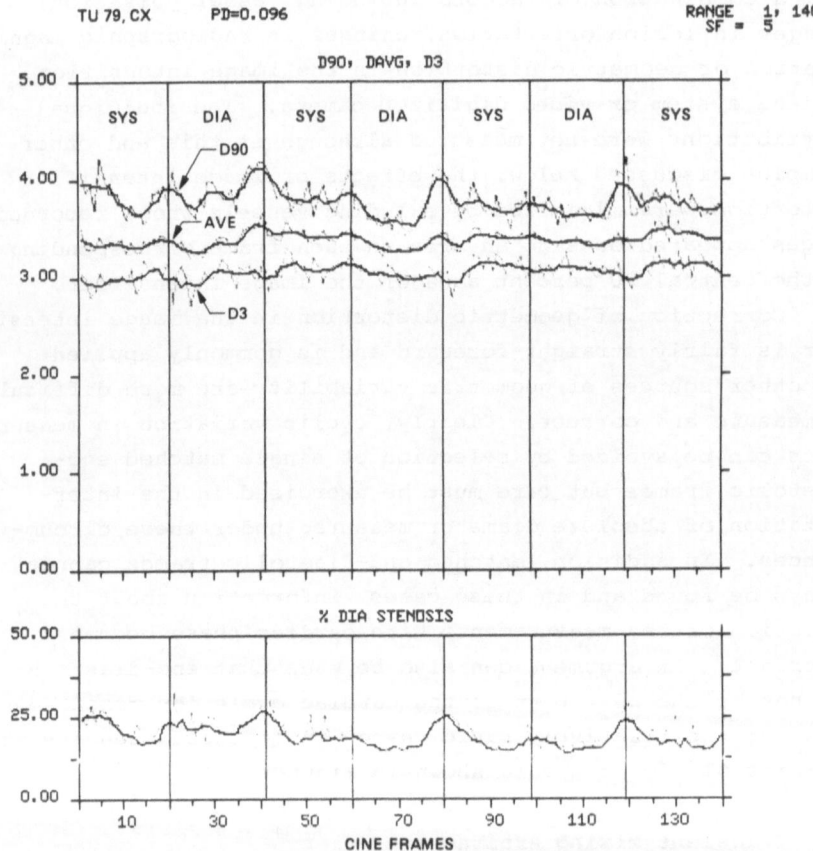

Figure 3. Plot of computer diameter and stenosis of 140
sequential frames circumflex segment. Note rapid change in
stenosis before and after end-diastole.

are visually apparent but not always. In one case, 135
frames of a right coronary bypass graft were visually screened
and believed to be uniformly opacified but the plot of average

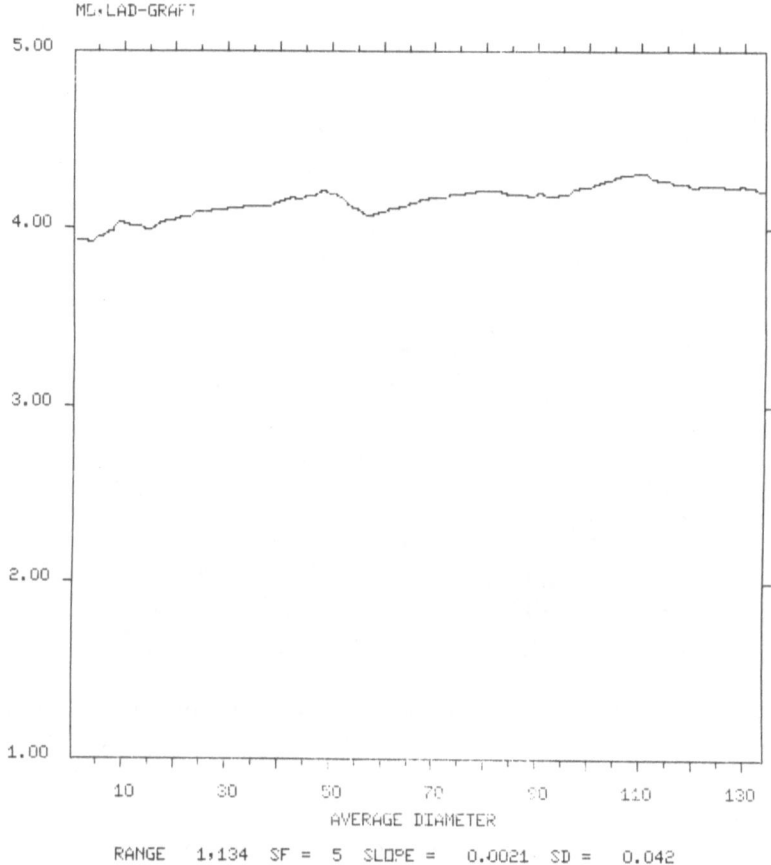

Figure 4. Plot of average diameter for 135 consecutive
frames for an LAD bypass segment showing an apparent increase
in diameter over two cardiac cycles.

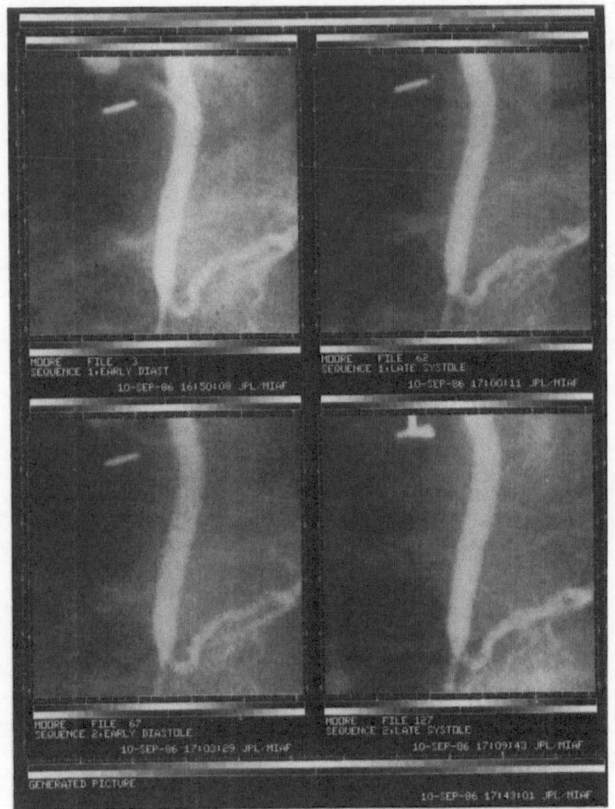

Figure 5. Selected frames from film used to generate Figure 4.

diameter, shown in Figure 4, shows a steadily increasing
measured diameter. The images for frames 3, 62, 67, and 127,
shown in Figure 5 do not indicate an obvious change in opaci-
fication. Detection of dilation or contrast artifacts of
this type may require processing of a sequence of frames which
will increase the cost and complexity of the analysis.

Film Quality

Large frame-to-frame variability in the lesion measurement can be demonstrated for cine or digital angiograms where
photon noise is high or where the relative contrast of the
vessel image compared to the surrounding areas is low.
Relatively small differences in film contrast or noise can
cause substantial measurement change. Consider the sample

frames shown in Figures 6 and 7. These frames are from the same subject but Figure 6 is taken from a 1982 angiogram and the frame in Figure 7 from a 1984 angiogram. The corresponding diameter measurements are shown in Figures 8 and 9. Measurement variability indicated in the earlier film is clearly lower while the film quality difference is relatively small.

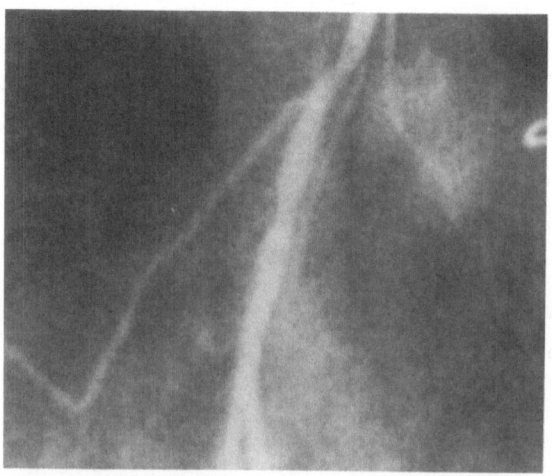

Figure 6. Frame from 1982 angiograms of patient BRO showing relatively good contrast.

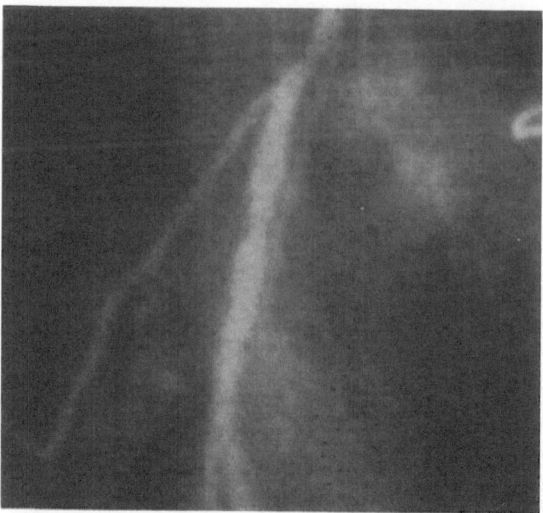

Figure 7. Frame from 1984 angiogram of patient BRO showing relatively poor contrast and increase in quantum mottle, as compared to the 1982 angiogram.

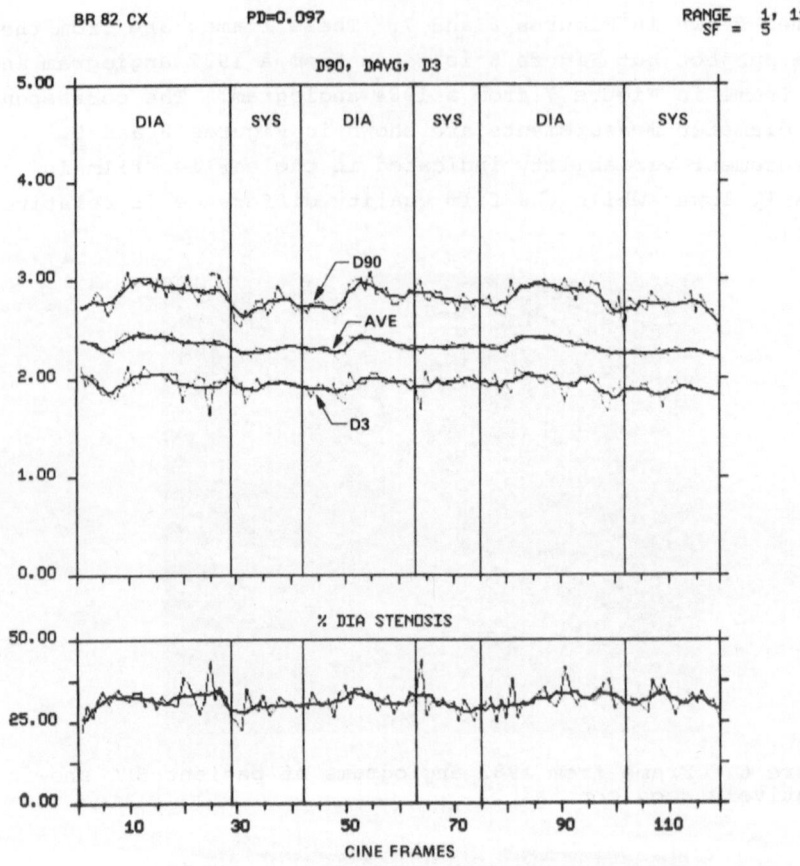

Figure 8. Diameter plots for subject BRO, 1982 angiogram.

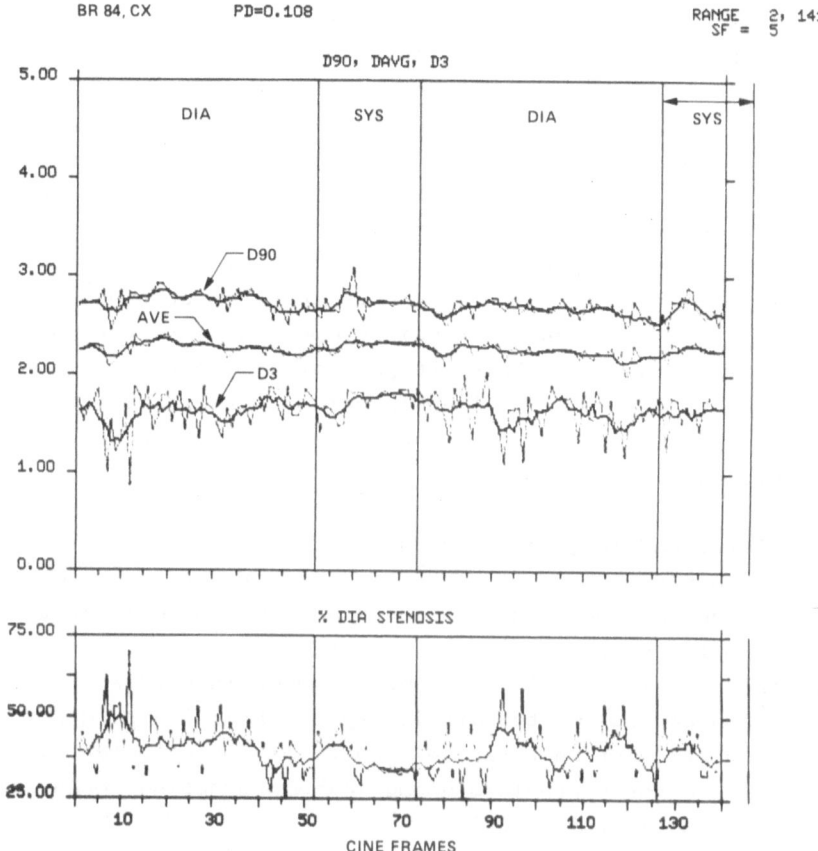

Figure 9. Diameter plots for subject BRO, 1984 angiogram.
Note increase in variability of the diameter measurements for
the 1984 angiogram.

Control of Measurement Variability

Currently, five to ten minutes are required to process each frame. This includes time to find and digitize the frame, to indicate to the computer the segment to be analyzed, to track the edges, to indicate the exact extent of the segment to be included in the measurement and to compute stenosis. If the required number of frames to be processed is very large (20 or more frames per segment is not out of the question), it will be essential to develop very much faster processing methods. If the amount of required operator intervention, which now accounts for 70 to 80 percent of the total processing time, can be decreased by development of more sophisticated algorithms, the prospects for development of a fast system are very good.

Ultrasound Image Processing

Automated methods to assess lesions from ultrasound images have not been widely used because of the difficulty in developing boundary tracking algorithms that function well with the high levels of image noise common in ultrasound images and because of the difficulty of obtaining precise image registration in serial examinations. Some potential solutions to these problems using image processing techniques are discussed in this section.

Boundary Detection in Ultrasound Images

Most boundary finding methods employ some type of image smoothing followed by a grey-level threshold detection or a gradient calculation. Because of the speckle noise in ultrasound images, the degree of required smoothing is large and boundaries become obscured. We have found that a modification of a non-linear filter called the variance filter, developed Kuwahara and his associates (21) to enhance boundaries in radioisotope images, effectively restores edges in ultrasound images after smoothing. Application of this filter is shown in Figures 10-12. Figure 10 shows an unprocessed transverse image of a carotid artery and figure 11 shows the effect of a 21 by 21 pixel averaging filter. Application of the Kuwahara variance filter is shown in Figure 12. This filter examines square sectors of pixels in each of four quadrants surrounding a point and sets the value of the point in the output

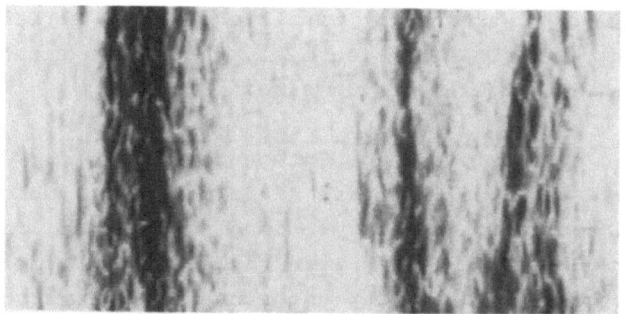

Figure 10.   Ultrasound image of the carotid artery.

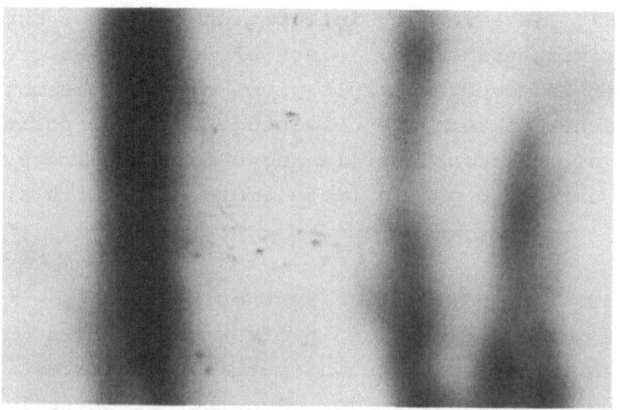

Figure 11.   Result of applying 21 by 21 pixel smoothing
filter to the image in Figure 10.

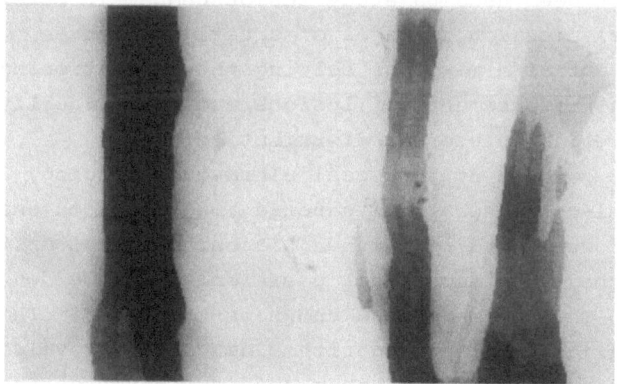

Figure 12.   Result of applying 5 by 5 variance filter to the
image in Figure 11.

picture to the mean of the sector with the smallest variance. For the carotid image shown in Figure 11, the sector size was chosen to be 5 by 5 elements in size.

Enhancement by Multiple Image Integration

Improvements in signal-to-noise ratio may be possible if the redundant information in multiple images can be utilized. If the noise in ultrasound images were truly random, simple frame averaging could be used, but unfortunately, ultrasound speckle has non-random components that are dependent on the object being imaged and on the position and direction of the ultrasound signal. As a result, integration of frames obtained from a fixed-position transducer is not effective. However, if the transducer is moved, multiple views of the same object with varying speckle pattern are obtained and if the position and orientation of the transducer is known for each image, the possibility exists to obtain image improvement with signal integration.

Image Integration and 3D Image Synthesis

One form of image integration involves combining a sequence of planar images with known spatial coordinates into a synthetic three-dimensional image. A number of investigators have employed spatial locating devices with ultrasound trans- ducers to generate 3D images of the ventricles (22-25) but the technique has not been used to study lesion change in arteries. Three-dimensional ultrasound images of arteries could be extremely important as a means of solving the repositioning problem in serial measurements of lesions and could facilitate measurement of lesion volume and distribution.

To test the concept of 3D vessel ultrasound imaging, 20 mutually parallel-cross-sectional carotid images spaced one millimeter apart were obtained with a Diasonics ultrasound transducer attached to a mechanical positioning device developed at U.S.C. (25). The 20 images are shown in Figure 13. The smoothing and variance filter algorithms described above were applied to these images and a maximum gradient detector then used to locate the arterial boundaries. Figure 14 shows the filtered images prior to edge detection.

After the arterial edges were determined in the 2D images, a 3D image was constructed and displayed using a shaded surface

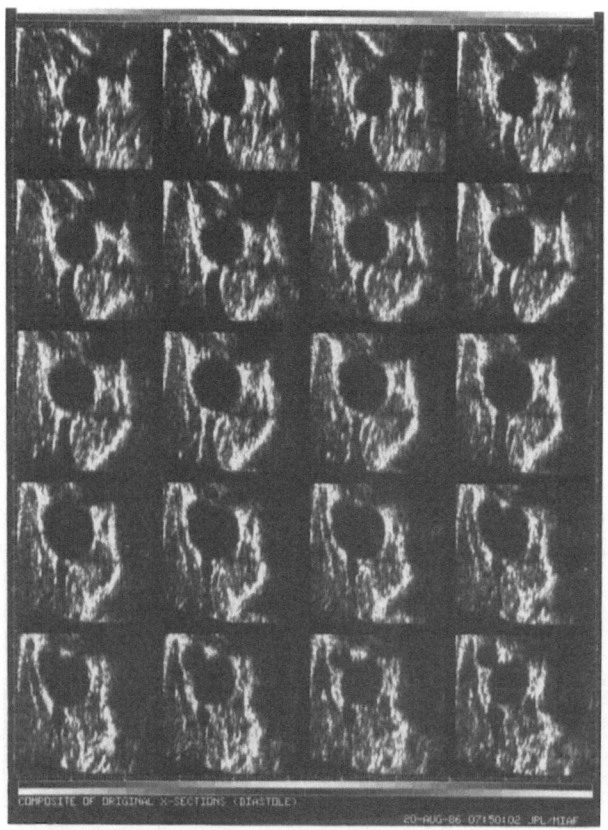

COMPOSITE OF ORIGINAL X-SECTIONS (DIASTOLE)

20-AUG-86 07:50:02 JPL/MIAF

Figure 13. Sequence of unprocessed carotid ultrasound images spaced one millimeter apart. Upper left image is most distal and lower right is most proximal.

algorithm as shown in Figure 15. A polar transform could be used to effectively open the artery and lay it flat. This type of representation, shown in Figure 16 for a simulated vessel, could provide a convenient geometry to map lesion size and distribution.

Feasibility of 3D Reconstruction for Non-Parallel Images
The use of a mechanical parallel-place positioning device is too restrictive for general 3D arterial imaging. Instead a spatial locating device is required that can be attached to the ultrasound transducer to track its position freely in space. Mechanical locaters have been available for ultrasound transducers for some time but are cumbersome to use. An acoustic (spark gap) spatial locater device manufactured

by Science Accessories Corporation and an electromagnetic
system manufactured by McDonnel Douglas Electronics are also
available but both of these devices have serious shortcomings
for this application. The spark gap system comes close to
meeting the spatial resolution requirements but generates
RF noise that interferes with nearby electronic systems
including the ultrasound signal processing units. The electromagnetic systems do not have sufficient spatial resolution.

   Assuming the spatial locater problem can be overcome,
development of the 3D ultrasound image for non-parallel input
would be similar to that for the parallel plane case except
that the coordinates of the arterial boundaries for each
planar image would have to be transformed to three-dimensional
space using the position information from the spatial locater.
With the capability for unrestricted transducer positioning,
it becomes possible to improve the signal-to-noise in the 3D

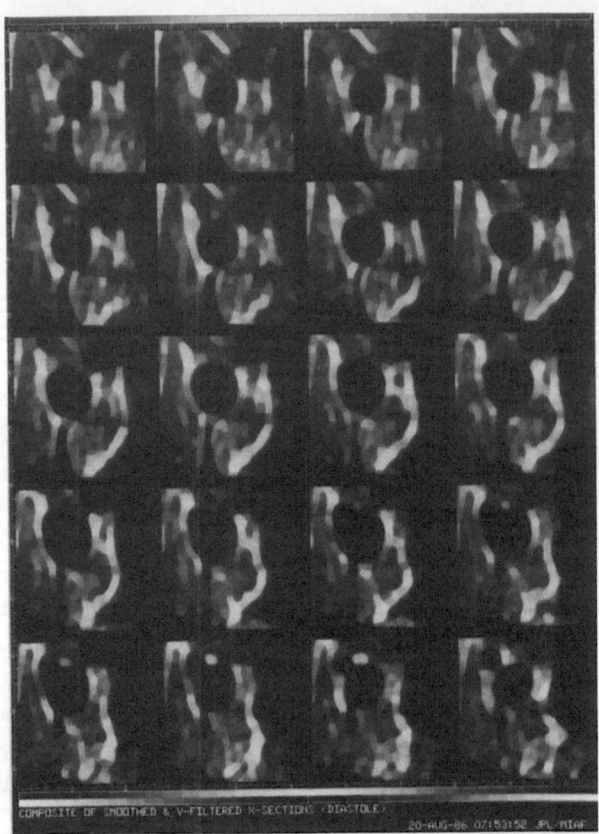

Figure 14. After application of smoothing and variance filter
to images in Figure 13.

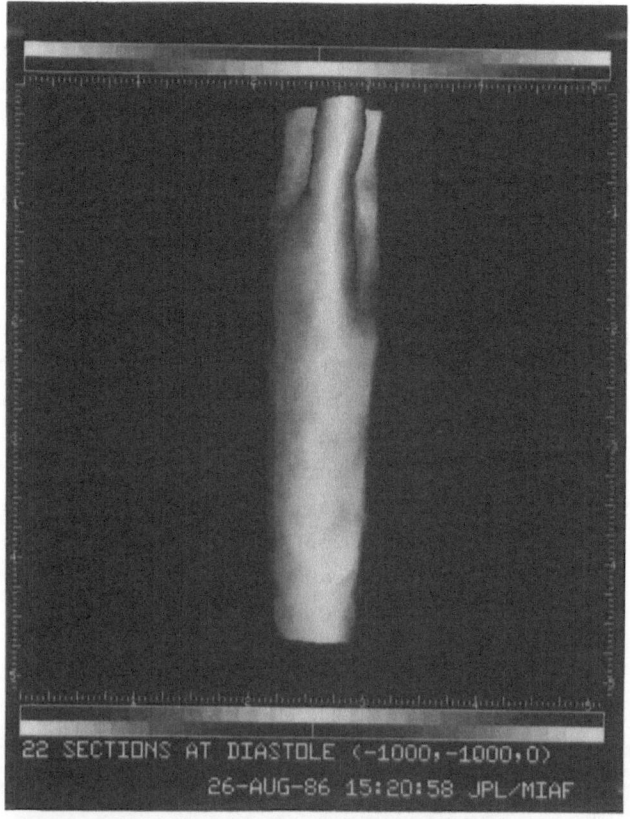

Figure 15. Three-dimensional ultrasound image of the carotid artery derived from the detected edges of the plane sections shown in Figure 14.

image using multiple image integration methods previously mentioned. With the boundary finding approach, the coordinates of the vessel in the 3D image would be obtained by averaging the coordinates derived from the various planar views. An alternate approach is first to assemble the unprocessed 2D grey-level images into a 3D grey-level image and then to find the arterial boundaries.

With the first approach, the time consuming filtering and edge detection must be applied to every frame and since the number of frames to be processed might be large, computing time might be very large. With the second approach, only a few filtering and boundary tracking operations are required but the amount of computer memory needed becomes very large.

For example, a three-dimensional image represented by 256
discrete picture elements in each dimension consists of 16.8
million picture elements (256 X 256 X 256). Since each
picture element requires at least two bytes to accumulate the
grey level values and another byte to count the number of
times a 2D image contributed to that 3D pixel, the required
memory storage becomes greater than 50 million bytes.

Implementation of 3D Ultrasound Imaging Systems
The 3D image synthesis can be implemented on virtually
any existing computer by accumulating the 3D image on magnetic
disk instead of in random access memory, but the increase in
computing time with a disk-based method may be excessive.
Furtunately, the astonishing improvements in computer hard-
ware in general and memory in particular combined with dropping
prices of the last 5-10 years continue and there is reason to
be optimistic that a practical and economic 3D ultrasound
computer system can be developed.

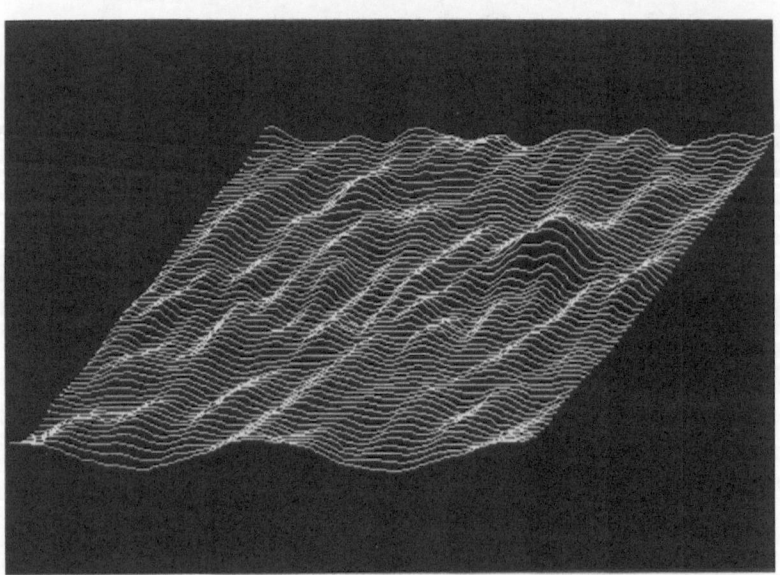

Figure 16. Results of applying a polar transformation to
a simulated 3D artery to obtain a "lesion map" representation
of luminal surface.

Current mid-size computers such as the DEC VAX 8600 can be configured with random access memory of 128 megabytes or more and so-called micro-computers such as the DEC MicroVax II or even an IBM PC/AT can be equipped with 16 megabytes of RAM at relatively modest cost. For example, this year, an 8 megabyte random access memory board for a DEC MicroVax II computer was purchased at JPL for $3200 (including tax). Ten years ago, $3000 bought 64 kilobytes of RAM.

Similar reduction in cost are available in other components required for an image processing system. For example, two years ago, at this meeting, we reported that the cost of a 512 X 512 byte refresh display memory dropped from $32,000 in 1974 to $4,000 in 1984. The same refresh display memory is today approximately $750. The cost of the memory chips required for a 512 X 512 byte memory, if purchased from a mail order discount store is $22.43. Similar reductions in computer processing chips have stimualted development of parallel architecture computer systems that utilize multiple processing chips to enhance performance. One system, the Connection Machine originally developed at M.I.T. and recently announced as a commercial product by Thinking Machines Corporation in Cambridge Massachusetts, utilizes 65,536 processors (26). Priced at 3 million dollars, this system is too expensive for application to the problems discussed above, but there is substantial reason to be optimistic that practical cost-effective computer systems that can solve these problems will become available in the next few years.

REFERENCES

1. Blankenhorn DH, Cashin WL, Selzer RH, and Brooks SH (1982) Coronary atherosclerosis regression studies with computer processed angiograms, In: Noseda G, Frangiacomo C, Furnagalli R, and Paoletti R, Eds, Lipoproteins and Coronary Atherosclerosis, Amsterdam, Elsevier Biomedical Press, pp 425-432.
2. Reiber JHC, Kooijman CJ, Slager JJ et al (1984) Computer assisted analysis of the severity of obstructions from coronary cineangiograms; a methodological review. Automedica, 5:219-238
3. Kirkeeide RL, Fung P, Smalling RW, and Gould KL (1982) Automated evaluation of vessel diameter from arteriograms. Comp in Card: 215-218
4. Brown BG, Bolson E, Frimer M, and Dodge HT (1977) Quantitative coronary arteriography. Estimation of

dimensions, hemodynamic resistance and atheroma mass of coronary artery lesions using the arteriograms and digital computation. Circulation 55:329-337

5. Sanders WJ, Alderman EL, and Harrison DC (1979) Coronary artery quantitation using digital image processing techniques. Comp in Card: 15-20

6. Collins SM, Skorton DJ, Harrison DG, White CW, Eastham CL, Hiratzka LF, Doty DB, and Marcus ML (1982) Quantitative computer-based videodensitometry and the physiological significance of a coronary stenosis. Comp in Cardiol 219-222

7. Sandor T, Als AV, and Paulin S (1979) Cine-densitometric measurement of coronary arterial stenoses. Cath Cardiovasc Diagn 5:229-245

8. Barth K, Faust U, Both A, and Wedekind K (1982) A critical examination of angiographic stenosis quantitation by digital image processing. First IEEE Comp Soc Int Symp on Medical Imaging and Image Interpretation. IEEE Cat No 82 CH1804-4:71-76

9. Kishon Y, Yerushalmi S, Deutsch V, and Neufeld HN (1979) Measurement of coronary arterial lumen by densitometric analysis of angiograms. Angiology 39:304-312

10. Vogel RA (1986) Digital coronary arterography, In: Rieber JHC and Serruys PW, State of the art in quantitative coronary arteriography, Dordrecht, Martinus Nijhoff, 17-31

11. Crawford DW, Brooks SH, Selzer RH, Barndt R, Beckenbach ES, and Blankenhorn DH (1977) Computer densitometry for angiographic assessment of arterial cholesterol content and gross pathology in human atherosclerosis. J Lab Clin Med 89:378-392

12. Ruhn G, Erikson U, Helminus G, and Hemmingson (1982) A computerized quantitation of atherosclerosis in an experimental model. Acta Radiologica Diagnosis 23:621-624

13. Toole JF and Berson A (1983) Multicenter trial for assessment of B-mode ultrasound imaging. In:Bond MG, Insull W, Glagov S, Chandler AB, and Cornhill JF, Clinical diagnosis of atherosclerosis, quantitative methods of evaluation, New York, Springer-Verlag, pp 389-397

14. Kaufman L (1986) Magnetic resonance imaging for the visualization of vasculature and atherosclerosis. In: Workshop on the Evolution of the Human Atherosclerotic Plaque, this volume, Chapter 59

15. Lees RL (1986) External imaging of active atherosclerosis with 99m Tc - LDL. In: Workshop on the Evolution of the Human Atherosclerotic Plaque, this volume, Chapter 58

16. Brooks SH, Blankenhorn DH, Chin HP et al (1980) Design of human atherosclerosis studies by serial angiography. J Chron Dis 33:347-359

17. Reiber JHC, Serruys PW, Kooijman CJ, et al (1985) Assessment of short-, medium-, and long-term variations in arterial dimensions from computer-assisted quantitation of coronary cineangiograms, Circ 71:280-288

18. Kirkeeidi R (1986) A controlled clinical trial of pharmacologic and environmental approaches to elevation of HDL cholesterol: effects evaluated by selective angiography, In: Workshop on the Evolution of the Human Atherosclerotic Plaque, unpublished data

19. Spears R and Sandor T (1986) Quantitation of coronary artery severity: Limitation of angiography and computer-ized information extraction. In: Reiber JHC and Serruys PW, State of the art in quantitative coronary arteriography, Dordrecht, Martinus Nijhoff

20. Selzer RH, Shircore A, Lee PL, Hemphill LL, and Blankenhorn DH (1986) A second look at quantitative coronary angio-graphy: Some unexpected problems. In: Reiber JHC and Serruys PW, State of the Art in Quantitative Coronary Arteriography, Dordrecht, Netherlands, Martinus Nijhoff, pp 125-143

21. Kuwahara M, Hachimura K, and Kinoshita M (1980) Image enhancement and left ventricular contour extraction techniques applied to radiosotope angiocardiograms, Automedica 3 107-119

22. Mortiz WE, Medema DK, Ainsworth M, McCabe D, and Pearlman AS (1980) Three-dimensional reconstruction and volume calculation from a series of nonparallel, real-time ultrasonic images. Circulation 62:111-143

23. Dekker DL, Piziali R, and Dong E (1974) A system for ultrasonically imaging the human heart in three dimensions. Comput Biomed Res 7:544

24. Skorton DJ, McNary CA, Child JA and Shah PM: Computerized image processing in cross-sectional echocardiography (abstr) Am J Cardiol 45:403

25. Geiser EA, Christie LG, Conetta DA, Conti CR and Gossman GS (1982) A mechanical arm for spacial registration of two dimensional echocardiographic sections. Cathet Cardiovas Diagn 8:89

26. Blankenhorn DH, Chin HP, Strikwevda S, Bamberger J, and Hestenes JD (1983) Common carotid artery contours reconstructed in three dimensions from parallel ultra-sonic images, Radiology148:533-537

27. Waldrop MM (1986) The connection machine goes commercial, Science 232:1090-1091

56

External Imaging of Active Atherosclerosis with ^{99m}Tc-LDL

Robert S. Lees, Ann M. Lees, Alan J. Fischman, and H. William Strauss

Atherosclerosis is usually thought of in anatomical or pathological terms. This is understandable since end-organ disease - myocardial infarction, stroke, peripheral vascular disease - is the result of obstructive lesions which impair arterial blood flow. In terms of atherogenesis and detection of early atherosclerosis, however, it may be more useful to think of the disease in metabolic, biochemical, or pathophysiological parameters. The early stages of athero-sclerosis are not associated with obstruction to flow, but are rather characterized by biochemical and metabolic changes in the arterial wall.

Low density lipoproteins (LDL), the major cholesterol transport proteins of the blood have been shown some time ago (1) to enter the normal arterial wall rapidly and inter-act with it. This interaction included both binding to the wall and degradation of the radiolabelled protein within the arterial wall (1). These studies were extended in 1983 (2) to the healing balloon de-endothelialized rabbit aorta, a commonly-used model of arterial injury, which resembles in some ways the changes of early atherosclerosis. Minick and colleagues demonstrated several years ago that cholesterol accumulates in foam cells in the healing aorta of the ballooned cholesterol-fed rabbit (3,4). Chow-fed rabbits were studied after balloon de-endothelialization of the aorta and at various times after injury, LDL labelled with ^{125}I was injected intra-venously. When the rabbits were placed in front of a standard

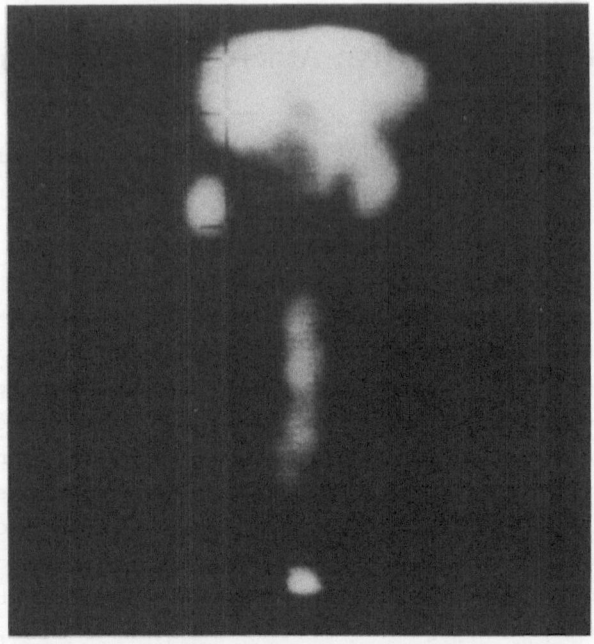

Figure 1. Anterior scintigram of the abdomen of a rabbit
injected with ^{125}I-LDL four weeks after balloon de-endothelialization of the abdominal aorta. The image was made 48 hours
after intravenous injection of 300 uCi of human ^{125}I-LDL (2).
The sequestration of the labelled lipoprotein by the liver
and kidneys at the top of the image is apparent, as is a
small amount of ^{125}I in the urinary bladder at the very
bottom medially. The healing aortic lesions can easily be
seen in mid-abdomen.

planar gamma scintillation camera (Figure 1) four to six
weeks after injury, the healing lesions, even though they were
only a few cell layers thick were able to be imaged and
localized. In addition, LDL metabolism in general was being
imaged externally, including hepatic and renal accumulation
of the labelled lipoprotein. Radioautography of the aortas
revealed marked accumulation of labelled LDL at the healing
edge of the balloon lesions.

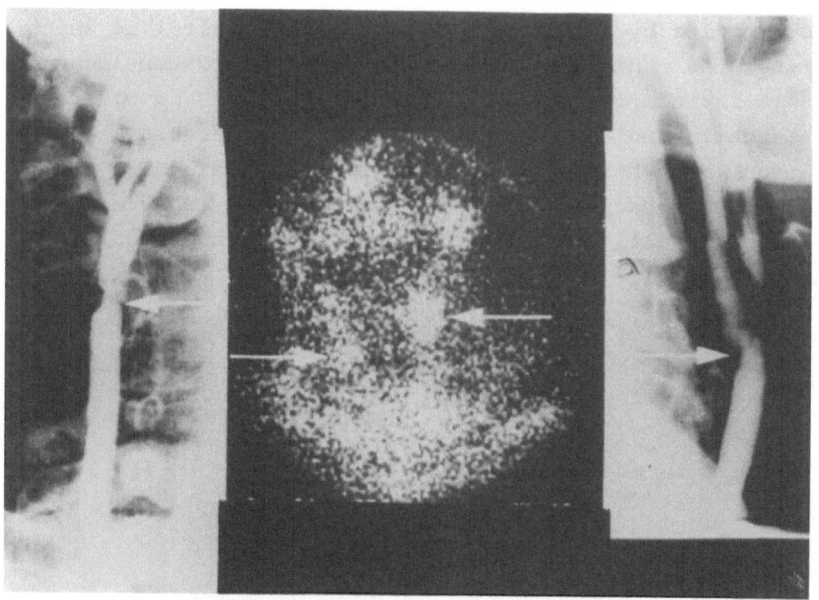

Figure 2. Comparison of bilateral carotid angiograms with
a 48-hour scintigram from a subject with bilateral carotid
stenosis. The thyroid gland is visible at the bottom of
the scintigram, and the blood pool in cerebral venous sinuses
at the top. The isolated right common carotid lesion (left
side of scintigram) sequesters I^{125}-LDL, while extensive
disease of the left common and internal carotids, which
extends much higher in the neck, accumulates far more
radiolabeled lipoprotein (right side of scintigram).
Reproduced with permission from Reference 5.

Encouraged by these results, patients who had been
injected intravenously with ^{125}I-LDL were imaged, since
this preparation was commonly used for kinetic and biochemical studies of LDL metabolism. Although ^{125}I is not a very
good isotope for imaging because the gamma rays emitted are
of low energy, nevertheless, with the cooperation of our
patients, who had to lie still for up to 20 minutes at a
time, both symptomatic and silent atherosclerotic plaques
were imaged and localized (Figure 2). Having shown that
LDL metabolism in general, and arterial LDL sequestration in
particular, could be imaged externally, a radiopharmaceutical
was designed which would allow more effective imaging of LDL
accumulation in tissue. The isotope, ^{99m}Tc, has a favorable
gamma emission which is excellent for external imaging, and

is accompanied by a relatively short 6-hour half-life which minimizes the radiation dose to the patient. Other advantages of ^{99m}Tc include low cost, ready availability, and wide acceptance in nuclear medicine. After considerable experimentation, a technique was devised for synthesis of ^{99m}Tc-LDL (6). This preparation is accumulated, as expected, in the arterial wall, the liver, kidneys, gut and adrenals (Figure 3) (6,7).

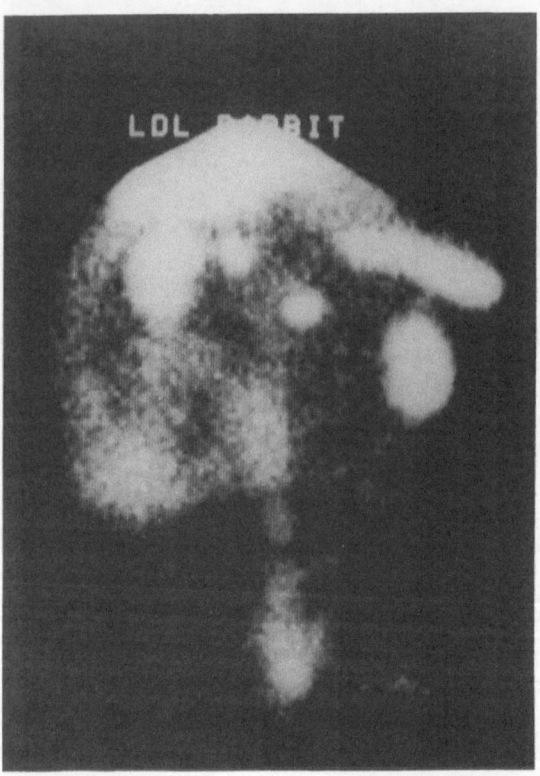

Figure 3. Anterior abdominal scintigram of a rabbit 16 hours after intravenous injection of 3 mCi of ^{99m}Tc-LDL. The rabbit had had balloon de-endothelialization of the abdominal aorta 4 weeks previously, as described elsewhere (6). Note the sequestration of radioactivity in the liver (top of the image), spleen (top left), kidneys, gut, aorta (midline) and some ^{99m}Tc in the bladder (midline at bottom of image). The two round "hot spots" on either side of the midline, just below the liver, are the adrenal glands. Their avid sequestration of radioactivity was confirmed by direct counting of the excised adrenals in a gamma well counter (6). Reproduced with permission from reference 6.

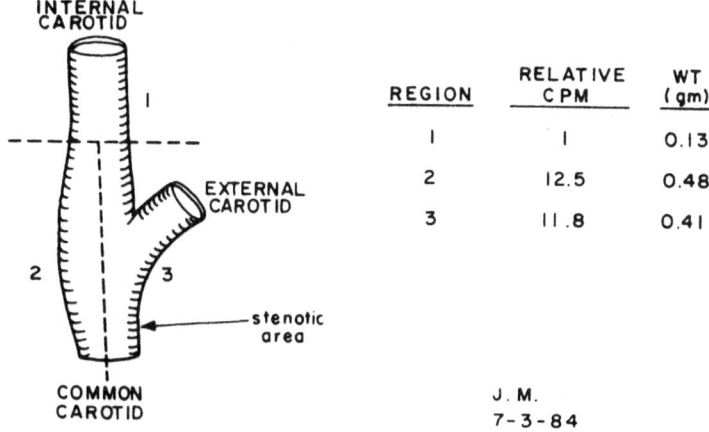

99mTc −LDL Uptake
RELATIVE CPM per REGION of SPECIMEN

INTERNAL CAROTID

REGION	RELATIVE CPM	WT (gm)
I	I	0.13
2	12.5	0.48
3	11.8	0.41

J. M.
7-3-84

Figure 4.   Relative distribution of radioactivity in the
carotid endarterectomy specimen of a 49-year-old patient
with a highly cellular rapidly progressive atherosclerotic
stenosis of the distal common carotid artery at the bifurcation.   The patient received 13 mCi of autologous LDL
labelled with 99mTc 16 hours before endarterectomy.   In
comparison with the minimally involved internal carotid
portion of the specimen (Region 1), the two halves (Regions
2 and 3) of the heavily involved part of the specimen, each
of which weighed 3-4 times as much as Region 1, had about
12 times the radioactivity.

99mTc-LDL shows many of the characteristics of a
"trapped label."   Once the technetium becomes intracellular,
much or all of it remains intracellular (8).   Thus, organs
which accumulate LDL avidly via the high-affinity LDL
receptor, such as the adrenal, retain the label even though
they may degrade LDL into oligopeptides and amino acids
(Figure 3).   They image well, and their radioactivity is a
direct reflection of total LDL uptake, as described by Pittman
et al (9) for 14C-tyramine cellobiose LDL.

      Preliminary clinico-pathological correlation in five
patients who had carotid endarterectomy after being imaged
with 99mTc-LDL seems to confirm the animal data that this

agent accumulates in highest amount where there is active atherosclerotic disease. Direct radioactivity measurement in the endarterectomy specimens showed the greatest counts in the most cellular specimen with active neovascularization and intramural hemorrhage, with a gradation towards the lowest radioactivity in an old fibrous minimally cellular specimen. In Figure 4 and 5 are shown the distribution of radioactivity in two such specimens.

It is evident from animal data, but must also be true for human subjects, that arterial LDL accumulation is indepen-dent of the high affinity LDL receptor. This has been shown to be true with two different modified LDL preparations, neither of which bind to any known protein or lipoprotein receptor. Both cyclohexanedione-modified LDL (10) and

$99mTc - LDL$ Uptake
RELATIVE CPM per REGION of SPECIMEN

REGION	RELATIVE CPM	WT (gm)
1	1	0.09
2	3.7	0.28
3	6	0.25

E. G.
5-15-85

Figure 5. Relative distribution of radioactivity in the carotid endarterectomy specimen of a 65-year-old patient with an asymptomatic fibrous paucicellular lesion. The endarter-ectomy was performed prophylactically before coronary bypass grafting; the patient had been known to have a carotid bruit for at least 2 years prior to surgery. The patient received 20 mCi of autologous LDL labelled with $99mTc$ 18 hours before carotid endarterectomy. Here the external carotid orifice (Region 1) was virtually uninvolved. The carotid bulb (Region 2) was highly fibrous and almost acellular; it was 3.1 times the weight of Region 1 and had 3.7 times as much radioactivity. Region 3, which contained the proximal internal carotid stenosis, was somewhat more cellular, but still highly fibrous, it had 2.8 times the weight of region 1 and was 6 times as radioactive.

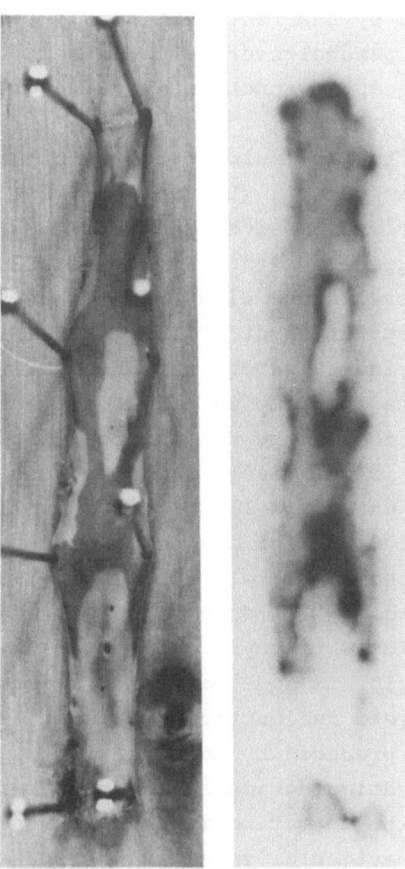

Figure 6.   Sequestration of CHD-LDL by the healing balloon-
de-endothelialized rabbit aorta.   The rabbit received 300
mCi of ^{125}I-labelled LDL which had been derivatized with
cyclohexanedione to abolish uptake by the high-affinity LDL
receptor, confirmed by *in vitro* lymphocyte assay.   The
^{125}I-CHD-LDL was injected intravenously 24 hours before
sacrifice.   The rabbit also received 50 mg of Evans Blue
dye 10 minutes before sacrifice, to stain the remaining
de-endothelialized aorta.   At the left is a photograph of
the pinned-out abdominal aorta.   The light areas are recovered with endothelium, while the dark, Evans Blue-stained
areas are bare.   At the right is the autoradiograph of the
same vessel.   There is extensive sequestration of radioactivity at the borders of the healing edge.   Since the
^{125}I-CHD-LDL does not bind to the LDL receptor, the arterial
accumulation is a receptor-independent process.

methylated LDL (11) are sequestered by the healing balloon
de-endothelialized rabbit aorta as well as or better than
native LDL (Figure 6).   That this is also true for human

arteries is attested by the fact that homozygous receptor-
negative familial hypercholesterolemic patients, who have
no detectable LDL receptor function, have severe atherosclerosis.

Experimental arterial lesions (2), rabbit adrenal LDL
uptake (8), and human carotid (5), coronary (9), and aorto-
femoral (9) atherosclerosis with radiolabelled LDL have been
imaged. Based on experience thus far, some of the drawbacks must be addressed along with the obvious promise of
this technique. Preparation of ^{125}I or ^{131}I LDL is relatively easy for the investigator, but the imaging is difficult
for the patient. Imaging time is long because of the poor
imaging characteristics of the radioisotope, and radiation
dose to the patient is relatively large because of the long
isotope half-life. Use of ^{123}I, which has excellent imaging
and dosimetric characteristics, is not a good solution at
present because of the relatively limited availability and
great expense of "clean" ^{123}I free of other, long half-life,
iodine isotopes. Even with thyroid blockage with "cold"
iodide, carotid imaging in some patients may be compromised
by even minimal thyroid radioactivity arising from uptake
of free radioiodide produced by deiodination of the radiolabelled LDL. This deiodination of iodine-labelled LDL may
give erroneous results in metabolic studies conducted with
such preparations, particularly in organs like the liver,
which have considerable deiodinase activity. Thus, a good
deal of apparent hepatic LDL "metabolism" may be deiodination rather than true metabolism of LSL, as suggested by
the much smaller percentage of ^{99m}Tc-LDL which appears to be
removed via the liver (6).

The disadvantages of ^{99m}Tc-LDL include the fact that
we have not yet learned how to remove the non-protein
bound technetium which is variably produced during the
coupling of pertechnetate to LDL (6). Although this does not
affect atherosclerotic imaging, it can have some effect on
metabolic studies, probably increasing the apparent LDL
removal by liver, spleen, and bone marrow.

One general problem with nuclear medicine must also be
mentioned. Although detection of radiopharmaceutical accumulation in lesions or organs of interest is easy and

sensitivity is great, spatial resolution in nuclear imaging
has been relatively poor - on the order of $\pm$ 1 cm. This
is in marked contrast to the $\pm$ 1 mm resolution of digital
radiography and the even higher resolution of analog angiography. However, limited resolution is not intrinsic to
radioactivity detection, and investigators can look forward
to dramatic improvements in resolution of gamma camera
imaging with the development of new detectors for imaging (12)
as well as to newer methods of tomography and signal processing.

Future directions seem fairly clear. The rapid development of improved techniques of external imaging must be
encouraged. While awaiting the improved spatial resolution
which is known to be possible (12), investigators can take
advantage of available technology for quantitation of radioactivity in gamma camera images (13,14). One can identify
a "region of interest" in an image, and can integrate the
counts in that region with moderate accuracy to estimate
the total uptake or radioactivity (13,14). Recent experiments with prosthetic arterial grafts as models of arterial
healing (15) suggest that total radioactivity as well as the
localization of radioactivity in a healing graft in the
rabbit can be related directly to the stage of healing.

Researchers must broaden their goals and must ask
what studies will be necessary to determine the sensitivity
and specificity of *in vivo* radiopharmaceutical imaging for
detecting early atherosclerotic changes and, perhaps, for
detecting active unstable advanced lesions (16,17). For
investigating the early lesion, animal studies, perhaps in
cholesterol-fed primates, will almost certainly be necessary,
since it is not feasible to image and then examine early
human lesions on a planned basis. Recent advances in angioscopy (16) should allow by contrast, imaging and then
identification of *in vivo* unstable lesions in human coronary
and peripheral arterial beds with this technique. The results
of such animal and human studies over the next several years
should allow us to place in proper perspective the role of
radiopharmaceutical arterial imaging in diagnosis and follow-
up of arterial disease by demonstrating its reliability in
localizing lesions and in detecting lesion growth or regression. Perhaps the most important element in that equation

is the need to improve radiopharmaceuticals for arterial imaging. Radiolabelled human LDL is far from an ideal agent. Investigators look forward to the possibility of designing and testing improved imaging agents in the near future, with greater and more rapid accumulation in the arterial wall, greater east of preparation,and longer shelf life. With such diagnostic drugs, radioisotope arterial imaging may help to solve some of the most troubling problems in the etiology, diagnosis, and treatment of arterio-sclerosis.

REFERENCES

1. Bratzler RL, Chisolm GH, Colton CK, Smith KA, Lees RS (1977) The distribution of labeled lipoproteins across the rabbit thoracic aorta *in vivo*. Atherosclerosis 28:289-307
2. Roberts AB, Lees AM, Rees RS, *et al* (1983) Selective accumulation of low density lipoproteins in damaged arterial wall. J Lipid Res 24:1160-1167
3. Minick CR, Stemerman MB, Insull W (1977) Effect of regeneration endothelium on lipid accumulation in the arterial wall. Proc Natl Acad Sci USA 74:1724-1728
4. Minick CR, Stemerman MB, Insull W (1979) Role of endo-thelium and hypercholesterolemia in intimal thickening and lipid accumulation. Am J Pathol 95:131-158
5. Lees RS, Lees AM, Strauss HW (1983) External imaging of human atherosclerosis. J Nucl Med 27:154-156
6. Lees RS, Garabedian HD,Lees AM, *et al* (1985) Technetium-99m low density lipoproteins: preparation and biodistri-bution. J Nucl Med 26:1056-1062
7. Isaacsohn JL, Lees AM, Lees RS, Strauss HW, Barlai-Kovach M, Moore TJ (1986) Adrenal imaging with technetium-99m-labelled low density lipoproteins. Metabolism 35: 364-366
8. Lees RS, Lees AM, Fischman AJ, Strauss HW (1986) Technetium-99m labelled low density lipoproteins (LDL), a new radiopharmaceutical for imaging LDL metabolism. Clin Invest Med 9:Suppl 1:A6
9. Pittman RC, Carew TE, Glass CK, Green SR, Taylor CA, Attie AD (1983) A radioiodinated, intracellularly trapped ligand for determining the sites of plasma protein degradation *in vivo*. Biochem J 212:791-800
10. Roberts AB, Lees AM, Fallon JT *et al* (1981) Determinants of low density lipoprotein (LDL) accumulation in the healing arterial wall. Circulation 64:Suppl 4:45
11. Fischman AJ, Lees AM, Lees RS, Barlai-Kovach M, Strauss HW (1987) Accumulation of native and methylated low density lipoproteins by healing rabbit arterial wall. Arteriosclerosis 7:361-366.
12. Kaufman L, Hosier K, Lorenz V *et al* (1978) Imaging characteristics of a small germanium camera. Invest Radiol 13:223-232.
13. Witztum KF (1985) Current methods of evaluating vascular disease with radionuclides. In: Bernstein E (ed) Non-invasive Diagnostic Techniques in Vascular Disease, 3rd Edition. St. Louis: C.V. Mosby Co., pp 182-211.

14. Sorenson JA and Phelps ME (1987) Physics in Nuclear Medicine, 2nd Edition, Grune and Stratton, New York, pgs 450-462

15. Miller A, Schoen FJ, Lees AM *et al* (1987) Low density-lipoprotein accumulation by PTFE grafts in the rabbit aorta, Trans. ASAIO 33:489-493

16. Sherman CT, Litvack F, Grundfest W *et al* (1986) Coronary angioscopy in patients with unstable angina pectoris. New Engl J Med 315:913-919

17. Davies, MJ and Thomas AC (1985) Plaque fissuring -- the cause of acute myocardial infarction, sudden ischaemic death, and crescendo angina. Br Heart J 53:363-373

57

Magnetic Resonance Imaging for the Visualization of Vasculature and Atherosclerosis

Leon Kaufman, Lawrence Crooks, Joseph Rapp, Gary Caputo, Phil Sheldon and James Hale

INTRODUCTION

Magnetic resonance imaging (MRI) offers a unique and extraordinary window into the body. Since 1983 the growth and acceptance of this modality as a diagnostic tool has been prodigious, and the enthusiasm with which it is received still grows. The original uses were centered on head imaging, and have since expanded to spine and extremities. Some acceptance is now being seen for body imaging, more for central portions of the chest and in the pelvis than in the abdomen. The routine use of MRI for cardiovascular work is generally limited to large centers. Because of the patient demand for MRI, and because of the desire to obtain revenue from the units, MRI has not been fully exploited in areas where the primary payoff is a contribution towards understanding disease processes. For this latter purpose, one of the most important characteristics of MRI is that it is non-invasive, and therefore ideally suited for both cross-sectional and longitudinal studies. There is an obvious match between MRI and the needs of those who aim to understand the evolution of the human atherosclerotic plaque.

Basic Principles

Hydrogen nuclei have magnetic dipole moments, as bar magnets do. Placed in a magnetic field, they gain a net

These investigations are supported in part by Contract N01-HV-38044 and Grant HL 34960 from the NHLBI (DHHS) and by Diasonics, Inc.

alignment with the field. Changes in alignment are associated with quanta of energy delivered in the form of
magnetic oscillation of a frequency that depends on the
strength of the magnetic field. These frequencies fall in
the radio, or RF range. In a uniform magnetic field, the
hydrogen nuclei flip into higher energy states when subject
to magnetic oscillations at resonant frequency. These
nuclei return to lower energy equilibrium by excitation due
to the random motion of molecules. That motion produces a
broad range of frequencies, some of which fall in the
resonant range. The time required to recover equilibrium
is characterized by the T1 exponential time constant. In
the process of returning to equilibrium the nuclei can give
off magnetic oscillations at the resonant frequency. In
tissues these radiations can be detected for a time shorter
than T1. The decay of this radiation is characterized by
an exponential time constant T2 (1).

Imaging
    There exist a plethora of imaging techniques. All of
them shape the magnetic field to encode position through
the unique relationship of magnetic field and resonant
frequency (2). Clinical work is done almost universally
using a technique called 2D-FT multi-section imaging.
First, a change of magnetic field (magnetic field gradient)
is established along one axis, e.g., the long axis of the
subject. The body is irradiated by an RF antenna for a
few milliseconds with a narrow range of frequencies. These
flip, or excite, nuclei in a plane that is at a magnetic
field strength corresponding to the resonant frequency.
The first gradient is turned off and a second gradient along
another axis, e.g., the front to back axis of the subject,
is turned on for a few milliseconds. This gradient encodes
back to front position of the nuclei. The original, section-
selecting gradient is turned on again at the nuclei subject
to a second RF pulse that serves to bring the radiation
from the nuclei back into coherence (coherence is lost
over time due to a number of effects). Finally, a magnetic
gradient is applied along the third axis, side to side in

this case. Due to this third gradient, nuclei reaching coherence radiate at different frequencies.

The location of the section and its width are encoded uniquely by the excitation pulse. Side to side position encoding is also uniquely determined by the third (readout) gradient. Unfortunately, the position encoding from front to back is not unique unless many different encodings are done. Each encoding requires a complete repetition of the sequence described above, only the second gradient changing slightly each time. The data thus produced can be turned into a representation of the object by a Fourier Transform along each of the two encoded axes, hence the name 2-D FT. The time between consecutive sequences is called TR. It is chosen on the basis of clinical and analytical experience (3-5), and it is on the order of T1. This is a very long time for imaging purposes. For instance, TR=2 sec. is quite common. If the sequence is repeated 250 times, this will require a time of 8 min. to form an image. Each sequence is quite short, a few tens of milliseconds. There- fore, during the TR interval the sequence can be applied sequentially to many sections. When the time TR is over, the cycle repeated. In this manner, if each sequence is 100 msec. long, for a TR of 2 sec. 20 sections can be fit into one TR. This process is called multi-section imaging, and makes MRI clinically viable.

The recovery of coherence produces a signal called a spin echo, measured at a time TE. The scale of TE is set by the values of T2, which in tissues are an order of magnitude shorter than T1. Therefore, there is time in a sequence to obtain images at more than one TE value. Two such spin echoes sample T2 on a pixel by pixel basis. T1 can be mapped from two sequences with different values of TR. Two kinds of images can be reconstructed from the 2-D FT process. One is called a magnitude image and shows signal intensity. The second is called a phase image. For stationaly objects the phase image is essentially feature- less except at some tissue interfaces.

Flow in MRI

The process of eliciting and spatially encoding an
NMR signal requires tens of milliseconds. The sequence is
designed to apply carefully timed RF and gradient pulses
that vary in their effect depending on the location of
nuclei. If nuclei move during the duration of the sequence,
they experience a different set of gradients. Therefore,
flow is detectable in MRI without the need for contrast
media. Broadly, flow effects can be taken advantage of by
two different means: incidental to an imaging sequence, or
by specialized flow sequences. The latter derive broadly
from work done by Singer in 1959 (6), and can be used to
quantitate flow. Incidental effects can be used to identify
the lumen of vessels (7,8). For studies where flow velocity
is not a needed parameter, 2-D FT multi-section imaging
techniques provide the data needed to perform this identification. There are three ways of assessing flow:

1. Effects on signal intensity. At slow velocities
the entrance sections of a multi-section sequence may show
elevated signal. This elevation is due to the wash in of
unexcited blood, which is fully magnetized. As velocity
increases, some of the nuclei in a section do not experience
the two selective RF pulses, and consequently do not produce
a signal. As velocity increases, more nuclei miss the co-
ordinated pulses and the signal from them disappears
(Figure 1). At high velocities the signal is zero (7,8).
Turbulent flow does not result in as large a loss of signal
(Figure 2). When flow is laminar, the patterns of signal-
producing regions can become quite complex (9), and care
must be taken in interpreting the images (Figure 3).

2. Effects on T2. When a double echo procedure is
used, the second echo looses signal much more slowly than
the first echo. As a consequence, the second echo gains
signal with respect to the first. T2 characterizes the
drop of signal between first and second echo, the shorter
T2 the faster the drop. As a result of flow, the drop
diminishes and T2 appears to increase. The value can
become extremely large, and even negative with more signal
in the second than in the first echo. In regions where

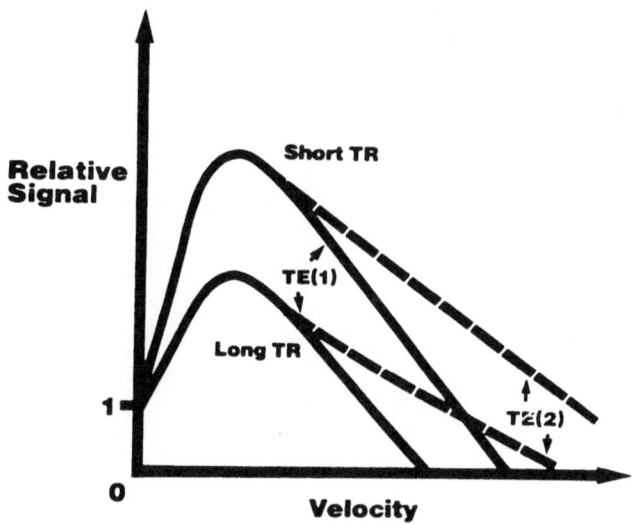

Figure 1. Compared with stationary blood, flowing blood can produce more or less NMR signal as velocity increases. In general, relative intensity is higher for the shorter values of TR. Also, the second echo is generally of more intensity than the first.

the blood is not flowing fast enough to drop the signal, T2 effects can highlight flow (Figure 4).

3. Effects on phase. As mentioned above, a phase image can be reconstructed from a 2-D FT data set. The magnetic vector is characterized by a magnitude (signal strength) and direction in which it points in space. This direction is ambiguous to within multiples of 360°, i.e., two regions of the sample where the phase has gone through whole rotations have the same phase. When nuclei move in a gradient field their phase changes. Therefore, in regions of the vessel where the flow is too slow or turbulent to produce unambiguous signal changes, the phase image will still show velocity (Figure 5). The phase change between moving nuclei and those that are stationary can be used to quantitate flow, except for two problems: a) If the sequence is not synchronized with the heart beat, then the individual spin echoes are

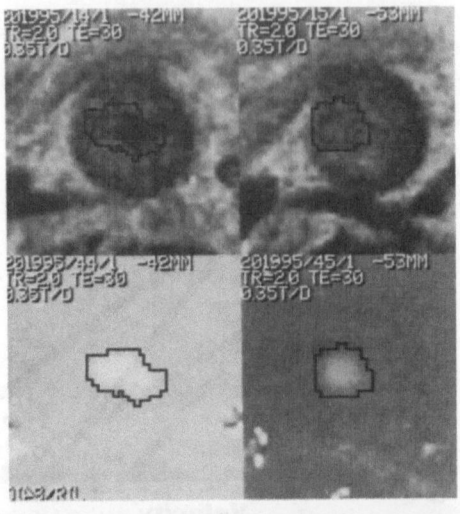

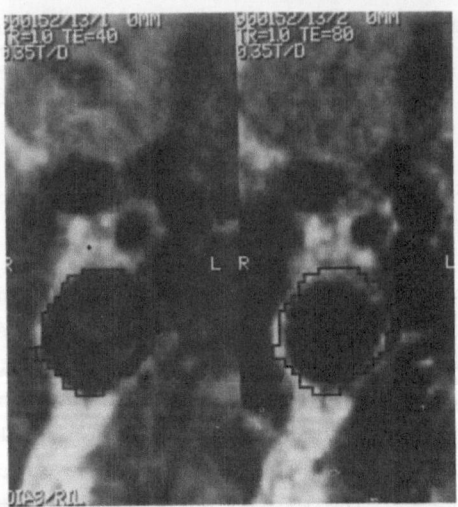

Figure 2.   Turbulent flow can result in signal indistinguishable from that of stationary tissues. At left some signal
loss due to flow is evident in the descending aorta of a
patient with plaque. One section closer to the feet, no such
difference is seen. At bottom, the corresponding phase images
provide information on flow.
Figure 3.   Right jugular in a normal volunteer. First echo
(left) and second echo (right). Note "bulls-eye" pattern in
the first echo, consisting of a central region with signal and
an outer ring. There is a dark region between the second and
the vessel wall. This could be misinterpreted as a ring of
plaque and calcification. In the second echo the inner
patterns disappear, but a ring appears next to the vessel
wall, making it seem smaller in area.

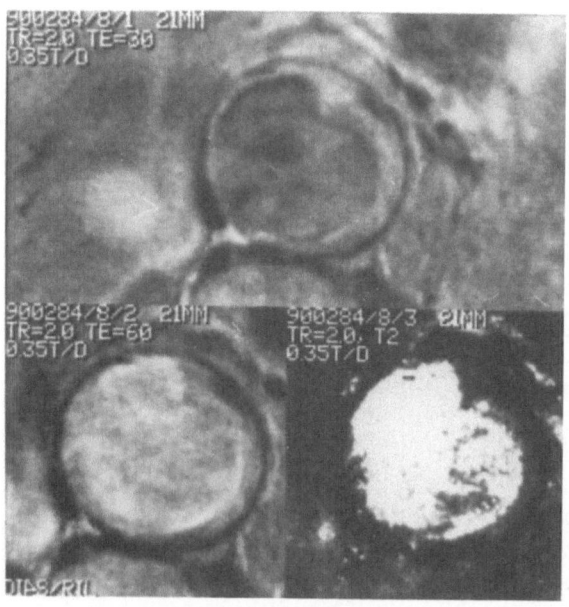

Figure 4. In a patient with a large aortic aneurysm and atherosclerosis, the first echo shows signals that could be interpreted as thrombus, especially in the second echo (bottom left). A T2 image (bottom right) clearly identifies the lumen with its long T2.

produced at different points in the cardiac cycle and the phase information can be garbled. To obtain flow volume from phase, images have to be produced at different points in the cardiac cycle, so as to obtain a velocity distribution; b) Even for a synchronized sequence, if the velocity is high enough, the phase may go through 360° one or more times, and velocity may not be measurable. There are ways of avoiding these ambiguities, but they interfere with the needs of efficient imaging techniques. In any event, phase is a reliable indicator of flow for lumen identification.

Imaging the Descending Aorta

MRI, because of its tomographic format, is ideal for studying lesions in vessels. A view transverse to the vessel measures the lumen and the location of the vessel wall, as well as the extent of lesions in between. The

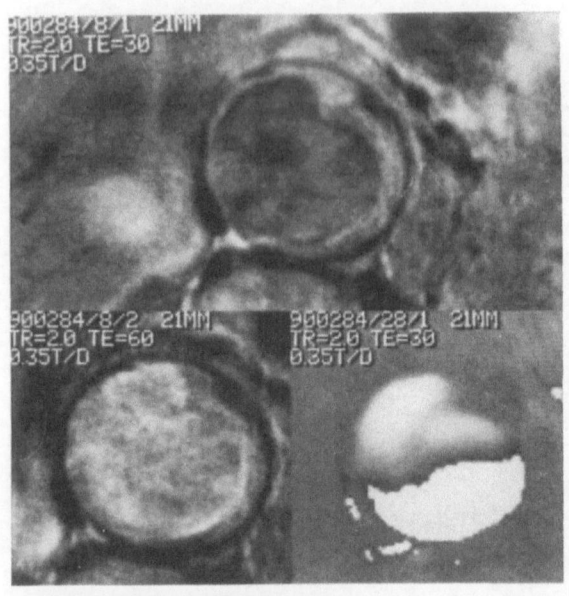

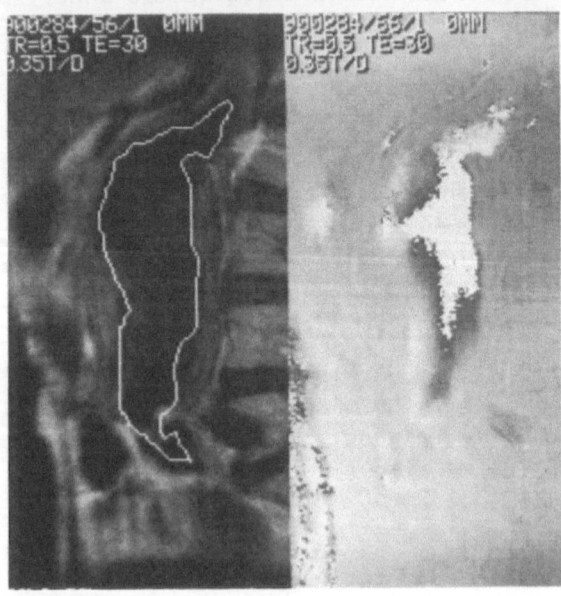

Figure 5. Above: In the patient of Figure 4, the phase image at bottom right shows the lumen. It also shows that flow in the bottom and top halves of the vessel is in opposite directions. Below: A large eddy current appears to exist in this patient; as evidenced in the sagittal view of the aorta.

transverse format, however, does not allow for easy visualization of the vessel. It could be argued that MRI, because
it can produce images along any plane, could visualize a
whole vessel as well. Unfortunately, the alignment of
vessels is not known a priori, and further, diseased vessels
can become quite tortuous. Also, where the vessel is tangential to the tomographic plane, partial volume effects make
it difficult to differentiate the various anatomic features
of interest. In our work we image the descending aorta in
the transverse plane, using 20, 1 cm-thick sections, covering
the region between the renal arteries and the bifurcation.
Initially, in-plane spatial resolution was 1.7 mm, and more
recently 0.9 mm. The lumen is identified by the flow signa-
ture, and computer programs are used to reconstruct the
vessel from a direction where its whole length is visible
(Figure 6). In these reconstructions the depth of the
vessel can be encoded in color. Also, the width of the lumen
can be made to represent the true cross section, by replacing
eccentric cross sections with circular ones of equal area (10)
(Figure 7). These vessel reconstructions compare well with
angiographic studies (11). Lesions can be superimposed on
these images, but, so far, they are shown in single highlight.
Nevertheless, more information can be provided in the future.
Because of the variations in relaxation times, some tissue
identification is possible in lesions. Extensively calcified
areas produce no signal. Vessel wall and connective tissues
are of low intensity. Plaque is next highest in intensity,
and thrombus tends to be brighter because ferromagnetic
substances in blood decrease relaxation times which increases
intensity (Figure 8).

Carotid Arteries

The geometry of the carotid arteries is in many ways
similar to that of the major abdominal vessels, in that the
carotids lie, in general, along the long axis of the neck.
The vessels are smaller, and there are more of them. But,
because of the smaller size of the neck, the spatial resolution used in MRI can be increased. For instance, section
thickness can be reduced to 5 mm for whole neck coverage,

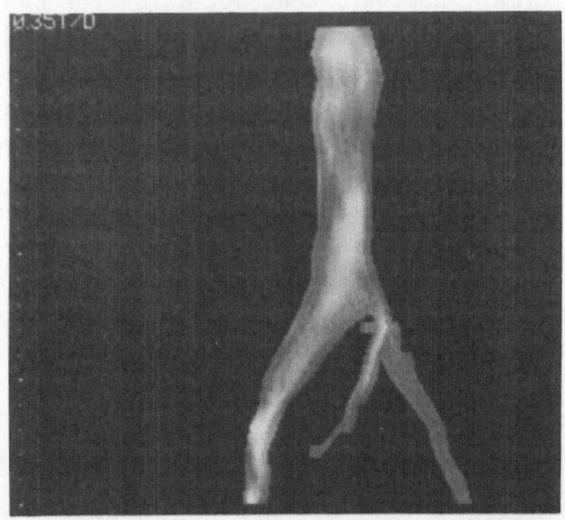

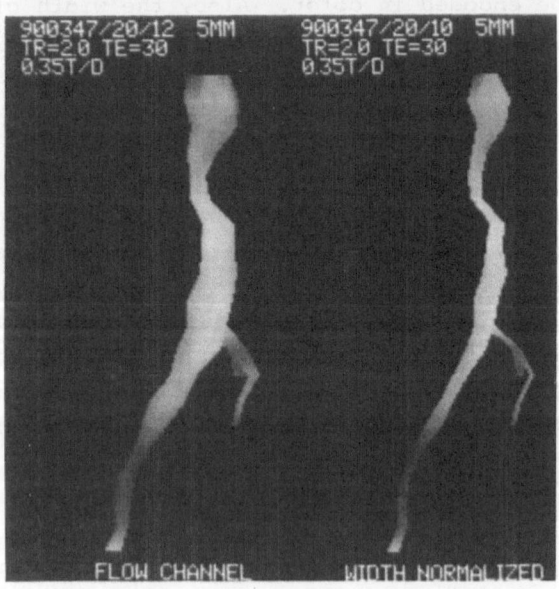

Figure 6. Reconstructed descending aorta. Flat gray areas represent plaque. Flow is shown with lower intensity as it becomes slower of more turbulent. Note streamline patterns.
Figure 7. For the vessel of Figure 6, at left is a reconstruction of the flow channel as seen in a frontal view. At right the displayed width has been normalized to represent cross-sectional area. In both images intensity represents distance from the viewer, with lower intensities being farther away (towards the patients back).

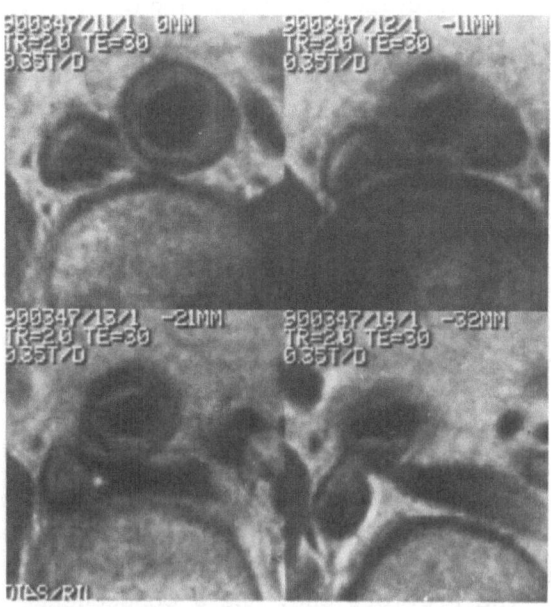

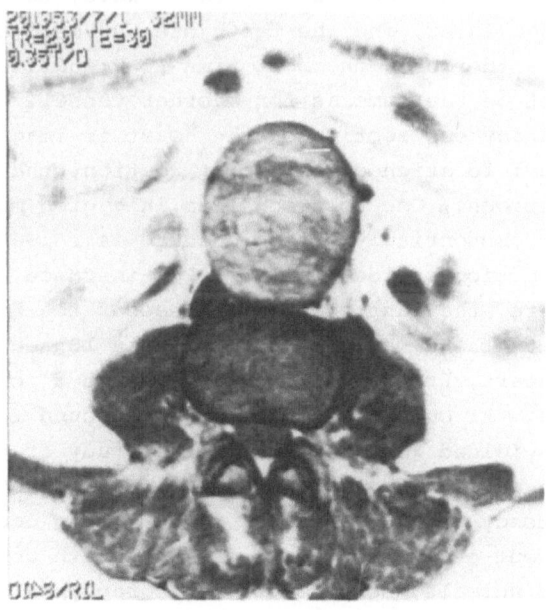

Figure 8. Above: Four consecutive sections through the
descending aorta at the level of bifurcation. Thrombus
is seen as regions of higher intensity at the edge of the
lumen. Below: A complex lesion showing layering, thrombus
and plaque.

and to 2.5 mm for studying a short region. In-plane resolution can be improved to 0.6 mm and better (Figures 9 and 10).
As a consequence, MRI of neck vessels can be very effective.
In this area, of course, it overlaps with ultrasound, which
is much less expensive. On the other hand, MRI can access
deeper portions of the vessel and yield improved characteri-
zations of lesions.

Coronary Arteries

The use of MRI for following coronary disease over long
periods of time and without hazards offers an exciting
potential. But, coronary imaging by MRI presents particular
challenges. The coronaries are small, tortuous and they move
during the cardiac cycle. The motion problem needs two
approaches to be solved. The first is cardiac synchronization
of the imaging sequence (12). But this by itself is not
sufficient. In multi-section imaging, each section is sampled
50 msec after the previous one. As a consequence, if the
first section is synchronized with the R-wave, the fifth one
occurs 250 msec later, and the tenth one 500 msec after the
first one. Furthermore, the best time to visualize one
vessel may not be the same as for another vessel. Since the
time at which any one section of the heart is imaged depends
on the physical location of the first section, the timing
problem is serious. One solution lies in cycled multi-section
imaging (13). Essentially, the procedure is repeated five
times, each section cycled in time. For instance, for the
fifth procedure, the last section instead of the first one
is in time with the R-wave. We thus obtain 10 sections
through the heart, from apex to base, each at 5 points in the
cardiac cycle. At our institution we have found that the
technique has yielded good results in the study of the patency
of coronary bypass grafts (where there is 90% accuracy in
detecting patency and 70% accuracy in detecting occlusions).

In a recent evaluation of 13 patients with coronary
lesions and 2 normals, compared to angiography, MRI correctly
visualized the normal left main, left anterior descending,
circumflex and right coronary arteries, and detected about
half of the lesions or occlusions shown by angiography in

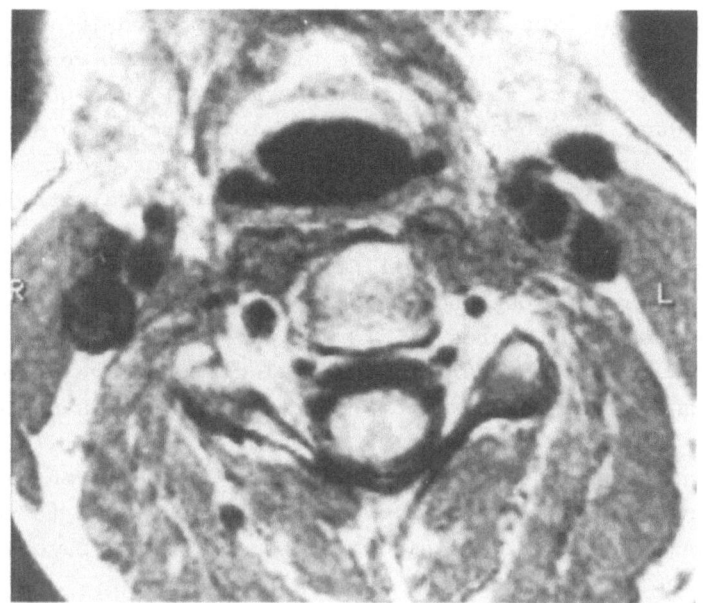

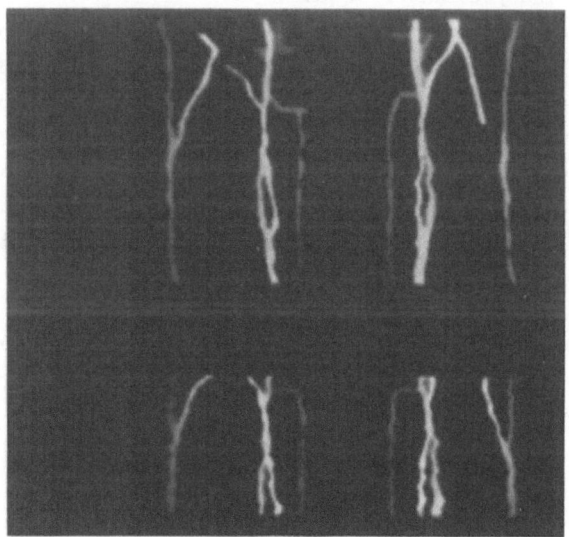

Figure 9. Neck vasculature at the level of carotid artery
bifurcation. Resolution is 0.6 mm.
Figure 10. Reconstructions of the neck arterial vasculature
from 5 mm thick slices (top) and 2.5 mm thick slices (bottom).
Note in the top set the missing section of the right carotid
above the bifurcation. The loss is probably due to partial
volume effects in the thicker slices.

these vessels. The results were almost as good in the posterior descending artery (one of eight normal vessels missed, one out of four obstructions missed), and poor in the diagonal branch of the left anterior descending and first obtuse artery, where it failed to detect about half of the normal vessels. This study was performed with 10 mm-thick sections and a 1.7 mm in-plane resolution. Advances in the equipment will allow us to repeat the study with thinner sections and a higher resolution. Examples are presented in Figures 11, 12 and 13.

While we do not believe that MRI will replace coronary angiography over the next few years, it may have a useful role in the heart. Certainly, it is of proved utility in assessing the patency of bypass grafts. It may eventually serve to screen patients prior to angiography, and to perform longitudinal studies in patients who have a baseline angiogram.

Viability of Longitudinal Studies

MRI is an expensive modality. The operating costs of a medium magnetic field strength unit range on the order of $1,000,000/year, including equipment depreciation costs, salaries, etc. Typical study costs are in the $700 plus range. These assume a 1 hour patient imaging time and professional fees. Imaging of the abdominal or neck vessels can be done in less than half an hour of machine utilization time, and we may reasonably expect costs to decrease as utilization improves. There will be some 500 units in operation in this county by the end of 1986 or early 1987. While not all of them have the same capabilities for vessel imaging, enough are available to allow for selected longitudinal studies for which this technique is ideally suited. With MRI we have the potential opportunity to study the progression of atherosclerosis in different vascular beds, and to monitor the impact to interventions designed to reduce plaque.

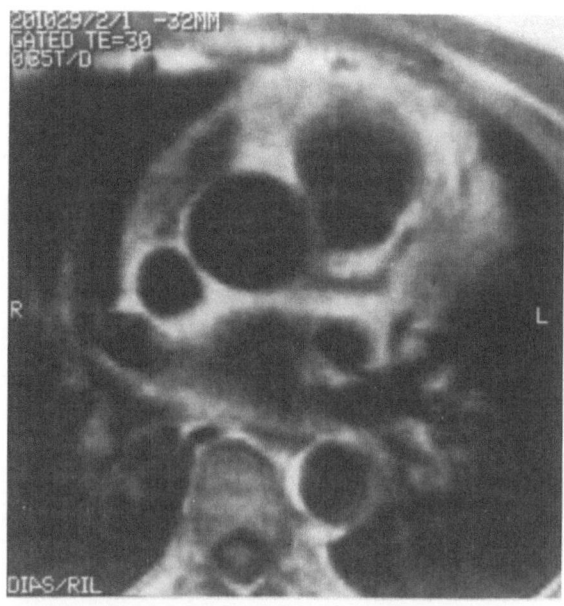

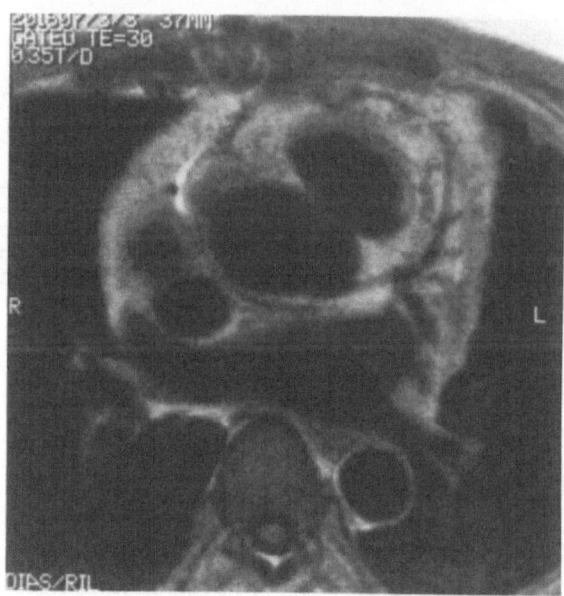

Figure 11.   Transverse cardiac section of a patient with a
fully occluded LAD.
Figure 12.   Proximal left coronary arteries.   On the right,
the bright feature is due to an iron marker left at surgery.
Next to it is an RCA bypass graft.

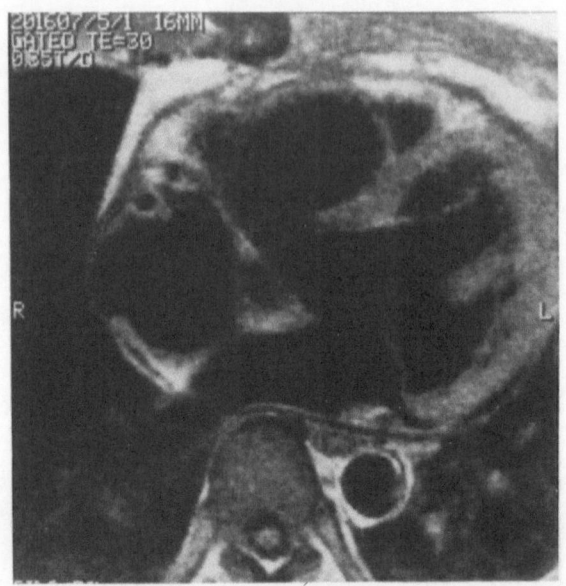

Figure 13. In a patient of Figure 12, we see the RCA and the bypass graft.

Acknowledgement. The work described in this paper was performed at the Jet Propulsion Laboratory, California Institute of Technology, and the University of Southern California School of Medicine and was supported by NIH/NHLBI Grant HL 23619 through an agreement with the National Aeronautics and Space Administration. Major contributions to the work described in this paper were made by Maria Siebes, Anne Shircore, Paul Lee, June Lee and Howard Freiden (Jet Propulsion Laboratory) and by David H. Blankenhorn, Linda Hemphill, H.P. Chan and Donna Conover (University of Southern California).

REFERENCES

1. Davis PL, Kaufman L, Crooks LE (1983) Tissue characteri-
    zation. In: Margulis A, Higgins C, Kaufman L, Crooks L
    (eds) Clinical Magnetic Resonance Imaging. San Francisco:
    University of California Press, Chapter 6.
2. Crooks LE, Kaufman L (1983) Imaging techniques. In:
    Margulis A, Higgins C, Kaufman L, Crooks L (eds) Clini-
    cal Magnetic Resonance Imaging. San Francisco: University
    of California Press, Chapter 3.
3. Brant-Zawadzki M, Normal D, Newton TH, et al. (1984)
    Magnetic resonance of the brain: The optimal screening
    technique. Radiology 152:71-77.
4. Ortendahl DA, Hylton NM, Kaufman L, Watts JC, Crooks LE,
    Mills CM, Stark D (1984) Analytical tools for MRI.
    Radiology 153:479.
5. Droege RT, Wiener SN, Rzeszotarski MS (1984) A strategy
    for MRI of the head: Results of semi-empirical model,
    Part II. Radiology 153:425-433.
6. Singer JR (1981) Blood flow measurements by MRI. In:
    Kaufman L, Crooks LE, Margulis AR (eds) NMR Imaging in
    Medicine. New York: Igaku Shoin, Chapter 7.
7. Kaufman L, Crooks LE, Sheldon PE, Rowan W, Miller T
    (1983) Evaluation of NMR imaging for detection and
    quantification of obstructions in vessels. Investi-
    gative Radiology 17:554.

8. Kaufman L, Crooks LE, Sheldon PE, Hricak H, Herfkens R,
    Bank W (1983) The potential impact of nuclear magnetic
    resonance imaging on cardiovascular diagnosis. Circula-
    tion 67:251.
9. Valk PE, Hale JD, Crooks LE, Kaufman L, Roos MS,
    Ortendahl DA, Higgins CB (1986) MRI of blood flow:
    Correlation of image appearance with spin echo phase
    shift and signal intensity. AJR 146:931.
10. Hale JD, Valk PE, Watts JC, Kaufman L, Crooks LE,
    Higgins CB, Deconinck F (1985) MR imaging of blood
    vessels using three-dimensional reconstruction:
    Methodology. Radiology 157:727.
11. Valk PE, Hale JD, Kaufman L, Crooks LE, Higgins CB
    (1985) MR imaging of the aorta with three-dimensional
    vessel reconstruction: Validation by angiography.
    Radiology 157:721.
12. Lanzer P, Botvinick EH, Schiller N, Crooks LE, Arakawa M,
    Kaufman L, Davis PL, Herfkens RF, Lipton MJ, Higgins CB
    (1984) Cardiac imaging using gated magnetic resonance.
    Radiology 150:121.
13. Crooks LE, Barker B, Chang H, Feinberg D, Hoenninger JC,
    Watts JC, Arakawa M, Kaufman L, Sheldon PE, Botvinick E,
    Higgins C (1984) Magnetic resonance imaging strategies
    for heart studies. Radiology 153:459.

58
Plaque Characterization—An Integrated Approach

Alan S. Berson

Considerable research and development effort is currently expended, with some success, to detect and quantify atherosclerotic plaque in human arteries using minimally invasive techniques. Evidence exists that definition of plaque characteristics may be equally as important as assessing the degree of lumen area reduction. In 1984, the National Heart, Lung, and Blood Institute solicited grant applications on this topic, lising a number of questions which were important to address:

Is the plaque surface irregular, with fissures or fractures?
Is the endothelium intact or denuded?
Is there evidence of platelet aggregation or of intramural plaque hemorrhage?
How much of a given plaque consists of connective tissue?
What is the lipid content of the plaque?
What is the calcium content of the plaque?
How much residual media is there?
Can mural thrombi be differentiated from plaque or occlusive thrombus be discerned?
Is the plaque structured in the laminar form?

These remain important unanswered questions; no existing minimally invasive techniques can reliably answer them.

However, they are theoretically answerable using several known modalities, and the two with the greatest potential for success are ultrasound and nuclear magnetic resonance (NMR). With both of these modalities, it is not yet clear how well they may be able to meet the requirements in terms of both spatial resolution and differentiation of lesion components. In fact, there is no clear quantitative goal, because the clinical significance of these changes has not been determined. For example, should it be possible to determine the relative volume of lipid vs collagen in a plaque to an accuracy of 10 percent, would this be of enormous value as against an accuracy of 30 percent? Until appropriate studies determine this, the best that can be done is to strive for greater accuracy and precision, recognizing that current resolution and differentiation capabilities are inadequate.

Ultrasound research in plaque composition focuses on the broad goal of differentiating lipid, collagen, and calcium content. The parameters considered to be important indicators are reflectivity, propagation velocity, attenuation, and backscatter characteristics. Tissue echogenicity is known to be related to biologic composition (1), but the precise relationship between echographic appearance and tissue or molecular organization remains unclear (2,3). What is lacking is a basic understanding of how echoes are produced in tissues. Many researchers believe that it is necessary to solve the backscattering problem for this basic understanding to come about, and that the quantitative scattering solution must account for attenuation in tissues (4). An exact solution to the inverse scattering problem may be necessary to develop quantitative images of density, velocity, and absorption. Such a theoretical solution has been reported (5). Spatial resolution is related to frequency but cannot be fully exploited without solving the backscatter problem. For B-scan systems currently available commercially, resolution may approach the theoretical limit of axial resolution but lateral resolution is almost always poorer.

One group of investigators has proposed and tested with phantoms a synthetic aperture technique which comes close to

achieving half wavelength resolution in both directions.
They have been able to obtain images of reflectivity with
0.15 mm resolution at 5 MHz (6). Inverse scattering imaging
using multiple frequency data may allow greater flexibility
in assessing plaque composition (7). Additional information
regarding plaque structure may be derived from flow patterns.
It has been suggested that radially directed flow in vessels
indicates the presence of stenosis and that the frequency
spectra of wall echoes may be useful indicators of wall
structure.

NMR research in plaque composition is currently
directed towards differentiation among water, lipid, and
collagen. Relaxation parameters are believed to be important
for accomplishing this since these values are different for
water and for lipid. NMR spectroscopy is also potentially
valuable in this regard since the frequency spectra may
allow determination of molecular constituents and their
relative concentration. A major problem is the lack of
good spatial resolution. Use of surface coils for vessels
close to the skin surface allows much improved resolution
but it is not yet clear whether this will be an adequate
solution for plaque characterization. Another problem is
the uniformity of magnetic field required for spectroscopy
if it is desired to resolve various lipid components and
collagen. A field uniformity to within one in ten (7) may
be required because NMR spectral lines are separated by just
a few parts per million (8). When imaging relaxation parameters, signal intensity can differentiate T_1 and T_2 but
proton density and motion also affect intensity and it
becomes difficult to discriminate between relaxation and wall
motion effects (9). A particular advantage for NMR methods
is that plaque shape may be outlined by imaging flowing blood,
utilizing measures of signal intensity, phase, and T_2 as
nuclei of flowing blood move into and out of gradient fields.

Ideally, instrumentation for plaque characterization
should be non-invasive. However, invasive techniques may be
justified if there is value in the additional information or
its accuracy. Some limitations of ultrasound, for example,
may be overcome if the ultrasound transducer is placed
closer to the target plaque. A transducer at the tip of an

arterial catheter can provide much greater resolution than
a transducer applied to the skin surface since the higher
frequency necessary for better resolution can interrogate
the plaque when ultrasound energy traverses only a few
millimeters. Engineering solutions for constructing small
transducers and forming good images are under study by
several investigators. A 25 MHz intraarterial probe has
been reported which may be able to achieve 60 μ axial resolution and 0.5 mm lateral resolution (10). Doppler displacement intraarterial probes are able to measure wall thickness
and perhaps range onto vessel wall layers. A one mm, 20 MHz
crystal has been reported for accomplishing this (11).

Use of light energy for spectroscopic analysis of
plaque composition has been proposed. Laser energy is transmitted through a fiberoptic arterial catheter, and reflected
energy of radiation striking the plaque may be analyzed.
Selective staining is possible to absorb specific wavelengths.
Transmission of light energy in the near infrared region
(650-270 nm) is under investigation as a method for identifying components such as hemoglobin, myoglobin, collagen, and
lipid. The mechanisms for tissue absorption of this radiation
are thought to be transitions of electrons to lower excited
states and overtones and combinations of vibrational
states (12). Fiberoptics allows delivery of sufficient
intensity for effective transmission of near infrared light
to tissues.

In some instances it may be possible to reduce the risk
associated with arterial catheters by introducing a catheter
through a vein. In the case of a carotid artery plaque, a
high frequency ultrasonic probe at the tip of a catheter
inserted into the jugular vein may permit placement close
enough to the plaque to attain high resolution. This may
also be a way to perform near infrared spectroscopy if
enough light can be transmitted through venous vessel walls
and directed to the artery wall at the site of the plaque.
Introduction of a coil through a venous catheter may also be
advantageous for improving spatial resolution in NMR imaging
and spectroscopy.

Tissue differences exist in dimensions other than
acoustic, visible light or magnetic resonance properties.

For example, electrical properties (permittivity) of tissues are very dependent upon frequency. As frequencies increase, dielectric constants decrease and conductivities increase. These properties may be exploited in the microwave range of frequencies when conductivity of fat and blood may differ by a factor of 20 and where dielectric constant may differ by a factor of 10 at 10,000 MHz (13). Microwave energy can penetrate deeply within tissues but the body is so complex with regard to tissue distribution that transmitted and reflected energy varies widely. Research efforts in this area are limited. Many more experimental studies will be needed to determine whether or not the large differences in permittivity of tissues at microwave frequencies can be exploited.

Future advances in characterizing plaque composition may rely on methods ranging from completely non-invasive to totally invasive and on combinations of technologies. Application of ultrasound or NMR from the body surface may permit locating and outlining plaques in many arterial beds; characterizing plaques at a relatively gross level may also be possible. For more detailed plaque characterization, invasive instruments using venous or arterial catheters may be required. A single catheter could possibly accommodate more than one modality for plaque interrogation, such as fiber-optics for light transmission and an ultrasonic probe or RF coil for NMR imaging. Combinations of technologies could permit exploiting one technology's advantages to complement another's. Even if no modality achieves a high level of precision by itself, plaque characterization using more than one technology offers a means of increased precision. Each method separates plaque components on the basis of different physical/chemical parameters, such as acoustic, magnetic resonance, or reflectivity of light. Improved classification of plaque may then be possible through multivariate analysis of these parameters. *In vivo* animal experimentation in this manner could also provide opportunities for cross validation of results from ultrasound, NMR, light spectroscopy, or other instrumentation.

REFERENCES

1. Field S, Dunn F (1973) Correlation of echographic
    visualizability of tissues with biological composition
    and physiological state. J Acoust Soc Am 54:809.
2. Abbott JG, Thurstone F (1979) Acoustic speckle:
    Theory and experimental analysis. Ultrasonic Imaging
    1:303.
3. Wagner RI, et al. (1983) Statistics of speckle in
    ultrasound B-scans. IEEE Trans Sonics Ultrasonics
    30:156.
4. Reid JM (1986) The measurement of scattering. In:
    Greenleaf J (ed) Tissue Characterization with Ultra-
    sound. CRC Press.
5. Johnson SA, Yoon TH, Ra JW (1983) Inverse scattering
    solutions of the scalar Helmholtz wave equation by a
    multiple source moment method. Electronic Letters
    19:130.
6. Johnson SA, et al. (1978) Quantitative synthetic
    aperture reflection imaging with correction for
    refraction and attenuation. Proc of San Diego
    Biomedical Symposium.
7. Berggren MJ, et al. (1986) Performance of fast inverse
    scattering solutions for the exact Helmholtz equation
    using multiple frequencies and limited views. Fifteenth
    Symposium on Acoustical Imaging. Halifax, Nova Scotia:
    Plenum Press.
8. Andrew ER (1986) NMR spectroscopy principles. In:
    Budinger TF, Margulis AR (eds) Medical Magnetic
    Resonance Imaging and Spectroscopy. Society of
    Magnetic Resonance in Medicine, p. 71.
9. Pohost GM (1986) Applications of NMR imaging to the
    cardiovascular system: Physiologic, pathologic, and
    angiographic studies. In: Budinger TF, Margulis AR
    (eds) Medical Magnetic Resonance Imaging and Spectro-
    scopy. Society of Magnetic Resonance in Medicine,
    p. 165.
10. Schmitt RM et al. (1983) Angular response of cut and
    uncut piezoelectric array receivers using low and
    high planer coupled ceramics. IEEE Ultrasonics
    Symposium Proceedings, p. 1030.
11. Hartley CJ et al. (1984) High frequency pulsed Doppler
    measurements of blood flow and myocardial dimensions
    in conscious animals. In: Herd JA, Gotto AM, Kaufman
    PG, Weiss SM (eds) Cardiovascular Instrumentation:
    Applicability of New Technology to Biobehavioral
    Research, NIH Pub. #84-1654, p. 95.
12. Jobsis FF (1977) Noninvasive, infrared monitoring of
    cerebral and myocardial oxygen sufficiency and circula-
    tory parameters. Science 198:1264.
13. Lin JC (1986) Microwave propagation in biological
    dielectrics with application to cardiopulmonary interro-
    gation. In: Larsen LE, Jacobi JH (eds) Medical Appli-
    cations of Microwave Imaging. IEEE Press, p. 47.

59
Atherosclerosis Risk in Communities (ARIC): A Follow-up Study of Early Arterial Lesions in the General Population

Gerardo Heiss and ARIC Investigators

The Atherosclerosis Risk in Communities (ARIC) Study is a prospective study sponsored by the National Heart, Lung, and Blood Institute, presently underway in four U.S. communities. Its goals are to 1) investigate the etiology of and natural history of atherosclerosis, 2) investigate the etiology of clinical atherosclerotic diseases, and 3) measure variation in cardiovascular risk factors, medical care and disease by race, sex, place, and time.

The ARIC Study takes place in four diverse communities. The communities are clearly defined geographical entities, have well delineated medical care referral patterns, and provide an opportunity to study blacks and whites, males and females in urban and rural settings.

The design was chosen so that data could be obtained for groups which differ by geography, race, and socio-economic status. The ARIC Study is not designed to select a representative sample of the entire U.S. population. Each community provides information on the occurrence of coronary heart disease in a unique environmental setting. The cohorts representing each community are studied so that inferences about risk factors and disease relationships can be made from

Supported by the National Heart, Lung and Blood Institute Contracts: University of North Carolina at Chapel Hill N01-HC-55018 and N01-HC-55015; University of Minnesota N01-HC-55018; Johns Hopkins University N01-HC-55020; University of Mississippi N01-HC-55021; University of Texas Health Science Center N01-HC-55022; and Baylor College of Medicine N01-HC-55016.

diverse population groups. This diversity permits the
evaluation of the consistency of any observed association.

The four communities studied are: Forsyth County,
North Carolina; Jackson, Mississippi; Minneapolis suburbs,
Minnesota; and Washington County, Maryland. Each community
serves as the framework for the cardiovascular epidemiologic
surveillance, and contributes a cohort of 4,000 men and
women between the ages of 45 and 64. The cohort in Jackson,
Mississippi was samples and recruited to have an all-black
population. The size and socio-economic characteristics of
the communities are summarized in Table 1.

These communities were selected using criteria which
included location, availability of census data, study population size, population stability, population characteristics
with respect to ischemic-heart disease, and the medical
facilities within the community. Table 2 describes age-
adjusted all-cause and ischemic heart disease mortality
rates for the ARIC communities.

The ARIC design incorporates two distinct design
features; a Cohort Component and a Community Surveillance
Component. The two arms of the study enhance the informativeness of the study as a whole in that a) the Community
Surveillance Component facilitates the generalizability of
the Cohort findings; and b) the Cohort Component validates
the profile of cardiovascular disease and of medical care
characteristics obtained from Community Surveillance.

In the Community Surveillance Component, the four
communities are under surveillance for the occurrence of
hospitalized myocardial infarction and coronary heart disease
death in men and women age 35-74 years. A review of hospital
records is done of all age-eligible residents of each
community with a discharge diagnosis of myocardial infarction
or one of several related screening diagnosis. A review is
done also of all age- and residence-eligible death certifi-
cates with various manifestations of coronary heart disease
coded as the cause of death. For deaths not occurring in a
hospital, the decedent's physician and next-of-kin are
querried about the circumstances around the time of death.

The aim of community surveillance is to estimate the
indicence and obtain a valid diagnostic classification of

Table 1. ARIC Study Communities: Demographic Characteristics, 1980

Study Community	Population		% Black	% Urban	Education 12+ yrs. (%)	Median Income
	Age 35-74	Total				
Forsyth County North Carolina	95,863	243,683	24	75	63	$16,600
Jackson, Mississippi	68,303	202,895	48	100	71	$14,800
Minneapolis Surburbs, Minnesota	69,338	192,004	1	100	85	$24,165
Washington County, Maryland	45,539	113,068	4	57	60	$16,623
Total	279,043	751,668				

Table 2. Age-Adjusted Mortality Rates[a] for Men and Women,
          Age 35-74, in the ARIC Study Communities, 1980

ARIC Communities	All-Cause Mortality		Heart Disease Mortality[b]	
	Men	Women	Men	Women
Forsyth County, North Carolina	16.3	8.7	6.7	2.7
Jackson, Mississippi (Black Only)	20.8	10.0	6.6	2.9
Minneapolis Suburbs, Minnesota	9.4	6.3	4.2	1.3
Washington County, Maryland	16.1	8.2	7.8	2.8
U.S. Total	14.4	8.0	5.7	2.6

[a] Indirect age-adjustment; annual rate per 1,000
[b] ICD-9, International Classification of Diseases, Ninth Edition; 390-398, 402, 404-429.

fatal CHD and hospitalized MI in residents aged 35 to 74 years in the four communities for the period January 1, 1987 to December 31, 1992. Community surveillance will provide measures of the geographical and temporal variation of athero-sclerosis and clinical CHD in the ARIC communities. The distributions of demographic characteristics, as well as the changes in these measurements, will suggest explanatory factors for the atherosclerosis and CHD profiles of the communities under surveillance.

In the Cohort Component, a random sample of 16,000 persons, age 45-64 years, is selected from the four communi-ties. They provide medical, social and demographic informa-tion and participate in two clinical examinations to study the etiology of atherosclerosis and its overt clinical sequelae. The Cohort Component will provide a baseline examination with a second examination three years later.

The baseline examination includes the measurement of
established cardiovascular risk factors, with the addition
of pulmonary function testing, ultrasound vascular imaging,
and measurement of lipids and hemostatic factors in the
blood. Storage of blood for future prospective case-control
analysis increases the chances that yet unsuspected precursors of cardiovascular disease will be discovered.

Central Lipid Laboratory measurement of lipids,
cholesterol in lipoprotein fractions, and apoproteins with
key roles in lipid metabolism permits ARIC to discriminate
among important hypotheses which relate lipid factors to
atherosclerosis. Total cholesterol and triglycerides, HDL
and HDL_3 cholesterols, lipoprotein Lp (a), and the apoproteins
A-I and B are measured directly; VLDL, LDL and HDL_2 cholesterols are derived quantities (Table 3). Each of these
determinations is made for all cohort participants on
frozen plasma. Additional, newer measurements are made on
selected cases and controls, using stored plasma.

In a study of atherosclerosis consideration of hemostasis may be critical both for the onset of clinical disease
(thrombotic occlusion leading to cerebral or myocardial
infarction) and for initiation and progression of the underlying atherosclerotic lesions. Since the hemostasis system
is highly reactive, prospective studies, rather than studies
of clinical cases, are necessary to test these hypotheses.
The specific measurements made at a central laboratory are
shown in Table 4.

Seven of these measurements (fibrinogen, factors VII
and VIII, von Willebrand factor antigen, aPTT, protein C
and AT-III) are made on blood from every cohort participant;
the remainder, on blood from selected cases and controls
only.

Atherosclerosis in the carotid and popliteal arteries
is assessed in the ARIC study by means of B-mode ultrasound imaging and through measurements of arterial distensibility. B-mode imaging will permit the standardized
quantification of morphologic characteristics of the
arterial wall, indicative of the extent and severity of
atherosclerosis, as well as of early arterial lesions.
These measurements are summarized in Table 5. Additional

Table 3. Measurements Performed at the ARIC Central
          Lipid Laboratory

---

1. Cholesterol and triglycerides by enzymatic method
2. HDL and HDL_3 cholesterol by enzymatic methods
   following sequential precipitation of VLDL + LDL
   and HDL_2 by magnesium and dextran
3. Apoproteins A-I and B by radioimmunoassay
4. Lp(a) by enzyme-linked immunosorbent assay

Table 4. Measurements Performed at the ARIC Central
          Hemostasis Laboratory

---

1. Platelets - plasma levels of BTG and PF-4, serum
   levels of TXB_2
2. Coagulation
   a. Coagulation factors - plasma levels of
      fibrinogen, factor VII, VIII activities,
      and von Willebrand factor antigen
   b. Coagulation activation - plasma levels
      of FPA.
3. Coagulation inhibitors - plasma levels of AT-III
   and protein C
4. Fibrinolysis - plasma levels of tPA and FPB-
   Beta (1-41)
5. General screen - aPTT.

Table 5. B-Mode Ultrasonographic Measurements Performed
          by the ARIC Ultrasound Reading Center

---

1. Near and far wall thickness in diastole and
   systole
2. Lumen diameter in diastole and systole
3. Maximal and mean lesion thickness (severity)
4. Length of lesion (extent)
5. Lesion area

---

measurements are performed on selected case-control studies.

These measurements are obtained on the ARIC cohort participants at baseline, and at the re-examination visits. As shown in Table 6, three types of measurements will be available to test various hypotheses relating to the pathogenesis and natural history of atherosclerosis. At baseline, the ultrasonographic measurements can be combined to provide a measure of extent and severity of arterial lesions. Other cardiovascular risk factors, putative as well as established ones, are measured concurrently. Also at baseline, clinically manifest ischemic disease is recorded. At re-examination changes relative to baseline will be measurable and permit statements on observed changes in extent and severity of atherosclerosis; on changes in other risk factors; and on the occurrence of newly developed cerebrovascular atherosclerotic disease.

Table 6. Role of the Ultrasound Measurements in the ARIC
         Study

Baseline	Re-Examination
Extent and Severity of Arterial Lesions	Change in Extent and Severity
"Other" Risk Factors	Change in Risk Factors
Manifest CHD or Stroke	Newly Developed Disease

Three principal modes of analysis will take advantage of these design features: cross-sectional, longitudinal, and case-control, as shown schematically in Table 7.

Analysis of the baseline measurements will provide distributional data on non-invasively determined extent and severity of atherosclerosis and early arterial lesions, in samples representative of four communities in the

Table 7. Role of the Ultrasound Measurements in the ARIC
Study According to Analysis Strategy

A. Cross-Sectional Analyses

Baseline   Re-Examination

Distribution of
Extent, Severity
of Atherosclerosis

        |
        v

-. Geographic
- By Race
- By Gender
- Other Baseline
  Characteristics

B. Longitudinal Analyses

Baseline   Re-Examination

Extent, Severity ————————> Changes in Extent
of Atherosclerosis   and Severity

Risk Factors at ————————> Changes in Extent
Baseline Exam   and Severity

Extent, Severity ————————> Newly Developed
of Atherosclerosis   CHD and Stroke

C. Case-Control Analyses

Baseline   Re-Examination

                                 Changes in Extent
                                 and Severity of
                                 Atherosclerosis,
                                 Clinical Events

Stored Blood.
Stored U-S Data, <————————
Special Studies

United States. Distributional patterns by demographic, geographic, biochemical, and life style characteristics will be examined.

Analysis of the prospective cohort data will permit statements on the natural history of early arterial lesions and of various measurements of atherosclerosis in free-living populations. Further, a range of baseline measurements can be examined as factors that influence and modify the observed course of this natural history. These constitute risk factors of the changes in arterial disease severity and extent. In addition to serving as the study outcome, ultrasonographic measures of atherosclerosis will also serve as predictor, or independent variables. This is represented in the row of Table 7 which relates arterial lesions recorded at baseline to the newly developed atherosclerotic disease observed in the course of the follow-up of the ARIC cohort.

The third major analysis strategy considered in the ARIC study is case control studies nested in the ARIC cohort. This feature is based on the storage of "raw" data collected at baseline for later analysis. In addition to blood specimens stored frozen, ultrasound videotapes, and arterial distensibility data are stored for this purpose. Cases for these efficient case-control studies will emerge from fatal or non-fatal clinical events that serve as study end points, but can also be selected from cohort members who exhibit notable changes in extent or severity of non-invasively determined atherosclerosis at re-examination. In either situation, suitable controls are selected from the ARIC cohort, and extensive, state of the art measurements of the data stored at baseline can be performed on this subset.

Without fear of exaggeration it can be stated that non-invasive techniques to measure arterial lesions have prompted a new generation of epidemiologic studies. Access to the work of previous investigators who have spearheaded the development and evaluation of non-invasive methodology has given the ARIC investigators an opportunity to introduce the ultrasonographic assessment of atherosclerosis as a central feature of the ARIC study. The resulting advantages are many.

As a qualtitative difference from previous epidemiologic studies, the ARIC study is significantly closer to studying the disease processes of atherosclerosis, instead of measuring it indirectly through its clinical sequelae. This enhances the specificity of the hypotheses and the informativeness of the study, but also changes dramatically the time frame of the epidemiologic inquiry. The latency period under consideration approaches that of atherogenesis, instead of the long latency that typically separates the development of arterial lesions and the clinically manifest ischemic event.

Clinical events are insensitive markers of the underlying atherosclerotic process, leading to errors in epidemiologic and clinical studies by virtue of the large proportion of "false negatives" that such an approach entails. Reliance on standardized ultrasonographic measurements of high quality improves the validity of our study outcomes as better measurements of atherosclerosis. Further, it improves considerably the accuracy of the study measurements as regards the measurement instrument, operator, and the reader.

Improvements in the variability with which the phenomenon under study is measured, on the other hand, translate into gains of statistical power. This is a particularly welcome development in population-based epidemiologic studies, which require large investments in sample size and follow-up time if the outcomes are the relatively rare clinical events.

One more consequence of the ability to examine arterial lesions non-invasively in epidemiologic studies is worthy of mention: the unique ability to carry out long-term, and repeated observations of the natural history of the atherosclerotic process. The ARIC study will be able to exercise this option in large, representative samples of four diverse communities, in an attempt to establish the patterns of progression/regression of plaques in the carotid and popliteal arteries, and the factors associated with these changes.

In conclusion, several unparalleled features of the ARIC study deserve to be highlighted. The prospective design permits identification of antecedent-consequent

relationships in the study of atherosclerosis risk factors
and clinical disease in populations. ARIC focused on
studying the disease process, as well as its manifestations,
in large scale community samples, and is the largest study
of its kind in terms of statistical power. This will make
it possible to study risk factor effects for various end
points, to examine the consistency of the observed associations across ARIC study communities, and to examine more
complex interactions between study variables. The effort
has drawn on modern biochemistry to study new cardiovascular
risk factors, introducing high quality measurements of lipoproteins and hemostasis, collected under standardized conditions in the field. Storage of blood specimens and
extensive ultrasonographic data will permit more detailed
case control studies in members of the ARIC cohort, as well
as access to new procedures and state of the art measurements in the future. Finally, the ARIC study draws on a
wealth of expertise that reflects the multidisciplinary
nature of this effort.

APPENDIX

List of Key ARIC Personnel in the Ultrasound Area

Members of the ARIC Steering Committee

Ralph Barnes, Ph.D., Bowman Gray School of Medicine
Aaron Folsom, M.D., University of Minnesota
Gerardo Heiss, M.D., University of North Carolina at
  Chapel Hill
Richard Hutchinson, M.D., University of Mississippi
Wolfgang Patsch, M.D., Baylor College of Medicine
A. Richey Sharrett, M.D., NHLBI
Moyses Szklo, M.D., Johns Hopkins University
O. Dale Williams, Ph.D., University of North Carolina
  at Chapel Hill
Kenneth Wu, M.D., University of Texas

ARIC Ultrasound Subcommittee

Ralph Barnes, Ph.D., Chairperson, Bowman Gray School
  of Medicine
Alan Berson, Ph.D., National Heart, Lung and Blood Institute
Gene Bond, Ph.D., Bowman Gray School of Medicine
David Christiansen, Ph.D., University of North Carolina
Kenneth Cram, M.D., University of Minnesota
Gerardo Heiss, M.D., University of North Carolina
Seshadra Raju, M.D., University of Mississippi
Ward Riley, Ph.D., ARIC Ultrasound Reading Center
Roger Saunders, M.D., Johns Hopkins School of Medicine
A. Richey Sharrett, M.D., National Heart, Lung and
  Blood Institute

888

ARIC Sonographers

Beverly Robertson, Washington County, Maryland
Dorrie Costa, Washington County, Maryland
Faye Blackburn, Mississippi
Shirley Willis, Mississippi
Amy Haire, Forsyth County, North Carolina
Danalee Furr, Forsyth County, North Carolina
Kate Provinzino, Minnesota
Gail Murton, Minnesota
Donna Ottenstroer, Minnesota

60

Atherosclerosis Risk in Communities—
Ultrasound Reading Center:
Quantitative B Mode Scanning Protocol

R.W. Barnes, M.G. Bond, W.A. Riley, and S.K. Wilmoth

INTRODUCTION

The Atherosclerosis Risk in Communities (ARIC) Study program is a multicenter epidemiological study. The cohort component of the ARIC study involves examination of 16,000 representative men and women from four communities: Forsyth County, North Carolina; Jackson, Mississippi; Suburban Minneapolis, Minnesota; and Washington County, Maryland - twice, at three-year intervals. A more detailed description of the rationale, goals and potential impact of this program is found in Chapter 61. One unique component of this program is B-mode ultrasound examinations of popliteal and extracranial carotid arteries. This noninvasive method has the ability, when used with detailed and standardized protocols, to detect and potentially monitor plaque evolution in asymptomatic subjects. We report here briefly the methods used in the B-mode imaging component of this study.

The examination of participants in a separate, designated ultrasound area in each of the four ARIC Field Centers consists of the following components: (1) B-mode ultrasound imaging of one popliteal artery and both extracranial carotid arteries; (2) measurement of common carotid artery distensibility; (3) automatic monitoring of blood pressure throughout the ultrasound examination; and (4) beat-to-beat

Supported by NIH Contract NO1-HC-55018 (Sub-contract University of North Carolina.

monitoring of heart rate with rapid sequential blood pressure monitoring during a postural change exam at the conclusion of the study. Interpretation of the ultrasound examination is performed at the ARIC Ultrasound Reading Center (URC) located at the Bowman Gray School of Medicine in Winston-Salem, North Carolina.

Selection of Ultrasound System

The ultrasound system selected for use in the ARIC study is the Biosound 2000 II sa. Selection was based on the results of a series of detailed studies of systems provided by four manufacturers, which included blinded, controlled *in vitro* tests on excised human arteries, measurement of transmitted pressure pulse waveform and intensity using a mineature hydrophone probe, routine system performance measurements on phantom test objects, and *in vivo* arterial evaluations which included ease of use by the sonographer.

Sonographer Training and Monitoring

The sonographer training program consists of a series of training sessions (120 hours) at the URC, followed by practice assignments at the Field Centers. The initial sessions (60 hours) consist of lectures, demonstrations and practical laboratory experience on (1) Ultrasonic Physics I, including basic physics concepts, units of measurement, and mathematics arising in the medical application of ultrasound; (2) Overview of Atherosclerosis and a detailed discussion of the normal artery wall; (3) Ultrasonic Physics II, including a discussion of the properties of ultrasonic waves, reflection at boundaries and scattering from small objects; (4) Ultrasonic Physics III, including the Doppler effect, ultrasound transducers and sound beams; (5) Pathology of Atherosclerosis including dissection of arterial specimens and the ultrasound of lesions; (6) Principles of Ultrasonic Instrumentation including pulse-echo imaging systems, pulsed Doppler systems, and spectral analysis; (7) Basic operation of the Biosound 2000 II sa; (8) Instrument Performance Monitoring and (9) Principles of Ultrasound Arterial Scanning.

The remaining sessions (total of 60 hours) consist of detailed arterial studies and practice of the ARIC Ultrasound protocol using the ancillary equipment, *i.e.*, Study Flow Panel (described below), IBM personal computer, Dinamap (Critikon) automated blood pressure instrument and an Arterial Wall Tracker for arterial distensibility studies. The training program concludes with a final exam to demonstrate mastery of the ARIC Ultrasound Scanning Protocol. Successful completion of this demonstration is the first step toward initial sonographer certification.

The first 15 ARIC participant studies performed by each sonographer after returning to the Field Centers are received and evaluated for protocol adherence. The criteria for successful completion of this phase for initial certification are the following: proper recording of a dimensional marker for calibration; vertical alignment of the 1.0 cm arterial segment being examined on the monitor screen; placement of the arterial segment within middle third (horizontal) of the image; correct identification of anatomic references within the carotid arteries; detection of arterial wall interfaces; proper sequential examination of arterial segments; correct placement of the cursor over specific anatomic references; audio labeling of the tape segment which demonstrates the best quality image; appropriate use of gain settings and field focus; and correct identification and recording of views from prescribed angles. The detailed results of these evaluations are sent to sonographers through electronic mail. If the sonographer is not certified, additional training and qualification studies are required.

The annual recertification procedure, in addition to the above described initial certification, requires detailed data analyses for each sonographer on lumen diameters and area, as well as combined intimal-medial thickness and area measurements. As the data base increases, acceptable quantitative standards for intra- and intersonographer variability will be determined, and comparison with these standards will be used for recertification.

Video Cassette Recording

Two video cassette recorders (VCR) are used with the
Biosound instrument. A SONY 3/4" VCR, which has high resolution, is used to record images sent to the Ultrasound
Reading Center. A PANASONIC 1/2" VCR is used to provide
backup at the Field Center. All of the examination results
recorded on the SONY VCR are also recorded on the PANASONIC
VCR. A RMI tissue mimicking ultrasound phantom (RMI Model
409) is used for weekly performance checks and quality control of the Biosound system. Results are recorded on the
VCR's and interpreted at the URC.

Study Flow Panel

The B-mode ultrasound examination consists of 11 steps
performed in a similar sequence for each participant. An
illuminated study flow panel assists the sonographer in
keeping track of these steps during the examination. This
panel has a series of small, labeled lights indicating the
current step being performed. When the best image for each
examination step is obtained, the sonographer presses a
footswitch. A digital code identifying the step is recorded
on one of the VCR audio channels, and then an audio tone is
recorded to identify the series of video frames for that
arterial site. Automatic sequencing is done upon release of
the footswitch. A manual override is available in case of
changes in the sequence, $i.e.$, to repeat or select a particular step, or for a quality control repeat.

Blood Pressure Instrumentation

A series of blood pressure measurements are made during
the ultrasound examination. The purposes are: (1) to provide baseline supine blood pressure measurements, (2) to
determine postural changes in blood pressure which occur
when participants stand up after the ultrasound examination
is complete, (3) to provide the pulse pressures required
for calculating artery distensibility, and (4) to estimate
an ankle-arm blood pressure index. Blood pressure is
measured using the Dinamap Model 1846 SX (Critikon), an
automated device which operates using oscillometric

techniques and is controlled by the computer. The Dinamap
Monitor displays the measured values of heart rate, systolic,
diastolic and mean arterial pressure in digital readouts.
Data are periodically collected and stored on floppy disk
by the IBM-PC.

Computer System IBM-PC

Data acquisition and storage, control of blood pressure
measurement in the Field Center ultrasound area and other
functions are performed using a personal computer modified
and programmed for this purpose. The computer interacts
with the ultrasound area equipment to perform the following
tasks: (1) obtains participant demographic data, such as
identification number, birthdata, race and gender;
(2) establishes data files and file extensions; (3) selects
the left or right popliteal artery for ultrasound examination
based on the participant identification number; (4) keeps
records from the study flow panel of the study steps performed and the time entailed, including quality control
repeat studies; (5) controls the Dinamap automated blood
pressure instrument during the popliteal and carotid artery
ultrasound examinations, the carotid artery distensibility
measurement and the postural change measurement; (6) controls
the analog-to-digital converter to digitize and store data
from the arterial wall tracker for distensibility calculations
and waveform processing; (7) calculates heart rate on a
beat-by-beat basis during the postural change examination
and (8) records all these data on hard disk for temporary
storage, and on the floppy disk that is sent to the Ultrasound Reading Center.

Arterial Wall Tracker

An arterial wall tracker is used to measure the change
in arterial diameter during the cardiac cycle for calculating
a measure of distensibility. The instrument is a dual
channel, zero-crossing tracker supplied by AUTREC in Winston-
Salem, North Carolina. Each channel is an analog system
with feedback to trace continuously the range of a zero

crossing in the near or far arterial wall echo complex.
The change in arterial wall diameter during the cardiac
cycle is determined from the time difference between the
selected zero crossing in the near wall echo complex and
the initial zero crossing from the far wall of the blood-
lumen interface echo complex.

Under typical operating conditions, continuous arterial
wall motion and diameter measurements are available on two
output channels. One output channel is a dc couples output,
calibrated for a 0 to 10 mm arterial diameter. The second
output channel is an ac coupled output calibrated for
arterial diameter changes of 0 to 1.0 mm, with diameter
resolution of less than .01 mm.

Participant Status

The participant is asked to refrain from smoking at
least one hour before the ultrasound examination, vigorous
exercise, coffee, tea and soft drinks containing caffeine
during the night preceding, and on the day of the ultrasound
examination, since these may alter heart rate or blood
pressure.

Popliteal Artery

One popliteal artery selected by the PC based on a
random sequence is examined by ultrasonography. The participant is prone during the examination on the popliteal
artery.

Criteria for Satisfactory Image Acquisition

The optimal B-mode ultrasound image of an arterial segment is defined on the basis of clear visualization of the
following arterial tissue interfaces at the site of an
external anatomical reference, (which, for popliteal artery)
is the skin crease at the back of the knee:

    (1)   Near Wall (artery wall nearest skin surface)

          (a)   adventitial - medial interface (Boundary 2)

          (b)   intimal - lumen interface (Boundary 3)

(2) Far Wall
    (a) lumen - intimal interface (Boundary 4)
    (b) medial - adventitial interface (Boundary 5)

Linear distances, calibrated on the basis of a recorded dimensional marker, are measured from B-mode images at the Ultrasound Reading Center. At 1 mm intervals along a 1.0 cm length of the popliteal artery, near wall thickness (the distance between B2 - B3), lumen diameter (B3 - B4) and far wall thickness (B4 - B5) are determined from video frames which contain peak systolic images.

The strongest and most reliably imaged interface echoes are B2 and B5, the medial-adventitial boundaries of the near and far walls, respectively. These interfaces are highly reflective and are apparent at very low gain settings. B3 and B4, lumen intimal boundaries, are smooth in normal arteries, and therefore usually less reflective and not as prominent at lower gain settings. If all four interfaces cannot be visualized, the sonographer attempts to obtain clear images of the boundary <u>pairs</u> in the following priority: (1) B4-B5; (2) B3-B4; (3) B2-B3. Arterial curvature, tortuosity, kinking, arterial mineral deposits or arteries more than 3.0 cm from skin surface may result in sub-optimal visualization of interfaces.

Carotid Artery Segment Definitions

Three anatomically defined segments of the extracranial carotid arteries are studied: (1) distal common carotid artery; (2) the carotid bulb; and (3) the internal carotid artery. The distal common carotid artery is defined as the distal 1.0 cm segment immediately proximal to the origin of the carotid bulb. The key anatomic feature required for reliable identification of this segment is the origin or crest of the carotid bulb, $i.e.$, the beginning of the dilatation associated with the bifurcation, at the transducer angle which best demonstrates the V-shape of the flow divider. This crest in normal arteries is usually elliptical in cross section with its greatest diameter being visualized from the angle which demonstrates the flow divider separating the internal and external carotid arteries. Visualization and recording of the distal 1.0 cm of the common carotid artery from an anatomic reference angle is required.

The carotid bifurcation segment is defined by two anatomic references which allow its reliable identification. The inferior extent of this segment is the origin of the carotid bifurcation. The superior extent is defined as the highest point in the arc of the flow divider. Usually, the angle which best demonstrates this segment is lateral or posterior-lateral, and is the same angle which is used to define the optimal angle of the distal common carotid artery segment. The length of the carotid bifurcation varies among subjects.

The internal carotid artery segment is defined as the proximal 1.0 cm of this vessel. The key anatomic feature in identifying this segment is the highest point in the arc of the flow divider.

The three segments of the carotid arteries are examined sequentially. The distal common carotid artery is viewed, and recorded, from three angles. The carotid bifurcation and internal carotid artery are interrogated from a single angle, the anatomic reference angle, defined as that which visualizes the flow divider, the origin of the bifurcation and as many of the four arterial interfaces as possible. The remaining two angles from which the distal common carotid artery is viewed are defined as posterior and anterior angles; -10°, and $+55^{\circ}$ from the horizontal, respectively.

Distal Common Carotid Artery (Right Side)

The subject is supine during the carotid artery examination. A triangular shaped, firm foam rubber wedge is used to position the head contralaterally at a 45° rotation angle. After scanning the popliteal artery, a longitudinal view of the distal common carotid artery is visualized, field focus is set in the appropriate range, $i.e.$, near, mid or far, depending on the depth of the artery from skin surface, and instrument gain settings are adjusted to the lowest settings that show as many of near and far wall interfaces as possible. The origin of the carotid bifurcation is identified and placed at the level of a cursor on the TV monitor. The artery images are then video taped. Optimum views are identified on the tape when the sonographer presses the footswitch. The transducer is then rotated first to the anterior angle position, and then to the posterior angle position in order to acquire B-mode images from those angles of interrogation. The transducer is then rotated back to the optimum angle and the probe moved superiorly until the carotid bifurcation with its anatomical references is visualized.

Carotid Bifurcation (Right Side)

The angle of interrogation that best demonstrates the carotid bifurcation is close to the anatomical reference angle used to examine the distal common carotid artery. Field focus is adjusted depending on the distance from skin surface to the artery wall. With the cursor identifying references on the monitor, the image of the bifurcation is optimized to demonstrate the required interfaces. The images are then recorded on video tape and identified by the audio tones when the sonographer pre-set the footswitch.

Internal Carotid Artery (Right Side)

The proximal 1.0 cm of the internal carotid artery is viewed from a single optimum angle. The method used to establish this view is to move the transducer superiorly after examining the carotid bifurcation. The transducer is rocked back and forth to differentiate internal from external carotid artery. Doppler ultrasound with spectral analysis is used to confirm correct arterial identification. The B-mode internal carotid artery image is then optimized and recorded as described in the other two carotid segments.

Carotid Artery Examination (Left Side)

At the completion of the studies on the right side of the neck, a similar series of evaluations is performed on the left side. Examination of the left side is identical to the right side with two exceptions: (1) the transducer probe is rotated 180 degrees when examining the left, and (2) arterial distensibility studies are performed only on the left common carotid artery.

SUMMARY

This paper briefly describes the general approach to B-mode ultrasound examination of popliteal and carotid arteries that is used in the ARIC study. The detailed protocols can be acquired by writing the Collaborative Studies Coordinating Center, University of North Carolina, NCNB Plaza, Suite 203, Chapel Hill, North Carolina 27514.

The B-mode ultrasound techniques and methods used in the ARIC study are based in part of validation studies in Chapter 50 and a recently published article (1) and reliability studies (2) as described in Chapter 46. The ultrasound research methods used in this epidemiological study should be clearly differentiated from those approaches to B-mode evaluation of symptomatic subjects that were used in the Clinical Centers within the United States Multicenter B-mode Assessment Trial. See Chapters 51-56, specifically regarding criteria of what is measured and how it is measured.

REFERENCES

1. Pignoli P, Tremoli E, Poli A, Oreste P, Paoletti R (1986) Intimal plus medial thickness of the arterial wall: A direct measurement with ultrasound imaging. Circulation 74:1399-1406.
2. Bond MG, Insull W Jr, Gardin JP, Wilmoth SK (1984) Reliability of B-mode ultrasound in measuring small carotid artery plaques. Circulation 70:II-162.

61

Ultrasound Measurement of Atherosclerosis: Directions for Epidemiology

Millicent W. Higgins and A. Richey Sharrett

In the past, philosophers searched for the elixir which would prolong life indefinitely and alchemists tried to transmute base metals into gold and silver. Epidemiologists may be their 20th Century counterparts looking for tests which will classify correctly persons with or without early disease and with or without characteristics which increase or decrease risk of developing disease in the future. So far, epidemiologists have been rather more successful than the ancient philosophers and alchemists, and recent technological advances provide a wealth of new opportunities to conduct epidemiological studies which were not possible in the past. Ultrasound measurement of atherosclerosis in peripheral arteries is one such recent advance which may be used to differentiate those with atherosclerosis from those without, or preferably, to quantify atherosclerotic involvement at specific sites. Alternatively, it may be used as a measure of risk for clinical manifestations including coronary heart disease, stroke and peripheral arterial disease.

Any test proposed for use in epidemiological studies of human populations must meet some established requirements. The first of these is that the test be a valid index of what it is supposed to measure. Those with lesions by ultrasound should have atherosclerosis, whereas those without lesions by ultrasound should be free of the condition. Ideally there should be no false negatives and no false positives, which is to say the test should be highly sensitive and highly specific. Extensive comparisons of findings from high frequency ultrasound examinations with results of angio- graphic and pathologic studies have been presented at this conference. They provide strong support for applying ultra- sound examinations to epidemiological research in the community. Other requirements are that the procedure be simple, safe and reproducible; it should be inexpensive, and it must be acceptable to the population under study. Sometimes tests which appear to fulfill most of these requirements in clinical studies of cases and controls turn out to be appreciably less useful when they are applied to the general population. The predictive value of a positive test depends in part on the prevalence of disease, which is lower in the general population than in the clinical setting, where contrived "prevalence rates" of 50 percent are assured by studying equal numbers of cases and controls. High specificity is of paramount importance in the epidemiological setting where false positive tests usually outnumber true positives and create serious problems for individual parti- cipants, for the procedure, for the study, and for those to whom these individuals are referred.

One important direction for epidemiology is to determine the prognostic significance of ultrasound lesions in longi- tudinal studies which measure incidence of fatal and non fatal manifestations of atherosclerosis. These studies should incorporate measurements of established risk factors and should be designed to provide estimates of risk for ultrasound lesions as an intermediate endpoint as well as for morbidity and mortality. We need to know whether adding ultrasound measurements improves risk estimates based on composite risk factor profiles. More accurate prediction would improve recognition of susceptible individuals and provide better opportunities for preventive approaches.

Ultrasound examinations offer new opportunities to make repeated measurements in apparently healthy persons as well as patients to detect early lesions, but also to observe progression or regression of lesions and to identify and measure associations between a variety of established and putative risk factors and the course of the underlying

disease process. Risk factors which predict clinical
events can be subdivided into those associated with atherosclerosis and those whose effect is mediated through another
mechanism. As a by-product of population based studies
using ultrasound, the frequency, range of severity, and
distribution of atherosclerotic lesions will be determined
and provide a new dimension to estimates of the magnitude
of the problem and of regional variation and trends over
time. From the epidemiologists perspective the most
exciting new opportunities are to identify causes and
precursors of atherosclerosis.

Ultrasound Studies of Factors Associated with Early Atheromata: Design Considerations

A. Richey Sharrett and Millicent Higgins

Arterial imaging of atherosclerotic lesions by ultrasound can be used in epidemiological studies of factors
associated with early atheromata. We believe that ultrasound
is ready for this application. However, prior to initiating
any major studies, the investigator should verify that
specific accuracy and precision requirements are met.

An Ultrasound Study of Early Atheromata

The design we wish to discuss has two parts: population
screening and case-control study. The interest is in early
lesions of typical atherosclerosis. Therefore, an age group
should be selected with an adequate prevalence of uncomplicated lesions - perhaps 35-50 years of age. Screening
consists of collecting simple baseline information (e.g.,
standard cardiovascular risk factors) and performing an
ultrasound arterial examination. The examination is relatively comprehensive, scanning bilaterally the accessible parts
of the carotid and femoro-popliteal systems, including major
sites of predilection for early atherosclerosis. Cases and
controls are selected from the screenees. Cases are selected
to have definite atheromata, and controls, matched to cases
by age and sex, to have no detectable lesions. The case-
control studies consist of tests and measurements of factors
hypothesized to be associated with early atheromata.

How much information relevant to the etiology of atherosclerosis can be gained by ultrasound studies of this general

design? How does this design compare with other studies of
human atherosclerosis? We will address this question with
respect to two types of non-ultrasound studies: prospective
and case-control studies of clinically overt disease. (For
completeness, we also mention non-ultrasound studies of
arterial lesions: using autopsy and angiographic measurements. Autopsy and angiographic studies have often had
problems involving selection of biases and small numbers of
subjects for investigation. In the future, like ultrasound,
other non-invasive methods may avoid such problems.) After
discussing some of the limitations of prospective and case-
control studies of clinical disease, we will compare these
with the ultrasound design we are describing.

Prospective Studies of Cardiovascular Diseases

The prospective study remains the design of choice for
identifying precursors of disease. When healthy persons are
examined for the presence of a factor and then followed over
the years for clinically apparent disease, it is clear which
came first, the clinical onset of disease or the factor. The
interpretation of this association is problematic, as in any
observational study: the precursor may or may not be a cause
of the disease.

A major limitation of prospective studies relates to
their cost. Thousands of persons must be examined and
followed for years before enough cardiovascular events occur
to assure that any associations observed are reliable. Only
one or two percent of the persons examined will have a stroke
or myocardial infarction (MI) in the next few years. Thus
there is a limit to the effort one is able to devote examining each participant. Therefore, many risk factors of possible importance are often not assessed in prospective studies.
Timed glucose tolerance tests, 24-hour urine collection for
catecholamines, blood pressure monitoring and collection of
careful dietary records are a few of many possible examples.
It is inconceivable that one would put each of thousands of
examinees through such complex investigations as measurement
of lipoprotein turnover rates or *in vivo* platelet survival
time.

Yet the predictability of stroke or MI from the simple
measurements typically made in prospective studies may be

limited. Diabetes is assessed better, not in fasting blood, but in blood collected while the body responds to a glucose challenge. The fibrinolytic capacity of endothelial tissues is evaluated after the challenge of vascular occlusion. Any dysfunction of a physiologic or biochemical system, including, we suspect, any dysfunction predisposing a person to cardiovascular events, is probably first detectable only when that system is challenged in some way.

Clinical Case-Control Studies

Clinical case-control studies, unlike prospective studies, are not limited to simple assessments. Patients are studied on metabolic wards, fed artificial diets, given tracers, endoscoped and biopsied, to find clues to their condition. The options are wide.

When cases and controls differ as hypothesized, the investigator infers that the factor studied is the clue he was looking for - a cause of the disease. But this is uncertain. The case-control study, unlike the prospective study, often provides no evidence that the factor found to be associated with the disease was its precursor. The patient with an MI may have shortened platelet survival or an altered lipoprotein metabolism because of his MI (or his hospital diet or the medications he has taken), rather than the other way around.

Advantages of the Ultrasound Study Design

Let us return to the design we described, using ultrasound screening of asymptomatic adults and performing special investigations on persons with and without atheromata. This design avoids some of the major shortfalls of both the prospective and clinical case-control designs.

The prospective study required so many participants that one could not perform definitive investigations on each one. Some of the investigations scientists suspect are most important are too complex or technically difficult. This is not so for the ultrasound design. A thousand participants may be screened, but the only cost is that of detecting atheromata. Perhaps a hundred cases and controls are selected for the detailed investigations. Methods of investigation can be just as complex as in clinical case-control studies.

But what advantage does this ultrasound study have over the clinical case-control study? The major advantage is that factors are studied in association with early athero-sclerosis, rather than with clinical events. The investigator is not trying to explain the complex etiology of end-stage disease. His task is simplified; his goals, more obtainable. He is closer to initial causes of the disease.

The ultrasound study has a second advantage over the clinical case-control study. Cases and controls should, in general, be quite comparable, except with respect to the specific factors under study. Clinical case-control studies typically have some difficulty selecting controls. The medical students, laboratory personnel and hospital controls often used are probably unlike MI patients in too many ways. The reason such controls are selected is that the clinician would have to double his work, do what epidemiologists do, to get comparable controls; identify the populations from which his hospital draws patients, recruit from these popu-lations, and account for volunteer biases. It is difficult to identify the appropriate populations. However, the ultrasound study we are describing does not encounter this problem. Once the population of interest is recruited and screened, cases and controls are both selected from the same population. There may be selection biases in screening, but these are unlikely to affect cases with and controls without occult atheromata differently.

There is a third advantage of the ultrasound study over the clinical case-control study. The clinician's controls may not be free of disease. The 60 year old MI patient may have extensive atherosclerosis, but so may his age-matched control. In the ultrasound study, controls are selected on the basis of evidence that they have minimal disease (no detectable disease in the arteries imaged), and ultrasound, we believe, is sensitive to very small lesions. If the ultrasound examination is sufficiently comprehensive, the differences between cases and controls are maximized, and the probability of finding factors associated with disease is maximized.

Let us return to the question of precursors of disease. In the ultrasound design, the factor and the disease are observed at the same time. The design is not prospective, but cross-sectional. Is a factor associated with athero-sclerosis in a cross-sectional study its precursor? Theoretically either the disease or the factor studied could have occurred first. But, are both of these theo-retical possibilities realistic? The answer will depend on the particular risk factor studied. If lipoprotein metabo-lism were found to be different in cases with early athero-mata and controls, it would seem unrealistic, contrary to scientific expectation, to suggest that atheromata altered the lipid metabolism. But do atheromata, with their roughened endothelial surfaces, shorten platelet survival? Possibly they do. The rule here is that the earlier in the disease process cases are selected, the more likely the factors found associated with disease are its causes; the later in the disease process, the more likely the factors are its effects.

One final methodological point relates to prevalence vs. incidence. The ultrasound study we are describing associates risk factors with the prevalence of atheromata, not incidence. Epidemiologists prefer to study incidence. There is a good reason for this preference. In a study of prevalent disease, factors associated with the duration of the disease may be thought, mistakenly to be associated with its incidence. But there is an equation epidemiologists use which is relevant. Under stable conditions, the pre-valence of a disease is a product of its incidence and its duration, (if a disease occurs frequently and lasts a long time it will be very prevalent). In the study we are describing, the prevalence vs. incidence issue is probably not a problem. It is true that a factor associated with the development of atheromata may also shorten a person's life (through atherosclerotic complications). If so, our design is conservative. But the life-shortening will be slight (the fatality rate for early atheromata is low) so that factors found associated with prevalence of early athero-mata are probably also associated with their incidence.

SUMMARY

Ultrasound screening of young adults and selection of
cases and controls with and without atheromata is a design
which has, in theory, a good chance of discovering factors
associated with atherosclerosis. If early lesions are
studied, the factors discovered are likely to be related to
the development of atherosclerosis. This has important
advantages over both traditional epidemiological approaches
to the study of human atherosclerotic diseases. It is more
efficient than the prospective study, permitting the kind
of test or measurement which is probably required to
investigate the etiology of atherosclerotic diseases.
Compared to the clinical case-control study, it has a
better chance of avoiding bias in selecting controls, and
it distinguishes more clearly between causes and effects.
By focusing on the disease process rather than the complex
end-stage of disease, it has an enhanced probability of
success.

Summary

63
Conclusions: Perspectives for Future Study of Human Plaques

Seymour Glagov

The contributions which form the basis for the present volume covered most aspects of the pathobiology of the human atherosclerotic plaque. A group of papers dealt with the identification, biology and possible roles of plaque cells. Others were concerned with the manner in which plaque components are organized and distributed. Several analyzed the particular pathobiologic processes which can be identified and characterized in plaques. Chemical, morphological and insudative phenomena which appear to preceed plaque formation received attention in extended studies. The role of the artery wall matrix as it interacts both with insudate and with artery wall cells was another major subject. The contributors presented what they considered to be the best operational working hypotheses concerning the relative roles of the various cell types, matrix elements and intimal deposits during the evolution of the human atherosclerotic plaque.

A series of presentations was devoted to validation studies of new techniques for vessel imaging and to recent information concerning plaque composition and evolution derived from such methods. Clinical studies applying these procedures to the evaluation of various treatment modalities are in progress and early results were presented. A number of presentations covered the responses of human plaques to clinical interventions, including risk factor control and direct invasive techniques. In all

of the clinical studies, attention was given to evaluations of
lesions in the major arterial beds at risk. It was clear from
these reports that practical clinical methods for following
plaque evolution and composition in the living subject and
for assessing local effects of plaques on blood flow are developing rapidly and that further advances in sensitivity and
specificity are likely to be forthcoming. Knowledge of human
plaque pathobiology and structure is therefore likely to become
increasingly available and practical prognostic indicators are
likely to be identified.

It was particularly evident from the presentations and
from the papers included in this volume that we must come to
understand and deal with the disease process in the context of
the hemodynamic and structural microenvironment. Both artery
wall and the plaque are composed of well organized, continuously interacting elements. Like other tissues in the body,
the reaction of the artery wall to injury is complex and
involves the mobilization of processes which tend to contain,
and if possible to remove injurious agents while preserving
adequate function. For the artery, maintaining function means
continuation of blood flow and preservation of mural integrity.
The plaque does not necessarily lead to morbid consequences in
all individuals, despite the presence of large and extensive
lesions. During most of the time, even with degrees of plaque
cross-sectional area and percent stenosis on cross-section far
exceeding that which develops in most experimental models,
lumen cross-sectional area and configuration remain adequate,
if not normal. The necrotic center tends to be isolated from
the lumen and the artery neither ruptures nor becomes obstructed
by the lesion or by thrombus formation.

We seem, therefore to be dealing with a chronic injury to
a highly integrated tissue which tends to adapt or accomodate
to the presence of the lesion by mechanisms we have only begun
to probe. We may not come to understand these mechanisms and
their limits sufficiently to be of clinical usefulness without
evaluating actual human arteries and plaques *in situ* in the
living subject and *in vitro* in suitably prepared excised
specimens. Since we are in the process of obtaining an

increasingly detailed grasp of the actual time-course of the
changes in the human plaque in the context of the actual
physical conditions of blood flow and pressure at the major
sites of plaque formation and complication, the time has
arrived to assess the relevance to human plaque formation of
the reactions we have characterized in artificially hyperlipidemic animals and in cultures of isolated cells. Conversely,
information obtained by studies of the human plaque should now
direct us to ask new and relevant specific questions of our
experimental models. The papers presented at the conference and
published here have not only summarized much of what we know
about human plaque pathobiology but have identified the approaches
which are likely to yield new information. The major specific
problems which are under study and which need to be addressed in
greater depth can be grouped, for purposes of discussion, into
two closely-related categories: 1) the nature or pathobiology
of the human atherogenic process and the possibilities for prevention and 2) the features of plaque evolution which may permit
us to evaluate existing plaques in living subjects, anticipate
morbid consequences and select appropriate therapies.

With respect to the first of these, the following questions
remain to be resolved. 1) What is the nature of the earliest
intimal change which can be considered to be a plaque? Can this
change be stabilized if not reversed? What is the sequence of
chemical, physical and cellular events during this early phase?
2) What is the nature of diffuse or focal intimal thickening
and of intimal hyperplasia? In what manner and to what extent
are these processes related to atherogenesis? Are they precursor
or predisposing states or are they non-atherosclerotic reactions
which may, for as yet unclear reasons, also occur in athero-
sclerosis-prone regions? What are the metabolic and/or hemodynamic determinants of possible transitions of these states to
plaque formation? 3) How do the identifiable hemodynamic and
metabolic clinical risk factors act to induce or predispose
such susceptible regions to atherogenesis? How do these same
factors and responses act to modify lesion structure and composition in such a manner as to favor or prevent symptom-producing
stenosis or plaque complication? 4) What is the nature of the

apparent differential atherogenic effects of the known clinical
risk factors on the major arteries? 5) How are the numerous
vasoactive and coagulation-related agents elaborated by the
cells of the artery wall and plaque related to the initiation,
progression, reversal or stabilization of the lesions? 6) How
are circulating blood cellular elements and coagulation factors
involved at various stages of lesion development? What is the
role of surface thrombogenesis in early plaque formation?
7) What are the roles of infectious agents, immunological
reactions and of associated cellular and inflammatory reactions
during lesion evolution? 8) What is the role of endogenous and
exogenous mitogenic agents, and 9) In addition to individual
blood lipid profiles, receptor-mediated responses, gender and
ethnicity, are there demonstrable genetically determined differences of artery wall reactivity?

With respect to the more directly practical aspects of
human atherosclerosis, those concerned with detection, characterization and treatment advances are rapid indeed. Several of the
following specific questions, though under study, require further
elucidation. 1) What is the status of our technology for
detecting and quantifying lesion size, composition and topography? 2) How can such data be used reliably to follow plaque
size and composition? 3) Can we identify and detect indicators
of vessel wall and lumen compensation for increasing plaque
volume and for containment of plaque complication? 4) Can we
arrive at a new classification of human plaques which deals with
pathogenesis rather than morphology? Can such a classification,
in conjunction with new methods of detection, provide a means
for assessing or predicting the stability of plaques? 5) Can
such data help to better individualize therapeutic approaches?
6) What are the determinants of the "catastrophic event",
i.e., plaque disruption and/or thrombosis, in particular with
respect to plaque composition, configuration or topography and
with respect to the mechanical stresses, both tensile and hemodynamic, in the region of the plaque? How do thrombi formed on
and about plaques or with aneurysmal dilations stabilize or
organize to maintain adequate circular lumens? What are the
determinants of thrombus incorporation into plaques and of the

modelling which tends to restore lumen configuration and maintain lumen patency? 7) To what extent does the severity of
lesions in one of the major vascular channels at high risk
correspond to severity in other high-risk regions? What
factors account for the discrepancies? 8) How do plaques
treated by direct intervention "heal" or "remodel"? What are
the determinants of recurrence of obstruction at sites of
direct intervention? The proceedings of the present workshop
indicate that these areas of study necessitate joint efforts
by radiologists, surgeons, cardiologists and pathologists.
The techniques and insights which have developed since the
Chicago Symposium of 25 years ago and which are summarized
in this volume provide assurance that we now have at least
provisional answers and that we have identified the means to
accelerate the detailed study of the disease in human arteries.
This perspective is based on the following considerations which
are detailed in the presentations of the workshop participants.

    1. <u>Methods of assessment in living subjects</u>. We are no
longer limited to visualization of the artery lumen. Angiography is undergoing continued refinement as a quantitative
tool and remains an extremely valuable diagnostic technique.
Angiographic evidence was presented which indicates that in
the same individual and even in the same artery, some plaques
are associated with a decrease in lumen diameter on interval
examination ("progressing"), some with an increase in lumen
diameter ("regressing") and others with no change in diameter
("stable"). Yet angiography provides only a limited estimate
of actual lesion size and degree of stenosis, since it relies
on comparisons of lumen diameters in adjacent segments and on
irregularities of contour on axial projections and may therefore not take sufficient account of compensatory enlargement
of arteries. Ultrasonic means for identifying the artery wall
and plaque while simultaneously assessing flow velocity and
other properties of the flow field have evolved rapidly. With
real time imaging and rapid ultrasonic techniques we can assess
wall compliance as well as plaque density. The application of
magnetic resonance imaging is developing more rapidly than
can be followed in a summarizing volume and promises to

markedly increase the precision of determinations of plaque
composition and topography as well as flow-field properties.
Detailed correlative studies of images and hemodynamics with
plaque composition are feasible and indicated and should begin
to reveal why some progress while others are stable. In conjunction with further studies of the nature of artery enlargement as plaques form and with characterization of limits of
this presumably adaptive mechanism, new information on human
plaque evolution will be forthcoming.

2. <u>Vascular surgery</u>. Techniques of vascular surgery have
developed rapidly. Direct measurements of flow velocity and
characterization of the mechanical properties of the artery
wall and of plaques are increasingly available. Excised
arterial lesions are now available for morphologic and chemical quantitative studies to compare with clinical findings,
including visualization and hemodynamic data gathered before
and after surgery. Endarterectomy specimens corresponding to
well characterized clinical studies and pre-operative interventions may be particularly useful. The use of autogenous
vessels as bypass grafts and the widespread use of other graft
materials, both biologic and synthetic, create measurable
alterations in conditions of pressure and flow in bypassed
native segments, in vessels proximal and distal to anastomoses,
and within the grafts. Corresponding morphologic and chemical
changes may be assessed in artery specimens in many instances,
obtained either at reoperation or at surgery. This material is
also being used for tissue culture studies, determinations of
cell types and for characterization of the biology of lesion
cells. Correlation of cell function and distribution with
plaque structure, plaque modelling and plaque complication are
shown to be feasible and essential undertakings. Cell proliferation and macrophage accumulation need not necessarily
be undesirable phenomena. In other tissues, particularly in
the presence of inflammation, these reactions tend to isolate
or remove pathogenic agents and/or to isolate regions of
necrosis and disruption. Although such phenomena are prominent
features of atherogenesis,they may be defensive at many stages
of lesion development and underlie regression or stabilization

of plaques. The "good guy" or "bad guy" controversy with regard to proliferation and inflammatory cell accumulation may therefore be misdirected. It may be more to the point to relate those reactions to plaque evolution without the presumption that we must necessarily seek to apply means for limiting proliferation and inflammatory cell accumulation at all stages of plaque development. Excised lesions also provide material for establishing the bases for plaque disruption. In this regard, detailed computer-assisted reconstructions should reveal the precise location of disruptions and other symptom-related plaque features. These may then be related to focal plaque composition and to processes which are likely to make plaques vulnerable to disruption. The technology is at hand to relate these foci to hemodynamic and other mechanical stresses which may cause the fissures and fractures described by several authors.

3. _Direct interventions_. In addition to bypass placements, direct interventions on plaques are sufficiently commonplace and varied to provide data concerning the reaction of arteries and plaques to pertubations of structure and flow. For example, percutaneous translumenal angioplasty creates disruptive injuries of plaques and of the artery wall. Subsequent _in situ_ assessment of the nature of the processes underlying restenosis, remodelling and actual plaque recurrence is possible in many instances. Surgical and autopsy material is available and should be collected and studied. Direct thrombolysis is in widespread use and experimental procedures such as laser endarterectomy and various modes of laser and mechanical plaque reduction are in advanced stages of development. Characterization of the rapidly advancing atherosclerosis which has been observed in transplanted hearts in relation to hemodynamic measurements and to the immunologic status of the patient will also yield new insights into the factors which determine lesion growth and configuration.

4. _Comparative studies of different vascular regions at_ _risk_. While morbidity due to disease at the carotid bifurcation is often attributable to embolization, presumably due to thrombi formed at the plaque, symptoms of coronary heart

disease arise when stenotic segments prevent adequate flow
under conditions of increased myocardial oxygen demand or are
suddenly occluded by thrombus. Lesions in different locations
also differ in composition corresponding to the manner in
which complications arise. Comparisons should reveal information regarding the manner in which local conditions modify
lesion evolution and produce symptoms. Differences in severity
and in types of complication may in large measure be related to
differences in such factors as flow division at bifurcations,
branch angles, relative diameters of branches, artery wall
compliance and motion, pulse wave velocity and pulse rate.
Such studies have already revealed that some of the previous
assumptions regarding the relationship of wall shear stress
to lesion localization have been incorrect. Some of these
studies are documented in the present volume. The evidence,
already derived from studies of human lesions in sites of
clinical importance would seem to indicate that regions where
wall shear stress is low and oscillating in direction are most
prone to plaque development. Regions of high, unidirectional
shear are relatively spared. The necessary technology for the
characterization of the clinical risk factors and the local
mechanical determinents is developed and more new insights into
plaque biology should be forthcoming.

5. <u>Better methods of morphologic study</u>. It has become
clear that accurate quantitative assessment of lesion and lumen
configuration and of cross-sectional areas of lumen and lesion
in excised arteries requires methods which restore *in vivo*
dimensions. Controlled-pressure distention or perfusion during
fixation along with maintenance of physiologic temperature
tends to restore lesion configuration. Corrections for shrinkage due to histologic processing help to establish accurate
quantitative data for comparison with *in situ* measurements.
The extended use of image analysis, including contour tracing
assisted by suitable computer programs for data storage and
analysis has greatly accelerated quantification procedures.
Morphometric studies, previously prohibitively cumbersome and
time-consuming, may now be undertaken with relative ease and
only a fraction of earlier costs for equipment and programs.

Histochemical and immunocytochemical techniques permit the
study of cell function in relation to cell distribution and
lesion composition. Such ongoing studies are described in this
volume. Extension of this work is likely to shed light on the
bases for lesion breakdown or lesion stabilization. Scanning
electron microscopy has permitted the study at fairly high
resolution of much more extensive sampling areas than have
been possible previously by transmission electron microscopy
and should be further applied to characterize surface micro-
injuries. The early phases of surface disruption of advanced
plaques have been shown to occupy very small areas. These
are likely to be the beginnings of serious complications and
can be studied systematically only when extended surfaces can
be examined at relatively high resolution. Although *in vivo*
visualization and surgical material are likely to continue to be
of great value, the systematic use of autopsy material should be
extended. Much has been learned and remains to be learned from
such studies. Recent investigations have already provided insights into the relationships among hemodynamics and plaque
location, the role of plaque fracture, the incidence of thrombosis, the precise location of plaques, the associated changes in
the endothelium and media and the possible precursors of plaques
in infants and yound adults.

 6. Staging of plaques. Classification of plaques according
to stage of development, configuration and complication, and
analysis in relation to lipid-related and matrix-related enzyme
activity will contribute a better operational understanding of
the nature of the processes which determine individual differences in plaque evolution. Such studies will provide further
insights into the relationships among plaque composition and
risk factor control and in relation to the administration of
pharmacologic agents which may arrest or retard plaque formation,
stabilize plaque composition or induce plaque regression. It
has been assumed, often by implication, that the same therapeutic
measures, including risk factor control as well as anti-atherogenic and anti-thrombogenic drugs, are potentially beneficial
at all stages of lesion development. This is not necessarily
the case. Some modes of intervention could even be harmful

at certain stages. As long ago as the previous plaque-evolution
meeting in 1963, Drs. Katz and Pick reported ulcerations of
experimental plaques during early phases of regression induced
by hormone administration. Such an effect, with serious consequences, could also occur when human plaques are exposed to
excessive hormone levels. For example, myocardial infarction
in young women taking estrogens for purposes of contraception
could be related to thromboses potentiated by plaque disruption.
It would be of value to be able to assess the extent to which
lesion composition determines the outcome of direct interventions
such as PTA, direct thrombolysis or laser or mechanical reduction of plaque volume. Whether a plaque is densely fibrous with
a well organized fibrous cap or has a soft semi-fluid, lipid
interior covered only by a thin, tenuous fibrous cap may make
a considerable difference to the outcome.

Research into the nature and causes of atherosclerosis must
of course continue as we attempt to develop better preventive
strategies. Knowledge concerning the evolution of the human
atherosclerotic plaque should however bring into sharper focus
perspectives for reducing morbidity in the subject with manifest advanced plaques. Until we can prevent the disease, a
major concern is to understand the nature of the process in
each of the major human vulnerable sites, i.e., coronary arteries, cerebrovascular sites and distal aorta and peripheral
arteries. Once the disease is evident in one or more of these
regions, we should like to know what kinds of plaques are present and what we can do to stabilize the process before it
causes stenosis or thrombosis.

The challenge is therefore not only to continue to perfect
methods of prevention and detection but also to find ways of
assessing and monitoring lesions *in situ* in order to anticipate
the effects of various modalities of risk factor control and
drug administration. This can be accomplished only by close
collaboration among the various specialists directly concerned
with the plaque. The broad representation of all of these
disciplines accounted in large part for the enthusiasm developed
at the workship and for the interest in the current publication.
Future meetings with broad participation should be focused on
the specific questions raised. Many answers are in the offing.

Index

922